THE ISCHEMIC EXTREMITY

ADVANCES IN TREATMENT

Edited by

James S.T. Yao, MD, PhD
Chief, Division of Vascular Surgery
Northwestern Memorial Hospital
Magerstadt Professor of Surgery
Northwestern University Medical School
Chicago, Illinois

William H. Pearce, MD
Division of Vascular Surgery
Northwestern Memorial Hospital
Professor of Surgery
Northwestern University Medical School
Chicago, Illinois

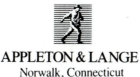

APPLETON & LANGE
Norwalk, Connecticut

Notice: The authors and the publisher of this volume have taken care to make certain that the doses of drugs and schedules of treatment are correct and compatible with the standards generally accepted at the time of publication. Nevertheless, as new information becomes available, changes in treatment and in the use of drugs become necessary. The reader is advised to carefully consult the instruction and information material included in the package insert of each drug or therapeutic agent before administration. This advice is especially important when using new or infrequently used drugs. The publisher disclaims any liability, loss, injury, or damage incurred as a consequence, directly or indirectly, or the use and application of any of the contents of the volume.

95 96 97 98 / 10 9 8 7 6 5 4 3 2 1

Prentice Hall International (UK) Limited, *London*
Prentice Hall of Australia Pty. Limited, *Sydney*
Prentice Hall Canada, Inc., *Toronto*
Prentice Hall Hispanoamericana, S. A., *Mexico*
Prentice Hall of India Private Limited, *New Delhi*
Prentice Hall of Japan, Inc., *Tokyo*
Simon & Schuster Asia Pte. Ltd., *Singapore*
Editora Prentice Hall do Brasil Ltda., *Rio de Janeiro*
Prentice Hall, *Englewood Cliffs, New Jersey*

Library of Congress Cataloging-in-Publication Data

The ischemic extremity : advances in treatment / edited by James S. T.
 Yao, William H. Pearce.
    p.   cm.
   ISBN 0-8385-4397-9
   1. Peripheral vascular disease—Treatment.   2. Ischemia—
Treatment.   I. Yao, James S. T.   II. Pearce, William H.
   [DNLM: 1. Extremities—surgery. 2. Ischemia—surgery. WE 800
I77 1995]
RC694.I82   1995
616.1'3106—dc20
DNLM/DLC
for Library of Congress   94-38434
                                                                              CIP

ISBN 0-8385-4397-9

Acquisitions Editor: Jane Licht
Production: Spectrum Publisher Services
Designer: Janice Bielawa

PRINTED IN THE UNITED STATES OF AMERICA   8/94

Contents

I. GENERAL CONSIDERATIONS

II. NEW ADJUNCTIVE TECHNIQUES IN MANAGEMENT OF
    LIMB ISCHEMIA

VI. THE BLUE TOE SYNDROME

VII. CORRECTION OF INFLOW LESIONS FOR LOWER EXTREMITY ISCHEMIA

VIII. INFRAINGUINAL REVASCULARIZATION FOR LOWER LIMB ISCHEMIA

Contributors

William M. Abbott, MD
Professor of Surgery
Harvard Medical School
Massachusetts General Hospital
Chief of Vascular Surgery
Boston, Massachusetts

John G. Adams, Jr, MD
Clinical Instructor in Surgery
Department of Surgery
University of Missouri–Columbia
Vascular Surgery Resident
University of Missouri Hospital &
  Clinics
Columbia, Missouri

Amine Bahnini, MD
Staff Surgeon
Pitié-Salpêtrière University Hospital
Paris, France

Hisham S. Bassiouny, MD
Assistant Professor of Surgery
The University of Chicago
Director, Vascular Laboratory
Chicago, Illinois

Michael Belkin, MD
Assistant Professor of Surgery
Vascular Surgeon
Harvard Medical School
Brigham and Women's Hospital
Boston, Massachusetts

Denis D. Bensard, MD
Assistant Professor of Surgery
University of Colorado Health Sciences
  Center
University Hospital
Denver, Colorado

Sven-Erik Bergentz, MD, PhD
Professor of Surgery
Lund University
Head Vascular Surgery
Department of Surgery
Malmö General Hospital
Malmö, Sweden

Eugene F. Bernstein, MD, PhD
Senior Consultant
Division of Vascular and Thoracic
  Surgery
Scripps Clinic and Research Foundation
La Jolla, California

Jan Brunkwall, MD, PhD
Associate Professor of Surgery
Lund University
Senior Vascular Surgeon
Department of Surgery
Malmö General Hospital
Malmö, Sweden

Elliot L. Chaikof, MD, PhD
Assistant Professor of Surgery
Emory University School of Medicine
Staff Surgeon

Emory University Hospital
Atlanta, Georgia

Benjamin B. Chang, MD
Assistant Professor
Albany Medical College
Albany Medical Center Hospital
Albany, New York

G. Patrick Clagett, MD
Professor
University of Texas
Head, Vascular Surgery Section
Southwestern Medical Center
Dallas, Texas

Lawrence B. Colen, MD, FACS
Associate Professor of Plastic Surgery
Eastern Virginia Medical School
Norfolk, Virginia

**John D. Corson, MB, ChB, FRCS
(Engl), FACS**
Professor of Surgery
The University of Iowa College of
  Medicine
Director, Vascular Surgery Section
The University of Iowa Hospitals and
  Clinics
Iowa City, Iowa

Jack L. Cronenwett, MD
Professor of Surgery
Dartmouth Medical School
Dartmouth-Hitchcock Medical Center
Lebanon, New Hampshire

Jacob Cynamon, MD
Associate Professor of Radiology
Albert Einstein College of Medicine
Associate Director of Vascular and
  Interventional Radiology
Montefiore Medical Center
New York, New York

Michael D. Dake, MD
Professor of Radiology and Medicine
Stanford University
Chief, Cardiovascular and
  Interventional Radiology
Stanford University Hospital
Stanford, California

R. Clement Darling, III, MD
Assistant Professor
Albany Medical College
Albany Medical Center Hospital
Albany, New York

Robert D. De Frang, MD
Assistant Professor of Surgery
University of New Mexico
Albuquerque, New Mexico

Magruder C. Donaldson, MD
Associate Professor of Surgery
Harvard Medical School
Surgeon, Department of Surgery
Division of Vascular Surgery
Brigham & Women's Hospital
Boston, Massachusetts

Joseph R. Durham, MD
Associate Professor Clinical Surgery
Northwestern University Medical
  School
Director, Blood Flow Laboratory
Northwestern Memorial Hospital
Chicago, Illinois

Janis Edwards, RN, RVT
Vascular Nurse Technologist
Medical College of Wisconsin
John Doyne Hospital
Milwaukee, Wisconsin

Calvin B. Ernst, MD
Clinical Professor of Surgery
University of Michigan Medical School
Head of Vascular Surgery
Henry Ford Hospital
Detroit, Michigan

Spencer W. Galt, MD
Instructor in Surgery
Northwestern University Medical
  School
Resident in Vascular Surgery
Northwestern Memorial Hospital
Chicago, Illinois

Dale N. Gerding, MD
Professor & Associate Chairman

Northwestern University Medical
 School
Chief, Medical Service
VA Lakeside Medical Center
Chicago, Illinois

Don P. Giddens, PhD
Professor and Dean of Engineering
Johns Hopkins University
Baltimore, Maryland

Seymour Glagov, MD
Professor of Pathology
University of Chicago Medical Center
Chicago, Illinois

Robert A. Graor, MD
Chairman
Department of Vascular Medicine
Cleveland Clinic Foundation
Cleveland, Ohio

Richard M. Green, MD
Associate Professor of Surgery
University of Rochester
Chief, Section of Vascular Surgery
Strong Memorial Hospital
Rochester, New York

**W. P. Hederman, MD, MCh, FRCS
 (Ireland)**
University College Dublin
Consultant Vascular Surgeon
Mater Misericordiae Hospital
Dublin, Ireland

Jamal T. Hoballah, MD
Assistant Professor of Surgery
University of Iowa College of Medicine
Staff Surgeon
University of Iowa Hospitals and Clinics
Iowa City, Iowa

Thomas Hölzenbein, MD
University of Vienna Medical School
AKH, General Hospital Vienna
Vienna, Austria

John William Joyce, MD
Professor of Medicine
Mayo Medical School

Consultant, Internal Medicine and
 Cardiovascular Diseases
Mayo Clinic/Mayo Foundation
Rochester, Minnesota

John A. Kaufman, MD
Instructor of Radiology
Harvard University
Vascular Radiologist
Massachusetts General Hospital
Boston, Massachusetts

Richard R. Keen, MD
Assistant Professor of Surgery
Rush Medical College
Attending Surgeon
Cook County Hospital
Chicago, Illinois

Edouard Kieffer, MD
Professor of Surgery and Chief,
 Department of Vascular Surgery
Pitié-Salpêtrière University Hospital
Paris, France

Fabien Koskas, MD
Staff Surgeon
Department of Vascular Surgery
Pitié-Salpêtrière University Hospital
Paris, France

Timothy F. Kresowik, MD, FACS
Associate Professor of Surgery
University of Iowa College of Medicine
Staff Surgeon
University of Iowa Hospitals and Clinics
Iowa City, Iowa

Georg J. Kretschmer, MD
Assistant Professor of Surgery
University of Vienna Medical School
AKH, General Hospital Vienna
Vienna, Austria

William C. Krupski, MD
Professor of Surgery
University of Colorado Health Sciences
 Center
Chief, Vascular Surgery Section
University Hospital
Denver, Colorado

Robert P. Leather, MD
Professor of Surgery
Albany Medical College
Head, Division of General Surgery
Albany Medical Center Hospital
Albany, New York

Marvin E. Levin, MD
Clinical Professor of Medicine
Washington University School of
  Medicine
St. Louis, Missouri

Frank W. LoGerfo, MD
Professor of Surgery
Harvard Medical School
Chief, Division of Vascular Surgery
New England Deaconess Hospital
Boston, Massachusetts

A. Loh, FRCS
Research Registrar
Department of Surgery
St. George's Hospital
London, England

Michael L. Marin, MD
Assistant Professor of Surgery
Albert Einstein College of Medicine
Attending in Surgery
Montefiore Medical Center
New York, New York

Mark A. Mattos, MD
Assistant Professor of Surgery
Section of Vascular Surgery
Southern Illinois University School of
  Medicine
Springfield, Illinois

Walter J. McCarthy, MD
Associate Professor of Surgery
Northwestern University Medical
  School
Active Staff
Northwestern Memorial Hospital
Chicago, Illinois

Robert B. McLafferty, MD
Vascular Research Fellow

General Surgery Resident
Oregon Health Sciences University
Portland, Oregon

Kenneth Ouriel, MD
Clinical Associate Professor of Surgery
University of Rochester Medical Center
Strong Memorial Hospital
Rochester, New York

Julio C. Palmaz, MD
S. R. Reuter Professor of Radiology
University of Texas Health Science
  Center at San Antonio
Chief, Cardiovascular and
  Interventional Radiology
University Hospital, Audie Murphy VA
  Hospital
San Antonio, Texas

Juan C. Parodi, MD
Chief of Vascular Surgery
Instituto Cardiovascular de Buenos Aires
Universidad Catolica Del Salvador
Buenos Aires, Argentina
Associate Professor of Surgery
Wake Forest University
Winston-Salem, North Carolina

William H. Pearce, MD
Professor of Surgery
Northwestern University Medical
  School
Attending Surgeon
Northwestern Memorial Hospital
Chicago, Illinois

Bruce A. Perler, MD
Associate Professor of Surgery
Johns Hopkins University School of
  Medicine
Director of Vascular Surgery Service and
  Vascular Noninvasive Diagnostic
  Laboratory
Johns Hopkins Hospital
Baltimore, Maryland

Frank B. Pomposelli, Jr, MD
Assistant Professor of Surgery
Harvard Medical School

Vascular Surgeon
New England Deaconess Hospital
Boston, Massachusetts

John M. Porter, MD
Professor of Surgery
Head, Division of Vascular Surgery
Oregon Health Sciences University
School of Medicine
Portland, Oregon

Carlo Ruotolo, MD
Staff Surgeon
Pitié-Salpêtrière University Hospital
Paris, France

Luis A. Sanchez, MD
Assistant Professor of Surgery
Albert Einstein College of Medicine
Assistant Attending in Surgery
Montefiore Medical Center
New York, New York

Marco Scoccianti, MD
Vascular Surgeon
Harbor–UCLA Medical Center
Torrance, California

Charles P. Semba, MD
Assistant Professor of Radiology
Department of Radiology
Stanford University
Stanford University Hospital
Stanford, California

Dhiraj M. Shah, MD
Professor of Surgery
Albany Medical College
Albany Medical Center Hospital
Albany, New York

William J. Sharp, MD, FACS
Associate Professor of Surgery
University of Iowa College of Medicine
Staff Surgeon
University of Iowa Hospitals and Clinics
Iowa City, Iowa

Alexander D. Shepard, MD
Clinical Associate Professor of Surgery

University of Michigan Medical School
Senior Staff Surgeon
Medical Director, Clinical Vascular
  Laboratory
Henry Ford Hospital
Detroit, Michigan

Cynthia K. Shortell, MD
Clinical Assistant Professor
University of Rochester
Attending Vascular Surgeon
Rochester General Hospital
Rochester, New York

Donald Silver, MD
W. Alton Jones Professor and Chairman
Department of Surgery
University of Missouri–Columbia
Chief of Vascular Surgery
Columbia, Missouri

Robert B. Smith III, MD
Professor of Surgery
Emory University School of Medicine
Head, General Vascular Surgery
Emory University Hospital
Atlanta, Georgia

James C. Stanley, MD
Professor of Surgery
University of Michigan Medical School
Head, Section of Vascular Surgery
University Hospital
Ann Arbor, Michigan

D. Eugene Strandness, Jr, MD
Professor
Chief, Division of Vascular Surgery
University of Washington School of
  Medicine
Seattle, Washington

David S. Sumner, MD
Distinguished Professor of Surgery
Chief, Section of Vascular Surgery
Southern Illinois University School of
  Medicine
Springfield, Illinois

Lloyd M. Taylor, Jr, MD
Professor of Surgery
Oregon Health Sciences University
Division of Vascular Surgery
Portland, Oregon

R. S. Taylor, MS, FRCS, FRCS (Edin)
Consultant Vascular Surgeon
Department of Vascular Surgery
St. George's Hospital
London, England

Jonathan B. Towne, MD
Professor, Vascular Surgery
Medical College of Wisconsin
Chairman, Vascular Surgery
Milwaukee County Medical Complex
Milwaukee, Wisconsin

William D. Turnipseed, MD
Professor, Department of Surgery
University of Wisconsin Medical School
Chief, Department of Surgery
University of Wisconsin Hospital and
  Clinics
Madison, Wisconsin

Mark R. Tyrrell, PhD, FRCS
Senior Registrar
Guys Hospital
London, England

Frank J. Veith, MD
Professor of Surgery
Albert Einstein College of Medicine
Chief, Vascular Surgical Services
Montefiore Medical Center
New York, New York

John V. White, MD
Professor of Surgery
Director of Surgical Research
Temple University School of Medicine

Temple University Hospital
Philadelphia, Pennsylvania

Rodney A. White, MD
Professor of Surgery
UCLA School of Medicine
Chief, Vascular Surgery
Harbor–UCLA Medical Center
Torrance, California

Anthony D. Whittemore, MD
Associate Professor of Surgery
Harvard Medical School
Chief, Vascular Surgery
Brigham & Women's Hospital
Boston, Massachusetts

Stephen P. Wiet, MD
Interventional Cardiology Fellow
Northwestern University Medical
  School
Chicago, Illinois

John H. N. Wolfe, MS, FRCS
Consultant Vascular Surgeon
St. Mary's Hospital Medical School
St. Mary's Hospital
London, England

James S. T. Yao, MD, PhD
Magerstadt Professor of Surgery
Northwestern University Medical
  School
Chief, Division of Vascular Surgery
Northwestern Memorial Hospital
Chicago, Illinois

Christopher K. Zarins, MD
Chidester Professor of Surgery
Stanford University
Chairman, Division of Vascular Surgery
Stanford University Hospital
Stanford, California

Preface

Ischemia of the extremities is common, and surgical procedures on peripheral blood vessels account for one-third of all reconstructive procedures performed in the United States. Vascular surgery began with simple suture of a lacerated peripheral artery and gradually evolved from arterial repairs of a divided artery to bypass grafting. Today, a wide variety of procedures are available to revascularize patients with an ischemic extremity. The primary objective of this volume is to provide vascular surgeons with an update on the current advances in this field.

The history of the modern surgical treatment of arterial problems of extremities encompasses nearly 90 years and nine countries. The first breakthrough in the treatment of atherosclerotic arterial occlusive disease came from an attempt in 1948 by Jean Kunlin of France, who used saphenous vein as a bypass conduit. The first saphenous vein bypass in the United States was performed by William Holden in 1950 in a patient with segmental occlusion of the superficial femoral artery.

By the mid-1950s, femoral bypass graft was confined to the popliteal artery. The use of femoral arteriography prompted Henry Haimovici and his colleagues to define operability of the bypass graft in relation to arteriographic pattern. In their report, Haimovici used the term *run-off* to define the possibility of the procedure's success. Run-off represents the patent major distal vessel below the site of segmental occlusion. This vascular channel is fed by a varying number of collaterals. The presence of an adequate outflow or run-off is the most decisive factor in the selection of patients for arterial grafting or thromboendarterectomy. When femoral bypass extended to the distal tibial arteries, the term *pedal arch,* coined by Anthony Imparato, offered a second set of arteriographic patterns to determine operability of femoral bypass graft.

The extension of bypass graft beyond the popliteal trifurcation began with an article by John McCaughan, Jr., who described the exposure of distal popliteal artery using the medial approach, which was favored at the time. Since then, bypass grafts have gradually extended to arteries at the ankle level to the plantar artery. Not only has the anatomic site for distal anatomosis changed dramatically, but also the increased use of autogenous vein has extended the operability of femoral graft. The chronology of development of femoral bypass from popliteal artery to distal arteries is shown in Table 1.

TABLE 1. CHRONOLOGY OF DEVELOPMENT OF FEMORAL BYPASS

Year	Surgeon	Vascular Development
1906	J. Goyannes (Spain)	In-situ popliteal vein—Popliteal aneurysm
1907	E. Lexer (Germany)	Saphenous vein—Axillary traumatic aneurysm
1913	J. H. Pringle, Hogarth (UK)	Saphenous vein—Popliteal aneurysm
1913	Soubbotitch (Serbia)	Vein graft—Arterial injury
1915	B. M. Bernheim (USA)	Saphenous vein—Popliteal aneurysm
1917	H. Warthmuller (Germany)	Saphenous vein—Traumatic aneurysm
1948	J. Kunlin (France)	Saphenous vein—Atherosclerotic occlusive disease
1950	W. Holden (USA)	Vein—Atherosclerotic occlusive disease
1951	E. Lowenberg (USA)	Saphenous vein (lateral approach)
1958	J. J. McCaughan (USA)	Distal popliteal artery exposure
1959	G. C. Morris et al. (USA)	Infrapopliteal (posterior tibial)—Posterior approach
1959	C. Rob (USA)	In-situ vein graft
1960	E. C. Palma (Argentina)	Vein graft to posterior tibial artery
1960	P. Cartier (Canada)	In-situ vein graft
1961	J. J. McCaughan (USA)	Vein graft to anterior and posterior tibial, calf level
1961	K. V. Hall (Norway)	In-situ vein graft
1962	W. A. Dale (USA)	Femoroproximal posterior tibial graft
1964	D. E. Szilagyi (USA)	Femorotibial vein graft
1964	J. A. Mannick and D. M. Hume (USA)	Femorotibial vein graft
1966	J. J. McCaughan (USA)	Femoroposterior tibial (ankle) vein graft
1966	H. E. Garrett et al. (USA)	Bypass to distal posterior tibial artery
1967	J. A. Mannick (USA)	Bypass to isolated popliteal artery
1967	J. J. Ochsner (USA)	Dorsalis pedis
1968	H. E. Garrett et al. (USA)	Tibial arteries at ankle level
1968	P. Martin, S. Renwick, and C. Stephenson (UK)	Profunda femoris artery
1969	V. V. Kakkar (UK)	Cephalic vein
1971	D. A. DeLaurentis and P. Friedman (USA)	Sequential graft
1972	W. A. Dale (USA)	Composite graft, Teflon-vein
1975	F. A. Reichle and R. Tyson (USA)	Peroneal artery
1988	E. Ascer, F. J. Veith, and S. K. Gupta (USA)	Bypass to plantar artery

During the early development of vascular surgery, many outstanding surgeons contributed significantly to the treatment of ischemic extremities. One of these pioneering surgeons is Dr. D. Emerick Szilagyi, former chairman of the Department of Surgery at Henry Ford Hospital, Detroit, Michigan. We have dedicated this volume to honor his multiple contributions in the field of vascular surgery, especially his critical approach to the evaluation of femoral bypass graft. As stated rightfully by Wiley Barker, D. Emerick Szilagyi is a "respected and honored teacher, investigator, clinician, friend, and superb craftsman; a critical voice who has served as the conscience of the world of vascular surgery throughout the majority of its active existence."

James S. T. Yao
William H. Pearce

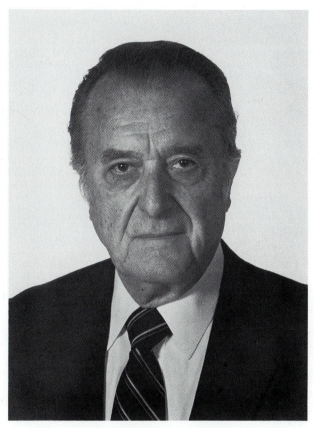

D. Emerick Szilagyi, MD

Introduction

D. Emerick Szilagyi:

The Student, Surgeon, Scientist, and Conscience of Vascular Surgery

James C. Stanley, MD

D. Emerick Szilagyi has been a dominant force in the discipline of vascular surgery since the midpoint of the 20th century. He is one of a small number of courageous and innovative physicians who established the foundation for the operative treatment of vascular diseases. He has witnessed the passing of this discipline through its adolescence to its position as a mature part of the medical profession. This brief biographical sketch of his life as a student, surgeon, scientist, and conscience of vascular surgery is offered as a measure of respect to this man to whom many patients and practitioners owe so much.

THE STUDENT

Dr Szilagyi's early education took place in Hungary. He was born in Nagykaroly in 1910, the second of three children, including a sister 2 years older and a brother 4 years younger. His father owned a small department store in their hometown of Szatmar that provided a comfortable living for the family during his childhood. When he was 7 years old, World War I ended and resulted in the partitioning of his native Hungary into four regions. His home became relegated to Rumania. Considerable political suppression of native Hungarians in this new country was commonplace. His father was contemplating moving his family to the United States or across the countryside to Hungary when he died in an accident. Emerick had just become a teenager. His mother subsequently met a fellow Hungarian who lived in the United States, and they were married. Shortly thereafter she emigrated with Emerick's sister to the United States, where her new husband had an established restaurant business in Detroit. Emerick and his brother remained in Europe to complete their education, living in a room rented by his mother. He was 14 years old.

Emerick was rambunctious as a young child and was intellectually precocious, being able to read newspapers by the age of 5. His education as a youth occurred in

Calvinist schools. He completed his gymnasium in Kolozavár, a community that he considers his hometown. His was a classical education in the true sense of the Austrian system, involving rigorous academic discipline. Emerick excelled in languages and mathematics. It should come as no surprise that Dr Szilagyi's first contribution to the literature came at age 12 in the form of poetry and prose published in a periodical for young people. Emerick led his classmates in academic achievement and finished his gymnasium education when he was 18 years old (Fig. I–1).

Dr Szilagyi subsequently enrolled as a student in medical sciences at the University of Kolozsvár in Rumania. He transferred 6 months later to the Sorbonne in Paris, where he attended science classes of more than 600 students. Each student wore a white coat with an identifying number so that he might be queried by the instructor, in what was a demeaning experience to Emerick. Given his strong-willed personality, Dr Szilagyi elected to return to Hungary, where he then attended the University of Debrecen as a medical student for an additional year. In late spring of 1931, he and his brother traveled to the United States at the request of his mother, crossing the Atlantic aboard the *Leviathan*.

His mother had persuaded him to undertake this trip with the intent that it would be a visit for a few months. Once in the United States, she convinced Emerick and his brother to stay. Unrest within European countries and the concern that their homeland might become the pawn in yet another world war underlay much of her concern. Her intuition proved correct.

As a new arrival in the United States and with American citizenship derived from his mother's having become a citizen earlier, Emerick set about to continue his education. His mother had made the acquaintance of an Irishman by the name of Beynon, who had established the Methodist church in their neighborhood and gave sermons in Hungarian. This rather unique individual helped Emerick, who spoke English haltingly, to obtain interviews for medical school at the City College of Detroit (the forerunner of Wayne State University) and at the University of Michigan in Ann Arbor.

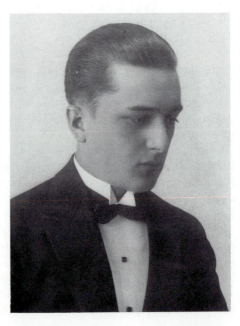

Figure I–1. D Emerick Szilagyi at the time of his graduation from the gymnasium in 1928.

At the University of Michigan, Dr Szilagyi pleaded his case to Frederick G. Novy, a world-reknowned bacteriologist. Dr Novy had been portrayed as a brilliant scientist in the novel *Arrowsmith*, written by Sinclair Lewis during his residence in Ann Arbor, and was a rather imposing individual in the university's medical community. Although Dr Szilagyi had a near-perfect academic record in Europe, he had not completed the prerequisite English course for admission to medical school. In recognition of his determination, Emerick was asked by Dr Novy to enroll in the literary school, where he could complete the required course in English. At the same time, he was permitted to take anatomy, physiology, biochemistry, and bacteriology with the entering freshman medical school class. Emerick received an A in English. Having passed muster for Dr Novy, he began his second year in Ann Arbor as a full-fledged sophomore medical student. Although the rest of the country was in the depths of the depression, Ann Arbor was a relatively protected academic and cosmopolitan community in which Dr Szilagyi flourished.

D. Emerick Szilagyi's student days at the University of Michigan Medical School from 1931 to 1935 were exemplary. The university at that time had a faculty who emulated the German system of medical education, with a scientifically based laboratory-oriented approach to teaching. Although Frederick A. Coller had been appointed Chairman of the Department of Surgery a few years before Dr Szilagyi started medical school, the faculty members who influenced him most were Henry K. Ranson, an elegant and excellent technical surgeon; Henry Field, a superb pulmonary specialist who was an accomplished diagnostician; Carl F. List, a Jewish refugee from Germany who made neurology exciting and later received further training to become a neurosurgeon; and Eugene Potter, another excellent clinical surgeon. At the conclusion of his medical school education, Emerick graduated with his medical degree cum laude and a clear commitment to become a surgeon.

THE SURGEON

Dr Szilagyi was accepted into the University of Michigan's Surgical Training Program in July 1935. He spent the next year as an intern at no pay, other than food and uniforms, rotating through the various medical specialties at the University Hospital. He spent his second year as a senior intern rotating through all the surgical disciplines of the day, at a salary of $20 a month (Fig. I–2). At the conclusion of his first 2 years of surgical training, Dr Szilagyi accepted an appointment as a teaching assistant in the Department of Pathology, working for the chairman, Carl Weller, a distinguished anatomic pathologist. The next 2 years, from 1937 to 1939, were very important in Dr Szilagyi's academic growth. He frequently cites Dr Weller as one of the most influential individuals in his development as a young physician. During this period he took part in more than 540 autopsies and became an expert microscopist, reviewing many slides with Dr Weller serving as a direct mentor. Emerick published two papers as a member of the Department of Pathology and received a Certificate of Performance in Pathology, but he did not heed Dr Weller's advice to pursue a career in this field. Dr Weller did, however, instill in him an understanding of the necessity to be thorough in one's investigative work in the search for scientific truth. Dr Szilagyi's professional career has been characterized by this sense of thoroughness.

Emerick Szilagyi applied for an appointment as an assistant resident in surgery at Henry Ford Hospital, a position he assumed in July 1939. Henry Ford Hospital was a different world from what he had experienced at the more public University

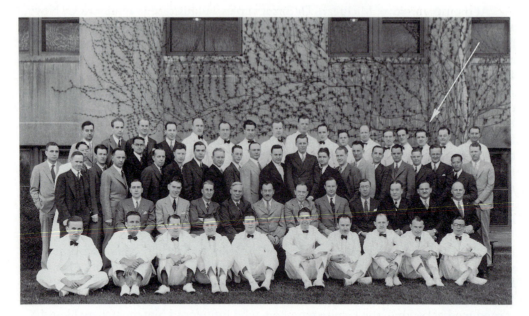

Figure I–2. The 1936–1937 University of Michigan Department of Surgery. D. Emerick Szilagyi, a senior intern, is in the top row (arrow).

Hospital as a student. Acute illnesses were more commonplace and nearly all the patients were private, representing the elite of Detroit society and its suburbs. Nevertheless, a strong academic atmosphere had been established by the Chairman of the Surgical Services, Roy D. McClure, who was a Johns Hopkins–educated and –trained surgeon and one of Halsted's famous "chosen 17." Emerick's experience at Henry Ford Hospital included rotations in orthopedics, obstetrics and gynecology, urology, and anesthesiology, as well as general surgery. During his early residency he wrote a thesis on pyloric stenosis in infants, which was the basis for his being awarded a Master of Science degree from the University of Michigan in 1940. The greatest influence during his surgical training at Henry Ford Hospital came from Lawrence S. Fallis, a Canadian who was trained in England and was an exceptional teacher of surgical technique.

At the completion of his surgery residency in 1942, Emerick took a 2-week vacation with the intent of reporting to active duty in the armed forces. However, Dr McClure requested that he consider replacing Dr Kenneth Waddell as Medical Director of the Ford Rubber Plantation in the Amazon valley of Brazil. The Ford Rubber Plantation was an essential source of rubber and an important aspect of the US military effort during World War II. Emerick's training and the fact that he was an experienced traveler made him an excellent choice for this assignment. He was reclassified from 3A to 2B, testimony to the fact that this civilian job was essential to the arms effort. To his mother's peace of mind, he accepted the medical directorship of the plantation. At the time, his brother was serving in the armed forces in the South Pacific. It is of historical note that when the time came for his departure to Brazil his visa was delayed. A young statesman by the name of Nelson A. Rockefeller working at the InterAmerican Affairs Office interceded with a telegram that allowed Emerick to leave the United States for the Amazon.

Henry Ford had established two rubber plantations in Brazil: a newer one in Belterra, approximately 20 miles along the Tapajós River, a major tributary to the

Amazon, and an older one located approximately 70 miles further upstream on the same waterway (Figs. I–3 and I–4). The latter plantation had been established nearly 15 years earlier and was known as Fordlandia.[1] Dr Fallis, Emerick's mentor during his residency, had been the first Henry Ford Hospital surgeon to serve at this plantation. When Dr Szilagyi arrived at the plantation, he was assisted by three Brazilian doctors whom he supervised. He learned Portuguese quickly and well.

Emerick performed nearly 600 operations during his 2½-year sojourn in Brazil, in a small hospital with one operating room and nearly 70 beds (Fig. I–5). The procedures were undertaken daily from 6 AM to 11 AM, when it became so hot that further work proved impossible. As Emerick notes, he "operated on all the organs except the brain and heart." Lest one question this, it should be noted that he performed 32 cataract extractions with the loss of only one eye, and became proficient at many surgical procedures within the abdomen, chest, and extremities.

Dr Szilagyi received his American College of Surgeons qualification by submitting 25 cases from his Henry Ford Hospital training as well as 25 new cases as a fledgling surgeon at the Brazilian plantation. Among the latter operations, no two were the same and his list encompassed many diverse procedures, including a cesarean section. Officials of the College contacted surgeons at Henry Ford Hospital and inquired as to whether this young fellow in Brazil was joking. They were informed that his list was indeed accurate and believable.

His surgical adventures in the jungle were clearly a competence and confidence builder unlike what many young surgeons of the day might ever experience. Emerick frequently consulted *Bigham's System of Surgery*, a six-volume text on the operative management of various illnesses. He developed such respect for being versatile that he rejected the establishment's traditional wisdom that a surgeon should do only what he had been trained to do. This was an irrational thought that his experience

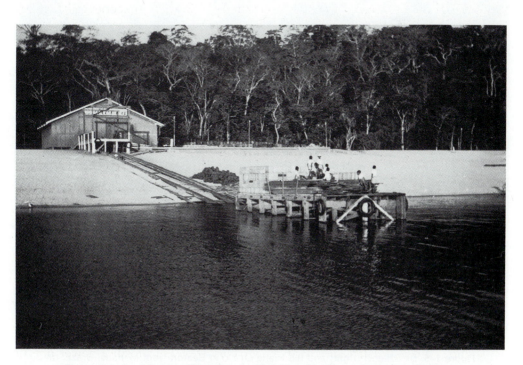

Figure I–3. Ford Rubber Plantation in 1943. Tapajós River approach to Belterra.

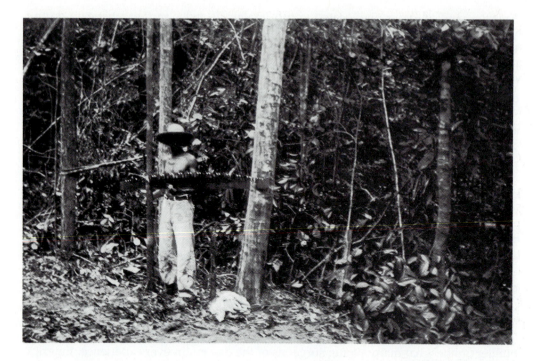

Figure I–4. Ford Rubber Plantation in 1943. Native tapper among rubber trees.

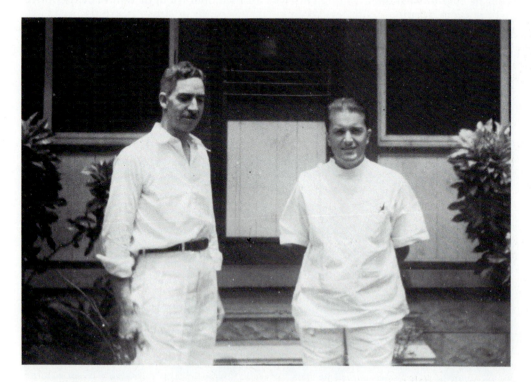

Figure I–5. Dr Szilagyi (**right**) and his friend Dr Colin Beaton from Manáos, Brazil, on whom he performed an appendectomy in Belterra in 1943.

refuted. Dr Szilagyi believed that a surgeon with reasonable training, a working knowledge of anatomy, and modest surgical skills should be able to "take on almost anything." The opportunity to try things when no one else was there to do it in the small hospital at Belterra clearly set the stage for many of his later contributions as a vascular surgeon.

In 1945 Dr Szilagyi returned from Brazil to Henry Ford Hospital, where he was appointed Assistant Surgeon and for 1 year served as chief surgical resident. Shortly thereafter, he organized the second of two surgical divisions within the Department of General Surgery. He served as chief of this division until 1966, when he became Chairman of the Department of Surgery at Henry Ford Hospital.

Dr Szilagyi's first vascular operation, other than a simple embolectomy, was performed in 1951 and consisted of a superficial femoral artery endarterectomy for a segmental occlusive lesion. He subsequently undertook major aortic reconstructive procedures, first with the use of homografts and later with fabricated prostheses. Emerick maintained a very large practice until his retirement from the operating theater in 1984. At that time he elected to devote his full energies to his past as operating editor of the *Journal of Vascular Surgery*. He was fortunate to have his faithful and most competent personal secretary of 16 years, Geri Fairchild, accompany him in this career change. Although the practice of surgery lost a stellar physician, the discipline of vascular surgery gained notably in his transition to this editorship.

THE SCIENTIST

Few vascular surgeons have made as many notable contributions to their profession as has Emerick Szilagyi. Perhaps his most lasting impact related to his very precise and complete documentation of outcomes following reconstructive arterial surgery. Although he was one of the leading pioneers in the performance of aortic surgery in the 1950s, it was his follow-up of these procedures that awakened the scientific community. His studies on the natural history of aortic aneurysms and their surgical treatment represent classics, as do his clinical publications on reconstructions of aortoiliac occlusive disease and femoropopliteal occlusive disease. Many of his contributions brought a sobering realism to our understanding of vascular surgery.

In fact, Dr Szilagyi's writings on the complications of aortic surgery, including colon ischemia and spinal cord injury, as well as his original observations on neointimal hyperplasia and the biological fate of vein grafts placed in the lower extremities, represent hallmark contributions to vascular surgery. Although his publications numbered more than 175, D. Emerick Szilagyi is best known for his application of statistics to outcome studies. This lent lasting credibility to his work. Prior to Dr Szilagyi's setting this standard, results were often simply labeled "early" or "late." The fact is that the Henry Ford Hospital Vascular Registry was the first comprehensive compilation of outcome data for vascular surgery patients in the United States. This effort, conceived and initiated by Emerick in 1956, clearly preceded computerized data bases familiar to today's practices, and epitomized his understanding of what it meant to be a scientific clinician.

THE CONSCIENCE

For more than half of his nearly 85 years, D. Emerick Szilagyi has been a familiar and resolute fixture at surgical meetings. Invariably, he sits in the front of the hall near the speaker's lectern and is a visible symbol of integrity in science. A survey of his presentations as the president of a number of prestigious surgical societies reflect on the breadth of his intellect: "In Defense of the Art of Medicine" (presidential address, North American Chapter, International Cardiovascular Society, 1965),[2] "The Physician: Savant, Saint or Servant?: Commentary on a Paradox" (presidential address, Central Surgical Association, 1967),[3] and "The Elusive Target: Truth in Scientific Reporting. Comments on Error, Self-delusion, Deceit and Fraud" (presidential address, Society for Vascular Surgery, 1983).[4] In these three contributions alone, he provided great insight into being a surgeon, the practice of surgery, and the importance of honesty in science. There is little question that Emerick's thoughts were molded in part by his indirect lineage to William S. Halsted,[5] whom he described as a surgeon whose "outlook was uncompromisingly altruistic and honest" and whose approach was "consistently original and rigorously scientific."[6] Vintage Halsted. Vintage Szilagyi.

In describing the art of medicine, Emerick notes: "It encompasses qualities of mind as well as precepts of conduct: the sentiments of compassion and forbearance and the imperatives of identification, sacrifice, and humility."[2] Emerick spoke further of the threat to these qualities we all seek in our own doctors and ourselves, regarding the regimentation of medicine: "No one who has practiced medicine with even a shred of social conscience can doubt that the economics of dispensing medical services needs some thoroughgoing reforms. I am convinced, however, that the scheme that our social planners have advocated to achieve the changes is not the correct answer, precisely because it would mean the ultimate destruction of the art of medicine."[2] Remarkable thoughts three decades ago from the conscience of a man of science.

In describing a physician's enigmatic image, Emerick noted: "Born of sick man's primitive instinct of self-preservation, the image of the physician as a man of learning, of superior moral obligations, and of devoted willingness to serve has brought forth a relationship between physician and patient that best fulfills the patient's needs and best rewards the physician."[3] Emerick believes that a physician must sustain his image. He stated: "He must live by the commandments of the method of a scientist, by the rules of a seeker of truth, while nurturing the gentle art of humanistic medicine and while rejecting the allure of the false world of mechanistic, regimented science. He must carry the burden of the ethical–moral dictates of his tradition while the appeal of moral laws in a libertine society around him is growing dimmer."[3] He knows this is a difficult task, and admonishes us: "In this world of ours, where so many are unfriendly to noble images, his labor to uphold this image may fall even shorter of the goal. But if the physician only sustains this endless battle, what he will accomplish cannot be a defeat, for through his trial he will have remained in part a scientist, in part a saint, and in part a servant."[3]

Dr Szilagyi, by example and query, has influenced at least three generations of physicians responsible for the management of patients with vascular disease. He has been the conscience of vascular surgery. Perhaps in no other period than when he served as editor of the *Journal of Vascular Surgery* from 1984 to 1990 was his influence on this discipline more resounding. His high standards were reflected in the visible success of this new periodical.

He also had some heady advice for those of our profession who may be unknowing recipients of untruthful reports in the literature when he noted that: "The reader of scientific publications has an effective way of reducing or canceling the impact of scientific falsehood. Scientific communication is a give-and-take affair. The listener or reader of these scientific reports, particularly those that claim to represent new and important information, should consider them with friendly but abiding skepticism and accept the conclusions after a leisurely interval of watchful waiting. Delay in acceptance of a worthy idea only postpones the day of its benefits. Prompt acceptance of a concept that is untrue, harmful, or both, enlarges the damage it may do."[7] Vascular surgery stands indebted to this wisdom. We must be responsible to ourselves.

CONCLUSION

Emerick Szilagyi has been recognized by his peers throughout the world with many honors. Those who know him also know of his devotion to his family. Emerick married his first wife, Evelyn (Eve), in 1951. She was an extraordinary artist whose medium was watercolor. Her illustrations of still life and her portraits were the product of exceptional intellect and talent. Eve's portrait of Emerick was remarkable for the character it captured (Fig. I–6). Dr Szilagyi has two daughters, Martha and Christine, one of whom is an expert in computer-based automotive research and the other is currently pursuing an advanced degree in clinical psychology. Emerick lost his first wife to cancer in 1981. He has spent his recent years with his second wife, Sally, who has an uplifting and vivacious spirit.

Dr Szilagyi has recently allowed a somewhat philosophical bent to encroach on his unyielding objective personality. He accepts the changing state of surgery from a dominant tool to treat disease, to a realization that molecular genetic approaches to many of today's common surgical diseases will make operative treatment obsolete. Emerick continues to be a voracious reader and clear thinker. As a student, surgeon, scientist, and conscience of vascular surgery he has no peer.

Acknowledgment
I wish to thank Dr Szilagyi for the many hours of conversation and photographs he contributed that made this biographical sketch possible.

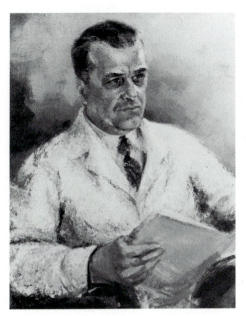

Figure I–6. Evelyn Szilagyi's portrait of her husband in 1978.

REFERENCES

1. Dempsey MA. Fordlandia. *Mich Hist*. 1994;78:24–33.
2. Szilagyi DE. In defense of the art of medicine. *Arch Surg*. 1965;91:707–711.
3. Szilagyi DE. The physician: savant, saint or servant?: commentary on a paradox. *Arch Surg*. 1967;95:325–331.
4. Szilagyi DE. The elusive target: truth in scientific reporting. Comments on error, self-delusion, deceit and fraud. *J Vasc Surg*. 1984;1:243–253.
5. Szilagyi DE. Report of a posthumous dialogue. *Arch Surg*. 1979;114:359–364.
6. McClure RD, Szilagyi DE. Halsted—teacher of surgeons. *Am J Surg*. 1951;82:122–131.
7. Smith RF. D. Emerick Szilagyi—in appreciation. *J Vasc Surg*. 1991;13:3–4.

I

General Considerations

1

New Understanding of the Pathophysiology of the Atherosclerotic Process

Seymour Glagov, MD, Christopher K. Zarins, MD, Hisham S. Bassiouny, MD, and Don P. Giddens, PhD

The evolution and complication of human atheromatous lesions are associated with modeling and remodeling processes that tend to promote stability with respect to wall shear stress and tensile stress. Healing and organizing reactions include both erosion and sclerosis beneath and within the plaque and the formation of a subendo-thelial fibrous cap. Ideally, these responses lead to outward sequestration of the plaque, resulting in isolation of potentially thrombogenic components from the artery lumen and preservation of a regular circular lumen contour, favoring continuation of stable laminar flow. The artery also undergoes enlargement where plaques form, such that the lumen cross-sectional area is preserved for extended periods. Early clinical detection of minimal asymptomatic plaques requires interrogation of precise locations at high risk for plaque induction in relation to flow field properties. Sequential changes in lumen contour and configuration of advanced plaques are associated with risk factor control and with direct interventions, often reflecting complicating and modeling processes as well as plaque progression, regression, or stabilization. Diagnosis of imminent, recent, or remote plaque disruption and fissuring depends on the clinical identification of a series of recognized microanatomic features. These are likely to become increasingly apparent as resolutions of clinical imaging methods improve. Restenosis of plaques that have been subjected to angioplasty or atherectomy is characterized by intimal hyperplasia, presumably induced by the mechanical disrup-tive injury. Modeling reactions related to the tendency to restore normal levels of wall shear and tensile stresses are likely to be major determinants of the outcome. Should baseline conditions of wall shear and tension be restored by the intimal model-ing and healing process following the procedures, the proliferative reaction would be expected to stop and patency to be maintained. Persistence of low-flow states would tend to induce continuation of the proliferative intimal adaptive response and lead to restenosis. It may prove to be more relevant to our understanding of human plaque morphogenesis and complication to identify and modulate the metabolic and flow-related processes and mechanisms that regulate the modeling responses during plaque formation and disruption than to find ways of suppressing cell proliferation and matrix production to prevent plaque formation, complication, or postinterventional restenosis.

Individual therapeutic decisions as well as meaningful interpretations of the outcomes of clinical trials designed to evaluate the effects of risk factor control or operative interventions on atherosclerotic arteries depend largely on knowledge of the morphogenesis of the atherosclerotic plaque under a variety of conditions and on an accurate appraisal of the corresponding images and hemodynamic measurements. Improvement in resolution and the advent of capabilities for three-dimensional image reconstruction are likely to permit increasingly detailed insights into the factors that determine the evolution of the atherosclerotic process in the principal vascular locations at high risk. This knowledge is of great clinical significance, for although mortality from cardiovascular disease seems to have diminished in recent years, the prevalence of cardiovascular disease has not decreased markedly. This discrepancy may be explained, at least in part, by great improvements in diagnostic and therapeutic measures, while preventive measures have not been as successful. In other words, individuals with manifest cardiovascular disease tend to survive to an older age than previously and succumb instead to other diseases. Until we can prevent or diminish the prevalence of atherosclerosis, precise information concerning the evolution of the atherosclerotic lesion is essential if we are to slow disease progression, select optimal therapies, and anticipate plaque complication and its consequences. Current specific areas of concern directly relevant to diagnosis and treatment include (1) detection of minimal, asymptomatic lesions, (2) recognition of the bases for changes in size, composition, and organization of advanced plaques, (3) clinical identification of the features indicative of plaque stability or instability, and (4) establishment of the morphologic and hemodynamic antecedents of restenosis following direct interventions. Clinicopathologic features related to each of these critical problems indicate that the mechanical stresses associated with blood circulation, wall shear stress and tensile stress, elicit adaptive modeling responses in artery wall and plaque which tend to preserve mural integrity and adequate flow for as long as possible. Our purpose here is to discuss each of the above categories in terms of the nature of the modeling reactions.

MODELING OF ATHEROSCLEROTIC PLAQUES

Detailed *ex vivo* studies of human atherosclerotic plaques have furnished a reasonably consistent morphologic classification of characteristic lesion types. The features and the usual transitions among these forms have been documented in recent reviews furnished by the Committee on Vascular Lesions of the American Heart Association.[1,2] The descriptive features imply a likely but not inevitable progression from the fatty streak to the complex conglomerate that defines the advanced plaque and its several morphologic variants. Structural morphogenesis during plaque induction and evolution are consistent with changes that suggest underlying adaptive modeling mechanisms. Lipid initially accumulates within a focal eccentric widening of the intima in relation to an intimal fibrocellular thickening containing smooth muscle cells. As the plaque progresses, reactions may be noted in the intima and in the underlying media (Fig. 1–1). Although erosion of the media can be noted, even in some advanced plaques, the intimal reaction immediately adjacent to the media is often characterized by sclerosis. Both collagen and elastin fibers are prominent. As the plaque progresses, a fibrocellular reaction is also evident at the luminal subendothelial aspect of the

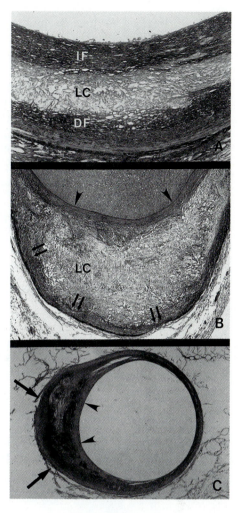

Figure 1–1. Sections of arteries that indicate the principal features of artery wall and plaque modeling during the evolution of a human atherosclerotic plaque. (**A**) As the plaque progresses from an initial fatty streak to stratified manifest plaque, fibrocellular tissue reactions occur within the intima adjacent to the underlying media (DF), often involving the media and beneath the endothelium (IF). In this manner lipid and necrotic debris (LC) are isolated from both the underlying media and the lumen. (**B**) The inner subendothelial fibrocellular region usually differentiates into a compact, layered structure consisting of smooth muscle cells and connective tissue fibers and resembling the structure and configuration of the media. This fibrous cap (arrowheads) isolates the underlying lipid core (LC) from the lumen. The deeper juxtamedial fibrous region may persist, enlarge, or show evidence of erosion of the underlying fibrous region or media (double arrows). (**C**) Cross-section of an artery with a typical advanced atherosclerotic plaque. The vessel wall bulges outward beneath a predominantly fibrous plaque (arrows). Portions of the fibrous cap are evident (arrowheads) as is a lipid core. (*C is from Glagov S, Weisenberg E, Zarins CK, et al. Compensatory enlargement of human atherosclerotic coronary arteries. Reproduced with permission from* N Engl J Med. *1987;316:1371–1375.*)

intima. The lipid and the associated products of tissue degeneration and necrosis (the lipid core) thus tend to be segregated to a mid-intimal zone by the deep and superficial fibrocellular reactions (Fig. 1–1A). The superficial zone often proceeds to differentiate into a compact fibrocellular structure, the fibrous cap (Fig. 1–1B), which is often similar in both thickness and architecture to the underlying media or to the media of the opposite uninvolved portion of the artery. These modifications result in stratification of the lesion and, in association with the changes in the media, bulging of the plaque outward into the adventitia. The plaque is thereby effectively sequestered from the lumen (Fig. 1–1C). In the absence of deforming complications by plaque disruptions, fissuring, hemorrhage, or thrombus deposition, the lumen surface remains smooth, the cross-sectional lumen contour remains more or less circular or oval, and the subendothelial fibrocellular fibrous cap reaction persists (Fig. 1–1C). Fibrosis and calcification progress and tend to become increasingly prominent as the lesion increases in size. Thus, large lesions tend to be complex, that is, composed of juxtaposed regions of contrasting composition.

Nevertheless, neither lesion size nor lesion composition necessarily corresponds to the degree of stenosis, for erosion of the media and/or plaque disruption or reorganization may result in a marked increase in vessel diameter, or ectasia. Furthermore, arteries enlarge as plaques form, tending to maintain a lumen of adequate cross-section even in the presence of relatively large intimal plaques.[3,4] Postmortem sections of the left anterior descending coronary artery taken at the same level in two individuals are shown in the upper portion of Fig. 1–2. The lumen cross-sectional area is about the same for each, but the lesion area is vastly different. If the artery on the left had not enlarged to compensate for the large plaque that formed, the lumen would have been totally occluded. That such artery enlargement is a consequence of plaque formation is indicated by the fact that in any given artery segment the lumen cross-sectional area is similar for involved and uninvolved segments. Enlargement occurs only where plaques are forming and lumen stenosis appears to be manifest, on the average for the left main coronary artery for example, when 40% or more of the potential lumen area, as defined by the area encompassed by internal elastin lamina, is occupied by plaque.[3] Since plaque enlargement is associated mainly with the outward bulging of the artery wall beneath the lesion (Fig. 1–1C) and the lumen contour tends to remain round and circular, the outer contour of the vessel becomes oval and deformed. Although there is evidence that plaques may stabilize at any stage of development or revert to a previous or simpler stage, new lesions may develop on an apparently previously stabilized plaque. The sequence of changes in the "new" superimposed plaque may be incomplete compared to the underlying plaque or may recapitulate the entire process. With advance of the disease, circumferential extension and extention into the lumen from the initial focus of involvement proceed, but the distribution of intimal lesion thickness tends, nevertheless, to remain eccentric. The features of the "defense" of an artery in the face of plaque development are summarized in Table 1–1. The healing and organizing reactions, modulated by the mechanical

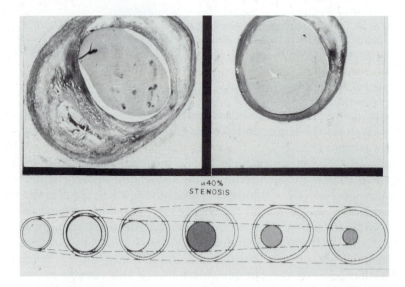

Figure 1–2. Sections from the same level of the left anterior descending coronary artery from two different individuals. The lumen cross-section is the same, but the plaque cross-section is markedly different. If the artery on the left had not enlarged as the plaque formed, the lumen would have been totally occluded. In the lower diagram the sequence of enlargement with increase in plaque size is shown diagrammatically, corresponding to a study of the left main coronary artery in 135 autopsies.[3] On the average, compromise of lumen diameter did not occur until 40% of the potential lumen area (ie, the area encompassed by the internal elastic lamina) was occupied by plaque.

TABLE 1–1. ARTERY DEFENSE AS PLAQUES ENLARGE

Maintainance of a circular lumen
Sequestration of plaque from lumen
  Fibrous cap
  Outward bulge
Compensatory enlargement

stimuli association with the circulation, occur in the face of a continuing, arrested, or resolving chemical–metabolic injury. The smooth muscle cells which are included in the fibrous cap in the subendothelial region may be presumed to become oriented and synthesize connective tissue fibers, in keeping with the imposed pulsatile stresses.[5] In the deeper reaches of the atheroma, these stimuli are likely to be dampened. We may thus define *modeling* of arteries with plaques as the manifestation of adaptive–reactive tissue responses that determine size, configuration, composition, and patency in relation to the interaction between atherogenic and mechanical factors. The modeling reactions as well as the tendency to complication appear to be not only patient specific but also site and lesion specific. In the same patient and over the same time interval, some plaques within a given vascular bed or in different vascular beds remain stable, some progress to greater stenosis, some show evidence of reduced stenosis, and some become complicated by ulceration and lumen distortion.

DETECTION OF MINIMAL ASYMPTOMATIC LESIONS

Clinical features that correspond to intimal lesion initiation or induction are considered to permit institution of clinical risk factor interventions at an early stage of plaque development. Detection of minimal intimal plaque formation usually depends on measurements of artery wall thickness (ie, intima plus media), changes in mural mechanical properties (compliance), or changes in wall composition with regard to matrix fiber content, lipid core deposits, cellularity, and calcification. In view of the usual focal and eccentric location of plaques and the relationship of plaque location to geometric transitions, particularly in regions of reduced and oscillating wall shear stress,[6,7] selection of precise regions to be interrogated is critical. For example, the sinus and the proximal internal carotid artery at the carotid bifurcation are common regions of detectable minimal plaque formation. The distribution of plaque formation in these regions tends to be helical, in keeping with the flow properties at each level.[8] Plaque distribution, however, is likely to correspond to individual geometric variations. Thus, any single direction of interrogation by ultrasound may not correspond to the maximal lesion thickness at that level, particularly for minimal or moderately advanced asymptomatic lesions (Fig. 1–3). Interrogation of a region at risk should therefore be examined over a range of incident angles whenever possible (Fig. 1–1B). The extent to which minimal asymptomatic atherosclerosis can be detected or quantified in various locations on the basis of calcification remains to be defined, but dystrophic calcium deposits often occur in plaques which have not yet resulted in stenosis and have not undergone disruption but may be absent from manifest plaques. The extent to which atherosclerosis is one of the locations at high risk may serve as a surrogate for detection of plaques in another site also awaits further investigation. Accruing evidence suggests that abdominal aortic and coronary atherosclerosis may precede the formation of thoracic aortic disease or cerebrovascular disease. On the other hand, metabolic abnormalities such as diabetes mellitus or other major risk

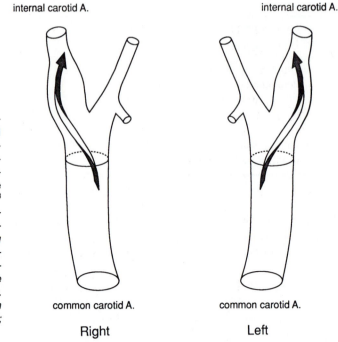

internal carotid A.

internal carotid A.

Figure 1–3. Diagrammatic representation of the circumferential
location of the region of maximum intimal thickening corresponding to minimal asymptomatic plaques in the region of the
human carotid bifurcation.[8]
(*From Masawa N, Glagov S, Zarins CK. Quantitative morphologic study of intimal thickening
at the human carotid bifurcation: II. The compensatory enlargement response and the role
of the intima in tensile support.
Reproduced with permission
from* Atherosclerosis. *1994:107;
138–147.*)

common carotid A.

common carotid A.

Right

Left

factors appear to be linked to certain patterns of preferential involvement and lesion
composition.

CHANGES IN SIZE, COMPOSITION, AND ORGANIZATION OF ADVANCED PLAQUES

On sequential studies increased, diminished, or unchanged plaque and wall thickness,
cross-sectional area, and lumen contour or diameter are likely to be indices of lesion
progression, regression, or stabilization, permitting evaluation of treatment options
in the presence of manifest established plaques. It should be noted, however, that
images of lumen diameter on angiograms may provide information regarding comparative degrees of lumen narrowing but may not provide an accurate appraisal of
lesion cross-sectional area or volume.[3,4,9] This limitation is due to the compensatory
enlargement of arteries where plaques form, changes in lumen size due to modifications of plaque modeling and composition, the occurrence of plaque disruptions and
ulcerations, erosions of the underlying media, and the formation and organization
of thrombi (Table 1–2). The relationship of plaque modeling to plaque composition
is discussed in the descriptive section on plaque evolution above.

FEATURES INDICATIVE OF PLAQUE STABILITY OR INSTABILITY

Features that indicate plaque stability or instability include modifications of lumen
contour, lesion configuration, lesion composition, and lumen surface integrity on
imaging studies. Lumen and plaque features that connote imminent, immediate,
recent, or remote plaque disruption, fissuring, hemorrhage, and thrombus deposition

TABLE 1–2. CHANGES IN WALL THICKNESS, INTIMA THICKNESS, LUMEN DIMENSIONS, AND LUMEN CONFIGURATION

Remodeling responses to changes in wall shear and tensile stresses

Plaque progression and regression

Artery enlargement during atherogenesis

Wall erosion by atherosclerosis

Ulceration of plaques

Formation of aneurysms

Organization of thrombi

Plaque hemorrhage

---

are likely to be closely related to the specific symptomatic manifestations of atherosclerosis. Problems of clinical interpretation of images arise in relation to artery and plaque modeling in response to alterations in both flow and wall tension; the rate and nature of component segregation and stratification during lesion induction, progression, or regression; and the healing and remodeling processes following plaque disruption, hemorrhage, or thrombosis. In addition, foci of symptom-producing plaque disruption may be quite small, limiting detection by most current imaging methods. At the histological level, the features of acute or subacute disruption of plaque organization that connote underlying plaque instability include (1) erosion of the fibrous cap, with or without an immediately adjacent lipid core or an associated inflammatory cellular infiltrate or thrombus deposition; (2) the presence of fissuring or ulceration, with or without evident thrombus deposition; (3) the presence of manifest hemorrhage within the plaque, that is, blood dissecting into the plaque by way of a focal surface disruption or from vasa vasorum within the plaque, or the presence of clusters of siderophages, suggesting previous resolved hemorrhage; (4) secondary lesion formation on an older stratified plaque, as indicated by foam cell and lipid core accumulations or focal inflammatory cell clusters within an underlying apparently stable plaque; and (5) the juxtaposition of regions of presumably different composition and elastic modulus associated with the above-mentioned features, especially when calcifications are in close apposition to the lumen surface. An example is shown in Fig. 1–4. Predictions of plaque instability from images depend on accurate detection, identification, and quantitative appraisal of these features. Consistent citeria are likely to emerge as resolution, sensitivity, and specificty of clinical imaging modalities improve.[10]

The occurence of plaque complications is probably directly related to individual metabolic and tissue reactive factors that determine plaque architecture, composition, and consistency and therefore determine plaque fragility, and to mechanical and geometric factors that determine the distribution, magnitude, and variation in shear and tensile stresses exerted on plaques. The likely determinants of plaque consistency in relation to temporal factors are listed in Fig. 1–5. Possible relationships to the function of component cells are shown in Fig. 1–6. The metabolic–atherogenic determinants and the likely mechanical determinants of the disruption of susceptible fragile plaques are listed in Table 1–3.

MORPHOLOGIC AND HEMODYNAMIC ANTECEDENTS OF RESTENOSIS

Plaque disruption or partial excision by intravascular instrumentation or intraoperative endarterectomy creates marked changes in lumen and lesion configuration and

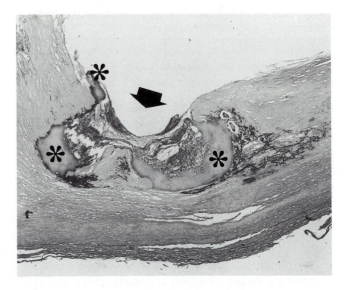

Figure 1–4. A region of plaque complication, such as this ulceration (arrow) at the proximal sinus of a carotid bifurcation. The close juxtaposition of components with contrasting physical properties, such as lipid and cell debris or foam cells and calcifications (asterisk), especially when these are close to the lumen surface as in this instance, often corresponds to focal lesion disruptions.

thereby in the distribution of flow- and tension-related physical stresses. Subsequent changes in image appearances correspond both to the degree of lesion modification by the intervention and to the subsequent healing–remodeling proliferative and differentiating processes initiated by the injury. Interpretation of these features in relation to clinical determinations of flow and to progression of the atherosclerotic process may be expected to identify factors that could establish the bases for and the predictors of eventual long-term patency or the development of secondary obstructions (restenoses) at sites of intervention.[11]

The restenosing process is characterized by a type of smooth muscle proliferation and matrix formation, usually termed *intimal hyperplasia*, in the vicinity of the disrupted plaque. It is presumably initiated by the mechanical disruptive injury. Lesions that reocclude have presumably been exposed to degrees of trauma similar to those applied to lesions that do not restenose, and no definite relationship has been established among underlying plaque composition, extent of disruption, and therapeutic outcome. The histological features of the intimal reactive proliferative response following angioplasty are similar to those that occur about surgically produced anastomoses in association with revascularization procedures, in vessels with markedly reduced flow, in saphenous veins or other vessels used as bypass grafts, and in vascular constructions for dialysis access.[12,13] It may, however, also be found in atherectomy specimens without previous intervention[14] and probably reflects a focal adaptive healing modeling reaction following plaque fissuring or other alterations in configuration due to changes in plaque composition or thrombosis.

Rapid Progression ⟶ "Soft" Plaque

Malleable, plastic, sharp gradients of compliance

Slow Progression ⟶ "Hard" plaque

"Fixed", inflexible-rigid, fibrotic calcific

Secondary rapid growth ⟶ "Fragile" plaque

Disruptible, fibrous cap dissolution, hemorrhage(?)

Figure 1–5. The temporal clinical aspects of plaque formation which are likely to affect plaque composition, consistency, and mechanical properties and determine susceptibility to disruption.

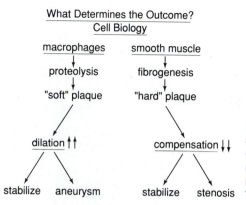

Figure 1–6. Cell composition is likely to have a strong effect on lesion composition. The relative contributions of smooth muscle cells and macrophages shown in this diagrammatic representation probably change considerably during plaque evolution and differ from region to region.

In specimens of nonatherosclerotic intimal thickening obtained from many human vessels, we have noted two prinicipal forms of the reaction: *intimal hyperplasia* and *intimal fibrocellular hypertrophy*.[15] We have suggested that the term *intimal hyperplasia* be reserved for tissue appearances that connote an ongoing predominantly proliferative response. The component cells tend to be fairly widely separated without any definite common orientation. The intervening matrix, although abundant, contains few distinct elastin or collagen fibers. We have utilized the term *intimal fibrocellular hypertrophy* for appearances that connote structural differentiation and stabilization. In this form, common orientation of the component cells is a prominent feature, as is the reduction in the relative proportion of matrix to cells but with formation of commonly oriented and prominent elastin and collagen fibers. The morphologic characteristics of the two forms of reactive intimal modeling are shown in Fig. 1–7. We consider the intimal response to be primarily a reaction that tends to narrow the lumen or to focally remodel the lumen surface and alter local flow patterns to restore wall shear stress to the normal baseline value of approximately 15 dynes/cm^2.[16,17] The intimal adaptive–reactive response after angioplasty appears initially as the mainly proliferative form, that is intimal hyperplasia. If baseline wall shear stress is reestablished, the predominantly proliferative phase is curtailed and transition to the archectecturally differentiated intimal fibrocellular hypertrophy response occurs, most likely closely modulated by local tensile stress conditions.[18] Transitional or superimposed forms, connoting intermediate changes, presumably in response to preceding modulations of

---

TABLE 1–3. LIKELY DETERMINANTS OF MODELING REACTIONS

Atherogenic

  Episodic progression and healing

  Age of onset

  Individual susceptibility

  Changes in lifestyle, diet, smoking

  Superimposition of hypertension, diabetes

Hemodynamic (Mechanical)

  Local differences in hemodynamic risk

  Individual differences in hemodynamic risk

  Individual differences in tissue response to physical stresses

  Changing mechanical properties of plaques

  Changing hemodynamics as plaque enlarges

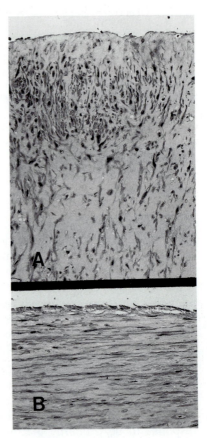

Figure 1–7. The two forms of nonatherosclerotic intimal thickening are shown in this photomicrograph. (**A**) Intimal hyperplasia consists of smooth muscle cells in no particular spatial orientation in an abundant matrix but with few formed connective tissue fibers. (**B**) With intimal fibrocellular hypertrophy the cells are aligned, matrix is less abundant, and formed and oriented fibers, collagen and/or elastin, are evident. (*From Glagov S. Intimal hyperplasia, vascular modeling and the restenosis problem. Reproduced with permission from* Circulation. *1994;89:2888–2891.*)

mechanical stresses, are often noted in surgical and autopsy material. The organizing intimal reaction then tends to merge with the adjacent artery wall and may exhibit structural features of media. The factors preventing stabilization and persistence of a patent lumen after angioplasty or atherectomy would therefore include the presence or creation of irreducible deformities associated with dense plaque fibrosis and/or calcification as well as the persistence of low-flow states due to proximal or distal atherosclerotic stenoses or to reduced cardiac output. The proposed role for mechanically induced modeling reactions as determinants of restenosis or patency and the relationship of the forms of intimal thickening to the possible outcomes are outlined in Table 1–4.

CONCLUSION

Thus far, our tissue culture experiments and our cholesterol-fed animal models have failed to provide clinically useful insights into the nature and regulation of the defensive modeling responses or the limits of the compensatory reactions, nor have they helped us to understand why some plaques break down when they do while others remain stable or how images and hemodynamic measurements could help us distinguish between the two. Nor do we have much clarity on the manner in which the tissue responses are elicited and regulated in relation to the mechanical stresses

TABLE 1–4. MECHANICALLY INDUCED MODELING IN RELATION TO PATENCY AND RESTENOSIS[a]

Stenosis → Intervention → Proliferative Healing Response

Persistent or Subsequent Progressive Low Flow (WSS ↓)

WSS ↓ → IH → r↓ → WSS ↑
Baseline WSS not restored
→ Continuing IH → *Restenosis*

Postinterventional Low Local Flow (WSS ↓)

WSS ↓ → IH → r↓ → WSS ↑
Baseline WSS restored
→ Stabilization (arrest of IH)
→ IFH → *Patency*

Higher than Baseline Local Flow (WSS ↑)

WSS ↑ → r↑ → WT ↑ → TS ↑
TS ↑ → SMC response (media ± intima ± IH)
→ Stabilization (appropriate TS and baseline WSS)
→ IFH → *Patency*

---

[a]The possible outcome, patency or restenosis, of an angioplasty or atherectomy procedure in relation to the proliferative reaction, intimal hyperplasia (IH), and to the subsequent stabilizing differentiating response, intimal fibrocellular hypertrophy (IFH), emphasizing the central role of the modeling adaptations to wall shear stress (WSS) and tensile stress (TS). r indicates radius; WT, Wall tension; SMC, Smooth muscle cell.

Reproduced with permission from Glagov S. Intimal hyperplasia, vascular modeling and the restenosis problem. *Circulation.* 1994;89:2888–2891.

attendant on blood flow or how mechanical stresses and plaque composition interact to provoke or prevent disruptions or to induce or prevent restenoses. These considerations indicate that quantitative clinicopathologic coorelative studies of the variations in the natural history of human plaques, in direct relation to clinical symptoms, imaging studies, and therapeutic outcomes, are essential and indispensable. Morphometric, histochemical, immunocytochemical, chemical, and molecular studies of the functional state of human lesion cells, in conjunction with methods for visualizing lesions, assessing lesion composition, and quantifying associated local hemodynamic conditions are likely to reveal the differential effects on lesions of various modes of risk factor control and help us to develop criteria to discern which plaques are likely to cause trouble. Although these findings should in turn direct us to ask specific questions about our experimental animal and tissue culture models, we must then return to the functional microenvironment of the actual human artery wall and plaque if we are to gain accurate and clinically applicable insights likely to permit anticipation, prevention, and management of complications. It may therefore prove to be more relevant to our understanding of plaque morphogenesis, and of the processes which underlie the development of plaque complications, to explore the controlling mechanisms of proliferation in relation to vessel wall adaptation to plaque formation and disruption than to find ways of entirely suppressing cell proliferation as a treatment or preventive measure of atherogenesis, plaque complication, or postinterventional stenosis.

Acknowledgment

The work covered in this report was performed under grants HL15062 (SCOR-Atherosclerosis) and HL41267 of the National Institutes of Health.

REFERENCES

1. Stary HC, Blankenhorn DH, Chandler AB, et al. A definition of initial, fatty streak and intermediate lesions of arteriosclerosis. *Circulation*. 1994:89;2462–2478.
2. Stary HC, Blankenhorn DH, Chandler AB, et al. A definition of advanced atherosclerotic lesions and a classification of atherosclerosis. *Arterioscler Thromb*. In press.
3. Glagov S, Weisenberg E, Zarins CK, et al. Compensatory enlargement of human atherosclerotic coronary arteries. *N Engl J Med*. 1987;316:1371–1375.
4. Zarins CK, Weisenberg E, Kolettis G, et al. Differential enlargement of artery segments in response to enlarging atherosclerotic plaques. *J Vasc Surg*. 1988;7:386–394.
5. Leung DYM, Glagov S, Mathews MB. Cycling stretching stimulates synthesis of matrix components by arterial smooth muscle cells in vitro. *Science*. 1976;191:475–477.
6. Zarins CK, Giddens DP, Bjaradaj BK, et al. Carotid bifurcation atherosclerosis: quantitative correlation of plaque localization with flow velocity profiles and wall shear stress. *Circ Res*. 1983;53:502–514.
7. Ku DN, Zarins CK, Giddens DP, et al. Pulsatile flow and atherosclerosis in the human carotid bifurcation: positive correlation between plaque localization and low and oscillating shear stress. *Arteriosclerosis*. 1985;5:292–302.
8. Masawa N, Glagov S, Zarins CK. Quantitative morphologic study of intimal thickening at the human carotid bifurcation. I. Axial and circumferential distribution of maximum intimal thickening in asymptomatic uncomplicated plaques. *Atherosclerosis*. 1994:107;126–137.
9. Masawa N, Glagov S, Zarins CK. Quantitative morphologic study of intimal thickening at the human carotid bifurcation: II. The compensatory enlargement response and the role of the intima in tensile support. *Atherosclerosis*. 1994:107;138–147.
10. Glagov S, Masawa N, Bassiouny H, et al. Morphologic bases for establishing end-points for early plaque detection and plaque instability. *Int J Cardiac Imaging*. 1944;10:in press.
11. Glagov S. Intimal hyperplasia, vascular modeling and the restenosis problem. *Circulation*. 1994;89:2888–2891.
12. Glagov S, Giddens DP, Bassiouny H, et al. Hemodynamic effects and tissue reactions at graft to vein anastomoses for vascular access. In: Sommer BG, Henry ML, eds. *Vascular Access for Hemodialysis—II*. Chicago, WL Gore and Associates/Precept Press; 1991;3–20.
13. Bassiouny H, White MS, Glagov S, et al. Anastomotic intimal hyperplasia: mechanical injury to flow induced. *J Vasc Surg*. 1992;15:708–717.
14. Miller MJ, Kuntz RE, Friedrich SP, et al. Frequency and consequences of intimal hyperplasia in specimens retrieved by directional atherectomy of native primary coronary artery stenoses and subsequent restenosis. *Am J Cardiol*. 1993;71:652–658.
15. Glagov S, Zarins CK. Is intimal hyperplasia an adaptive response or a pathologic process? *J Vasc Surg*. 1989;10:571–573.
16. Kamiya A, Togawa T. Adaptive regulation of wall shear stress to flow change in the canine carotid artery. *Am J Physiol*. 1990;239:H14–H21.
17. Zarins CK, Zatina MA, Giddens DP, et al. Shear stress regulation of artery lumen diameter in experimental atherogenesis. *J Vasc Surg*. 1987;5:413–420.
18. Dobrin PB, Litooy FN, Endean ED. Mechanical factors predisposing to intimal hyperplasia and medial thickening in autogenous vein grafts. *Surgery*. 1989;105:393–400.

2

Hematologic Factors in Arterial Thrombotic Disease

G. Patrick Clagett, MD

Prothrombotic or hypercoagulable states occur when deficiencies of serine proteases or natural anticoagulants exist, when imbalances occur in the fibrinolytic system, when substances are present that accelerate coagulation or platelet reactions, and when diffuse endothelial dysfunction exists. Hypercoagulable states can be classified into two broad categories: hereditary and acquired[1] (Table 2–1). The hereditary or congenital coagulation abnormalities, of which antithrombin III and protein C and S deficiencies are examples, are often referred to as inherited thrombophilic disorders. The biochemical abnormalities are generally fixed and persistent, and yet the clinical thrombotic events are episodic. Acquired hypercoagulable states, such as the antiphospholipid syndrome and heparin-associated thrombocytopenia, often accompany another illness. In addition, there is a group of less well-defined acquired hypercoagulable states in which multiple complex hemostatic aberrations accompany diverse clinical conditions; examples include malignancy, pregnancy, and the postoperative state. Acquired hypercoagulable states are far more common than congenital thrombophilias.

Inherited thrombophilic disorders are frequently characterized by venous thrombosis, especially in unusual sites, whereas acquired hypercoagulable states may present with venous or arterial thrombosis. Suspicion of an underlying congenital hypercoagulable disorder should be aroused by any of the following characteristics: unexplained venous thrombosis in a person younger than 45 years of age; recurrent venous thromboembolism; thrombosis of mesenteric, hepatic, portal, renal, or cerebral veins or the inferior vena cava; diffuse cutaneous microvascular thrombosis; and a positive family history of thrombosis.[2]

Arterial thrombosis is a much less common manifestation of hypercoagulable syndromes, and when it does occur it is usually in patients over 50 years of age who have risk factors. In contrast to venous thrombi, which are caused primarily by sluggish blood flow in the presence of hypercoagulable disorders, arterial thrombi result from elevated shear stress at sites of vessel wall injury and are composed predominantly of platelets. Platelet function and vessel wall disorders characterized by endothelial dysfunction are the hallmarks of disorders associated with a propensity to arterial thrombosis. Abnormalities of platelets are associated with myeloproliferative disor-

TABLE 2–1. PROTHROMBOTIC OR HYPERCOAGULABLE CONDITIONS

Hereditary

Antithrombin III deficiency
Protein C deficiency
Resistance to activated protein C (factor V defect?)
Protein S deficiency
Congenital fibrinolytic disorders
Dysfibrinogenemia
Homocystinuria (cystathionine synthase deficiency)
Lipoprotein(a)

Acquired

Antiphospholipid antibodies
Heparin-induced thrombocytopenia
Myeloproliferative disorders
Malignancy
Inflammatory disorders and postoperative state
Pregnancy
Oral contraceptives
Elevation of fibrinogen and factor VII levels
Nephrotic syndrome

ders, and vessel wall abnormalities include homocystinuria and inflammatory vasculopathies.[3,4] Heparin-induced thrombocytopenia and the antiphospholipid antibody syndrome are examples of hypercoagulable states associated with both platelet and vessel wall abnormalities. Thrombin is the most potent physiological stimulus for platelet aggregation and secretion, and classic hereditary hypercoagulable syndromes that lead to generation of thrombin are being increasingly recognized as causing arterial thrombosis as well as venous thrombosis.[3] In addition, arterial thromboembolism is sometimes associated with venous thrombosis and may develop from paradoxical embolism across a patent foramen ovale. In one study 40% of patients under the age of 55 presenting with ischemic stroke had a patent foramen ovale by microbubble echocardiography in comparison to 10% of age-matched controls without stroke.[5] This is an increasingly recognized entity and should be considered in patients presenting with "cryptogenic" arterial emboli because clinically occult deep venous thrombosis is common and paradoxical embolism across a patent foramen ovale can occur in the absence of pulmonary embolism and high pulmonary arterial pressures when there is reversal of the normal interatrial pressure gradient that can occur spontaneously during ventricular systole or from coughing or Valsalva's maneuver.

HYPERCOAGULABLE STATES IN VASCULAR SURGERY PATIENTS

Multiple groups have reported an alarming incidence of hypercoagulable syndromes in patients undergoing vascular surgery. In studies in which patients were prospectively screened, the overall incidence varies from 10% to 25% and increases to about 50% in patients with special risk factors (Table 2–2) such as age less than 50 years, history of systemic lupus erythematosus, and a history of unexplained thrombotic events, including multiple failed vascular reconstructions.[6–10] Although all hypercoagulable states, hereditary and acquired, are uncovered in these surveys, the antiphospholipid antibody syndrome is the most frequently encountered abnormality among vascular surgery patients.[7,8,10] It is important to identify these patients preoperatively because the acute and intermediate-term failure of vascular reconstructions is reported to be

TABLE 2–2. RISK FACTORS FOR HYPERCOAGULABLE STATES IN VASCULAR SURGERY PATIENTS

Young patients (less than 50 years of age)
Patients with systemic lupus erythematosus
History of unexplained arterial and/or venous thrombotic events
Multiple failed previous vascular reconstructions
Unexplained prolongation of the activated partial thromboplastin time
Strong family history of thrombotic events

as high as 27% to 50%.[8,9,11] Although not proven, it is possible that careful perioperative anticoagulation with heparin and long-term treatment with warfarin and possibly aspirin will improve these patients' outlook. Recently, a multicenter prospective study of patients with the antiphospholipid syndrome demonstrated that long-term warfarin therapy did not prevent recurrent arterial thrombosis.[12] In patients undergoing vascular reconstructions with a history of systemic lupus erythematosus and antiphospholipid antibodies, perioperative steroid therapy may have a role.[11]

Reports of arterial thrombosis occurring in patients with hereditary hypercoagulable states are increasing. Protein S deficiency appears to represent a particular risk for arterial thrombosis.[3] In a large study of patients with proteins S deficiency who had no other risk factors for atherothrombosis, the incidence of arterial thrombosis involving the cerebral or coronary arteries was 14%.[13] There have also been many reports of patients with protein C or antithrombin III deficiency who develop arterial thrombosis manifested by transient cerebral ischemic attacks, stroke, myocardial infarction, and peripheral arterial occlusion.[14–19]

One of the problems with many reports of vascular surgical patients with hypercoagulable states is that there are no control populations for comparison to determine whether the overall incidence is increased among patients with vascular disease. In an ongoing study at the University of Texas Southwestern Medical Center in young patients (age less than 50 years) presenting with peripheral arterial disease, the incidence of hypercoagulable states was 33%, a figure consistent with other surveys in similar patients.[20] However, 22% of age-matched controls also had positive screening tests for hypercoagulable states and this incidence is not significantly different from that of patients with vascular disease.

Despite the uncertainty of whether these conditions are more frequently associated with vascular disease and arterial thrombosis, the presence of a hypercoagulable state as a comorbid condition in a patient undergoing vascular surgery clearly places that patient at special risk for a thrombotic complication. Does this justify the additional expense of screening all patients undergoing vascular operations for hypercoagulable states? Because of the varying incidence depending on the referral population, the added time and expense, and the uncertainty as to whether therapy would be altered in many cases, the answer is no. A more selective approach reserving screening for patients with special risk factors is appropriate.[9,10] These risk factors are listed in Table 2–2.

HEREDITARY HYPERCOAGULABLE STATES

Antithrombin III Deficiency

Congenital antithrombin III deficiency is inherited as an autosomal dominant trait with equal expression in males and females.[21] The estimated prevalence in the general population is between 1 in 2,000 and 1 in 5,000 individuals. Antithrombin III deficiency is found in about 3% of patients presenting with deep vein thrombosis. Heterozygous patients have antithrombin III levels between 30% and 70% of normal; homozygous antithrombin III deficiency is lethal *in utero*. The major clinical features of antithrombin III deficiency include young age at onset of clinical thrombosis; idiopathic venous thrombosis with no identifiable clinical predisposing conditions, such as prolonged immobility; family history of venous thromboembolism; recurrent venous thromboembolism; thrombosis at an unusual site; thrombosis during pregnancy; and thrombosis resistant to heparin therapy.[2] Thrombosis of superficial or deep veins of the leg occurs in over 90% of patients with thromboembolic episodes, and pulmonary emboli are reported in about half of these. Clinical manifestations are somewhat age dependent, with the risk of thrombosis increasing dramatically after age 15. The overall prevalence of venous thromboembolism proven by objective tests is about 20% among adult heterozygotes.[22] It has been estimated that by the age of 55 years, venous thrombosis develops in up to 85% of carriers. Although approximately 50% of episodes of deep venous thrombosis occur without clinically obvious provocation, the remainder are precipitated by factors that may cause thrombosis in nondeficient patients, particularly trauma, surgery, pregnancy, use of oral contraceptives, and infection. Treatment usually entails long-term warfarin therapy.

Two major types of antithrombin III deficiency have been described, one caused by decreased synthesis and the other by synthesis of a defective molecule.[23] The most common abnormality is due to the former problem that stems from various gene mutations. Antigenic and functional antithrombin III levels are reduced in these individuals. Less frequently, functional deficiencies associated with specific molecular abnormalities occur and are diagnosed by reduced antithrombin III biological activity in functional assays.

Protein C Deficiency

Like antithrombin III deficiency, protein C deficiency is inherited as an autosomal dominant trait, with heterozygotes suffering recurrent venous thromboembolism.[24] However, there are two key differences between deficiency of antithrombin III and that of protein C. One is the variable expression of thrombosis in carriers and the other is the existence of a homozygous state. Homozygous protein C deficiency causes neonatal purpura fulminans that is extremely difficult to treat and almost always fatal. As with antithrombin III, a moderate reduction to about half of normal levels can cause devastating thrombotic complications among heterozygotes.[25] The clinical manifestations (young age at onset, venous thrombosis at unusual sites) are similar to those of antithrombin III deficiency. The incidence of venous thromboembolism is 60% to 80% among protein C deficiency kindreds.[26] Although the prevalence of this disorder is unknown, protein C levels below 50% have been found in 0.3% of blood donors. In patients presenting with deep vein thrombosis, protein C deficiency may be more common than antithrombin III deficiency.

Warfarin-induced skin necrosis has occurred in some patients with protein C or protein S deficiency.[27] In this disorder necrosis and skin infarction appear on the trunk, breasts, extremities, or tip of the penis within a few days of initiating warfarin therapy. The mechanism is probably due to marked reductions in protein C levels from warfarin. Treatment includes immediate heparin, plasma or protein C infusions, and discontinuance of warfarin. Because of the possibility of warfarin-induced skin necrosis in individuals with unrecognized protein C deficiency, heparin should always be administered with warfarin until the prothrombin time is in therapeutic range.

Resistance to Activated Protein C

Deficiencies of antithrombin III, protein C, and protein S are present in 9% to 21% of patients presenting with unexplained venous thromboembolism.[28,29] The frequency of other biochemically defined hypercoagulable states is even smaller. Thus, no molecular abnormality has been identified in 60% to 80% of these thrombophilic patients. Recently, a new and potentially important genetic risk factor was suggested by the identification of families with thrombosis and inherited resistance to activated protein C.[30] Subsequent studies have shown that approximately 40% of consecutive patients presenting with venous thromboembolic disease have resistance to activated protein C.[31,32] Thus, this condition is highly prevalent and, in all likelihood, represents the most common hypercoagulable syndrome yet defined. The condition is due to a deficiency in a previously unrecognized anticoagulant factor that functions as a cofactor to activated protein C. The cofactor appears to be inactivated factor V that most likely has a molecular defect unrelated to its other functions in coagulation pathways.[33] The defect is inherited as an autosomal dominant and appears to be at least 10 times more common than any of the other known inherited deficiencies of anticoagulant proteins.

Protein S Deficiency

Protein S, the vitamin K–dependent cofactor of activated protein C, is also associated with thromboembolic disease when deficiency states exist.[24] The clinical manifestations of protein S deficiency are similar to those of deficiencies of antithrombin III and protein C. In addition to deep vein thrombosis and pulmonary embolism, cerebral venous thrombosis, mesenteric venous thrombosis, portal vein thrombosis, purpura fulminans, subclavian vein thrombosis, and arterial thrombosis have been reported in congenital deficiency of protein S.[2]

About 60% of protein S circulates in an inactive form bound to C4b-binding protein.[24] The remaining 40% is free and is the active form. Increased plasma levels of C4b-binding protein decrease the levels of free protein S and can influence thrombotic events.[25] Since C4b-binding protein is an acute phase reactant that increases during inflammatory states and the postoperative period, relative decreases in free protein S may result, predisposing the patient to thrombotic complications. Levels of total protein S in deficient heterozygotes range from 30% to 65% and levels of free protein S range from 15% to 50% of normal.[25] Those with free protein S levels of less than 5% of normal are considered homozygous. Patients with protein C and S deficiencies who have thromboembolic episodes are best managed with lifelong warfarin therapy.

Congenital Fibrinolytic Disorders

Impaired fibrin digestion due to abnormalities in the fibrinolytic system can lead to thrombotic complications.[1] Familial deficiencies and functional abnormalities in plasminogen, defective release of plasminogen activator from vessel walls stemming from defective endothelial synthesis of plasminogen activator, and the presence of excess circulating inhibitors to plasminogen activators have been described.[34] These disorders are rare and the prevalence is unknown. As with the other congenital disorders, fibrinolytic abnormalities are usually manifested clinically as venous thromboembolism, and treatment for recurrent thrombosis involves lifelong anticoagulant therapy.

Dysfibrinogenemia

Impaired fibrinolysis may be due to the formation of fibrin that is pathologically resistant to plasmin. Congenital functional abnormalities of fibrinogen exist that cause a hypercoagulable state complicated by thrombosis and the process is transmitted in an autosomal dominant fashion. Patients with dysfibrinogenemia and thrombosis respond to anticoagulant therapy.

Homocystinuria (Cystathionine Synthase Deficiency)

The development of premature atherosclerosis, as well as arterial and venous thrombo-embolism, is a prominent clinical feature of homocystinuria.[35] Homocysteine causes endothelial damage and dysfunction.[36] It down-regulates endothelial thrombomodulin function and may also impair endothelial plasmin generation by inhibiting binding of tissue plasminogen activator to its endothelial cell surface receptor.[37] In patients with homozygous cystathionine synthase deficiency, severe vascular disease may appear in childhood and most of these have thromboembolic events before the age of 40 years. Patients with heterozygous homocystinuria (estimated to be 1 in 70 of the normal population) may develop premature atherosclerosis. It has been estimated that 20% to 40% of patients presenting with premature peripheral vascular disease or stroke have heterozygous homocystinuria.[38] Pyridoxine treatment reduces the incidence of thromboembolic events in homozygous patients. It is not known whether treatment with pyriodoxine or other vitamins that influence homocysteine metabolism influences the course of premature atherosclerosis in heterozygotes.

Lipoprotein(a)

Lipoprotein(a) consists of a low-density lipoprotein (LDL) particle enveloped by a unique apolipoprotein, apolipoprotein(a) [apo(a)], disulfide linked to the apolipoprotein B-100 moiety of LDL.[39] Apo(a) shows remarkable homology with plasminogen, especially in the tandemly repeated sequences that resemble the kringle form of plasminogen.[40] Because of its homology with plasminogen, it has been reported that lipoprotein(a) may compete for binding with fibrin and endothelial cell surface plasminogen, thereby blocking fibrinolysis and creating a thrombogenic microenvironment.[41] Lipoprotein(a) is demonstrable in atherosclerotic plaques, where it colocalizes with fibrin. Recently, homocysteine was found to enhance the binding of lipoprotein(a) to fibrin, thus providing a biochemical link among thrombosis, atherogenesis, and homocystinemia.[42] Epidemiological studies have shown increased levels of lipoprotein(a) in approximately 20% of the population and that these elevations, genetically determined, represent a major risk factor for coronary heart disease, occlusion of the saphenous vein bypass graft, and stroke.[40] It appears to be a special risk factor for premature atherosclerosis.[39] Studies at the University of Texas Southwestern Medical Center indicate that elevated lipoprotein(a) occurs in approximately one-third of patients under 50 years of age with symptomatic peripheral atherosclerosis and is more common than any of the other hypercoagulable states studied.[20]

Other Inherited Disorders Less Clearly Associated with Thrombosis

A variety of other inherited disorders have been reported to be associated with thrombotic manifestations, but evidence of a true association is lacking.[1] Factor XII deficiency and deficiency of α_2 macroglobulin are among these. In addition, heparin co–factor II (a circulating plasma protein that inhibits thrombin but not factor Xa and whose action is enhanced by heparin) deficiency was thought to be a cause of thrombophilia, but recent studies suggest that this is not the case. Altered levels of endothelial plasminogen activator inhibitor–1 (PAI-1) and tissue plasminogen activator have been reported to be associated with thrombosis, but a prospective study of levels of these substances concluded that these components of fibrinolysis were not predictive of thrombosis. Histidine-rich glycoprotein binds heparin and complexes with fibrinogen. Increased levels of this material could potentially lead to thrombotic complications. Although increased levels of this substance have been observed in some patients with thrombosis, the association is uncertain. Sickle cell anemia produces obstruction of microvessels by stiff, deformed red blood cells, but thrombosis does not appear to play a major role in this process.

ACQUIRED HYPERCOAGULABLE STATES

Lupus Anticoagulant and Related Antipholipid Antibodies

The lupus anticoagulant is an antibody that prolongs phospholipid-dependent coagulation tests such as the activated partial thromboplastin time (aPTT) by binding to phospholipid. Although initially described in patients with systemic lupus erythematosus, hence its name, the antibody is more frequently encountered in patients without lupus. The paradoxical nature of the term is further compounded by the fact that patients with lupus anticoagulant appear to have a thrombotic, not hemorrhagic, diathesis. Interest has been directed toward a related antiphospholipid antibody: anticardiolipin antibody. Evidence indicates that lupus anticoagulant and anticardiolipin antibody define two distinct but related patient populations, each associated with an increased risk of arterial and venous thromboses.[43] It has become clear that the lupus anticoagulant and anticardiolipin antibodies are two separate entities; many individuals with anticardiolipin antibodies do not have a lupus anticoagulant, and many with lupus anticoagulant do not have anticardiolipin antibodies. About 1% to 2% of individuals in the general population and higher percentages of patients with autoimmune disorders produce a family of circulating antibodies directed against anionic phospholipids.[12] The true incidence and risk of thrombosis are unknown because there are too few prospective longitudinal studies on patients with these antibodies to determine how many will develop thrombosis. The clinical manifestations are diverse and include venous thromboembolism, stroke, myocardial infarction, postoperative thrombosis of arterial reconstructions, and obstetric complications due to thrombosis of placental vessels.[44] Antiphospholipid antibody syndrome is one of the most common causes of transient cerebral ischemia and stroke in young individuals.[45]

Various potential mechanisms have been proposed to explain the increased risk of thrombosis, including decreased plasma levels of free protein S, a plasma inhibitor of endothelial activation of protein C, a plasma inhibitor of protein C, a plasma inhibitor of factor Va degradation, increased levels of PAI-1, and inhibition of endothelial cell release or production of prostacyclin.[46–52] All of these biological activities of the antibodies have been demonstrated *in vitro*, but it is not clear which mechanisms are responsible for promoting thrombosis *in vivo*. Diagnostic tests include various coagulation tests (aPTT, the kaolin clotting time, and the dilute phospholipid test), the test for antibodies against cardiolipin, and other assays for antibodies against phospholipids. No single test has been demonstrated to be the best predictor of thrombosis, and because the tests may be transiently positive, a positive test result should be repeated after a period of weeks. In patients with systemic lupus erythematosus, persistently positive assays are predictive of thrombosis. In patients who have experienced arterial or venous thrombosis, long-term oral anticoagulant therapy is usually indicated; however, recent evidence suggests that warfarin therapy does not protect against recurrent thrombosis.[12] Antiplatelet therapy with aspirin or ticlopidine may also be useful.

Heparin-induced Thrombocytopenia and Thrombosis

Heparin-induced thrombocytopenia is uncommon and occurs in about 6% of patients receiving heparin.[53] Unlike thrombocytopenia due to other drugs, bleeding seldom occurs; instead, these patients suffer arterial and venous thromboses. Thrombotic complications occur in fewer than 1% of patients having a decreased platelet count while on heparin therapy. Neither the dose nor the source (porcine versus bovine) of heparin is related to the severity of the thrombocytopenia or the severity of thrombotic complications.[54] Thrombocytopenia has been reported with all routes of administration of heparin, including intravenous, subcutaneous, and even heparin bonded to indwelling venous catheters. The thrombotic complications are diverse and include venous thromboembolism, stroke, myocardial infarction, and peripheral arterial thromboembolism. The mortality from thrombotic complications ranges from 20% to 40% and the morbidity in the form of limb loss is 60% to 75%.[55] Peripheral thrombosis will frequently be manifested in an artery or vein previously damaged by catheterization or instrumentation. The pathogenesis of the disorder appears to be related to the development of a heparin-dependent immunoglobulin G antibody that attaches to platelets via the Fc receptor and triggers platelet secretion and aggregation.[56] In addition, heparin-induced antibody binds to endothelial cells and is associated with the expression of tissue factor on the endothelial cell surface. The combination of a potent stimulus for platelet aggregation and secretion, which also alters the thrombogenicity of endothelium, may be the underlying mechanism for thrombosis in some patients with this disorder.

All patients receiving heparin should be monitored with frequent platelet counts.[55] If severe thrombocytopenia or thrombosis develops, heparin should be discontinued. Alternative methods of anticoagulation are necessary in most patients. Substituting a heparin-like compound can be useful.[56] For example, Lomoparan is a combination of heparan sulfate and dermatan sulfate that cross-reacts very little with most antiheparin antibodies. Iloprost, a prostacyclin analog, has been used to inhibit platelet activation during short periods of heparin administration, such as during cardiopulmonary bypass or during vascular reconstructions. Success has also been reported with the use of ancrod, a rapidly acting defibrinogenating agent. In patients presenting with venous thromboembolism as a complication of heparin therapy, placement of a Greenfield filter, systemic thrombolytic therapy, and warfarin therapy are useful.

Myeloproliferative Disorders

The myeloproliferative disorders are a group of related diseases of narrow stem cells and include polycythemia vera, chronic myelogenous leukemia, myeloid metaplasia, and essential thrombocythemia. Arterial and venous thromboses occur with these diseases and, paradoxically, bleeding complications are prominent.[57] Along with common sites of arterial and venous thromboses, patients with myeloproliferative disorders may develop thrombosis at unusual sites, such as the splenic, portal, hepatic, and mesenteric veins.[2] Cerebrovascular ischemia may present as stroke or transient cerebral ischemic attacks and peripheral gangrene from microvascular thrombosis may occur without loss of pulses.[58,59] These arterial complications are encountered particularly in polycythemia vera and essential thrombocythemia. In polycythemia vera elevated whole blood viscosity due to increased red blood cell mass contributes to the risk of thrombosis. The contribution of thrombocytosis, especially in essential thrombocythemia, is unclear. There is no apparent correlation between the platelet count and the risk of thrombosis, but reduction in the circulating number of platelets can dramatically improve symptoms of cerebrovascular or digital ischemia. A variety of morphologic, functional, and metabolic defects of platelets have been described in the myeloproliferative disorders and these arise from clonal abnormalities of megakaryocytes.[60] It is thought that these heterogeneous platelet abnormalities are important in the pathogenesis of arterial and venous thromboses in these patients as well as the pronounced tendency to bleed. Treatment of thrombosis in patients with myeloproliferative disorders usually involves phlebotomy and cytoreductive therapy to reduce the red blood cell mass and the number of platelets as well as aspirin therapy.

Malignancy

The overall incidence of thrombosis in patients with malignancy is about 5% to 15%, but may be as high as 50% with some tumors, notably pancreatic carcinoma.[61] Thrombosis is not equally common in all types of malignancies. The highest incidence of thrombotic manifestations is found in patients with acute promyelocytic leukemia, myeloproliferative disorders, primary tumors of the brain, and mucin-secreting adenocarcinomas of the pancreas (especially the body and tail of the pancreas), gastrointestinal tract, lung, and ovary. The overall incidence of thromboembolic manifestations in malignancy bears some relationship to the frequency of tumors of particular types. Thus, although an especially high proportion of patients with cancer of the pancreas develops clinically evident thromboembolic disease, cancer of the pancreas is relatively uncommon in comparison with carcinoma of the lung, which, because of its relatively greater frequency, is the tumor most commonly associated with clinically evident thromboembolic disease. Episodes of thrombosis, particularly migratory superficial thrombophlebitis, may antedate by months the clinical diagnosis of cancer in some patients and may be the first clinical indication of the underlying cancer. In addition to venous thromboembolism, arterial embolism from nonbacterial thrombotic endocarditis may develop.

Multiple coagulation abnormalities predisposing to thrombosis have been described in patients with malignancy. These include thrombocytosis, shortening of the prothrombin time and aPTT, elevation of plasma coagulation factors (increases in fibrinogen and factors V, VIII, IX, and XI) and fibrinogen–fibrin degradation products, shortened platelet and fibrinogen survival, decreased antithrombin III levels, and increased PAI-1 activity.[1,4] Many of these changes reflect generalized activation of the clotting system, resulting in chronic partially compensated disseminated intravascular coagulation. The clinical expression of these abnormalities may include bleeding and large vessel thrombosis in complex cases.[61] In addition to these hemostatic abnormalities, there is evidence for platelet activation by tumor cells, the expression of tissue factor by monocytes and macrophages stimulated by tumor antigens, endothelial cell expression of tissue factor by cytokines produced by tumors, and the production of procoagulants by tumors cells that activate factor X. Other procoagulants may be released, such as thromboplastic substances contained in the granules of leukemic progranulocytes. Cytotoxic chemotherapy can also cause release of thromboplastic substances from tumor cells and precipitate thrombotic events. An increased risk of thrombosis has been reported with chemotherapy for leukemias, breast cancer, and prostate cancer.[62] In some cases it appears that cytotoxic agents themselves may contribute to thrombosis.

Postoperative and Inflammatory States

After major surgery or trauma of any nature, several hemostatic changes occur that predispose the patient to thrombosis. These include elevations in coagulation factors (fibrinogen and factor VIII), moderate (20% to 30%) depression of antithrombin III levels, decrease in free protein S levels (due to increases in C4b-binding protein levels), thrombocytosis, increased platelet reactivity or stickiness, and release of tissue thromboplastin into the bloodstream.[4] In addition, defective fibrinolysis may occur 48 to 72 hours postoperatively because of elevations in α_2-macroglobulin and other inhibitory proteins. Recent evidence suggests that postoperative fibrinolytic shutdown is mediated by plasma factors that stimulate endothelial cell PAI-1 biosynthesis.[63] Increases in blood viscosity are also common and are related to fluid shifts and dehydration. When these changes are combined with immobilization and venous pooling in the lower extremities from anesthetics and narcotics, postoperative venous thromboembolism may result.

Inflammatory disorders such as inflammatory bowel disease, rheumatoid arthritis, and chronic infections are associated with an increased incidence of thrombosis. High levels of inflammatory mediators such as tumor necrosis factor and interleukin-1 that increase the expression of procoagulant properties of the endothelial surface may be involved. In addition, C4b-binding protein is elevated decreasing levels of free protein S.[27]

Pregnancy

Although pregnancy is associated with an increased risk of venous thromboembolism, the risk increases several-fold immediately after delivery. Multiple anatomic, physiological, and biochemical changes during pregnancy and the postpartum period predispose the patient to venous thromboembolism. Venous compression by the gravid uterus and increased intra-abdominal pressure along with venous smooth muscle relaxation induced by estrogen and other hormonal effects bring about venous pooling of blood in the lower extremities. Fibrinogen levels increase along with concentrations of factors VII, VIII, IX, X, and XII, while antithrombin III levels and protein S levels are mildly decreased.[1] Depression of fibrinolytic activity further enhances hypercoagulability.

Oral Contraceptives

An increased risk of mortality from cardiovascular disease and particularly venous thromboembolism is seen in women who use oral contraceptives. Use of newer low-dose estrogen combination pills reduces but does not eliminate this risk. The systemic effects induced by oral contraceptives are similar to those seen in pregnancy and include increased levels of clotting factors and decreases in antithrombin III levels.

Increased Levels of Fibrinogen and Factor VII

Multiple epidemiological studies have shown an association between elevated levels of plasma fibrinogen and increased levels of factor VII coagulant activity and the risk of ischemic heart disease, stroke, and peripheral vascular disease.[64–68] A recent meta-analysis suggests that fibrinogen is an independent cardiovascular risk factor.[66] Epidemiological studies show that smoking is a major determinant of the fibrinogen level and that dietary fat intake is related to factor VII coagulant activity. Thus, two major cardiovascular risks influence coagulation activity and the risk of thrombosis. Fibrinogen is a major determinant or blood viscosity, influences platelet aggregability, and interacts with the endothelial cell surface to generate fibrin in inflammatory states. The factor VII–tissue factor pathway is a crucial physiological variable controlling the basal activation state of coagulation.

Nephrotic Syndrome

Patients with nephrotic syndrome have lowered levels of antithrombin III due to loss in the urine and decreased levels of free protein S due to high circulating levels of C4b-binding protein. In addition, many of these patients have systemic lupus erythematosus and antiphospholipid antibodies.

REFERENCES

1. Nachman RL, Silverstein R. Hypercoagulable states. *Ann Intern Med.* 1993;119:819–827.
2. Kitchens CS. Thrombophilia and thrombosis in unusual sites. In: Colman RW, Hirsh J, Marder VJ, et al, eds. *Hemostasis and Thrombosis: Basic Principles and Clinical Practice.* 3rd ed. Philadelphia: JB Lippincott; 1994:1255–1273.
3. Schafer AI, Kroll MH. Nonatheromatous arterial thrombosis. *Annu Rev Med.* 1993;44:155–170.
4. DeLoughery TG, Goodnight SH. The hypercoagulable states: diagnosis and management. *Semin Vasc Surg.* 1993;6:66–74.
5. Lechat P, Mas JL, Lascault G, et al. Prevalence of patent foramen ovale in patients with stroke. *N Engl J Med.* 1988;318:1148–1152.
6. Eldrup-Jorgensen J, Flanigan DP, Brace L, et al. Hypercoagulable states and lower limb ischemia in young adults. *J Vasc Surg.* 1989;9:334–341.
7. Eldrup-Jorgensen J, Brace L, Flanigan DP, et al. Lupus-like anticoagulants and lower extremity arterial occlusive disease. *Circulation.* 1989;80(Suppl III):III-54–III-58.
8. Donaldson MC, Weinberg DS, Belkin M, et al. Screening for hypercoagulable states in vascular surgical practice: a preliminary study. *J Vasc Surg.* 1990;11:825–831.
9. Ahn SS, Kalunian K, Rosove M, et al. Postoperative thrombotic complications in patients with the lupus anticoagulant: increased risk after vascular procedures. *J Vasc Surg.* 1988;7:749–756.
10. De Frang RD, Edwards JM, Moneta GL, et al. Repeat leg bypass after multiple prior bypass failures. *J Vasc Surg.* 1994;19:268–277.
11. Shortell CK, Ouriel K, Green RM, et al. Vascular disease in the antiphospholipid syndrome: a comparison with the patient population with atherosclerosis. *J Vasc Surg.* 1992;15:158–166.
12. Vianna JL, Khamashta MA, Ordi-Ros J, et al. Comparison of the primary and secondary antiphospholipid syndrome: a European multicenter study of 114 patients. *Am J Med.* 1994;96:3–9.
13. Wiesel ML, Borg JY, Grunebaum L, et al. Influence of protein S deficiency on the arterial thrombosis risk. *Presse Med.* 1991;20:1023–1027.
14. Matsushita K, Kuriyama Y, Sawada T, et al. Cerebral infarction associated with protein C deficiency. *Stroke.* 1992;23:108–111.
15. Sacco RL, Owen J, Mohr JP, et al. Free protein S deficiency: a possible association with cerebrovascular occlusion. *Stroke.* 1989;20:1657–1661.
16. Coller BS, Owen J, Jesty J, et al. Deficiency of plasma protein S, protein C, or antithrombin III and arterial thrombosis. *Arteriosclerosis.* 1987;7:456–462.
17. Conard J, Samama MM. Inhibitors of coagulation, atherosclerosis, and arterial thrombosis. *Semin Thromb Hemostasis.* 1986;12:87–90.

18. Kohler J, Kasper J, Witt I, et al. Ischemic stroke due to protein C deficiency. *Stroke.* 1990;21:1077–1080.

19. De Stafano V, Leone G, Micalizzi P, et al. Arterial thrombosis as a clinical manifestation of congenital protein C deficiency. *Ann Hematol.* 1991;62:180–183.

20. Valentine RJ, Clagett GP. Unpublished observations.

21. Hirsh J, Piovella F, Pini M. Congenital antithrombin III deficiency. *Am J Med.* 1989;87:34S–38S.

22. Demers C, Ginsberg JS, Hirsh J, et al. Thrombosis in antithrombin-III–deficient persons. Report of a large kindred and literature review. *Ann Intern Med.* 1992;116:754–761.

23. Blajchman MA, Austin RC, Fernandez-Rachubinski F, et al. Molecular basis of inherited human antithrombin deficiency. *Blood.* 1992;80:2159–2171.

24. Comp PC. Hereditary disorders predisposing to thrombosis. In: Collier BF, ed. *Prog Hemostasis Thromb.* Orlando, Grune and Stratton; 1986;8:71–102.

25. Esmon CT. The protein C anticoagulant pathway. *Arterioscler Thromb.* 1992;12:135–145.

26. Allaart CF, Poort SR, Rosendaal FR, et al. Increased risk of venous thrombosis in carriers of hereditary protein C deficiency defect. *Lancet.* 1993;341:134–38.

27. Comp PC, Elrod JP, Karzenski S. Warfarin-induced skin necrosis. *Semin Thromb Hemostasis.* 1990;16:293–298.

28. Gladson CL, Scharrer I, Hach V, et al. The frequency of type I heterozygous protein S and protein C deficiency in 141 unrelated young patients with venous thrombosis. *Thromb Haemostasis.* 1988;59:18.

29. Pabinger I, Brucker S, Kyrle PA, et al. Hereditary deficiency of antithrombin III, protein C and protein S: prevalence in patients with a history of venous thrombosis and criteria for rational patient screening. *Blood Coagul Fibrinolysis.* 1992;3:547.

30. Dahlback B, Carlsson M, Svensson PJ. Familial thrombophilia due to a previously unrecognized mechanism characterized by poor anticoagulant response to activated protein C: prediction of a cofactor to activated protein C. *Proc Natl Acad Sci USA.* 1993;90:1004–1008.

31. Griffin JH, Evatt B, Wideman C, et al. Anticoagulant protein C pathway defective in majority of thrombophilic patients. *Blood.* 1993;82:1989–1993.

32. Svensson PJ, Dahlback B. Resistance to activated protein C as a basis for venous thrombosis. *N Engl J Med.* 1994;330:517–522.

33. Dahlback B, Hildebrand B. Inherited resistance to activated protein C is corrected by anticoagulant cofactor activity found to be a property of factor V. *Proc Natl Acad Sci USA.* 1994;91:1396–1400.

34. Bachmann F. The plasminogen–plasmin enzyme system. In: Colman RW, Hirsh J, Marder VJ, et al, eds. *Hemostasis and Thrombosis: Basic Principles and Clinical Practice.* 3rd ed. Philadelphia: JB Lippincott; 1994:1592–1622.

35. Rees MM, Rodgers GM. Homocysteinemia: association of a metabolic disorder with vascular disease and thrombosis. *Thromb Res.* 1993;71:337–359.

36. Nishinaga M, Ozawa T, Shimada K. Homocysteine, a thrombogenic agent, suppresses anticoagulant heparan sulfate expression in cultured porcine aortic endothelial cells. *J Clin Invest.* 1993;92:1381–1386.

37. Rodgers GM, Conn MT. Homocysteine, an atherogenic stimulus, reduces protein C activation by arterial and venous endothelial cells. *Blood.* 1990;75:895–901.

38. Taylor LM Jr, Porter JM. Elevated plasma homocysteine as a risk factor for atherosclerosis. *Semin Vasc Surg.* 1993;6:36–45.

39. Valentine RJ. Lipoprotein(a): a new risk factor for vascular disease. In: Goldstone J, ed. *Perspectives in Vascular Surgery.* St. Louis, Mo: Quality Medical Publishing; 1992:84–99.

40. Howard GC, Pizzo SV. Biology of disease. Lipoprotein(a) and its role in atherothrombotic disease. *Lab Invest.* 1993;69:373–386.

41. Hajjar KA, Gavish D, Breslow JL, et al. Lipoprotein(a) modulation of endothelial cell surface fibrinolysis and its potential role in atherosclerosis. *Nature (London).* 1989;339:303–305.

42. Harpel PC, Chang VT, Borth W. Homocysteine and other sulfhydryl compounds enhance the binding of lipoprotein(a) to fibrin: a potential biochemical link between thrombosis, atherogenesis, and sulfhydryl compound metabolism. *Proc Natl Acad Sci USA.* 1992;89:10193–10197.

43. Bick RL, Baker WF. Anticardiolipin antibodies and thrombosis. *Hematol/Oncol Clin North Am.* 1992;6:1287–1299.
44. Rosove MH, Brewer PMC. Antiphospholipid thrombosis: clinical course after the first thrombotic event in 70 patients. *Ann Intern Med.* 1992;117:303–308.
45. Ginsburg KS, Liang MH, Newcomer L, et al. Anticardiolipin antibodies and the risk for ischemic stroke and venous thrombosis. *Ann Intern Med.* 1992;117:997–1002.
46. Lellouche F, Martinuzzo M, Said P, et al. Imbalance of thromboxane/prostacyclin biosynthesis in patients with lupus anticoagulant. *Blood.* 1991;78:2894–2899.
47. Ginsberg JS, Demers C, Brill-Edwards P, et al. Increased thrombin generation and activity in patients with systemic lupus erythematosus and anticardiolipin antibodies: evidence for a prothrombotic state. *Blood.* 1993;81:2958–2963.
48. Marciniak E, Romond EH. Impaired catalytic function of activated protein C: a new in vitro manifestation of lupus anticoagulant. *Blood.* 1989;74:2426–2432.
49. Schorer AE, Wickham NWR, Watson KV. Lupus anticoagulant induces a selective defect in thrombin-mediated endothelial prostacyclin release and platelet aggregation. *Br J Haematol.* 1989;71:399–407.
50. Watson KV, Schorer AE. Lupus anticoagulant inhibition of in vitro prostacyclin release is associated with a thrombosis-prone subset of patients. *Am J Med.* 1991;90:47–53.
51. Oosting JD, Derksen RHWM, Bobbink IWG, et al. Antiphospholipid antibodies directed against a combination of phospholipids with prothrombin, protein C or protein S: an explanation for their pathogenic mechanism? *Blood.* 1993;81:2618–2625.
52. Chamley LW, McKay EJ, Pattison NS. Inhibition of heparin/antithrombin III cofactor activity by anticardiolipin antibodies: a mechanism for thrombosis. *Thromb Res.* 1993;71:103–111.
53. Becker PS, Miller VT. Heparin-induced thrombocytopenia. *Stroke.* 1989;20:1449.
54. Schmitt BP, Adelman B. Heparin-associated thrombocytopenia: a critical review and pooled analysis. *Am J Med Sci.* 1993;305:208–215.
55. Laster J, Cikrit D, Walker N, et al. The heparin-induced thrombocytopenia syndrome: an update. *Surgery.* 1987;102:763–770.
56. Warkentin TE, Kelton JG. Heparin and platelets. *Hematol/Oncol Clin North Am.* 1990;4:243–264.
57. Schafer AI. Bleeding and thrombosis in the myeloproliferative disorders. *Blood.* 1984;64:1–12.
58. Jabaily J, Iland HL, Laszlo J, et al. Neurologic manifestations of essential thrombocythemia. *Ann Intern Med.* 1983;99:513–518.
59. Michiels JJ, Abels J, Steketee J, et al. Erythromelalgia caused by platelet-mediated arteriolar inflammation and thrombosis in thrombocythemia. *Ann Intern Med.* 1985;102:466–471.
60. Schafer AI. Essential thrombocythemia. *Prog Hemostasis Thromb.* 1991;10:69–96.
61. Dvorak HF. Abnormalities of hemostasis in malignant disease. In: Colman RW, Hirsh J, Marder VJ, et al, eds. *Hemostasis and Thrombosis: Basic Principles and Clinical Practice.* 3rd ed. Philadelphia: JB Lippincott; 1994:1238–1254.
62. Levine MN, Gent M, Hirsh J, et al. The thrombogenic effect of anticancer drug therapy in women with stage II breast cancer. *N Engl J Med.* 1988;318:404–407.
63. Kassis J, Hirsh J, Podor TJ. Evidence that postoperative fibrinolytic shutdown is mediated by plasma factors that stimulate endothelial cell type I plasminogen activator inhibitor biosynthesis. *Blood.* 1992;80:1758–1764.
64. Cortellaro M, Boschetti C, Cofrancesco E, et al. The PLAT study: hemostatic function in relation to atherothrombotic ischemic events in vascular disease patients. Principal results. *Arterioscler Thromb.* 1992;12:1063–1070.
65. Nordoy A. Haemostatic factors in coronary heart disease. *J Intern Med.* 1993;233:377–383.
66. Ernst E, Resch KL. Fibrinogen as a cardiovascular risk factor: a meta-analysis and review of the literature. *Ann Intern Med.* 1993;118:956–963.
67. Qizilbash N, Jones L, Warlow C, et al. Fibrinogen and lipid concentrations as risk factors for transient ischaemic attacks and minor ischaemic strokes. *Br Med J.* 1991;303:605–609.
68. Ernst E. Fibrinogen: an important risk factor for atherothrombotic diseases. *Ann Med.* 1994;26:15–22.

3

Cardiac Evaluation in Patients with Lower Extremity Ischemia

William C. Krupski, MD, and Denis D. Bensard, MD

Perioperative adverse cardiac events remain a major problem for vascular surgeons. Numerous strategies to prevent morbidity after peripheral vascular surgery have been proposed, and their proper application is the subject of much controversy. Moreover, what to do with the information obtained by preoperative screening is even *more* uncertain. This analysis explores the prevalence of coronary artery disease (CAD) in patients with ischemic extremities and discusses current tactics to avoid adverse cardiac outcomes in patients who are operated on for peripheral vascular disease.

SCOPE OF THE PROBLEM

Cardiovascular disease affects one in four Americans.[1] The annual mortality from cardiovascular disease in the general population of the United States is 1 million, accounting for one of every two deaths in the United States.[2] The annual morbidity exceeds 2.5 million: 1.5 million myocardial infarctions (MIs), 600,000 strokes, and 400,000 cases of congestive heart failure (CHF). Total morbidity and mortality costs per year surpass $83 billion.[3]

Atherosclerotic cardiac and peripheral vascular disease will continue to be a major problem, despite recent evidence that cardiovascular death *rates* have decreased by 20% to 30%.[3] The prevalence of cardiovascular disease increases with age, and the US population is aging rapidly. Twenty-five million people are now over the age of 65, including 2.7 million older than 85.[4] By the middle of the next century, the population over 65 is expected to reach 66 million (Fig. 3–1). It is estimated that nearly 9 million people over the age of 65 will develop symptomatic atherosclerosis by the year 2010 (Table 3–1).

In addition, asymptomatic CAD producing silent myocardial ischemia has come to be recognized as a frequent manifestation of CAD. Silent ischemia carries a prognosis similar to that of symptomatic myocardial ischemia and its incidence is frequently underappreciated. Cohn estimated that 2 to 5 million individuals have subclinical CAD, indicating that current statistics for CAD may not reflect the true prevalence

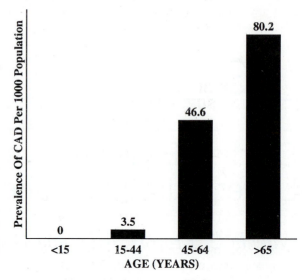

Figure 3–1. Prevalence of CAD in four age groups in the United States. *(From the National Center for Health Statistics, US Public Health Service, Department of Health and Human Services, 1988.)*

in the general population.[5] He concluded that silent ischemia occurs in (1) 2.5% to 10% of middle-aged men never having signs or symptoms of CAD, (2) 18% of asymptomatic patients after MI, and (3) 40% of patients with classic angina pectoris.

Patients with peripheral vascular disease are at particular risk for cardiac complications. The commitment of vascular surgeons to limb salvage notwithstanding, the risk of death in patients with ischemic extremities is greater than the risk of amputation, owing to the systemic nature of atherosclerosis.[6] Most late deaths in patients undergoing vascular reconstruction are caused by heart disease (40% to 60%), malignancy (7% to 23%), and cerebrovascular disease (2% to 15%).[7] In 1960 Boyd reported that 39% of individuals with intermittent claudication sustained a nonfatal MI or stroke within 10 years of developing extremity symptoms; strikingly, only 22% of patients were alive 15 years after the onset of claudication.[8] Likewise, Kallero found that patients 55 to 69 years of age with abnormal segmental limb pressure measurements had a twofold increased risk for death and a 14-fold increased risk for MI at 10 years compared with persons having normal lower extremity perfusion.[9] By extrapolation of findings from the classic 1984 Cleveland Clinic study in which coronary angiograms were routinely obtained in 1,000 patients under consideration for elective peripheral vascular reconstruction, approximately half of patients with *severe* CAD at the time

TABLE 3–1. INCIDENCE AND PREVALENCE OF CORONARY ARTERY DISEASE IN THE UNITED STATES

Year	Incidence	Prevalence
1980	692,117	5,977,405
1985	729,235	6,700,639
1990	759,583	7,230,904
1995	792,006	7,625,001
2000	834,522	7,973,869
2005	888,438	8,385,046
2010	953,750	8,939,816

Reproduced with permission from Weinstein MC, Coxson PG, Williams LW, et al. Forecasting coronary heart disease incidence, mortality, and cost. *J Am Coll Cardiol.* 1988;12:840.

of diagnosis of peripheral vascular disease will suffer a fatal cardiac complication in the ensuing 5 years.[6,10]

INCIDENCE OF PERIOPERATIVE CARDIAC MORBIDITY IN VASCULAR SURGERY

Perioperative cardiac morbidity, generally defined as MI, unstable angina, CHF, serious arrhythmias, and cardiac death, is the leading cause of death after anesthesia and surgery.[2] However, assessment of such morbidity is complicated. For example, most postoperative MIs are silent and many are subendocardial.[2,11–14] Perioperative arrhythmias require continuous monitoring of electrocardiograms (ECGs), making detection difficult.[15–17] The diagnosis of CHF in the postoperative period can be confused with pulmonary congestion precipitated by decreased osmotic pressure or pulmonary capillary leak owing to sepsis, pre-existing pulmonary disease, or overhydration. Thus, the reported rates of adverse cardiac outcomes vary markedly.

Comparison of cardiac morbidity among studies can be misleading because the reported incidence of perioperative cardiac complications depends on the methods of screening. Not surprisingly, more intensive surveillance leads to the detection of increased numbers of patients who either possibly or definitely have sustained adverse cardiac outcomes. Retrospective reviews of vascular operations generally report perioperative MI rates of about 3%, while more meticulous prospective surveillance discloses rates of 10% to 15%.[18] In a prospective study of 232 mostly high-risk patients undergoing noncardiac operations, Charlson and associates showed that postoperative MIs are substantially underestimated unless cardiac enzymes and ECGs are routinely obtained for several postoperative days.[19]

As noted previously, silent myocardial ischemia also plays an important role in determining the incidence of perioperative cardiac morbidity. Fifty to ninety percent of postoperative ischemic events detected by Holter monitoring are silent.[15,20–22] In a 1989 study Ouyang and colleagues studied 24 patients with stable CAD undergoing peripheral vascular reconstructions using Holter monitoring.[21] Fifteen (63%) developed clinically silent postoperative myocardial ischemia, and 8 (53%) of these patients subsequently experienced a significant postoperative adverse cardiac outcome (MI, CHF, or unstable angina). In contrast, only 1 of 9 (11%) patients had postoperative clinical ischemic events. Mangano and the Study of Perioperative Ischemia Research Group at the University of California–San Francisco showed that during the 2-year interval after an operation, the risk of an acute MI is increased twofold in patients who develop postoperative myocardial ischemia, most of which is silent.[23] Seventy percent of all long-term adverse outcomes were heralded by in-hospital postoperative ischemia.

Predictably, the occurrence of postoperative cardiac morbidity depends on the presence of defined CAD and the patient population. The Coronary Artery Surgery Study (CASS) revealed that the risk of postoperative cardiac death after noncardiac operations in the general population is 0.5% but increases nearly fivefold (2.4%) in patients with significant CAD.[24] In this group of 1,600 individuals in the CASS registry, 8.7% of patients with known CAD experienced postoperative chest pain, nearly double the number of patients without CAD or with previous coronary artery bypass grafting (CABG). Of note, the patients with postoperative chest pain represent a minority of total ischemic events, because most postoperative ischemia is silent (see above). The incidence of MI after all noncardiac surgery varies from 0% to 0.7%, but postoperative

MIs occur in 2% to 6.4% of patients having elective vascular operations, and nearly half of these are fatal.[18] Others have described even greater cardiac morbidity after vascular reconstructions. For example, Pasternack et al reported eight MIs in 50 high-risk patients having abdominal aortic aneurysm repair—an overall incidence of 16%.[25]

Detection of CAD in vascular patients is confounded by impaired ambulation caused by the disorders suffered by this population: limb ischemia, strokes, and dyspnea.[26] Gage and associates found that standard exercise stress tests were falsely positive for significant CAD in 40% of patients and falsely negative in 15%. One of four patients in this report were unable to undergo stress testing because of shortness of breath or claudication.[27] However, it is clear that CAD is distressingly common in patients with peripheral vascular disease. In the Cleveland Clinic study cited previously, only 4% of those with and 14% of those without clinically suspected CAD had normal coronary arteriograms.[10]

THE VALUE OF RISK STRATIFICATION

Theoretically, determination of risk for perioperative cardiac morbidity allows either invasive treatment of CAD or selection of alternative methods of therapy (eg, longer observation in the intensive care unit, radiological endovascular procedures, extra-anatomic bypasses, and additional invasive monitoring). Operative treatment of limb ischemia may be averted entirely in patients with less than compelling indications.

However, controversy exists regarding the value of extensive evaluation of cardiac risk in vascular patients. In 1992 Taylor and colleagues at the Oregon Health Sciences University reported excellent results using minimal preoperative cardiac screening in 491 consecutive patients.[28] A total of 534 vascular procedures were performed in these patients (105 aortic, 87 carotid, 297 infrainguinal, 51 extra-anatomic, and 84 other.[28] Basic cardiac evaluation consisted of history, physical examination, and resting ECG. A small fraction (5.8%) of patients with severe symptomatic CAD had additional studies, which included cardiology consultation, dipyridamole thallium scintigraphy (DIS), evaluation of cardiac ejection fraction, and/or coronary arteriography. This frugal use of resources to evaluate cardiac risk resulted in an overall postoperative MI rate of only 3.9%. Whereas 8.2% of patients having *emergent* procedures suffered MIs, only 2.8% of patients having *elective* vascular operations had postoperative MIs. Critics of this "minimalist" approach cite the following: (1) one-fifth of the patients in the study had previously undergone myocardial revascularization, (2) patients were studied for only the first 72 postoperative hours, and (3) almost one-third of patients did not have cardiac enzymes obtained for the full 3 days of the postoperative period studied.

In contrast, Bunt[29] described an aggressive approach for assessing perioperative cardiac risk in patients with peripheral arterial disease. He studied 630 consecutive patients considered for elective peripheral vascular procedures who were prospectively entered into a protocol for determination of risk for cardiac morbidity. All patients had detailed history and physical examination, resting ECG, and radionuclide cardioangiography. Thirty-two percent of patients had no abnormalities on initial examination and did not undergo further work-up; 68% (428/630) had clinical evidence of CAD as demonstrated by positive history or ECG, and stress thallium testing (STT) was performed. Of the patients undergoing STT, 93% had no perfusion defects and proceeded to surgery, whereas 7% (44/630) with fixed or reversible perfusion defects underwent coronary angiography. This stringent protocol resulted in an *overall* perioperative MI rate of only 0.7%, ranging from 0% in patients undergoing aortic or carotid surgery to 1.6% in patients undergoing infrainguinal revascularization. The results of Bunt's study are exemplary, but, like the Oregon publication, several features warrant caution. First, cardiac enzymes were routinely obtained only for the first 48 hours, so some MIs may have been missed. Second, the outcomes of the 44 patients with positive STTs (41 of whom had cardiac catheterizations) are not described; if these patients had a high rate of mortality from CABG, for example, the prudence of Bunt's algorithm is questionable. Finally, the cost-effectiveness of such an aggressive policy bears scrutiny in view of the high rate of negative studies (93%) and the expense of DTS (averaging about $1,500 in most medical centers).

Bunt and Taylor et al demonstrated that a low rate of cardiac morbidity is attainable in vascular surgery patients, even though they suggest very different strategies.

WHAT SHOULD BE DONE WHEN CORONARY ARTERY DISEASE IS IDENTIFIED?

The adage that a test should not be obtained unless it will change management of the patient holds great relevance with respect to screening vascular patients for CAD. Hertzer at the Cleveland Clinic is an advocate of coronary revascularization prior to peripheral vascular operations, not only to enhance safety of the vascular procedure, but also potentially to prolong life expectancy and quality of life in these patients. In the Cleveland Clinic study previously cited, CABG was performed in 70 of 250 patients (28%) with infrarenal abdominal aortic aneurysm, 63 of 295 (21%) with cerebrovascular disease, and 70 of 381 (18%) with lower extremity vascular insufficiency before vascular reconstruction.[10] Of these 216 patients with surgically correctable CAD who underwent CABG, 72% were alive at 5 years postoperatively. In striking contrast, only 15 of 35 candidates (43%) for CABG who refused the operation and 12 of 54 (22%) patients with severe uncorrectable CAD remained alive at 5 years.

In support of the protective effect of CABG prior to vascular surgery, Ennix et al[30] reported outcomes in 1,546 consecutive carotid endarterectomies in 1,238 patients over a 10-year period. Whereas the overall rate of perioperative MI was only 1.6%, MIs occurred in 12.9% of 85 patients with symptomatic CAD. In contrast, the MI incidence was reduced to 2.6% in 155 patients with symptomatic CAD with prior or simultaneous CABG.

Although the Cleveland Clinic results are particularly impressive, it must be remembered that whereas the cardiac catheterizations were performed consecutively and prospectively, the results of prophylactic CABG were retrospectively analyzed. Moreover, comparison of patients eligible for CABG with those having unreconstructable CAD is not equitable. Recommendation of prophylactic CABG or angioplasty must be tempered by recognition of potential hazards of this strategy. For example, the operative mortality of a CABG before elective vascular surgery in the Hertzer study was 5.2%.[10] Thus, the benefit of risk reduction by prophylactic coronary revascularization is realized only by those who survive bypass surgery *and* subsequent vascular reconstruction.

Cutler and Leppo have also shown the potential downside of prophylactic CABG.[31] They performed DTS scans in 116 patients scheduled for aortic surgery; 6% of patients were referred for CABG based on DTS results. No operative deaths occurred in the patients undergoing aortic surgery without CABG. However, there was one death in the 6 patients referred for CABG—a mortality rate of 16.7% attributable to precautionary CABG. Routine preoperative cardiac catheterization and prophylactic bypass is unrealistic due to the expense and the risks of the procedure. However, the optimal approach to assessing and treating patients with severe CAD and peripheral vascular disease sufficient to warrant multiple surgical procedures is unresolved.

Little has been published about the role of prior coronary angioplasty on the outcome of noncardiac operations. Huber and colleagues at the Mayo Clinic performed percutaneous transluminal coronary angioplasty (PTCA) in 55 patients in preparation for noncardiac surgery.[32] Five of 50 patients had an unsuccessful angioplasty and were excluded from subsequent analysis (thus potentially skewing the study by not following "intention to treat" statistical rules). All 5 patients had either emergent or elective CABG. Fifty-four operations were subsequently performed in the 50 patients who had successful preliminary PTCA. The overall frequency of postoperative MI was 5.5% (3/54) and operative mortality was 1.9%. When one compares these figures with the MI and death rates reported above using the minimalist approach of Taylor and coworkers in Oregon,[28] the prudence of prophylactic revascularization is called into question.

HOW TO PREDICT PERIOPERATIVE CARDIAC MORBIDITY: CLINICAL VARIABLES

Age

Data supporting the predictive value of age[11,25,30,33,34] are about equal to those negating it.[12–14,35,36] Although age does depress cardiac response to different forms of stress, such as exercise and exogenous catecholamines, it does not affect resting ejection fraction, left ventricular volume, or regional wall motion per se.[35] A recent prospective long-term study of 474 veterans having noncardiac operations found that even in elderly patients at high risk for cardiac complications, MI is not the leading cause of death after noncardiac surgery.[36] In this report hypertension, severely limited activity, and renal insufficiency—not age—were predictors of in-hospital mortality. Carliner and colleagues[33] demonstrated a 38% incidence of myocardial ischemia, MI, or cardiac death in patients older than 70 compared with 7% in those aged 40 to 49. In the Goldman series the risk of perioperative cardiac death was increased 10-fold for patients older than 70.[11] Likewise, Eagle et al found that age was an independent variable that predicted perioperative cardiac morbidity by multivariate analysis.[34] Most recently, Baron and associates in Paris prospectively studied 457 consecutive patients undergoing elective abdominal surgery and found that age greater than 65 years, definite CAD, and an ejection fraction below 50% were the predictors of postoperative MI.[37] Age greater than 65 years was the *only* characteristic associated with postoperative mortality in the multivariate analysis.

Angina Pectoris

Angina is usually associated with angiographically significant coronary artery stenosis. Ninety percent of men older than 40 years old and woman older than 60 who have angina have significant CAD.[38] Surprisingly, up to one-fifth of similarly aged *asymptomatic* patients have significant coronary artery stenoses.[38] In Goldman's oft-quoted studies[11,39] stable angina was conspicuously absent as a predictor of perioperative cardiac morbidity even by univariate analysis. One explanation for this apparent paradox may be that 75% or more of ischemic episodes in patients with CAD are clinically silent.[5,15,17] In contrast to Goldman, Eagle and associates[40] concluded that angina was one of five major predictors of perioperative cardiac morbidity.

Previous Myocardial Infarction

In a classic study 30 years ago Topkins and Artusio showed that both the history of a previous MI and its temporal relationship to the planned operative procedure determine susceptibility to postoperative adverse cardiac events.[41] The incidence of postoperative MI in patients without a documented prior MI was 0.66%, compared to 6.5% in patients with antecedent MI. The mortality of a postoperative MI in patients without antecedent MI was 26.5%, rising to 72% in those with prior MI. Reinfarction was at 54.5% when a previous MI had occurred within 6 months of surgery compared to 4.5% in patients who sustained an MI more than 6 months earlier. Rao and associates confirmed these findings, reporting reinfarction rates of 36% when prior MIs had occurred at up to 3 months, 26% at 3 to 6 months, and 5% at over 6 months.[42] Vascular surgery patients have a 15% average incidence of reinfarction, increasing to 37% if the past MI was recent.[2]

Recent MI was highly predictive in Goldman's classic study of cardiac risk in noncardiac surgical procedures.[11] Of the 1,001 patients studied, 22 had a recent MI (within the preceding 6 months); of these, 3 (14%) had a life-threatening but nonfatal cardiac event and 5 (23%) suffered cardiac death. Of the variables in the Goldman cardiac risk index (GCRI; see below), only CHF was assigned more points than recent MI (11 versus 10, respectively). Recently, however, Rivers and colleagues from Montefiore Medical Center have challenged this dogma.[43] They treated 30 patients requiring urgent or emergent vascular procedures in the first 6 weeks after MI (median, 11 days). Although there were four postoperative deaths (three cardiac-related) and two nonfatal reinfarctions, 20 of 24 patients survived. The overall cardiac complication rate was 17% (5/30).

Congestive Heart Failure

Clinical or radiological evidence of left ventricular failure is associated with a poor prognosis in patients with CAD. CHF may be the most important predictor of short- and long-term mortality in patients with acute MIs. The 5-year survival of patients with CHF is less than 50%.[2] Patients with an ejection fraction of less than 30% have a 1-year cumulative mortality rate as high as 30%.[44-46] Using data from the Multicenter Postinfarction Research Group, Dwyer et al reported that individuals in the general population who retain normal left ventricular function after MI have a 7% 1-year mortality rate, but annual mortality increases to 44% in those whose ejection fraction was below 30%.[47] The extent of myocardial dysfunction may contribute to perioperative mortality even more than the interval from MI or the extent of CAD.[46,48] In most cardiac risk indexes CHF is heavily weighted.[11,49] However, CHF is a constellation of clinical symptoms rather than a specific entity, and the predictive value of specific signs is controversial. The following signs have been proposed as predictors: jugular venous distention[39,49]; alveolar pulmonary edema[24]; pathological heart sounds (S_3–S_4 gallop)[11]; and dyspnea on exertion, left ventricular wall motion abnormalities, and left ventricular ejection fraction under 50%.[50,51]

Valvular Heart Disease

The prognosis for patients with valvular heart disease depends on which valve is diseased and the extent of disease. Because of confounding factors associated with valvular heart disease, such as left ventricular dysfunction, the perioperative risk caused by valvular disease per se is difficult to quantitate. Limited data suggest that the presence of aortic stenosis is associated with excessive perioperative mortality. In their classic study, Goldman and associates reported a 14-fold increased perioperative morality in patients with aortic stenosis who undergo noncardiac surgery.[11] Notably, the diagnosis of aortic stenosis was made largely by physical examination without objective measurement of the degree of stenosis. Although the incidence of postoperative CHF was increased by the presence of mitral stenosis or insufficiency in this study, only aortic stenosis was associated with increased mortality.

Dysrhythmias

Dysrhythmias are common and are usually benign in healthy patients without known heart disease. In the presence of significant CAD or poor left ventricular function, rhythm disturbances become ominous.[44] Few studies have rigorously addressed the importance of preoperative dysrhythmias. The available data suggest that frequent premature ventricular contractions or rhythms other than normal sinus rhythm on preoperative ECG are independent predictors of outcome in patients undergoing noncardiac surgery.[30,37,38] Particularly dangerous are arrhythmias that occur after acute MI or those associated with hypokalemia and ischemia causing sudden death.[52,53] In contrast, the presence of bifascicular or even trifascicular block, right bundle-branch block, or left anterior hemiblock does not appear to increase perioperative risk, unless they occur in the setting of an acute MI.[2]

Cigarette Smoking

Cigarette smoke causes numerous adverse endothelial, serologic, and hematologic effects, influencing myocardial oxygen supply and demand. Acutely, it produces increased coronary vascular resistance (particularly in the presence of preexisting stenosis) and increased carboxyhemoglobin levels; the raised rate–pressure product results in increased myocardial oxygen demand.[54] Chronically, smoking causes endothelial injury, vasoconstriction, increased serum fibrinogen levels (with consequent adverse effects on blood viscosity), increased hematocrit, increased low-density lipoprotein levels, enhanced platelet aggregation, and others.[55] Thus, intuitively, cigarette smoking would seem to be a risk factor for perioperative cardiac morbidity. However, Foster and associates, reporting findings from the CASS registry, found that cigarette smoking was neither a univariate nor multivariate predictor of adverse cardiac outcome after noncardiac operations.[24] Few other data are available.

Diabetes Mellitus

Diabetes is a major risk factor for the development of atherosclerosis, and MI is the leading cause of death in patients with diabetes.[56,57] In the CASS and other studies the presence of diabetes heralded increased cardiac risk following noncardiac surgery.[24,26] Diabetics are at increased risk for late mortality after peripheral vascular procedures.[58] They are also at increased risk for silent ischemia, in part because visceral neuropathy may contribute to a lack of pain from myocardial ischemia.[5]

HOW TO PREDICT PERIOPERATIVE CARDIAC MORBIDITY: SCREENING TESTS

Because vascular patients have impaired walking imposed by vascular disease, they may not report symptoms of exertional angina or CHF, producing risk scores that do not accurately reflect the degree of cardiac disease present. For example, Lette et al[59] reported that 10.4% of vascular surgery patients classified as low risk (ie, Goldman or Detsky class I; see below) sustain perioperative cardiac complications, emphasizing these limitations.

Consequently, recent approaches have focused on the development of objective preoperative tests to better predict adverse cardiac outcomes. Patients who have either symptomatic CAD or extensive left ventricular dysfunction are generally considered to be at greatest risk for perioperative cardiac complications and can usually be identified by clinical evaluation as described above.[2,11,29,49] Other patients may be at substantial risk due to *occult* cardiac disease unmasked only by the stress of surgery.[29] There has been a proliferation of special tests to identify patients who are at high risk for cardiac complications after peripheral vascular operations. However, additional cardiac studies are often expensive, of questionable validity, and sometimes risky, either as a direct result of the procedure or due to how the information is subsequently used.[32]

The literature concerning which preoperative tests should be used for stratifying cardiac risk is voluminous.[6,25,29,34,51,60,61] In practice, however, fewer than 5% of patients undergoing noncardiac operations who are clinically determined to be at low risk will suffer adverse cardiac events, most of which are nonfatal. Conversely, up to one-half of patients identified as intermediate or high clinical risk may sustain perioperative cardiac complications. Some patients with clinically symptomatic CAD warrant special evaluation irrespective of the need for noncardiac surgery. Patients with high scores on clinical cardiac risk indexes (GCRI score over 12 or Detsky score over 15; see below) or more than three of the five Eagle criteria (age over 70, diabetes, angina pectoris, Q waves of ECG, or ventricular arrhythmias; see below) are at greatest risk for MI or cardiac death following vascular surgery.[11,34,40,61-63] Additional tests in patients determined clinically to be at low cardiac risk are unlikely to provide information that would alter management. Alternatively, patients considered high risk by clinical criteria are unlikely to benefit from further risk stratification, because evidence for increased perioperative cardiac morbidity is overwhelming.[49] Most high-risk patients will require specific intervention for their heart disease (eg, invasive treatment of CAD, intense perioperative monitoring, or change in operative plan) before an elective peripheral vascular procedure. Intermediate-risk patients (according to clinical risk indices) will benefit most from additional cardiac evaluation.

Resting Electrocardiogram

The predictive value of preoperative resting (ECGs) is unsettled, but this is one objective test that should be routinely obtained in all patients undergoing vascular operations.[64] As noted previously, ventricular arrhythmias and Q waves on ECG (ie, history of MI, particularly recent) are widely accepted predictive variables. Postoperative cardiac complications are increased as much as threefold in the presence of an abnormal preoperative ECG.[14,33,64] In the Cleveland Clinic series 44% of patients with clinical findings of cardiac disease *and* abnormal ECG (ST-T segment changes and evidence of previous MI) had *severe* CAD by angiography (over 70% stenosis of one or more coronary arteries), in comparison to only 22% of those with normal ECGs.[10] von Knorring prospectively studied 12,654 patients undergoing noncardiac surgery and found that 214 patients had ECG patterns suggestive of previous MI, left ventricular hypertrophy or strain, or myocardial ischemia.[14] Of these 214 patients, 17.7% suffered a postoperative MI, with a cardiac mortality rate of 32%.

There is a poor negative predictive value for the resting ECG. Whereas an abnormal ECG usually indicates underlying CAD, a normal resting ECG may be deceptive. Up to one-half of previous MIs are missed on ECG because they are misread or lack the typical findings of an old MI. Although Hertzer showed an excellent *positive* predictive value of abnormal resting ECGs for CAD, he also reported that 37% of vascular patients with normal resting ECGs had significant stenosis (70% or above) of one or more coronary arteries (ie, poor *negative* predictive value).[10]

Stress Electrocardiogram (Exercise Treadmill Testing)

In patients who are able to exercise, the stress ECG is an inexpensive, noninvasive, and accurate method of predicting postoperative cardiac morbidity. Obviously, this test is rarely applicable to patients with severely ischemic lower extremities. Arm ergometry can be substituted for the treadmill, but the maximal level of exercise generated by this technique is generally far lower than for standard exercise treadmill testing protocols. ST segment abnormalities on ECG during exercise and/or inability to exercise at low cardiac workloads predicts perioperative cardiac morbidity. Gerson et al[65] reported that inability to exercise was 80% sensitive and 53% specific for predicting adverse postoperative cardiac outcomes in geriatric patients undergoing noncardiac surgery. Cutler and coworkers showed that perioperative MIs occurred in 37% of vascular patients with positive stress ECGs compared to 1.5% with normal studies.[66]

Normal exercise treadmill tests were found in two-thirds of men and one-third of women with angiographically documented significant CAD in 2,045 patients in the CASS registry with a history of angina pectoris.[66] When men and women were matched for age and presence or extent of CAD, the false-positive (approximately 50%) and false-negative (approximately 13%) rates were the same, irrespective of gender. Thus, in a population in whom the prevalence of CAD is high, a positive ETT only slightly increases the likelihood of CAD, whereas a negative ETT correlates poorly with the absence of CAD.[66]

Holter Monitoring (Ambulatory Electrocardiogram)

Holter monitoring, which is most commonly used to detect cardiac arrhythmias, also has utility for assessment of cardiac risk in patients before noncardiac operations.[15,17,20,22,67–69] The period of monitoring for silent ischemia is typically 24 hours, but shorter or longer intervals can be used. Eighteen to 40% of patients with or at risk for CAD experience ischemic episodes during the 48 hours preceding surgery. Over 75% of ischemic episodes are clinically silent.[70] Raby and colleagues found that ischemia on preoperative ambulatory ECG was the most reliable predictor of postoperative cardiac events by multivariate analysis even after all other preoperative risk factors were controlled.[61] Fewer than 1% of patients without detectable Holter ischemia sustained perioperative cardiac complications. Pasternack and coworkers[22] confirmed the frequency and importance of silent ischemia detected by Holter monitoring. In the absence of preoperative Holter evidence of ischemia, no patient had perioperative cardiac complications. In 1988 Mody and associates compared ETT, Holter monitoring, and cardiac catheterization in patients with stable angina pectoris.[71] Patients with positive Holter monitoring had a greater likelihood of having multivessel CAD; however, negative Holter monitoring results were of less predictive value.

Holter monitoring was particularly useful in the patients we studied prospectively for cardiac morbidity at the San Francisco Veterans Administration Medical Center.[15,17,70] Preoperative ischemia by Holter was present in 28% of patients having noncardiac operations, and the incidence of ischemia almost doubled in the postoperative period. Ninety-four percent of ischemic episodes were silent and peaked in severity on the third postoperative day. Ischemia occurred throughout the first postop erative week, emphasizing the importance of routine surveillance for perioperative cardiac morbidity in order to obtain accurate statistics on its frequency.

Advantages of Holter monitoring to identify patients at high risk for cardiac complications include its wide availability, ease of interpretation (because of computer enhancement) and relatively low cost. Its disadvantages are that 10% or more of patients have pre-existing ECG abnormalities that confound interpretation of ST segment depression, and ECG patterns such as left ventricular hypertrophy may lead to false-positive evidence of ST segment depression unrelated to CAD.[34]

Radionuclide Angiography (Measurement of Ejection Fraction)

Left ventricular dysfunction can be measured by determination of ejection fraction. Pasternack and associates at New York University showed that in patients having either aortic or lower extremity operations, the degree of left ventricular dysfunction as measured by radionuclide angiograms (gated blood pool studies) identified those patients at greatest risk for postoperative MIs.[25,51] Eighty percent of patients having aortic and 70% of patients having infrainguinal operations sustained an adverse perioperative cardiac event when ejection fraction was below 30%.[25,51] Although not all studies have substantiated the New York University results,[31,60] Bunt used measurement of ejection fraction as the index test to predict perioperative cardiac complications and identify those patients who should have additional studies.[29]

Dipyridamole Thallium Scintigraphy (Stress Thallium Imaging)

Radionuclide determination of cardiac perfusion by injection of thallium performed when coronary blood flow is increased by exercise or injection of dipyridamole (Persantine) is more sensitive than imaging under resting conditions.[72,73] It can detect stenoses beginning at 50% cross-sectional narrowing.[40] Thallium 201 is taken up by myocardial cells in proportion to blood flow. Dipyridamole inhibits the reuptake and transport of endogenously produced adenosine, a potent coronary vasodilator. Adenosine accumulates in the interstitium and causes coronary vasodilation. Intravenous dipyridamole effectively dilates coronary vessels, doubling or tripling coronary artery blood flow to myocardium supplied by nonstenotic vessels.[74,75] Thus, intravenous dipyridamole produces a *steal* phenomenon because nonstenotic arteries have increased flow, whereas stenotic vessels cannot vasodilate. On scanning performed later in the day, this poorly visualized area reappears on the scan if viable myocardium is present, suggesting a region of myocardium potentially at risk for ischemia. This later normalization of thallium 201 uptake in myocardium initially hypoperfused is termed *redistribution*.[74] In contrast, myocardium supplied by occluded vessels does not take up thallium 201 and produces a fixed deficit that does not change on later scanning.

Boucher and associates in Boston evaluated DTS in 48 patients prior to vascular operations.[6] They concluded that DTS accurately predicts perioperative cardiac morbidity. Normal DTS results in patients scheduled for vascular operations indicate low risk for cardiac complications (ie, good *negative* predictive value).[31,34,40,50,60,74,76] The prognostic implication of an abnormal scan is less well established.

The accuracy of DTS remains controversial. We reported the only prospective blinded study of DTS assessment of perioperative risk.[16] DTS was performed preoperatively in 60 patients who were undergoing elective vascular surgery patients. Planar images were acquired following a standard protocol. The thallium studies were not analyzed until the patient was discharged; therefore, the entire surgical team was blinded to the results. The overall rate of adverse cardiac outcomes was 22%. Of the patients suffering cardiac complications, 37% had redistribution, 30% had fixed defects, and 33% had normal studies. Most ischemic cardiac events (54%) occurred in patients without reversible defects. No correlation could be found between redistribution defects and adverse cardiac outcomes or risk of perioperative ischemia (Holter, ETT). Both positive and negative predictive values of DTS were poor.

In a study from the University of Iowa by Kresowik and coworkers, DTS was performed in 190 patients before elective vascular surgery with ($n = 78$) and without ($n = 112$) clinical CAD.[77] Thallium redistribution defects (about 45%) were equally distributed in the two groups; and severe three-vessel or left main coronary disease was found with similar frequency in those with and without clinical findings suggesting CAD. This investigation was not designed to evaluate the utility of DTS for predicting perioperative cardiac complications, but the authors conclude that *routine* DTS screening should not be performed; instead, they recommended selection of patients for DTS based on whether or not documentation of the extent of CAD would influence therapy.

Baron and colleagues in Paris recently reported the largest and probably the best evaluation of DTS in vascular surgery patients.[37] Clinical and scintigraphic information was collected prospectively in 457 consecutive patients undergoing elective abdominal aortic surgery. Variables potentially predictive of adverse cardiac outcomes were evaluated by multivariate analyses. In brief, as previously discussed, definite CAD and age were the only statistically significant markers predictive of adverse cardiac outcomes. Of note, DTS did *not* predict adverse cardiac outcomes.

The expense of DTS must be factored into the algorithm. Bry et al[78] reported that the positive predictive value of DTS was 19% for all patients with reversible defects, 12% for patients with one reversible defect, and 36.7% for patients with two or more reversible defects. The total cost of screening averaged $3,092 per patient, including DTS in 237 patients, cardiac catheterizations in 51 patients, CABG in 6 patients, coronary angioplasty in 3 patients, MI in 14 patients, and cardiac death in 3 patients. According to this study, $392,253 was spent per life saved and $181,039 was spent per MI averted.

Thus, DTS for preoperative evaluation of vascular surgery patients is controversial. It seems to add little to the work-up of patients at low and high risk for cardiac morbidity, because accurate cardiac risk assessment can be achieved by clinical criteria alone. The identification of an intermediate-risk group by clinical criteria may allow the selective application of DTS and permit additional stratification, at least according to Eagle et al.[40]

Dobutamine Stress Echocardiography

Two-dimensional echocardiography can detect regional wall abnormalities resulting from myocardial ischemia produced by dobutamine infusion and is a potentially useful method for detection of CAD.[79] Lalka and colleagues at the University of Indiana recently studied 60 patients undergoing elective aortic surgery using this technique.[80] Eleven adverse cardiac events occurred in 38 patients with an abnormal dobutamine stress echocardiograph; in contrast, only 1 of 22 patients with a normal study had a cardiac event. The difference in event rates between patients with positive and negative studies (29% versus 4.6%) was statistically significant ($P < .025$). The average cost of dobutamine stress echocardiography was stated to be $600. In comparison, the costs for other screening studies were as follows: DTS, $1,200; radionuclide ventriculography, $900; stress ECG, $450; 24-hour Holter monitor, $280; and coronary angiography, $2,400.

Coronary Angiography

Indications for coronary angiography before vascular surgery are unclear; some recommend it for each vascular surgery patient with clinical or noninvasive evidence of CAD, whereas others believe it is rarely necessary.[6,10,26,28] Again, obtaining coronary angiography presupposes that some intervention will be performed for positive findings. The controversy over prophylactic CABG or PTCA has been discussed previously. In addition to enhancing the safety of peripheral vascular surgery, CABG or PTCA may improve late survival in selected patients. The CASS proved that left main or multivessel CAD correlates with both early and late mortality.[81] In the Cleveland Clinic study severe correctable CAD was present in 34% of patients with clinical evidence of CAD ($n = 511$).[10] In addition, severe surgically correctable CAD was present in 14% of those with *no* clinical indication of CAD ($n = 415$). Of note, only 8% of patients in this series had normal coronary arteries, but CAD was limited to a mild or moderate degree in another 32%. However, the presence of significant coronary stenosis does not necessarily indicate that MI is unavoidable or that invasive intervention is required, because the involved artery may supply an area of myocardial scar or its stenosis may be compensated for by collaterals.

CARDIAC RISK INDICES

Numerous authors have attempted to identify clinical risk factors most predictive of perioperative cardiac risk.[2] Stratification of risk seeks to identify patients in whom (1) cardiac risks outweigh the potential benefits of operations; (2) abnormalities can be corrected before surgery; and (3) risk-reducing interventions are most likely to provide benefit. In 1977 Goldman and associates[11] were among the first to estimate perioperative cardiac risk based on information from history and physical exam. Of the clinical variables examined, the strongest predictors of adverse cardiac outcome were (1) recent MI and (2) CHF; additional factors identified included (in decreasing order of importance) (3) abnormal rhythm; (4) more than five premature ventricular contractions per minute; (5) intra-abdominal, intrathoracic, or aortic surgery; (6) age over 70 years; (7) significant aortic valvular stenosis; (8) emergency operation; and (9) poor general medical condition. Goldman's group ascribed a different number of points to each of nine variables and retrospectively used multivariate analysis to correlate cardiac outcome with the total score, thereby deriving the GCRI.[11] Ten of 19 cardiac deaths (53%) among the 1,001 patients occurred in those with more than 26 points.

The history and physical examination are the cornerstones of all clinical risk indexes. For example, characteristics determined by the history and physical examination account for 35 of the total 53 points in the GCRI, with the remaining points derived from laboratory tests and resting ECGs.[11] The GCRI has subsequently been substantiated in other studies.[19,62,63,82,83] Shah and colleagues,[82] for example, retrospectively analyzed 24 preoperative variables in 688 patients with heart disease undergoing noncardiac surgery. Six of eight variables predictive of perioperative cardiac morbidity were present in the GCRI. In this study the overall postoperative MI rate was 4.7% (32/688) and 7 of these 32 patients (21.9%) died a cardiac death. Detsky et al[63] also validated and modified Goldman's original index, adding categories for angina and past history of pulmonary edema.

Although these indices estimate cardiac risk for the general population undergoing noncardiac surgery, they are less accurate when applied to patients having vascular operations. Eagle and associates developed a simple risk index that he combined with a thallium imaging technique to predict ischemic events after vascular surgery.[34] Of 254 consecutive patients referred for evaluation before peripheral vascular operations, 30 (12%) had early postoperative cardiac ischemic events, 6 (2%) had cardiac deaths, and 9 (3.5%) had nonfatal MIs. The Eagle criteria for clinically identifying patients at high risk for cardiac events are (1) age, (2) history of angina, (3) Q wave on ECG, (4) history of ventricular ectopic activity, and (5) diabetes. Forty-four patients had surgery canceled or postponed on the basis of the preoperative evaluation, thus weakening the conclusions of the study by potentially enhancing the positive predictive value of their protocol.

Uniform opinion is lacking concerning the efficacy of a preoperative predictive risk index when applied to vascular surgery patients. Lette et al[59] evaluated 125 consecutive patients undergoing vascular reconstruction using cardiac risk indexes and DTS. No clinical scoring systems they studied (GCRI,[11] Dripps–American Society of Anesthesiologists,[84] Detsky,[63] Eagle,[40] Cooperman,[85] and Yeager[86]) reliably predicted major adverse cardiac perioperative outcomes. In contrast, Wong and Detsky[49] reexamined Lette's report and concluded that a high Goldman score accurately determined increased perioperative cardiac risk. Nonetheless, all clinical risk indices lack sufficient sensitivity to identify very low-risk subsets of patients. Thus, they are most useful for identifying intermediate- or high-risk patients.

DIFFERENCES IN CARDIAC RISK BETWEEN AORTIC AND INFRAINGUINAL OPERATIONS

The reported incidence of MI after vascular surgery varies enormously, ranging from 0% to 16%, but rates are not uniformly dependent on the type of procedure performed[25,28,29] (Tables 3–2, 3–3, and 3–4). The criteria for diagnosing an MI play an important role in this disparity in reported MI rates, in addition to the importance

TABLE 3–2. INCIDENCE OF PERIOPERATIVE MYOCARDIAL INFARCTION IN AORTIC OPERATIONS

Year	Authors	Patients (n)	Incidence (%)
1986	Johnson et al	459	2.0
1986	Szilagyi et al	1,748	5.0
1986	Peck et al	270	2.6
1988	Perry and Calcagno	160	3.7
1988	Bernstein et al	123	0.8
1989	Wilson et al	126	1.6
1990	Cappeler et al	349	2.9
1990	Ameli et al	105	1.9
1990	Clark et al	200	1.5
1990	Mason et al	144	4.2
1990	Isaacson et al	102	2.0
1990	McEnroe et al	95	5.2
1990	Prendiville et al	114	2.6
1990	Golden et al	500	3.0
1991	Shah et al	280	2.5
1991	Asurahman	332	3.0
1992	Bunt	156	0

From Bunt TJ. The role of a defined protocol for cardiac risk assessment in decreasing perioperative myocardial infarction in vascular surgery. Reproduced with permission from *J Vasc Surg.* 1992;15:626. (Specific references to the authors listed are contained in the original article.)

TABLE 3–3. INCIDENCE OF PERIOPERATIVE MYOCARDIAL INFARCTION IN FEMOROPOPLITEAL OPERATIONS

Year	Authors	Patients (n)	Incidence (%)
1986	Taylor et al	239	1.7
1988	Parker et al	223	2.0
1989	Whittemore et al	300	3.0
1990	Petrovic et al	132	2.3
1991	Towne et al	361	2.2
1991	Bunt	159	0.6

From Bunt TJ. The role of a defined protocol for cardiac risk assessment in decreasing perioperative myocardial infarction in vascular surgery. Reproduced with permission from *J Vasc Surg*. 1992;15:626. (Specific references to the authors listed are contained in the original article.)

of the vigor with which the diagnosis is pursued (as discussed previously). In a comprehensive review of the literature, Yeager estimated that when the diagnosis of MI was made by retrospective review, the incidence of MI following vascular surgery averaged 3%.[18] When the diagnosis of MI was made prospectively using ECG changes *and* cardiac enzyme elevation, the incidence of MI rose to 9.7% on average. Finally, when the diagnosis of MI was made prospectively using MB isoenzyme elevation as the only criterion, postoperative MI rates were a striking 14.7%.

Most articles on preoperative cardiac screening have described patient cohorts considered for aortic surgery, either for occlusive disease or abdominal aortic aneurysms. The frequent occurrence of adverse cardiac events was usually attributed to the stress on myocardium as a consequence of anesthetic induction, aortic clamping, declamping hypotension, washout acidosis, blood loss, large shifts, and metabolic abnormalities.[70] Because infrainguinal vascular operations generally produce such profound hemodynamic and physiological alterations, they might be expected to cause fewer cardiac complications.

To address this question, we prospectively compared cardiac morbidity in 140 patients undergoing aortic (n = 53) and infrainguinal reconstructions (n = 87).[70] Presumably because coronary disease was even higher in patients having less stressful infrainguinal procedures, we observed that the number of postoperative cardiac events (cardiac death, MI, unstable angina, CHF, and ventricular tachycardia) was similar to that in patients undergoing major abdominal procedures. Further, 57% of patients undergoing infrainguinal operations had documented ischemia by ambulatory ECG

TABLE 3–4. INCIDENCE OF PERIOPERATIVE MYOCARDIAL INFARCTION IN FEMOROTIBIAL OPERATIONS

Year	Authors	Patients (n)	Incidence (%)
1984	Rutherford et al	156	3.2
1988	Andros et al	224	5.4
1988	Flinn et al	75	2.6
1988	Patel et al	78	2.6
1988	Ascer et al	24	8.3
1989	Kent et al	266	2.6
1990	Klamer et al	65	4.6
1992	Bunt	90	3.3

From Bunt TJ. The role of a defined protocol for cardiac risk assessment in decreasing perioperative myocardial infarction in vascular surgery. Reproduced with permission from *J Vasc Surg*. 1992;15:626. (Specific references to the authors listed are contained in the original article.)

monitoring compared to 31% of patients undergoing aortic reconstruction ($P = .005$). Interestingly, the ischemia was clinically silent in nearly all (98%) patients, consistent with previous reports which suggest that most postoperative ischemia is asymptomatic.[15,17]

Late cardiac outcomes in patients having operations for infrainguinal occlusive disease is even worse than for patients having aortic operations. A later follow-up of the patient cohort described above revealed that at 2 years a full 25% of all patients had died, about half due to cardiac disease.[58] Twenty of 81 (25%) patients who had infrainguinal procedures compared with 4 of 48 patients (8%) who had aortic operations suffered adverse cardiac events in late follow-up ($P = .04$) (Fig. 3–2). Multivariate analysis showed that a history of diabetes ($P = .001$) and definite CAD ($P = .01$) were independently associated with adverse outcomes after both types of peripheral vascular operations.

From a practical standpoint, however, preoperative cardiac work-up must also take into account the indication for surgery. Patients with threatened limbs often cannot afford the time involved for obtaining additional tests such as Holter monitoring, DTS, or cardiac catheterization. Moreover, the question of what to do with the information provided by special studies is problematic in such instances. For example, if DTS shows marked redistribution in a patient with asymptomatic CAD and a gangrenous foot, what is gained by the long delay in ultimate lower extremity revascularization by prophylactic CABG? As emphasized throughout this analysis, reports supporting prophylactic CAD intervention are nonrandomized and uncontrolled.[30,87–92]

CONCLUSION

CAD is present in most patients with peripheral arterial disease and is the leading cause of morbidity and mortality after vascular surgery. Several clinical features and special tests are useful to estimate perioperative cardiac risk. Eagle's clinical risk index consisting of (1) age, (2) history of angina, (3) Q wave on ECG, (4) history of ventricular ectopic activity, and (5) diabetes is easy to remember and perhaps one of the best available. Risk assessment attempts to identify those patients at low, intermediate,

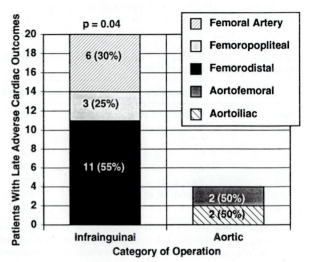

Figure 3–2. Late adverse outcomes in patients undergoing infrainguinal versus aortic operations. Statistical significance was achieved ($P = .04$) when all infrainguinal operations were compared with all aortic operations. *[Reproduced with permission from Krupski WC, Layug EL, Reilly LM, et al. Comparison of cardiac morbidity between aortic and infrainguinal operations; Two Year Follow Up. Study of Perioperative Ischemia (SPI) Research Group. J Vasc Surg. 1993;18:609–617.]*

or high cardiac jeopardy for adverse cardiac outcomes. Although estimates of *low* risk do not preclude perioperative complications, further testing adds little additional information to the estimates obtained by clinical scoring. Conversely, patients with *high* cardiac risk scores are clearly at increased risk of experiencing postoperative complications, but further investigations are needed only if knowledge of the functional severity or degree of myocardial ischemia will alter subsequent management. In general, *high* risk patients should proceed to coronary angiography, intensive perioperative monitoring, alteration in the planned operation, or avoidance of surgery altogether if indications are less than compelling. Those patients identified as *intermediate* risk by clinical scoring benefit most from additional tests. In these patients ambulatory ECG, DTS, or coronary arteriography *may* be useful if the vascular surgery can be delayed until myocardial revascularization is completed.

Despite its popularity, recent studies have questioned the accuracy of DTS. Holter monitoring or dobutamine stress echocardiography provide reasonable and less expensive alternatives.

Despite suggestive evidence from uncontrolled nonrandomized studies of prophylactic CABG, coronary artery bypass surgery should be recommended only on the merits of the patient's cardiac symptoms and anatomy, not necessarily to enhance safety of the proposed vascular procedure. Recent advances in surgical and anesthetic techniques as well as intraoperative and postoperative monitoring have resulted in lower morbidity and mortality of elective noncardiac surgery, but, as always, treatment must be individualized.

REFERENCES

1. Frye RL, Higgins MW, Bellar GA, et al. Major demographic and epidemiologic trends affecting adult cardiology. *J Am Coll Cardiol.* 1988;12:840.
2. Mangano DT. Perioperative cardiac morbidity. *Anesthesiology.* 1990;72:153.
3. Weinstein MC, Coxson PG, Williams LW, et al. Forecasting coronary heart disease policy model. *Am J Public Health.* 77:1417–1426.
4. Current population reports. US Department of Commerce, Bureau of the Census Series 138. 1987;23.
5. Cohn PF. Silent myocardial ischemia. Dimensions of the problem in patients with and without angina. *Am J Med.* 1986;89(suppl 4C):1.
6. Hertzer NR. The natural history of peripheral vascular disease: implications for its management. *Circulation.* 1991;83(suppl I):I12.
7. Bergan JJ, Wilson SE, Wolf G, et al. Unexpected, late cardiovascular effects of surgery for peripheral artery disease. *Arch Surg.* 1992;127:1119.
8. Boyd AM. The natural course of arteriosclerosis of the lower extremities. *Angiology.* 1960;11:10.
9. Kallero KS. Mortality and morbidity in patients with intermittent claudication as defined by venous occlusion plethysmography: a ten year follow-up study. *J Chronic Dis.* 1981;34:455.
10. Hertzer NR, Beven EG, Young JR, et al. Coronary artery disease in peripheral vascular patients: a classification of 1000 coronary angiograms and results of surgical management. *Ann Surg.* 1984;199:223.
11. Goldman L, Caldera DL, Nussbaum SR, et al. Multifactorial index of cardiac risk in noncardiac surgical procedures. *N Engl J Med.* 1977;297:845.
12. Steen PA, Tinker JH, Tarhan S. Myocardial reinfarction after anesthesia and surgery. *JAMA.* 1978;239:2566.
13. Tarhan S, Moffitt E, Taylor WF, et al. Myocardial infarction after general anesthesia. *JAMA.* 1972;220:1451.

14. von Knorring J. Postoperative myocardial infarction: a prospective study in a risk group of surgical patients. *Surgery.* 1981;90:55.

15. Mangano DT, Hollenberg M, Fegert G, et al. Perioperative myocardial ischemia in patients undergoing noncardiac surgery—I: incidence and severity during the 4 day perioperative period. The Study of Perioperative Ischemia (SPI) Research Group. *J Am Coll Cardiol.* 1991;17:843.

16. Mangano DT, London MJ, Tubau JF, et al. Dipyridamole thallium-201 scintigraphy as a preoperative screening test: a reexamination of its predictive potential. *Circulation.* 1991;84:493.

17. Mangano DT, Wong MG, London MJ, et al. Perioperative myocardial ischemia in patients undergoing noncardiac surgery—II: incidence and severity during the 1st week after surgery. *J Am Coll Cardiol.* 1991;17:851.

18. Yeager RA. Basic data related to cardiac testing and cardiac risk associated with vascular surgery. *Ann Vasc Surg.* 1990;4:193.

19. Charlson ME, MacKenzie CR, Ales K, et al. Surveillance for postoperative myocardial infarction after noncardiac operations. *Surg Gynecol Obstet.* 1988;167:407.

20. McCann RL, Clements FM. Silent myocardial ischemia in patients undergoing peripheral vascular surgery: incidence and association with perioperative cardiac morbidity and mortality. *J Vasc Surg.* 1989;9:583.

21. Ouyang P, Gerstenblith G, Furman WR, et al. Frequency and significance of early postoperative silent myocardial ischemia in patients having peripheral vascular surgery. *Am J Cardiol.* 1989;64:1113.

22. Pasternack PF, Grossi EA, Baumann FG, et al. The value of silent myocardial ischemia monitoring in the prediction of perioperative myocardial infarction in patients undergoing peripheral vascular surgery. *J Vasc Surg.* 1989;10:617.

23. Mangano DT, Browner WS, Hollenberg M, et al. Long-term cardiac prognosis following noncardiac surgery. *JAMA.* 1992;268:233.

24. Foster ED, Davis KB, Carpenter JA, et al. Risk of noncardiac operation in patients with defined coronary disease: the Coronary Artery Surgery Study (CASS) registry experience. *Ann Thorac Surg.* 1986;41:42.

25. Pasternack PF, Imparato AM, Bear G, et al. The value of radionuclide angiography as a predictor of perioperative myocardial infarction in patients undergoing abdominal aortic aneurysm resection. *J Vasc Surg.* 1984;1:320.

26. Hertzer NR. Myocardial ischemia. *Surgery.* 1983;83:97.

27. Gage AA, Bhayana JN, Balu V, et al. Assessment of cardiac risk in surgical patients. *Arch Surg.* 1977;112:1488.

28. Taylor LJ, Yeager RA, Moneta GL, et al. The incidence of perioperative myocardial infarction in general vascular surgery. *J Vasc Surg.* 1992;15:52.

29. Bunt TJ. The role of a defined protocol for cardiac risk assessment in decreasing perioperative myocardial infarction in vascular surgery. *J Vasc Surg.* 1992;15:626.

30. Ennix CL, Lawrie GM, Morris GC, et al. Improved results of carotid endarterectomy in patients with symptomatic coronary disease: an analysis of 1,546 consecutive carotid operations. *Stroke.* 1979;10:122.

31. Cutler BS, Leppo JA. Dipyridamole thallium 201 scintigraphy to detect coronary artery disease before abdominal aortic surgery. *J Vasc Surg.* 1987;5:91.

32. Huber KC, Evans MA, Bresnahan JF, et al. Outcome of noncardiac operations in patients with severe coronary artery disease successfully treated preoperatively with coronary angioplasty. *Mayo Clin Proc.* 1992;67:15.

33. Carliner NH, Fisher ML, Plotnick GD, et al. Routine pre-operative exercise testing in patients undergoing major non-cardiac surgery. *Am J Cardiol.* 1985;56:51.

34. Eagle KA, Coley CM, Newell JB, et al. Combining clinical and thallium data optimizes preoperative assessment of cardiac risk before major vascular surgery. *Ann Intern Med.* 1989;110:859.

35. Port S, Cobb FR, Coleman RE, et al. Effect of age on the response of left ventricular function to exercise. *N Engl J Med.* 1980;303:1133.

36. Browner WS, Li J, Mangano DT, et al. In-hospital and long-term mortality in male veterans following noncardiac surgery. *JAMA*. 1992;268:228.

37. Baron JF, Mundler O, Bertrand M, et al. Dipyridamole–thallium scintigraphy and gated radionuclide angiography to assess cardiac risk before abdominal aortic surgery. *N Engl J Med*. 1994;330:663.

38. Diamond GA, Forrester JS. Analysis of probability as an aid in the clinical diagnosis of coronary artery disease. *N Engl J Med*. 1979;300:1350.

39. Goldman L. Cardiac risks and complications of noncardiac surgery. *Ann Intern Med*. 1983;98:504.

40. Eagle KA, Singer DE, Brewster DC, et al. Dipyridamole–thallium scanning in patients undergoing vascular surgery. Optimizing preoperative evaluation of cardiac risk. *JAMA*. 1987;257:2185.

41. Topkins MJ, Artusio JF. Myocardial infarction and surgery: a five-year study. *Anesth Analg*. 1964;43:716.

42. Rao TL, Jacobs KH, El-Etr AA. Reinfarction following anesthesia in patients with myocardial infarction. *Anesthesiology*. 1983;59:499.

43. Rivers SP, Scher LA, Gupta SK, et al. Safety of peripheral vascular surgery after recent acute myocardial infarction. *J Vasc Surg*. 1990;11:70.

44. Bigger JT, Fleiss JL, Kleiger R, et al. The relationship among ventricular arrhythmias, left ventricular dysfunction, and mortality in the 2 years after myocardial infarction. *Circulation*. 1984;69:250.

45. Multicenter Postinfarction Research Group. Risk stratification and survival after myocardial infarction. *N Engl J Med*. 1983;309:331.

46. Sanz G, Castaner A, Betriu A. Determinants of prognosis in survivors of myocardial infarction. *N Engl J Med*. 1982;306:1065.

47. Dwyer EMJ, Greenberg HM, Steinberg G. Clinical characteristics and natural history of survivors of pulmonary congestion during acute myocardial infarction. The Multicenter Postinfarction Research Group. *Am J Cardiol*. 1989;63:1423.

48. Dirksen A, Kjoller E. Cardiac predictors of death after non-cardiac surgery evaluated by intention to treat. *Br Med J*. 1988;297:1011.

49. Wong T, Detsky AS. Preoperative cardiac risk assessment for patients having peripheral vascular surgery. *Ann Intern Med*. 1992;116:743.

50. Lazor L, Russell JC, DaSilva J, et al. Use of the multiple uptake gated acquisition scan for the preoperative assessment of cardiac risk. *Surg Gynecol Obstet*. 1987;167:234.

51. Pasternack PF, Imparato AM, Riles TS, et al. The value of radionuclide angiogram in the prediction of perioperative myocardial infarction in patients undergoing lower extremity revascularization procedures. *Circulation*. 1985;72(suppl II):II13.

52. McGovern B. Hypokalemia and cardiac arrhythmias. *Anesthesiology*. 1985;63:127.

53. Schultz RAJ, Strauss HW, Pitt B. Sudden death in the year following myocardial infarction: relation to ventricular premature contractions in the late hospital phase and left ventricular ejection fraction. *Am J Med*. 1976;62:192.

54. Nicod P, Rehr R, Winniford MD, et al. Acute systemic and coronary hemodynamic and serologic responses to cigarette smoking in long-term smokers with atherosclerotic coronary artery disease. *J Am Coll Cardiol*. 1984;4:964.

55. Krupski WC. The peripheral vascular consequences of smoking. *Ann Vasc Surg*. 1991;5:291–304.

56. Kannel WB, McGee DL. Diabetes and cardiovascular risk factors: the Framingham study. *Circulation*. 1979;59:8.

57. Waller BF, Palumbo PJ, Lie JT, et al. Status of the coronary arteries at necropsy in diabetes mellitus with onset after age 30 years: analysis of 229 diabetic patients with and without clinical evidence of coronary heart disease and comparison to 183 control subjects. *Am J Med*. 1980;69:498.

58. Krupski WC, Layug EL, Reilly LM, et al. Comparison of cardiac morbidity rates between aortic and infrainguinal operations: two-year follow-up. Study of Perioperative Ischemia (SPI) Research Group. *J Vasc Surg*. 1993;18:609.

59. Lette J, Waters D, Lassonde J, et al. Multivariate clinical models and quantitative dipyridam-ole–thallium imaging to predict cardiac morbidity and death after vascular reconstruction. *J Vasc Surg*. 1991;14:160.

60. Boucher CA, Brewster DC, Darling RC, et al. Determination of cardiac risk by dipyridam-ole–thallium imaging before peripheral vascular surgery. *N Engl J Med*. 1985;312:389.

61. Raby KE, Goldman L, Creager MA, et al. Correlation between preoperative ischemia and major cardiac events after peripheral vascular surgery. *N Engl J Med*. 1989;321:1296.

62. Detsky AS, Abrams HB, Forbath N, et al. Cardiac assessment for patients undergoing noncardiac surgery: a multifactorial clinical risk index. *Arch Intern Med*. 1986;146:2131.

63. Detsky AS, Abrams HB, McLaughlin JR, et al. Predicting cardiac complications in patients undergoing non-cardiac surgery. *J Gen Intern Med*. 1986;1:211.

64. Velanovich V. The value of routine preoperative laboratory testing in predicting postopera-tive complications: a multivariate analysis. *Surgery*. 1991;109:236.

65. Gerson MC, Hurst JM, Hertzberg VS, et al. Cardiac prognosis in noncardiac geriatric surgery. *Ann Intern Med*. 1985;103:832.

66. Cutler BS, Wheeler HB, Paraskos JA, et al. Applicability and interpretation of electrocardio-graphic stress testing in patients with peripheral vascular disease. *Am J Surg*. 1981;141:501.

67. Boucher CA, Brewster DC, Darling RC, et al. Correlation between preoperative ischemia and major cardiac events after peripheral vascular surgery. *N Engl J Med*. 1989;321:1296.

68. Gardine RL, McBride K, Greenberg H, et al. The value of cardiac monitoring during peripheral arterial stress testing in the surgical management of peripheral vascular disease. *J Cardiovasc Surg*. 1985;26:258.

69. Raby KE, Goldman L, Creager MA, et al. Predictive value of preoperative electrocardio-graphic monitoring. *N Engl J Med*. 1990;322:931.

70. Krupski WC, Layug EL, Reilly LM, et al. Comparison of cardiac morbidity between aortic and infrainguinal operations. Study of Perioperative Ischemia (SPI) Research Group. *J Vasc Surg*. 1992;15:354.

71. Mody FV, Nademanee K, Intarachot V, et al. Severity of silent myocardial ischemia on ambulatory electrocardiographic monitoring in patients with stable anginal pectoris: relation to prognosis determinants during exercise stress testing and coronary angiography. *J Am Coll Cardiol*. 1988;12:1169.

72. Franco CD, Goldsmith J, Veith FJ, et al. Resting gated pool ejection fraction: a poor predictor of perioperative myocardial infarction in patients undergoing vascular surgery for infrain-guinal bypass grafting. *J Vasc Surg*. 1989;10:656.

73. McEnroe CS, O'Donnell TF Jr, Yeager A, et al. Comparison of ejection fraction and Goldman risk factor analysis to dipyridamole–thallium 201 studies in the evaluation of cardiac morbid-ity after aortic aneurysm surgery. *J Vasc Surg*. 1990;11:497.

74. Eagle KA, Strauss HW, Boucher CA. Dipyridamole myocardial perfusion imaging for coro-nary heart disease. *Am J Cardiac Imaging*. 1988;2:292.

75. Mays AE, Cobb FR. Relationship between regional myocardial blood flow and thallium 201 redistribution in the presence of coronary artery stenosis and dipyridamole-induced vasodilatation. *J Clin Invest*. 1984;73:1359.

76. Cutler BS, Hendel RC, Leppo JA. Dipyridamole–thallium scintigraphy predicts periopera-tive and long-term survival after major vascular surgery. *J Vasc Surg*. 1992;15:972.

77. Kresowik TF, Bower TR, Garner SA, et al. Dipyridamole thallium imaging in patients being considered for vascular procedures. *Arch Surg*. 1993;128:299.

78. Bry JDL, Belkin M, O'Donnell TF Jr, et al. An assessment of the positive predictive value and cost-effectiveness of dipyridamole myocardial scintigraphy in patients undergoing vascular surgery. *J Vasc Surg*. 1994;19:112–124.

79. Berthe C, Pierard LA, Hiernaux M, et al. Predicting the extent and location of coronary artery disease in acute myocardial infarction by echocardiography during dobutamine infu-sion. *Am J Cardiol*. 1986;58:1167.

80. Lalka SG, Sawada SG, Dalsing MC, et al. Dobutamine stress echocardiography as a predictor of cardiac events associated with aortic surgery. *J Vasc Surg*. 1992;15:831.

81. Myers WO, Gersh BJ, Fisher LD, et al. Medical versus early surgical therapy in patients with triple vessel disease and mild angina pectoris: a CASS registry study of survival. *Ann Thorac Surg*. 1987;44:471.

82. Shah KB, Kleinman BS, Rao TL, et al. Angina and other risk factors in patients with cardiac diseases undergoing noncardiac operations. *Anesth Analg.* 1990;70:240.
83. Zeldin RA. Assessing cardiac risk in patients who undergo noncardiac surgical procedures. *Can J Surg.* 1984;27:402.
84. Dripps RD, Lamont A, Eckenhoff JE. The role of anaesthesia in surgical mortality. *JAMA.* 1961;178:261.
85. Cooperman M, Pflug B, Martin EW, et al. Cardiovascular risk factors in patients with peripheral vascular disease. *Surgery.* 1978;84:505.
86. Yeager RA, Weigel RM, Murphy ES, et al. Application of clinically valid cardiac risk factors to aortic aneurysm surgery. *Arch Surg.* 1986;121:278.
87. Arous EJ, Baum PL, Cutler BS. The ischemic exercise test in patients with peripheral vascular disease. *Arch Surg.* 1984;119:780.
88. Edwards WH, Mulherin JL, Walker WE. Vascular reconstructive surgery following myocardial revascularization. *Ann Surg.* 1978;187:653.
89. Jamieson WR, Janusz MT, Miyagishima RT, et al. Influence of ischemic heart disease on early and late mortality after surgery for peripheral occlusive vascular disease. *Circulation.* 1982;66(suppl I):I92.
90. Mahar LJ, Steen PA, Tinker JH, et al. Perioperative myocardial infarction in patients with coronary disease with and without aorta-coronary bypass grafts. *J Thorac Cardiovasc Surg.* 1978;76:533.
91. Toal KW, Jacocks MA, Elkins RC, et al. Preoperative coronary artery bypass grafting in patients undergoing abdominal aortic reconstruction. *Am J Surg.* 1984;148:825.
92. Gersh BJ, Rihal CS, Rooke TW, et al. Evaluation and management of patients with both peripheral vascular and coronary artery disease. *J Am Coll Cardiol.* 1991;18:203.

4

The Definition of Critical Ischemia:

Current Criteria for Clinical Application

Eugene F. Bernstein, MD, PhD

Current medical use of the word *critical* implies a crisis or turning point, or a level of disease beyond the ordinary or stable condition.[1] Thus, for the vascular surgeon, the concept of *critical ischemia* has evolved to describe the most extreme degree of lower extremity signs and symptoms suggesting a limb-threatening condition. In parallel efforts in Europe and the United States, a more quantitative and useful expanded definition of critical limb ischemia has been developed over the past few years.

A history of the modern classification of ischemic disease of the lower extremities should include the classification of Fontaine, which has been in general use in Europe for many years (Table 4–1). In this system both stage III and stage IV are considered limb salvage situations.[2,3] However, the Fontaine system, although very useful, was based entirely on clinical signs and symptoms. Newer methods of quantitating the anatomic and functional levels of occlusive arterial disease have permitted the creation of more precise criteria.

INTERNATIONAL WORKING PARTY

Credit for the contemporary approach to this issue must go to the first international "Working Party," which reported a classification that included both acute and chronic ischemia in 1982.[4] In this brief paper it was suggested that critical ischemia include not only the traditional signs and symptoms of persistent and severe rest pain, gangrene, or necrosis, but also an objective measurement, including (1) an ankle pressure lower than 40 mm Hg systolic or (2) an ankle pressure lower than 60 mm Hg systolic in the presence of necrosis, ulceration, or gangrene (Table 4–2).

A major justification of this more quantitative definition was the hope that worldwide adoption of common criteria would result in comparable reporting information regarding the natural history of the condition, results of a particular treatment, and

TABLE 4–1. FONTAINE CLASSIFICATION OF ARTERIAL DISEASE

Stage	Characteristic
I	Without objective signs or symptoms of disease
II	Intermittent claudication
III	Rest pain
IV	Gangrene

Adapted from Bollinger A. *Funktionelle Angiologie*. Stuttgart, Germany: Georg Thieme Verlag; 1979;70.

data from clinical trials. Thus, existing problems with apparently conflicting data might be resolved. These authors also recommended excluding or separating diabetic patients, as well as those with intermittent claudication, from patients with "critical ischemia."

SOCIETY FOR VASCULAR SURGERY/INTERNATIONAL SOCIETY FOR CARDIOVASCULAR SURGERY STANDARDS COMMITTEE REPORT

In 1986 the North American SVS/ISCVS Standards Committee report recommended terms and criteria dealing with lower extremity ischemia which have subsequently become the accepted standard for publications in the *Journal of Vascular Surgery* and for presentations of data in North America.[5] Jamieson participated in this committee in an effort to coordinate the American and European efforts.

Regarding *acute* limb ischemia, three levels of disease progression were defined: viable, threatened, and irreversible (Table 4–3). Chronic ischemia was divided into four grades and seven categories, with both a clinical description and vascular laboratory objective criteria for each (Table 4–4). Categories 4, 5, and 6, which include ischemic rest pain and tissue loss, are analogous to those patients described originally by the Working Party as critical limb ischemia, both clinically and by laboratory criteria.[4]

The SVS/ISCVS Standards Committee report included a plea to abandon the term *limb salvage*, preferring *chronic critical ischemia* or *foot salvage*. Furthermore, specific exclusions that may not qualify as "foot salvage" are detailed, including operations for blue toe syndrome or atheromicroembolism, and Syme's amputation, which involves shortening of the leg. The SVS/ISCVS report also includes a scale of clinical and vascular laboratory criteria for clinical improvement and for vascular graft patency, details regarding Life Table analysis of data, and scales for grading runoff arteries,

TABLE 4–2. DEFINITION OF CRITICAL ISCHEMIA OF THE LOWER LIMB: WORKING PARTY OF THE FIRST INTERNATIONAL VASCULAR SYMPOSIUM, 1981

1. Acute critical ischemia
   Persistent motor or sensory loss
2. Chronic critical ischemia
   A. Rest pain for 4 weeks impairing sleep and requiring regular analgesia
   B. Necrosis involving the base of a digit or superficial skin necrosis involving part of the foot
   Ankle pressure lower than 60 mm Hg
3. Diabetic patients to be grouped separately in view of the complexity of their ischemic/septic diathesis

Adapted from Bell PRF, Charlesworth D, DePalma RG, et al. The definition of critical ischaemia of a limb. *Br J Surg*. 1982;69(suppl):S2.

TABLE 4–3. CLINICAL CATEGORIES OF ACUTE LIMB ISCHEMIA (SVS/ISCVS)

Category	Description	Capillary Return	Muscle Weakness	Sensory Loss	Doppler Signals Arterial	Doppler Signals Venous
Viable	Not immediately threatened	Intact	None	None	Audible (AP[a] >30 mm Hg)	Audible
Threatened	Salvageable if promptly treated	Intact, slow	Mild, partial	Mild, Incomplete	Inaudible	Audible
Irreversible	Major tissue loss, amputation regardless of treatment	Absent (marbling)	Profound, paralysis (rigor)	Profound, anesthetic	Inaudible	Inaudible

[a] AP indicates ankle pressure.
Adapted from Rutherford RB, Flanigan DP, Gupta SK, et al. Suggested standards for reports dealing with lower extremity ischemia. *J Vasc Surg.* 1986;4:80–94.

TABLE 4–4. CLINICAL CATEGORIES OF CHRONIC LIMB ISCHEMIA (SVS/ISCVS)

Grade	Category	Clinical Description	Objective Criteria[a]
0	0	Asymptomatic—no hemodynamically significant occlusive disease	Normal treadmill/stress test
I	1	Mild caludication	Completes treadmill exercise[b]; AP after exercise <50 mm Hg but >25 mm Hg less than BP
	2	Moderate claudication	Between categories 1 and 3
	3	Severe claudication	Cannot complete treadmill exercise; AP after exercise <50 mm Hg
II	4	Ischemic rest pain	Resting AP <40 mm Hg, flat or barely pulsatile ankle or metatarsal PVR; TP <30 mm Hg
III	5	Minor tissue loss—nonhealing ulcer, focal gangrene with diffuse pedal ischemia	Resting AP <60 mm Hg, ankle or metatarsal PVR flat or barely pulsatile; TP <40 mm Hg
	6	Major tissue loss—extending above the TM level, functional foot no longer salvageable	Same as category 5

[a] AP indicates ankle pressure; BP, brachial pressure; PVR, pulse volume recording; TP, toe pressure; TM, transmetatarsal.
[b] Five minutes at 2 mph on a 12% incline.
Adapted from Rutherford RB, Flanigan DP, Gupta SK, et al. Suggested standards for reports dealing with lower extremity ischemia. *J Vasc Surg.* 1986;4:80–94.

types of operations, and complications of surgery. These have rapidly become the standard for reporting experience with lower extremity ischemia in North America.

EUROPEAN CONSENSUS

Shortly thereafter, in 1988, the European consensus process began. Initially, small workshops were held, culminating in a 3-day European Consensus Meeting in Berlin in 1989, with more than 100 participants. The initial consensus document was circulated and then reviewed in 34 medical journals and at many specialist meetings. This process was much more ambitious than the SVS/ISCVS approach, and included collecting and editing information concerning pathophysiology, methods of diagnosis, channels of referral, and details of management, including risk factor management, medical therapy, thrombolysis, and surgery. Following this initial review, an effort was made to obtain suggestions for improvement and supportive endorsements from many related specialties and societies, such that the broadest acceptance of these definitions and management algorithms would rapidly alter the management of patients with occlusive arterial disease of the lower extremities (Table 4–5). Accordingly, suggested improvements with very specific recommendations regarding management were incorporated into the next version of the document. A Consensus Meeting sponsored by the World Health Organization was held in 1991, and a Second European Consensus Document that deals only with the chronically ischemic limb was published in 1991.[6]

The final description offered in the Second Consensus statement is: "Chronic critical leg ischemia, in both diabetic and nondiabetic patients, is defined by either of the following two criteria: persistently recurring ischemic rest pain requiring regular adequate analgesia for more than two weeks, with an ankle systolic pressure ≤ 50 mm Hg and/or a toe systolic pressure ≤ 30 mm Hg; or ulceration or gangrene of the foot or toes, with an ankle systolic pressure of ≤ 50 mm Hg or a toe systolic pressure ≤ 30 mm Hg."[6]

The definition is followed by detailed suggestions for workup, which include angiography and a local microcirculation evaluation involving capillary microscopy, transcutaneous oxygen tension, or laser Doppler. Data are included regarding the reported incidence of critical ischemia in a variety of patient populations and regarding

TABLE 4–5. ENDORSING AND COLLABORATING SOCIETIES IN THE SECOND EUROPEAN CONSENSUS DOCUMENT, 1991

The European Regional Office of the World Health Organization
l'Accademia dei Lincei
The Royal Society of Medicine
Le Collège Français de Pathologie Vasculaire
Cardiovascular and Interventional Radiological Society of Europe
European Diabetic Group
European Society of Cardiology
European Society for Microcirculation
European Society for Vascular Surgery
European Thrombosis Research Organization
International Union of Angiology
European Chapter of the International Society for Cardiovascular Surgery

the outlook of such patients for both limb salvage and survival. For example, in a United Kingdom review, within 1 year 25% of such patients underwent a major amputation, and 20% died. The consensus statement also specifically recommends a course of specialist referral, diagnostic tests, and both general principles and specific details of management.

DISCUSSION

One criticism of the two definitions detailed above relates to their lack of consistency. In the European report 50 mm Hg is the cutoff ankle pressure, while in the SVS/ISCVS study it is 40 mm Hg with rest pain and 60 mm Hg with ulceration and gangrene. In the European report 30 mm Hg is the toe pressure cutoff, while in the SVS/ISCVS document it is the same for rest pain, but 40 mm Hg for ulceration and gangrene. Therefore, study proposals and clinical reports prepared for presentation are likely to differ depending on the geographic area of origin and the academic affiliation of the investigators. Neither the European nor the North American group has indicated that it plans to sponsor meetings to create a joint definition to which all parties can agree.

Other areas of concern regarding the two definitions include the absence of any agreement regarding stress testing. Available alternatives include use of the exercise treadmill test (at a precisely stated angle and speed), postocclusive reactive hyperemia, or the toe pulse reappearance time. The latter two have the advantages of being objective, evaluating each leg independently, avoiding the need for cardiac monitoring, and easily separating out those patients whose symptoms are secondary to cardiac, bone, joint, nerve, or muscle pathology. Some form of precisely defined and standardized stress test is important both for a more complete characterization of the functional limitation of the patient and for analyzing the results of treatment.

Another important consideration relates to the introduction of new noninvasive technology which has appeared subsequent to the publication of the critical ischemia definition reports. For example, real-time Doppler color flow imaging is currently one of the earliest examinations performed in patients with lower extremity ischemia, and may provide information which is more important in predicting outcome than any of the items currently included in the definitions. Such Doppler information includes identifying the specific site, length, and character of both proximal and distal lesions. The data of Moneta and colleagues[7] document the improved detection rates for over 50% stenosis when Doppler-derived data were compared with segmental pressure information (Table 4–6). Since invasive technology can effectively deal with many of these lesions, the location, number, and composition of the obstructing pathology lesions may well be critical in determining the outcome of treatment in a given individual.

Whether the strong support for tests of the microcirculation in the European Consensus Document is warranted is still not certain, and must await an analysis of therapeutic trials currently under way. Thus, one of the benefits of the large-scale use of the proposed definitions will be information that will permit further refinement of the truly important items in both the definition and the suggested subsequent workup and management. Perhaps the most important benefits of the widespread use of the current plans will be the generation of data against which newly proposed treatments may be measured. An example of such information is shown in Table 4–7, which summarized the available data concerning infrainguinal bypass for "limb

TABLE 4–6. ACCURACY OF DETECTION OF STENOSIS >50% BY SEGMENTAL PRESSURES AND BY DUPLEX MAPPING[a]

| No. of Arterial Segments (151) | Detection of >50% Stenosis | | | | P Value |
| | Correct | | Incorrect | | |
	Segmental Pressure	Duplex Mapping	Segmental Pressure	Duplex Mapping	
Superficial femoral artery	113	146 (97%)	38	5	.0001
Popliteal artery	82	137 (91%)	69	14	.0001

[a] Note: No difference was seen with diabetes.
Adapted from Moneta GL, Yeager RA, Antonovic R, et al. Accuracy of lower extremity arterial duplex mapping. *J Vasc Surg.* 1992;15:275–284.

salvage."[8] Presumably, all of these patients would meet the current definitions of critical ischemia, although many of these series were reported prior to the publication of the definitions. The universal use of consistent criteria is critical for such data to be useful.

For all the reasons stated above, it seems clear that a new World Conference on the Classification of Peripheral Arterial Disease is necessary. First, the conflicts between the existing European and North American definitions must be resolved. Second, new technology and information must be evaluated, and modification of the definitions must be performed accordingly. Third, a mechanism for a continuing process of review and modification should be developed. Precisely these functions are currently performed by other health groups, most notably in the malignant diseases. It is time for those interested in vascular disease to catch up.

CONCLUSION

Two separate efforts to define chronic critical ischemia of the lower extremity have been completed with generally similar wording and criteria, and one of these also

TABLE 4–7. DATA SUMMARY OF LIMB SALVAGE WITH INFRAINGUINAL REVASCULARIZATION: 1981–1990

	Limb Salvage at 3 Years (%)	No. of Reports
Below-Knee Femoropopliteal Bypass		
Reversed vein	86	3
In situ vein	83	3
PTFE[a]	No data	—
Infrapopliteal Bypass		
Reversed vein	82	7
In situ vein	83	2
PTFE	56	3

[a] PTFE indicates polytetrafluoroethylene graft.
Adapted from Dalman RL, Taylor LM Jr. Basic data related to infrainguinal revascularization procedures. *Ann Vasc Surg.* 1990;4:309–311.

classifies acute limb ischemia. The differences between the definitions appear relatively minor, but remain as a source of confusion for investigators and reporters. Utilization of the SVS/ISCVS reporting system is recommended for authors in North America at the present time. A worldwide consensus, which includes new technology and continues to review newer information, is an extremely important step for the future.

REFERENCES

1. *Webster's Medical Dictionary*. Springfield, Mass., Merriam; 1977:270.
2. Fontaine R. Resultats des operations hyperemisantes dans les obliterations arterielles chroniques spontanees des membres. *Rev Chir*. 1953; 72:204–230.
3. Bollinger A. *Funktionelle Angiologie*. Stuttgart, Germany: Georg Thieme Verlag; 1979;70.
4. Bell PRF, Charlesworth D, DePalma RG, et al. The definition of critical ischaemia of a limb. *Br J Surg*. 1982;69(suppl):S2.
5. Rutherford RB, Flanigan DP, Gupta SK, et al. Suggested standards for reports dealing with lower extremity ischemia. *J Vasc Surg*. 1986;4:80–94.
6. Second European Consensus Document on Chronic Critical Leg Ischemia. *Circulation*. 1991;84(suppl 4).
7. Moneta GL, Yeager RA, Antonovic R, et al. Accuracy of lower extremity arterial duplex mapping. *J Vasc Surg*. 1992;15:275–284.
8. Dalman RL, Taylor LM Jr. Basic data related to infrainguinal revascularization procedures. *Ann Vasc Surg*. 1990;4:309–311.

II

New Adjunctive Techniques in Management of Limb Ischemia

5

Carbon Dioxide Angioscopy

John V. White, MD

Endovascular intervention is being used to treat increasing numbers of patients with peripheral arterial occlusive disease. The appropriate application of endovascular techniques, including balloon angioplasty, atherectomy, and stents, requires clear definition of the location, composition, and size of the arterial lesion. Angiography, the current imaging standard, provides little information about lesion composition. Most arterial occlusive lesions, especially atherosclerotic plaque, embolic debris, and thrombus, have the same angiographic appearance. Each, however, requires a different form of endovascular intervention for successful treatment. More sensitive methods of intraluminal visualization, therefore, must be utilized. Real-time arterial imaging with the angioscope permits the direct inspection of the arterial lumen, determination of the causes of occlusive disease, and improved application of endovascular therapies. With the aid of the angioscope, directed thrombectomy, guide wire and catheter placement, pseudointimal resection, and postprocedural luminal evaluation are all possible.[1-4]

To definitively evaluate the flow surface and perform such procedures during angioscopy, clear visualization of the vessel lumen is required. This is most commonly achieved by standard vascular control of inflow and the elimination of backflow bleeding by saline irrigation. Coaxial fluid administration through the angioscope can be delivered by simple hand injection or through an infusion pump connected to the working channel of the scope. Fluid overload and tissue edema can, however, be associated with such maneuvers. Additionally, cold fluid infusions induce vasospasm, and bubbles within the injectate may pose a problem during irrigation of sensitive arterial beds, such as those within the intracranial and mesenteric circulation. To expand the usefulness of angioscopy and avoid these potential complications, we have begun to explore the use of CO_2 gas for evacuation of blood from the lumen and maintenance of clear visualization of the flow surface.

Few, if any, systemic changes occur with the infusion of small amounts of CO_2 into the vascular tree. The clinical administration of intra-arterial CO_2 was reported more than 3 decades ago. Durant and colleagues, using CO_2 as a contrast medium for the evaluation of the heart and great vessels, found that doses of 0.5 to 2.0 mL/kg injected into the right or left ventricle of patients were well tolerated.[5,6] Over the past 10 years, CO_2 has been increasingly utilized as a contrast medium for the performance of angiography. Numerous investigators have reported the infusion of

50 to 100 mL of CO_2 gas directly into the peripheral arterial tree without complication.[7-10] Few clinically significant cardiopulmonary, embolic, renal, or acid–base complications have been reported. Indeed, to evaluate graft patency in patients who had undergone renal artery bypass grafting, Harward and colleagues injected 70 mL of CO_2 into the aorta just above the graft origin.[11] Despite the fact that patients were studied in the immediate postoperative period, there were no episodes of deterioration of renal function or other complications. These clinical applications suggest that in most patients small infusions of CO_2 are readily tolerated and easily excreted.

PHYSICAL BEHAVIOR OF CARBON DIOXIDE GAS

The safe use of CO_2 gas within the body requires an understanding of some basic physical principles of gas behavior. CO_2 gas demonstrates many of the physical properties of an idealized monoatomic gas. For an idealized gas the properties of pressure, volume, and temperature are interrelated. The relationship is described by:

$$pV = nRT$$

where p is the absolute pressure expressed in atmospheres, V is the volume of gas, n is the number of moles of the gas, R is the gas constant (8.31 J/mol K), and T is the temperature expressed in Kelvin units.[12]

Although this equation may appear complex, it does help to provide an understanding of the behavior of CO_2 gas both as it travels from the metal cylinder to the patient and within the vasculature. Simply stated, the equation suggests that the volume of a constant amount of gas at a constant temperature will increase as the pressure exerted on the gas is reduced. Conversely, at a constant pressure, the volume of a gas will increase as the temperature of the gas increases. These concepts have direct application to the intravascular infusion of CO_2 gas.

A metal cylinder of medical-grade CO_2 gas is pressurized to 2250 psi or 153 atm. This pressure is considerably higher than the sea-level atmospheric pressure of 760 mm Hg to which the body is exposed. Direct release of CO_2 from the metal cylinder at 153 atm to sea-level pressure of 1 atm causes a dramatic increase in gas volume. Similarly, CO_2 cannot be introduced into the vasculature from medically available fluid injectors, such as arterial contrast injectors used by radiologists, because of the tendency of these devices to initially compress the gas prior to delivery. If this rapid increase in volume were to occur within the vasculature, it would be capable of causing catastrophic injury. Therefore CO_2 cannot be directly infused from its container into a patient without a step down in pressure. A gas regulator is required that permits both the staged reduction of gas pressure and controlled expansion in gas volume. Pressure regulators are commonly found in insufflators, such as those used for the performance of laparoscopic surgery. Currently available insufflators permit the steady infusion of CO_2 into the patient at pressures of only 10 to 50 mm Hg. Substantially below physiological blood pressure, these insufflation pressures are well tolerated by blood vessels.

The relationship among the properties of pressure, volume, and temperature also predicts that the gas volume will increase as it is warmed in the body. Because the temperature gradient between the operating room and the interior of the body is not great and the process of warming is slow, the increase in gas volume is modest and not precipitous. This physical principle provides one of the benefits of CO_2 angioscopy. Once the gas is infused into the arterial tree, the CO_2 begins to warm and slowly increase in volume. This expansion continues to gently displace blood backward from the point of gas infusion and thus permits the use of less gas.

Finally, gases and fluids are not immediately miscible. Within a controlled system, such as an artery with a proximal cross-clamp in place, the infusion of CO_2 will form a gas–blood interface (Fig. 5–1). Although CO_2 is readily soluble in blood, the process of dissolution occurs only at the gas–blood interface. The surface area of this interface is small relative to the volume of CO_2 present within the blood vessel. Therefore, a clear field of vision can be maintained with the infusion of only small amounts of gas. Upon completion of angioscopy, this gaseous environment can be easily eliminated by either releasing the gas into the environment or restoring inflow and allowing the gas to dissolve in the blood. These physical properties underscore the safe application of CO_2 for the displacement of blood within the vasculature. The appropriate use of CO_2 for the performance of angioscopy also requires a clear understanding of the physiological behavior of CO_2 within the body.

PHYSIOLOGICAL BEHAVIOR OF CARBON DIOXIDE

Although CO_2 composes only 0.03% of the earth's atmosphere and is nearly absent in inspired air, it is virtually ubiquitous within the body. CO_2 is produced with water as an end product of aerobic metabolism. Once produced, CO_2 is released from cells

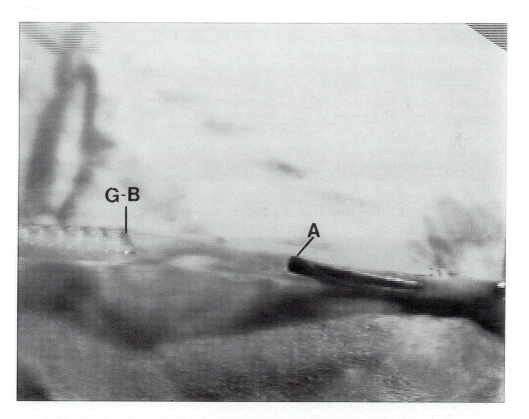

Figure 5–1. Laboratory demonstration of the gas–blood interface (G-B) that forms upon the infusion of CO_2 gas through an angioscope (A) into a blood-filled polyethylene tube. As the gas warms, it expands and continues to move the interface in a retrograde direction.

TABLE 5–1. PHYSIOLOGICAL EFFECTS OF ELEVATED BLOOD LEVELS OF CARBON DIOXIDE

Systemic
  Increased pulse rate
  Increased stroke volume
  Increased cardiac output
  Bronchodilation
  Increased respiratory rate
  Transient mild acidemia
Local
  Vasodilation
  Enhanced oxyhemoglobin dissociation

into the bloodstream, where it is dissolved and transported to the lungs. Because there is little CO_2 in inspired alveolar air, there is a large chemical gradient driving CO_2 from the blood into the lungs so that it may be excreted during expiration. The diffusion gradient permits the pulmonary excretion of CO_2 even in the presence of lung dysfunction and a reduction in oxygen exchange.[13] This simple cycle of CO_2 production and excretion belies the significant impact of this gas as a mediator of numerous body mechanisms (Table 5–1).

As an end product of metabolism, CO_2 has a significant effect on local and systemic vascular tone. As might be expected, rises in pco_2 in the absence of respiratory disease indicate an increase in metabolic rate and produce changes in the cardiovascular system to accommodate the increase in metabolism. Systemically, elevations in pco_2 lead to an increase in pulse rate and cardiac output.[14] These changes appear to arise from both a direct effect on the myocardium and the triggering of chemoreceptors near the aortic arch and the carotid bifurcations. Locally, increases in pco_2 cause vasodilation in most vascular beds.[15] This vasodilation increases local blood flow, brings more oxygen and metabolic substrate to the tissues, and enhances the clearance of CO_2, water, and other end products of metabolism. The locally high CO_2 concentrations also enhance the release of hemoglobin-bound oxygen by red blood cells in the region. All these responses act in concert to sustain the increase in metabolism that occurs during muscular exercise.

CO_2 also significantly influences respiratory function. The compound is the most vigorous stimulant of respiratory function in the nonexercising patient.[16] Increasing blood levels of CO_2 results in a significant increase in respiratory minute ventilation. Because elevation of pco_2 in the resting individual is most often associated with pulmonary disease and hypoxemia, it was previously believed that the combination of hypoxemia and hypercarbia was required to drive respiration. Studies in which normal volunteers inhaled high concentrations of CO_2 (1% to 30%) have clearly demonstrated, however, that there is an increase in minute ventilation with each increase in pco_2 despite normal ranges of po_2.[17] This increase in respiration is also associated with bronchodilation. The relationship between pco_2 and respiratory drive links the rate of metabolism and CO_2 production with the mechanism of pulmonary excretion. Thus, as the metabolic rate increases, so does the respiratory drive, with an increase in oxygen intake and CO_2 excretion.

The intermediate step between the cellular production and pulmonary excretion of CO_2 is that of blood transport of the compound. Introduction of CO_2 into the blood transiently impacts on the bicarbonate blood buffer system. The process of acid–base equilibrium within the blood is described by:

$$H_2O + CO_2 \quad H_2CO_3 \quad H^+ + HCO_3^-$$

During normal metabolism, much of the CO_2 produced is hydrated to form carbonic acid, which serves to replenish the blood buffer system.[18] The carbonic acid establishes an equilibrium with bicarbonate. The H^+ ion is accepted by deoxygenated hemoglobin to maintain blood pH.

The above equation also predicts that the infusion of larger amounts of CO_2 into the blood will result in a rapid shift of the equation to the right. Accommodation of excessive CO_2 will result in the transient production of excessive H^+ ions, which cannot be accepted by deoxygenated hemoglobin. The hydrogen ions become bound to bicarbonate. This is reflected by a transient decrease in blood pH and a fall in bicarbonate levels. The elevation in Pco_2 causes a significant increase in respiratory rate, which promotes clearance of CO_2, a shift of the blood buffer equilibrium to the left, and restoration of normal blood pH and bicarbonate levels. The accommodation of transient rapid increases in blood levels of CO_2 is only limited by the ability of the lungs to increase minute ventilation and excrete the gas.

These changes are frequently seen during the performance of laparoscopic surgery, during which more than 60 L of CO_2 gas may be infused into the peritoneal cavity. As with most compounds instilled into the peritoneal cavity, there is rapid absorption of CO_2 into the blood and an elevation of pco_2 levels. Most of the physiological changes desribed above become clinically apparent. A recent study documented the magnitude of changes in 16 patients.[19] End-tidal CO_2 levels increased from 31.4 ± 0.7 to 42.1 ± 1.6 mm Hg and pco_2 levels increased from 33.3 ± 0.7 to 43.7 ± 1.2 mm Hg. This was associated with a fall in blood pH from 7.43 ± 0.01 to 7.34 ± 0.01. The bicarbonate concentration did not change significantly. Despite these changes, there was no significant alteration in cardiac output. Increases in minute ventilation can rapidly return blood pco_2 and blood pH to normal levels.

CARBON DIOXIDE ANGIOSCOPY: EXPERIMENTAL OBSERVATIONS

The use of CO_2 gas to facilitate angioscopy requires the fulfillment of three conditions: (1) the ability of the gas to displace blood, (2) patient tolerance of rapid large-volume infusions, and (3) the absence of gas embolization and capillary bed obstruction. Each of these conditions has been evaluated experimentally and supports the use of CO_2.

In a canine hindlimb model Silverman and associates compared the ability of CO_2 to that of saline for the displacement of blood during angioscopy.[20] They found that CO_2 successfully cleared blood from the field of vision in 80% of attempts. The field remained clear for a mean of 9 ± 1 seconds after the infusion of gas was terminated. These results were better than those achieved with saline, which was initially successful in only 14% of attempts and preserved a clear field of vision for only 6 ± 1 seconds. These initial observations have been confirmed and extended.[21]

Our laboratory at Temple University Hospital has attempted to determine the safety of large-volume intra-arterial CO_2 injection sufficient to displace blood for angioscopy, and to assess circulatory and systemic responses to such infusion.[22] To accomplish this, a branch of rabbit superior mesenteric artery with its intestinal perfusion bed was isolated. The inflow artery was cannulated for infusion and blood sampling. After baseline measurements arterial inflow was occluded and 60 mL of room air or pure CO_2 was injected to clear the entire isolated vascular bed of blood. This volume was sufficient to displace approximately 20% of the blood volume. Heart and respiratory rate, blood pH, pco_2, bicarbonate, and O_2 saturation were recorded prior to gas infusion and periodically after blood reperfusion. The isolated bowel segments were harvested for histology.

There were no deaths in animals infused with CO_2, whereas all animals receiving room air died shortly after infusion, presumably from embolization. The infusion of CO_2 effectively displaced blood from both the arteries and veins within the isolated portion of the mesenteric arcade in approximately 10 seconds and maintained clearance until the proximal vascular clamp was removed (Fig. 5–2A). Although no direct evaluation of the capillary beds was performed, it was presumed that the microvasculature between CO_2-filled arteries and veins was also gas filled. After removal of the proximal vascular clamp, there was rapid inflow into the visible arterial tree, followed shortly thereafter by the appearance of blood in the draining veins (Fig. 5–2B and C). The pattern of reperfusion demonstrated filling of the arteries first, soon followed by the appearance of blood in the draining veins. There was no evidence of mixing blood and gas. The gas–blood interface persisted throughout the experiment and the gas moved through the vasculature as a column, not as bubbles. There was no evidence of persistent gas emboli or vascular occlusion. As measured by laser Doppler, there was no significant inhibition to reperfusion. By 20 minutes postinjection blood flow had returned to a mean value of 128 mL/min from a mean baseline value of 138 mL/min preinjection. The histological sections demonstrated no tissue ischemia. Blood-filled arterioles were present within the bowel wall (Fig. 5–3).

The process of blood displacement by CO_2 did not have a significant effect on heart rate. The baseline heart rate was 172 ± 16 beats per minute, with a mean of

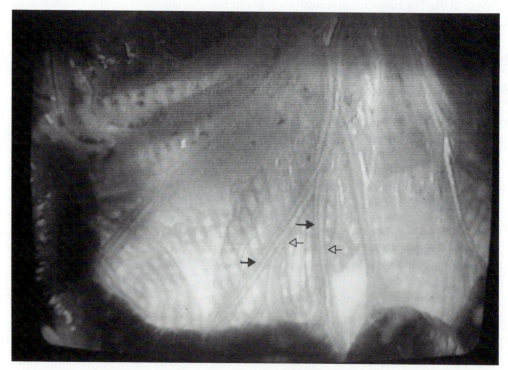

A

Figure 5–2. (A) Injection of CO_2 into the superior mesenteric artery completely cleared both arteries (solid arrows) and veins (open arrows) within the isolated bowel segment. The intervening capillary bed within the bowel wall was also presumably blood free. (*Figure continues*)

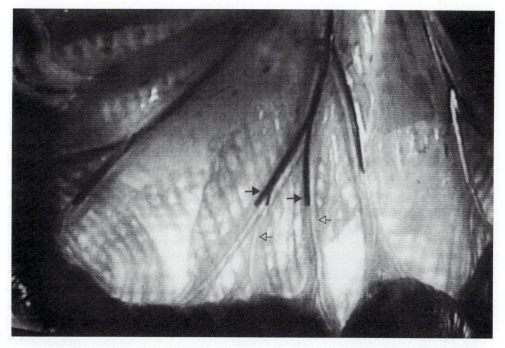

B

Figure 5–2. (*continued*) (**B**) After removal of the proximally occluding vascular clamp, blood flow restoration occurred promptly. Blood returned into the arteries (solid arrows) as a column without mixing or bubbling. The veins (open arrows) remained blood free during arterial reperfusion. (*Figure continues*)

164 ± 12 beats per minute after CO_2 injection. Blood transport of this large amount of CO_2 did not significantly reduce oxygen saturation of the blood. The mean oxygen saturation prior to CO_2 administration was $95\% \pm 1\%$ and was $94\% \pm 3\%$ after CO_2. There was no significant change in respiratory rate despite the CO_2 load, most likely because of respiratory suppression from general anesthesia. The baseline respiratory rate was 33 ± 8 breaths per minute, with a mean of 32 ± 6 breaths per minute at all time periods after gas infusion. These alterations in heart and respiratory rates and oxygen saturation were not statistically significant ($P > .05$).

The large volume of CO_2 did induce alterations in acid–base balance (Table 5–2). Arterial pco_2 increased from a baseline value of 39.27 ± 4.98 mm Hg to a maximum level of 48.38 ± 10.15 mm Hg at 1 minute after injection and fell to 45.25 ± 8.56 mm Hg by 30 minutes postinjection. There was a concomitant decrease in arterial pH from a baseline of 7.36 ± 0.08 to a nadir of 7.21 ± 0.06 at 30 minutes postinfusion. This fall in pH was proportional to the rise in pco_2. Bicarbonate concentration decreased steadily from a preinfusion value of 22.35 ± 5.42 mm Hg to 15.65 ± 5.44 mm Hg 30 minutes following CO_2 administration. The mild decrease in bicarbonate levels suggests a shift in the equilibrium of the carbonic acid–bicarbonate blood buffer system that could have been modified by an increase in respiratory rate during infusion.

Tolerance of CO_2 has also been demonstrated for the intracranial circulation. In an animal model Shifrin and associates infused CO_2 into the carotid artery without any adverse changes in electroencephalogram or neurological function.[23] Similarly, using a cranial window to monitor intracranial blood flow in a small animal model,

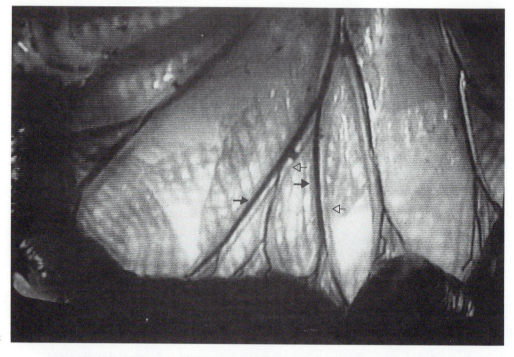

C

Figure 5–2. (*continued*) (**C**) There was complete reperfusion of the arterial segment (solid arrows) within 10 seconds after release of the proximally occluding clamp. After a brief pause the columns of blood refilled the venous tree (open arrows), displacing the gas into the superior mesenteric vein. Note the small bubble of blood within the vein being advanced by the pressure of reperfusion.

our laboratory has documented that CO_2 injected directly into the carotid artery is quickly cleared and does not result in occlusive gas emboli.[24]

The results of these many experimental studies demonstrate that even large-volume infusions of CO_2 gas are well tolerated, that the gas ultimately dissolves in blood without causing vascular occlusion, and that it is transported to the lungs for excretion. Based on these results, we have begun a clinical trial of CO_2 angioscopy.

CLINICAL APPLICATIONS OF CARBON DIOXIDE ANGIOSCOPY

Equipment and Technique

While the overall process of angioscopy is unchanged, the use of CO_2 rather than saline to displace blood and maintain a clear field of vision requires minor changes in equipment and technique. The major components of the angioscopy system, including the light source, video camera, and monitor, are unchanged. Although CO_2 angioscopy may be performed with any angioscope, it is most convenient to use a scope with a working channel that permits coaxial infusion of gas. Delivery of the gas through the distal end of the scope is not only more effective in displacing blood but also more helpful in keeping the tip of the scope free from blood.

A fluid infusion system is not used. Instead, a CO_2 insufflator, such as that used for the performance of laparoscopic surgery, is utilized to infuse the gas. These insufflators can be either volume or pressure regulated. Volume-regulated mechanical insufflators will infuse a set volume of CO_2 over a rather wide range of pressures.

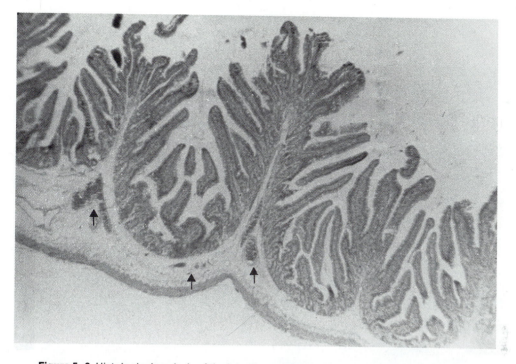

Figure 5–3. Histological analysis of the bowel segments demonstrated normal blood-filled arteries and arterioles within the bowel wall (arrows). The bowel wall was normal in appearance without areas of ischemic necrosis.

These devices can infuse gas even in the presence of significant backflow, but gas delivery must be interrupted to refill the gas reservoir each time it is emptied. The pressure-regulated electronic insufflator is the most common type of CO_2 delivery system available (Fig. 5–4). This device ceases to deliver gas when a set backpressure is reached. Therefore, gas flow must be augmented in the presence of significant arterial backflow. This can be accomplished by connecting a three-way stopcock to the working channel port and attaching the CO_2 infusion tubing to one port and a 60-mL syringe to the other. When gas flow ceases because of high backpressure, CO_2 can be infused with the syringe until backflow is controlled.

For the performance of CO_2 angioscopy, distal vascular control is achieved with a Silastic vessel loop so that a gastight seal can be obtained after introduction of the scope. If the vascular control cannot be accomplished with a Silastic loop, then an introducer sheath with hemostatic valve is placed to permit angioscopy without blood

TABLE 5–2. BLOOD CHEMISTRY CHANGES INDUCED BY INTRA-ARTERIAL CARBON DIOXIDE INFUSION

	Mean Values (CO_2-treated Animals)			
	Pre-CO_2	1 min	10 min	30 min
pH	7.36	7.23[a]	7.22[a]	7.21[a]
pCO_2	39.3	48.4[a]	42.4[a]	45.8[a]
HCO_3^-	22.4	19.2[a]	16.8[a]	17.5[a]
O_2 saturation	95.7	92.8	94.2	91.9

[a] $P < 0.05$ compared to pre-CO_2 values.

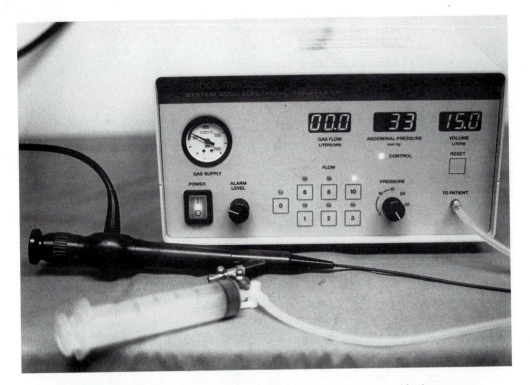

Figure 5–4. The high-flow electronic CO_2 insufflators, such as those used for laparoscopy, can be adapted for angioscopy. The abdominal pressure gauge reads the pressure at the tip of the angioscope. The pressure limit determines the level at which cessation of gas flow occurs. The outflow port of the insufflator is connected to a stopcock on the working channel of the angioscope with standard Silastic tubing.

loss. The outer surface of the scope may be wiped with heparinized saline to promote smooth movement of the instrument within the vessel, but the working channel is not flushed with saline. The rate of CO_2 infusion through the working channel of the angioscope may be decreased after the channel becomes filled with saline because of increased backpressure. Prior to the insertion of the angioscope, the CO_2 insufflator is set to deliver 6 to 9 L/min at a pressure of 30 to 50 mm Hg. Because of the length of the scope and the small diameter of the working channel, the ejection pressure of gas at the tip of the scope is rarely greater than 20 mm Hg. This is considerably lower than the exit pressure of saline at the tip of the angioscope when delivered by a high-flow infusion pump.

Gas flow is initiated and confirmed by lowering the tip of the scope into saline and observing vigorous bubbling. The angioscope is inserted into the vessel and a 30- to 60-mL bolus of CO_2 is injected to establish a gas–blood interface. Maintenance CO_2 insufflation is then begun. In a leak-free system a clear field of vision is usually evident. The gas–blood interface can be seen to move away from the tip of the scope as the gas slowly warms and expands. Occasionally, bubbling of blood at the interface is observed (Fig. 5–5). These bubbles may smear the lens of the angioscope with blood and decrease light transmission and image quality. The impact of these bubbles on light transmission can be reduced by wiping the lens of the angioscope with a small amount of an antifogging compound prior to its use. Should backflow of blood increase and the field of vision be reduced, such as when passing a patent tributary

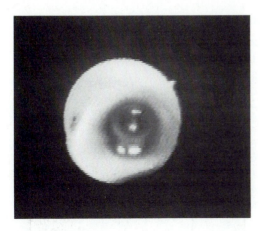

Figure 5–5. The appearance of a CO_2 bubble at the gas–blood interface during angioscopy of the superficial femoral artery.

orifice, supplemental gas can be administered by hand injection. Once past the orifice, the maintenance flow of CO_2 can be resumed. Vasoconstriction around the scope, which occurs more commonly in the saphenous vein than in diseased segments of the arterial tree, can be treated with CO_2 in the same fashion that it is treated with saline irrigation. Gentle compression of the vessel a short distance beyond the tip of the scope and continued low-pressure insufflation of CO_2 through the working channel enhances vascular relaxation and release of the angioscope. Upon completion of angioscopy, the scope is removed from the vessel and gas is allowed to escape from the arteriotomy site. Gas flow through the angioscope is maintained for several seconds after withdrawing the scope to ensure complete clearance of blood from the working channel.

The anesthesiologist should be informed that intra-arterial CO_2 is to be administered so that end-tidal CO_2 and other physiological parameters can be carefully monitored during the angioscopic examination. If an increase in end-tidal CO_2 greater than 12 mm Hg occurs, the patient's respiratory rate should be increased to enhance CO_2 clearance. Failure to reduce end-tidal CO_2, the development of a persistent acidemia, or a persistent reduction in oxygen saturation should be considered indications to terminate CO_2 administration.

Clinical Experience

We have performed 14 CO_2 angioscopic examinations in eight patients over the past 8 months (Table 5–3). Patients who were undergoing peripheral vascular reconstruction with an established need for intraoperative angioscopy, had limited patient fluid tolerance (eg, those with mild chronic congestive heart failure or renal insufficiency), and had clinical evidence of pulmonary disease associated with preoperative CO_2 retention were considered suitable candidates for CO_2 angioscopy. All studies were performed with the patient under general anesthesia, intubated, and mechanically ventilated. End-tidal CO_2, blood pH and pco_2 levels, oxygen saturation, and cardiac rhythm were carefully monitored in addition to the usual physiological parameters.

The studies were performed using a 2.3-mm-diameter angioscope (Karl Storz Endoscopy, Culver City, Calif). This scope has a working channel of 1 mm. A color chip video camera was connected to the ocular of the angioscope and the image was displayed on a color video monitor. A 150-W xenon light source that automatically adjusts the lighting level based on the intensity of reflected light was used to provide illumination. An electronic pressure-regulated laparoscopic CO_2 insufflator (Laparo-

TABLE 5–3. CLINICAL SUMMARY OF CARBON DIOXIDE ANGIOSCOPY

Patients (*n*)	8
Studies (*n*)	14
Scope diameter	2.3 mm
Vascular segments examined	Common femoral artery
	Superficial femoral artery
	Profunda femoris artery
	Popliteal artery
	Proximal tibial arteries
	Greater saphenous vein
Mean study time	10 min
Mean gas infusion	400 mL
Complications	None

flator, Karl Storz Endoscopy) was used to deliver the gas to the patient. The peak gas delivery pressure was set at 45 mm Hg and the peak gas flow rate was set at 9 L/min. The gas delivery tubing was connected to a port of the stopcock on the working channel of the angioscope, gas flow was initiated, and angioscopic evaluation was begun.

Of the studies performed, 6 were arterial evaluations after thrombectomy, 4 were inspections of the distal outflow tract after vascular reconstruction, and 4 were examinations of the greater saphenous vein during *in situ* bypass grafting. Arterial segments studied included the common femoral, superficial femoral, deep femoral, popliteal, and proximal tibial arteries and the greater saphenous vein from the saphenofemoral bulb to the proximal calf. In all cases proximal vascular occlusion was accomplished with a vascular clamp, and distal vascular control around the angioscope was achieved with Silastic vessel loops. Introducer sheaths were not used.

Angioscopy was successfully completed in all attempts using only CO_2 to displace blood from the field of vision. No saline infusions were required or administered. The visual quality of the angioscopic image generally equaled or exceeded that obtained with saline infusions (Fig. 5–6). There was rapid establishment of the gas–blood interface, which permitted immediate visualization of the lumen. There was no haziness of the initial images caused by swirling of red blood cells during the rapid injection of saline into the blood vessel (Fig. 5–7A and B). Intermittent image deterioration, which was experienced during our early applications of CO_2 angioscopy, was found to be due to rapid advancement of the scope into the gas–blood interface.

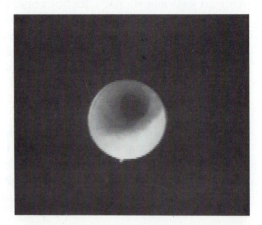

Figure 5–6. CO_2 angioscopy provided an excellent depth of vision and clear delineation of the lumen even with scopes as small as 1.4 mm in diameter.

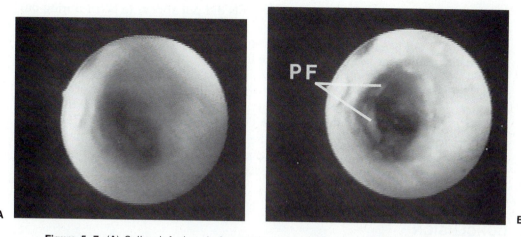

Figure 5–7. (A) Saline infusion during angioscopy of this polytetrafluoroethylene graft causes swirling of the red blood cells, which obscures luminal detail. **(B)** CO_2 angioscopy of the same graft. Because the gas rapidly displaced blood from the lumen of the vessel without mixing, the field of vision is immediately clear and luminal details, such as pseudointimal flaps (PF), are readily apparent.

This caused blood smearing of the distal lens. The problem was easily rectified by withdrawing the scope and wiping the tip with a saline-moistened cloth and was prevented by wiping the distal lens with a small amount of antifogging agent and slowing the advancement of the scope.

The time required to perform a CO_2 angioscopic study of the common, superficial femoral, and popliteal arteries averaged 10 minutes. This compares favorably to our usual saline angioscopy time of 8 minutes. The relative ease of examining this segment of the arterial tree results from the lack of branches contributing to the amount of backflowing blood. Evaluation of the deep femoral and tibial arteries was occasionally somewhat slower in the presence of multiple backflowing branches. Angioscopic examination of the greater saphenous vein was easily accomplished because of the low pressure of blood within this vessel and the ease with which it could be displaced despite multiple tributaries.

The total amount of CO_2 infused to completely evaluate the common, superficial femoral, and popliteal arteries averaged 400 mL (300 to 600 mL) as measured by the insufflator. Interestingly, this amount is comparable to the range of 439 to 467 mL reported for saline by Miller and colleagues for angioscopic examination of the same segment. The insufflation of even 600 mL of CO_2 directly into the arterial tree caused no discernible systemic effects. There was no sustained increase in end-tidal CO_2, rise in pco_2, or fall in blood pH or oxygen saturation. This lack of systemic manifestation may be due in part to the fact that much of the CO_2 is released into the environment upon the removal of the scope and is not transported to the lungs for excretion.

COMPLICATIONS

There were no local or systemic complications related to the infusion of CO_2 in any of the patients. All patients tolerated the angioscopic examination well, without evidence of systemic physiological alterations induced by the infusion of CO_2. Care should be taken when using CO_2 during the preparation of the greater saphenous vein because of the theoretical possibility that the gas may travel through tributaries and enter the deep venous system directly. This did not appear to occur during our clinical applications and can be avoided by maximizing vascular control and minimizing the amount of gas insufflated during vein preparation.

Despite the absence of fluid within the lumen during angioscope advancement, there were no instances of intimal injury. The gas did not appear to induce any significant vasoconstriction within arteries or veins. There was one instance of vasoconstriction of a greater saphenous vein immediately upon introduction of the angioscope. CO_2 infusion was continued and the vasoconstriction was resolved. Overall, it appeared that insufflation of CO_2 into the vasculature, especially into the greater saphenous vein, appeared to cause significant vasodilation. There were no episodes of arterial or graft thrombosis in the immediate postoperative period.

CONCLUSION

As vascular surgeons seek more sensitive methods of evaluating the lumen of blood vessels, the utilization of angioscopy will continue to increase. Angioscopy provides an unequaled view of the flow surface and can serve as a guide to modification of this surface. Visualization at this time is dependent on clearance of blood from the lumen. CO_2 insufflation of segments of the arterial tree appears to be an excellent method of displacing blood. More information about the impact of CO_2 gas infusions on the function of endothelial cells is needed before widespread use of this gas in blood vessels is recommended.

In addition, equipment specifically designed for CO_2 angioscopy is necessary. Current techniques involve the adaptation of laparoscopic insufflators, designed to deliver large amounts of gas into the peritoneum. New methods of gas delivery which permit the well-controlled and safe infusion of gas into all arterial beds are under development. As these devices are incorporated into the performance of angioscopy, the ability of the vascular surgeon to perform endovascular intervention through this imaging modality will be enhanced. This will permit vascular surgical interventions to become more specific and less invasive with a more durable result.

REFERENCES

1. Segalowitz J, Grundfest WS, Treiman RL, et al. Angioscopy for intraoperative management of thromboembolectomy. *Arch Surg.* 1990;125:1357.
2. Miller A, Marcaccio EJ, Tannenbaum GA, et al. Comparison of angioscopy and angiography for monitoring infrainguinal bypass vein grafts: results of a prospective randomized trial. *J Vasc Surg.* 1993;17:382.
3. White GH, White RA, Kopchok GE, et al. Endoscopic intravascular surgery removes intraluminal flaps, dissections, and thrombus. *J Vasc Surg.* 1990;11:280.
4. White JV, Haas KS, Comerota AJ. An alternative method of salvaging occluded suprainguinal bypass grafts with operative angioscopy and endovascular intervention. *J Vasc Surg.* 1993;18:922.
5. Oppenheimer MJ, Durant TM, Stauffer HM, et al. In vivo visualization of intravascular structures with gaseous carbon dioxide: cardiovascular effects and associated changes in blood chemistry. *Am J Physiol.* 1956;186:325.
6. Durant TM, Stauffer HM, Oppenheimer MD, et al. The safety of intravascular carbon dioxide and its use for roentgenologic visualization of intracardiac structures. *Ann Intern Med.* 1957;47:191–201.

7. Miller F, Mineau DE, Koehler PR, et al. Clinical intra-arterial digital subtraction imaging. Use of small volumes of iodinated contrast material or carbon dioxide. *Radiology.* 1983;148:273–278.

8. Weaver FA, Pentecost MJ, Yellin AE, et al. Clinical applications of carbon dioxide/digital subtraction angiography. *J Vasc Surg.* 1991;13:266–272.

9. Weaver FA, Pentecost MJ, Yellin AE. Carbon dioxide digital subtraction arteriography: a pilot study. *Ann Vasc Surg.* 1990;4:437.

10. Seeger JM, Self S, Harward TR, et al. Carbon dioxide gas as an arterial contrast agent. *Ann Surg.* 1993;217:688.

11. Harward TR, Smith S, Hawkins IF, et al. Follow-up evaluation after renal artery bypass surgery with use of carbon dioxide arteriography and color-flow duplex imaging. *J Vasc Surg.* 1993;18:23–30.

12. Halliday D, Resnick R, eds. *Fundamentals of Physics.* 3rd ed. New York: John Wiley & Sons; 1988;484–508.

13. Dantzker DR. Pulmonary gas exchange. In: Kelley WN, ed. *Textbook of Internal Medicine.* Philadelphia: JB Lippincott Co; 1992;1684–1688.

14. Marshall RJ, Sheperd JT. *Cardiac Function in Health and Disease.* Philadelphia: WB Saunders Co; 1968.

15. Milnor WR. Autonomic and peripheral control mechanisms. In: Mountcastle VB, ed. *Medical Physiology.* St Louis, Mo: CV Mosby Co; 1980;1047–1060.

16. Lambertsen CJ. Chemical control of respiration at rest. In: Mountcastle VB, ed. *Medical Physiology.* St Louis, Mo: CV Mosby Co; 1980;1774–1827.

17. Lambertsen CJ. Therapeutic gases: oxygen, carbon dioxide, and helium. In: DiPalma JR, ed. *Drill's Pharmacology in Medicine.* 4th ed. New York: McGraw-Hill Book Co; 1971.

18. Gamble JL Jr. *Acid–Base Physiology.* Baltimore: The Johns Hopkins University Press;1982.

19. Liu S-Y, Leighton T, Davis I, et al. Prospective analysis of cardiopulmonary responses to laparoscopic cholecystectomy. *J Laparoendosc Surg.* 1993;1:241–246.

20. Silverman SH, Mladinich CJ, Hawkins IF, et al. The use of carbon dioxide gas to displace flowing blood during angioscopy. *J Vasc Surg.* 1989;10:313–317.

21. Mladinich CR, Akins EW, Weingarten KE, et al. Carbon dioxide as an angioscopic medium. Comparison to various methods of saline delivery. *Invest Radiol.* 1991;26:874–878.

22. Kozar RA, Harada R, Jaffe F, et al. Carbon dioxide angioscopy: hemodynamic and hemorrheologic responses to large volume CO_2 insufflation of the arterial tree. Presented at Eighth Annual Meeting of the Eastern Vascular Society; 1994; Montreal, Quebec, Canada.

23. Shifrin EG, Plich MB, Verstandig AG, et al. Cerebral angiography with gaseous carbon dioxide CO_2. *J Cardiovasc Surg.* 1990;31:603.

24. Salehi H, White JV, Vasthare US, et al. CO_2 embolization of cerebral microcirculation. *Proc Annu Meet Microcirc Soc.* 1994.

6

Intravascular Ultrasound as an Adjunct to Vascular Interventions

Marco Scoccianti, MD, and Rodney A. White, MD

Patients with limb ischemia frequently require vascular interventions to alleviate symptoms. Operative procedures are associated with significant postoperative morbidity and mortality from concomitant coronary and carotid artery disease. Endovascular techniques, either alone or in combination with conventional vascular operations, have emerged as an attractive option to surgical therapy with the potential to revascularize ischemic tissues with minimal postoperative morbidity. Endoluminal procedures are particularly appealing for the vascular surgeon in three areas: as a treatment for discrete lesions in high-risk patients, as a means to establish an adequate inflow before distal reconstructions, and as a treatment for failing bypasses.

An understanding of the distribution and morphology of occlusive vascular disease is essential in selecting the appropriate therapeutic strategy, and for positioning the interventional device to effectively treat the lesion. Although an ideal guidance system is not currently available (Table 6–1), intravascular ultrasound (IVUS) has been shown to be complementary to angiography for performing successful procedures and for assessing the outcome of interventions by providing a detailed image of the transmural anatomy of vessels before, during, and after endovascular interventions, including balloon angioplasty,[1,2] mechanical atherectomy,[3,4] laser ablation,[5] intravascular stent deployment,[6-8] and endoluminal graft deployment.[9,10]

INTRAVASCULAR ULTRASOUND IMAGING DEVICES

Several types of IVUS catheters are currently available. When introduced into the lumen of the vessel being evaluated, they produce a 360° transmural cross-sectional image. Piezoelectric transducers at the tip of the catheters with a frequency of 10 to 30 MHz are used to generate the ultrasound images. The entire circumference of the vessel is visualized either by mechanically rotating the imaging element or by using electronically switched arrays. Mechanical transducers have two basic configurations in which either the rotating element is the transducer or it is an acoustic mirror that deflects the ultrasound beam produced by a distally placed fixed transducer.

TABLE 6–1. IDEAL GUIDING SYSTEM FOR ENDOVASCULAR PROCEDURES

1. Expedite passage through tight stenoses and obstructions.
2. Identify the target lesion in a diffusely diseased vessel.
3. Define lesion morphology.
4. Provide data useful in choosing the appropriate therapeutic modality.
5. Guide the therapeutic device to the target site.
6. Provide on-line information during the endovascular procedure with a sensitivity equivalent to the thickness of the lesion or of the treated vessel.
7. Evaluate the effects of the various endovascular procedures providing data useful in establishing prognostic factors of success and of early or late recurrence of lesions.

Electronically switched array IVUS catheters have multiple transducer elements placed circumferentially at the tip of the catheter along with a miniaturized integrated circuit. Circumferential images of the vessel are then produced by electronically switching single transducer units in a sequential fashion.

Three-dimensional reconstructions can also be obtained by staking a longitudinally aligned set of consecutive two-dimensional IVUS images. These are obtained by withdrawing the catheter at a uniform rate length of the vessel being examined. Three-dimensional reconstructions make certain aspects of visualization and interpretation of the two-dimensional images easier, facilitating clinical decisions.[11]

CLINICAL UTILITY OF INTRAVASCULAR ULTRASOUND

The clinical utility of IVUS in the management of patients with limb ischemia is both diagnostic and therapeutic (Table 6–2). By providing precise localization of lesions and accurate characterization of morphology, IVUS may suggest a particular endovascular approach and/or help determine the appropriate interventional device. In addition, IVUS is being used to guide the angioplasty catheter to the chosen target, to assess the effect of the procedure, and to provide data useful for establishing prognostic factors of success or failure.

Diagnostic Applications

Several studies have demonstrated that angiography underestimates the extent of disease when the atherosclerotic process is diffuse or is eccentrically positioned in the vessel.[12–14] In addition, the percentage of stenosis is more accurately validated by IVUS than by angiography, since the reference vessel may appear relatively normal angiographically while containing significant disease when examined by IVUS[15,16] (Fig. 6–1). By visualizing both the lumen and the arterial wall, IVUS can differentiate plaque from thrombus and define the volume, position, and type of lesion as well as the presence and extent of intimal flaps or medial dissections[12,17] (Figs. 6–2 and 6–3).

The information obtained by IVUS is critical from several aspects. Precise calculation of lesion volume before and after the procedure permits evaluation of the efficiency of different therapeutic devices and provides a reference value to assess the recurrence of lesions. The spatial distribution of the lesion in a concentric or eccentric pattern and the presence of a soft (fibrous) or hard (calcific) plaque may suggest the best therapeutic device for each specific lesion as well as predict the risk of immediate or late complications (perforation, thrombosis, or restenosis).[2,4,18]

TABLE 6–2. APPLICATIONS OF INTRAVASCULAR ULTRASOUND

Diagnostic
    A. Assess the reference segment disease.
    B. Assess plaque geometry (concentric vs eccentric).
    C. Assess plaque morphology (fibrous vs calcific).
    D. Assess the presence and extension of vessel wall dissection.
    E. Differentiate plaque from thrombus.
    F. Measure vessel cross-sectional dimensions.
    G. Measure the percentage of luminal stenosis.
    H. Measure plaque volume.

Therapeutic
    A. Match the interventional method with the lesion characteristic.
    B. Define the procedural strategy.
    C. Define the procedural end points.
    D. Determine the device size.
    E. Guide the device to the target lesion.
    F. Assess the mechanism of action of the procedure.
    G. Assess the effects of the procedure.
    H. Provide accurate control data.
    I. Confirm the proper device (stent or endoluminal graft) deployment.
    J. Identify postprocedural complications.
    K. Define the appropriate corrective measures.

Therapeutic Applications

Endovascular therapeutic modalities are in rapid evolution. IVUS is essential both as a guidance system for endovascular devices and for immediate postprocedural assessment of the effects of intervention.

Percutaneous Transluminal Angioplasty (PTA)

The et al studied 16 patients with lesions of the superficial femoral artery before and after angioplasty.[19] In this study IVUS was able to discriminate soft from hard plaques and concentric from eccentric lesions. After the procedure IVUS accurately detected the presence of dissections, plaque fractures, and internal elastic lamina ruptures with thinning of the media. This study also showed that the increase in luminal dimensions after PTA is produced by overstretching of the arterial wall while the volume of the lesion remains constant. These authors also suggested that embolization of thrombotic material adherent to the lesion is often associated with balloon angioplasty.

Losordo et al performed a similar study in 40 patients with iliac artery lesions and determined that plaque fracture and displacement contributed to 71.9% of the final luminal cross-sectional area following PTA, with "stretching" providing an additional increase of 17.9%.[20] Honye et al found a correlation among the morphometric characteristics of the plaque, the mechanisms of coronary PTA, and the risk of restenosis.[21] In their study calcified plaques (detected in 83% of cases by IVUS but in only 14% by angiography) were more prone to dissection and were associated with a wider postprocedural residual lumen than fibrous plaques. Fibrous and concentric lesions that did not show signs of fracture or dissection following angioplasty were at highest risk of late restenosis secondary to elastic recoil. This observation has been confirmed by Tobis et al.[2]

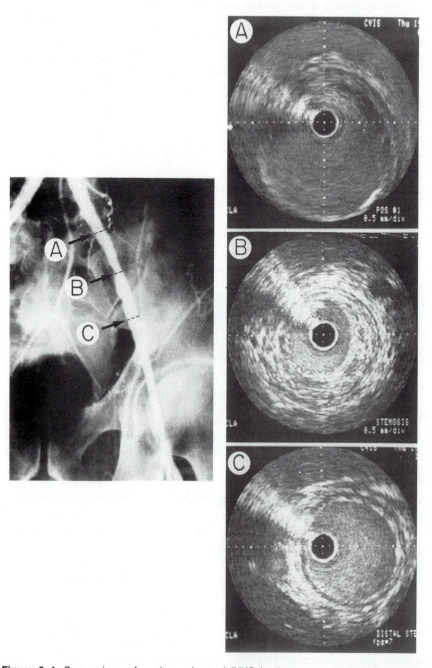

Figure 6–1. Comparison of angiography and IVUS in the common and external iliac arteries. (**A**) Normal lumen; (**B**) severe stenosis in the external iliac artery; (**C**) a normal vessel distal to the lesion. Note the three-layer appearance of this muscular artery wall in the normal segments. Note in B a cross-sectional area stenosis of 77% by IVUS, estimated at 40% by angiography. (*Reproduced by permission from Tabbara MR, White RA, Cavaye DM, et al. J Vasc Surg. 1991;14:496–504.*[14])

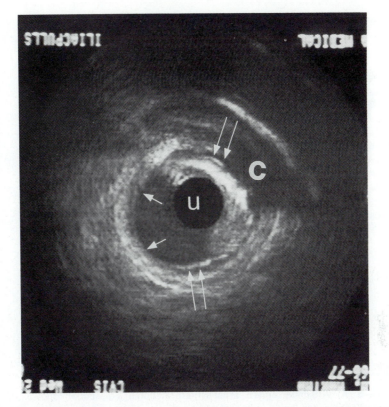

Figure 6–2. IVUS image of an iliac artery lesion. Single arrows outline vessel lumen; double arrows highlight the echolucent media of the artery. c indicates superficial calcification of the vessel wall; u, ultrasound probe. (*Reproduced by permission from Tabbara MR, Mehringer CM, Cavaye DM, et al. Ann Vasc Surg. 1992; 6:179–184.*)

Recent studies[22–24] have indicated that choosing balloon sizes for angioplasty using angiography alone frequently leads to misjudgment of the appropriate-sized balloon for the lesion. This is postulated as a cause of early or late angioplasty failure. IVUS provides a more accurate method to optimally size balloons to match the vessel lumen. The incorporation of an IVUS transducer into an angioplasty balloon is being evaluated as a method to monitor procedures real-time with the potential to correct complications or inadequate dilatations.

Intravascular Stents

Intravascular stents have been introduced to optimize the results and to treat the complications of endovascular interventions. Common indications for stent deployment are to treat arterial dissections, elastic recoil of the vessel wall, residual stenosis, or the presence of a hemodynamic pressure gradient following intervention.[25] While stenting has improved the angioplasty results of both coronary and peripheral vessels, inaccurate stent selection or maldeployment can lead to acute thrombosis, stent migration, or vessel perforation.

IVUS has proved to be particularly effective for assessing the result of primary intervention, for establishing the need for stenting, and for guiding stent deployment.[9,26,27] Precise measurement of the arterial diameters permits selection of the appropriate stent size, while visualization of the lesion and of the stent–wall interface

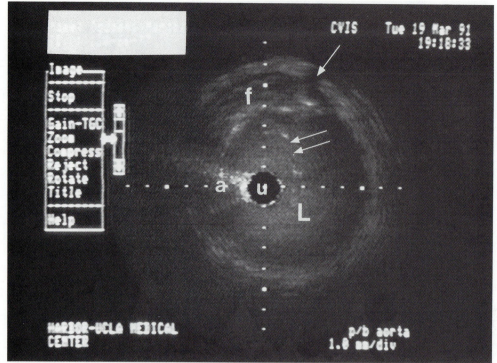

Figure 6–3. (A) IVUS image and **(B)** artist's interpretation of a dissection following balloon angioplasty of an iliac lesion, demonstrating an intimal flap (double arrows), disruption of the arterial media (single arrow), vessel lumen (L), and fibrous plaque (f). a indicates image artifact; u, ultrasound probe. Dots are at 1.0-mm intervals. (*Reproduced by permission from Tabbara MR, Mehringer CM, Cavaye DM, et al. Ann Vasc Surg. 1992;6:179–184. (Figure continues)*)

allows exact stent position and expansion.[2,6–9,27] Three-dimensional reconstruction is particularly useful in this setting, as incomplete stent deployment is visualized as a "lattice" pattern on the reconstructed images at the site of deployment[27] (Fig. 6–4).

It has been shown that IVUS demonstrated adequate stent expansion in only 13% of cinefluoroscopy-guided treatment of coronary lesions.[2] Katzen et al have reported that angiography-guided stent deployment of peripheral lesions resulted in incorrect positioning or expansion in 20% of procedures.[8] Postdeployment interrogation of the stented vessel by IVUS allows further dilatation or sequential stenting in 73% of procedures.[4]

Atherectomy

IVUS has provided important information regarding the utility of different atherectomy devices. The most striking feature is related to the significant plaque burden left after both directional and high-speed rotational atherectomy. While angiography reveals a satisfactory result with both types of devices, IVUS evaluations following the intervention demonstrates residual plaque volumes of 48% and 74%, respectively.[4,28] These studies confirm the inaccuracy of angiography in the evaluation of postprocedural vessel wall morphology and the determination of mechanisms of lesion recurrence.

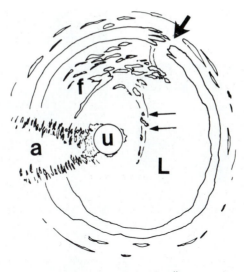

B

Figure 6–3. (*continued*)

IVUS studies of plaque ablation using directional atherectomy have demonstrated that the luminal enlargement produced by plaque removal is enhanced by stretching of the arterial wall, which contributes an additional 18% increase in cross-sectional area.[2] Studies on the effect of high-speed rotational atherectomy[3,28,29] have confirmed that rotational atherectomy causes an increase in the vessel lumen by selective ablation of the calcific portion of the plaque, and that the residual lumen is usually free of dissections. These data suggest the use of directional atherectomy for eccentric fibrous lesions and rotational atherectomy for superficially calcific plaques. Figure 6–5 demon-

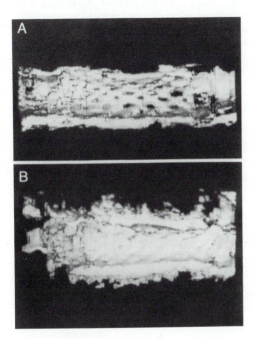

Figure 6–4. Three-dimensional IVUS image of a deployed stent. (**A**) A "lattice" pattern of stent struts is seen, suggesting incomplete expansion. (**B**) Following further balloon expansion the stent is deployed fully, with all struts abutting the vessel wall, and a smooth luminal contour is seen. (*Reproduced by permission from Cavaye DM, Diethrich EB, Santiago OJ, et al.* Int Angiol. *1993;12:212–220.*[27])

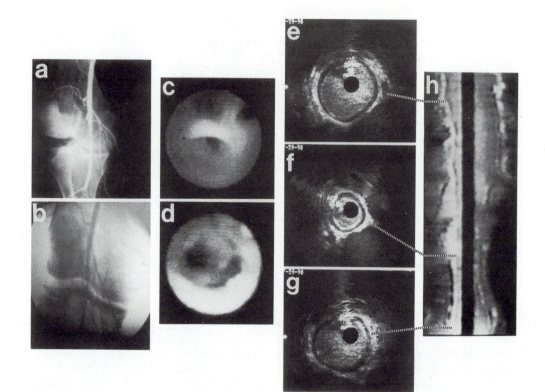

Figure 6–5. (Left to right) Cineangiograms, angioscopy IVUS, and longitudinal reconstruction of the IVUS images acquired along the length of a popliteal artery treated by a 3-mm–diameter high-speed rotational atherectomy (Rotoblator) device. Angiogram (**A**) and angioscopy (**C**) prior to the intervention demonstrate an occlusive lesion observed following the intervention by angiography (**B**), angioscopy (**D**), and IVUS (**E–G**). Angiography underestimated the lesion removal while IVUS demonstrated a 3-mm lumen with complete removal of the plaque. Longitudinal gray-scale IVUS (**H**) confirmed narrowing of the recanalized segment but no residual lesion. Based on the combined angioscopy and IVUS imaging, the procedure was terminated without further treatment that had been indicated by angiography alone. Follow-up duplex examination of the popliteal artery at 1 year confirmed patency with triphasic flow through the popliteal artery, which had dilated to 7 mm at the site of the prior lesion. (*Reproduced by permission from Scoccianti M, White RA, Kopchok G, et al. J Endovasc Surg. 1994;1:71–80.*)

strates the utility of IVUS during atherectomy for quantitating the lesion and for assessing the outcome of procedures.

The role of IVUS in coronary revascularization has also been demonstrated by the GUIDE trial (guidance by ultrasound imaging for decision endpoints), in which IVUS changed the therapeutic decision in 48% of all revascularization procedures.[30]

Endoluminal Graft

A novel and exciting evolution of endovascular technology is the treatment of occlusive peripheral lesions by stented grafts. This approach, initially used to exclude aortic and peripheral aneurysms,[31–33] has recently been applied to relieve ischemic symptoms in high-risk patients with iliac and femoral artery lesions. Cragg et al first reported placement of a percutaneous femoropopliteal graft in 8 patients with ongoing patency at 6-month follow-up.[34] Marin et al have similarly treated 17 patients with an endoluminal aortofemoral or iliofemoral graft with an initial success rate of 83%.[35] This approach has been advocated to treat long dissections complicating PTA or long stenosis and obstructions that usually have poor long-term patency rate following either PTA or stenting. The rationale is to exclude the luminal surface of the treated vessel from the blood flow, thereby lessening the chance that intimal hyperplasia will produce recurrence.

It is clear that the complexity of this procedure and the level of accuracy required for successful endoluminal graft deployment demand a versatile guiding system capable of providing information presently not attainable with angiography. IVUS has been used to acquire critical data before, during, and after deployment of endoluminal grafts.[10] By accurately measuring the luminal cross-sectional area, IVUS can help select the appropriate graft size. By detecting the various components of the vessel wall anatomy, IVUS can be used to determine the position and the full expansion of the fixation device (Fig.6–6). After deployment IVUS confirms proper alignment of the graft and the presence of folds or kinks that might predispose the patient to graft thrombosis (Fig. 6–7).

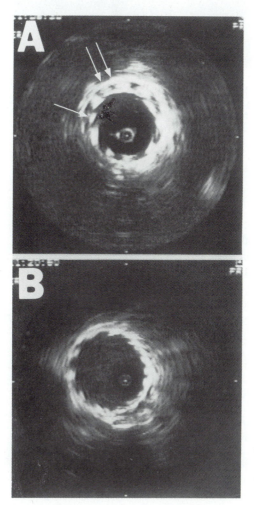

Figure 6–6. (A) IVUS image of a stent in an artery that appeared fully deployed by fluoroscopic examination. **(B)** The same stent after further balloon inflation using real-time IVUS, showing full deployment. The single arrow indicates stent struts; double arrows, artery wall. (*From White RA, Verbin CS, Kopchok GE*, J Vasc Surg. *In press.*)

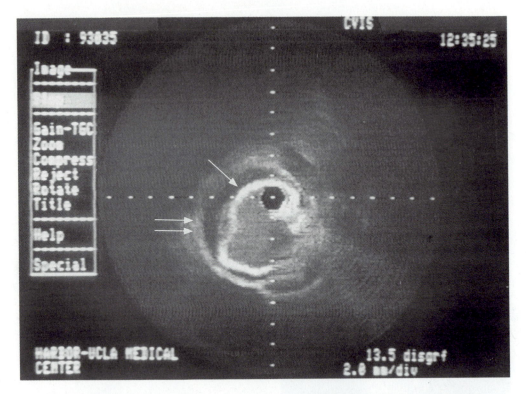

Figure 6–7. IVUS image of an endoluminal vascular prosthesis (single arrow) deployed in the lumen of a canine aorta (double arrows). IVUS demonstrates an irregular contour and a large fold in the prosthesis that moved freely with pulsatile blood flow, while the angiogram displayed normal luminal contours and suggested no deformity.

CONCLUSION

IVUS is a rapidly developing technology that is redefining the interpretation and the role of cinefluoroscopy during interventional procedures. Not only does IVUS offer a nonionizing method of catheter-based imaging, it provides accurate information regarding the pathophysiology of lesions and the utility of devices. Current investigations are also demonstrating the utility of this method to guide interventional devices. In the future IVUS may play an increasing role in the development, evaluation, and utility of endovascular methods.

REFERENCES

1. Gerritsen GP, Gussenhoven EJ, The SHK, et al. Intravascular ultrasonography before and after intervention: in vivo comparison with angiography. *J Vasc Surg.* 1993;18:31–40.
2. Tobis JM, Mahon DJ, Goldberg SL, et al. Lessons from intravascular ultrasonography: observations during interventional angioplasty procedures. *J Clin Ultrasound.* 1993;21:589–607.
3. Mintz GS, Potkin BN, Keren G, et al. Intravascular ultrasound evaluation of the effect of rotational atherectomy in obstructive atherosclerotic coronary artery disease. *Circulation.* 1992;86:1383–1393.

4. Fitzgerald PJ, Yock PG. Mechanisms and outcomes of angioplasty and atherectomy assessed by intravascular ultrasound imaging. *J Clin Ultrasound*.1993;21:579–588.

5. Itoh A, Miyazaki S, Nonogi H, et al. Angioscopic and IVUS imaging before and after percutaneous holmium–YAG laser coronary angioplasty. *Am Heart J*. 1993;125:556–558.

6. Colombo A. Coronary stenting without anticoagulation. Presented at Seventh International Congress on Endovascular Interventions; February 13–17, 1994; Phoenix, Ariz.

7. Laskey WK, Brady ST, Kussmaul WG, et al. Intravascular ultrasonographic assessment of the results of coronary artery stenting. *Am Heart J*. 1993;125:1576–1583.

8. Katzen BT, Benenati JF, Becker GJ, et al. Role of intravascular ultrasound in peripheral atherectomy and stent deployment. *Circulation*. 1991;84(suppl II):2152. Abstract.

9. White RA, Donayre CE, Scoccianti M, et al. Ultrasound guidance in peripheral interventions. Presented at Seventh International Congress on Endovascular Interventions; February 13–17, 1994; Phoenix, Ariz.

10. White RA, Verbin CS, Kopchok GE, et al. Role of cinefluoroscopy and intravascular ultrasound in evaluating the deployment and healing of experimental endovascular prostheses. *J Vasc Surg*. In press.

11. Cavaye DM, White RA, Kopchok GE, et al. Three dimensional intravascular ultrasound imaging of normal and diseased canine and human arteries. *J Vasc Surg*. 1992;16:509–519.

12. Waller BF, Pinkerton CA, Slack JD. Intravascular ultrasound: a histological study of vessels during life. The new "gold standard" for vascular imaging. *Circulation*. 1992;85:2305–2310.

13. Tabbara MR, Kopchok GE, White RA. In-vivo and in-vitro evaluation of intraluminal ultrasound in normal and atherosclerotic arteries. *Am J Surg*. 1990;160:556–560.

14. Tabbara MR, White RA, Cavaye DM, et al. In-vivo comparison of intravascular ultrasound and angiography. *J Vasc Surg*. 1991;14:496–504.

15. Nissen SE, Gurley JC, Grines CL, et al. Intravascular ultrasound assessment of lumen size and wall morphology in normal subjects and patients with coronary artery disease. *Circulation*. 1991;84:1087–1099.

16. Cavaye DM, White RA. Intraluminal ultrasound and the management of peripheral vascular disease. In: Whittemore AD, ed. *Advances in Vascular Surgery*. St Louis, Mo: Mosby–Year Book; 1993;1:137–158.

17. Gussenhoven WJ, Essed CE, Frietman P, et al. Intravascular echographic assessment of vessel wall characteristics: a correlation with histology. *Int J Cardiac Imaging*. 1989;4:105–116.

18. Hodgson JM, Mecca WL. Impact of new ultrasound imaging technologies. In: Vlietstra RE, Holmes DR, eds. *Coronary Balloon Angioplasty*. Boston: Blackwell Scientific Publications; 1994;452–473.

19. The SHK, Gussenhoven WJ, Zhong Y, et al. Effect of balloon angioplasty on femoral artery evaluated with intravascular ultrasound imaging. *Circulation*. 1992;86:483–493.

20. Losordo DW, Rosenfield K, Pieczek A, et al. How does angioplasty work? Serial analysis of human iliac arteries using intravascular ultrasound. *Circulation*. 1992;86:1845–1858.

21. Honye J, Mahon DJ, Jain A, et al. Morphological effects of coronary balloon angioplasty in vivo assessed by intravascular ultrasound imaging. *Circulation*. 1992;85:1012–1025.

22. Roubin GS, Douglas JS Jr, King SB III, et al. Influence of balloon size on initial success, acute complications, and restenosis after percutaneous transluminal coronary angioplasty: a prospective randomized study. *Circulation*. 1988;78:557–565.

23. Nichols AB, Smith R, Berke AD, et al. Importance of balloon size in coronary angioplasty. *J Am Coll Cardiol*. 1989;13:1094–1100.

24. Cacchione J, Nair R, Hodson J. Intracoronary ultrasound: better than conventional methods for determining optimal PTCA balloon size. *J Am Coll Cardiol*. 1991;17:112A. Abstract.

25. Busquet J. The current role of vascular stents. *Int Angiol*. 1993;12:206–213.

26. Diethrich EB. Endovascular treatment of abdominal aortic occlusive disease: the impact of stents and intravascular ultrasound imaging. *Eur J Vasc Surg*. 1993;7:228–236.

27. Cavaye DM, Diethrich EB, Santiago OJ, et al. Intravascular ultrasound imaging: an essential component of angioplasty assessment and vascular stent deployment. *Int Angiol*. 1993;12:214–220.

28. Kovach JA, Mintz GS, Pichard AD, et al. Sequential intravascular ultrasound characterization of the mechanisms of rotational atherectomy and adjunct balloon angioplasty. *J Am Coll Cardiol.* 1993; 22:1024–1032.

29. Fitzgerald PJ, Muhlberger VA, Moes NY, et al. Calcium location within plaque as a predictor of atherectomy tissue retrieval: an intravascular ultrasound study. *Circulation.* 1992;86(suppl I):I-516. Abstract.

30. The GUIDE trial investigators. Impact of intravascular ultrasound on device selection and end-point assessment of intervention: phase I of the GUIDE trial. *J Am Coll Cardiol.* 1993;21:134A. Abstract.

31. Parodi JC, Palmaz JC, Barone HD. Transfemoral intraluminal graft implantation for abdominal aortic aneurysms. *Ann Vasc Surg.* 1991;5:491–499.

32. Marin ML, Veith FJ, Panetta TF, et al. Transfemoral endoluminal stented graft repair of a popliteal artery aneurysm. *J Vasc Surg.* 1994;19;754–757.

33. Diethrich EB, Papazoglou CO, Lundquist P, et al. Early experience with aneurysm exclusion devices and endoluminal bypass prostheses. Presented at Seventh International Congress on Endovascular Interventions. February 13–17, 1994; Phoenix, Ariz.

34. Cragg AH, Dake MD. Percutaneous femoropopliteal graft placement. *JVIR.* 1993;4:455–463.

35. Marin ML, Veith FJ, Panetta TF, et al. Minimally invasive aorto-iliac reconstruction: the use of stented grafts for limb salvage in patients with co-morbid medical illnesses. Presented at 22nd Annual Symposium on Vascular Surgery of the Society for Clinical Vascular Surgery; March 2–6, 1994; Tucson, Ariz.

7

Preliminary Experience with Stent/Graft Technology in Lower Extremity Bypass

Michael D. Dake, MD, and Charles P. Semba, MD

The exciting development and widespread use of endovascular procedures for managing peripheral vascular disease are explained by several factors, including rising health care costs, postoperative morbidity, advances in percutaneous catheter technology, and a high level of acceptance by patients of nonoperative interventions, such as percutaneous transluminal angioplasty (PTA). PTA, by virtue of its long-term success, has set the standard by which other modes of percutaneous vascular intervention must be judged. It represents the optimal method of treatment, surgical or nonsurgical, for focal iliac, femoral, and popliteal lesions. Late restenosis, however, is clearly a problem following PTA of long-segment stenotic disease and total occlusions. In the femoral artery in particular, it has been shown that PTA of segments longer than a few centimeters has poor long-term patency.[1,2]

In an effort to increase both initial technical and long-term clinical success rates in peripheral vascular disease not adequately handled by PTA, several new interventional devices were investigated. Examples of this newly introduced technology include laser and laser-assisted angioplasty,[3,4] atherectomy,[5,6] and stents.[7] Initial and midterm patient data with these adjunctive devices have not significantly improved on the results established with PTA.

Currently, most vascular specialists recommend femoropopliteal bypass surgery for the treatment of long-segment or diffuse superficial femoral and/or popliteal artery disease. Among vascular surgeons some disagreement exists regarding the use of autologous or prosthetic graft material; however, many believe that prosthetic above-knee femoropopliteal bypass represents a good initial approach to the treatment of diffuse disease.[8] In 1993 we reported our initial experience with a technique for percutaneous or femoropopliteal graft placement using conventional polytetrafluoroethylene (PTFE) graft material and a variety of implantation techniques for long-segment femoropopliteal revascularization. The hypothesis that serves as the basis for this procedure is to isolate a segment of the femoral artery by "endoluminal bypass," thereby lessening the chance that intimal hyperplasia will occur and produce restenosis.

In our clinical experience we have used three different implantation techniques corresponding to the idiosyncratic deployment procedures for three types of vascular stents. These stents include (1) a rigid balloon-expandable stainless steel Palmaz stent (Johnson & Johnson Interventional Systems, Warren, NJ), (2) a flexible self-expanding nitinol Cragg stent (Mintech, Inc, Cassis, France), and (3) a flexible self-expanding Elgiloy Wallstent (Schneider, Inc, Plymouth, Minn).

In all cases the percutaneously delivered graft consisted of standard thin-walled PTFE graft material (Gore, Inc, Flagstaff, Ariz). The diameter of the graft in all cases was 6 mm.

In the future it is likely that similar stent/graft combinations will be developed for percutaneous expansion in the femoral and popliteal arteries. Many of these devices will clearly represent significant improvements over our initial prototypes. It is unlikely that any of the devices outlined in this chapter will enjoy widespread clinical use. This is due to a number of idiosyncratic design problems that became apparent during our initial experience. The nature of these problems will be discussed subsequently. Rather, it is our intent to emphasize the feasibility and potential of this technique rather than monopolize the discussion with promotion of one particular design or device.

We have performed the procedure of percutaneous femoropopliteal graft placement in 18 patients. In patients in whom the Palmaz or Cragg stent was used to construct the stent/graft device, the graft material was secured to the underlying metallic endoskeleton 5-0 with polypropylene suture. In the cases utilizing the Wallstent for mechanical support, the 6-mm PTFE graft was first advanced into position using a series of tethers; it was then initially expanded with a 6-mm balloon before stenting its length with the Wallstent.

At this point a brief synopsis of the specific technical details regarding the use of the three stent/grafts should be presented.

RIGID BALLOON-EXPANDABLE STENT

In the rigid balloon-expandable stent design each end of a 6-mm–diameter thin-walled PTFE graft was attached to a 10-mm–long Palmaz 104 stent. The graft was secured to the middle of each stent with two interrupted polypropylene sutures. In this manner the graft overlapped about half the length of each stent. The stent/graft combination was coaxially mounted on a 6-mm–diameter, 10-cm–long, 5 French balloon angioplasty catheter. All stent/grafts were 10 cm long or less. The stents were hand-crimped over the balloon and loaded into a Teflon tube to facilitate introduction through the hemostatic valve of an angiographic sheath, which was placed antegrade in the ipsilateral femoral artery.

After the site of disease was defined with road-mapping guidance techniques, the stent/graft assembly was advanced over a 0.035-in guide wire to a position bridging the involved segment. The balloon was then inflated and the stent/graft was deployed with anchoring of each stented end by means of a friction seal.

FLEXIBLE SELF-EXPANDABLE NONFORESHORTENING NITINOL CRAGG STENT

A standard 6-mm–diameter thin-walled PTFE graft was attached to a self-expanding nitinol stent with a series of interrupted polypropylene sutures. The stent is constructed of a monofilament of nitinol wire. It has a thermal memory with longitudinal and radial flexibility and minimal foreshortening during deployment.[9] In this design the graft forms the flow-contacting surface since it lines the inside of the stent.

This stent/graft was delivered by compressing it in a tubular loading cartridge and advancing it through an angiographic sheath using a solid polyethylene mandrel as a pusher. After positioning the graft across the length of the diseased arterial segment, the sheath was withdrawn while maintaining the pusher in a stationary position to deploy the graft. After self-expansion the graft was dilated to 6 mm with an angioplasty balloon.

FLEXIBLE SELF-EXPANDING FORESHORTENING ELGILOY WALLSTENT

The procedure utilizing this stent in combination with the 6-mm thin-walled PTFE graft material was the most complex (Fig. 7–1A through I). This was because of the

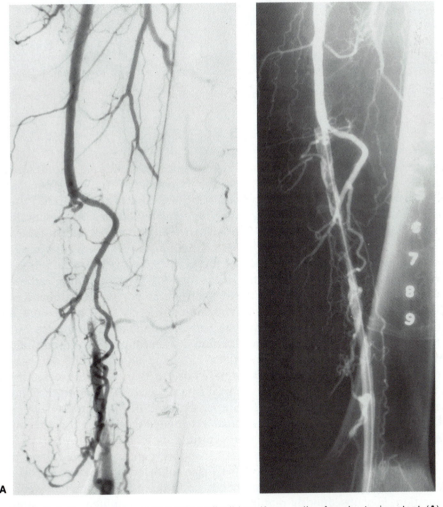

Figure 7–1. Stent/graft procedure using a flexible self-expanding foreshortening stent. (**A**) A left leg arteriogram demonstrating complete occlusion of the distal superficial femoral artery in the region of the adductor canal. (**B**) Irregularly narrowed lumen after recanalization with guide wire and catheter techniques followed by balloon angioplasty. (*Figure continues*)

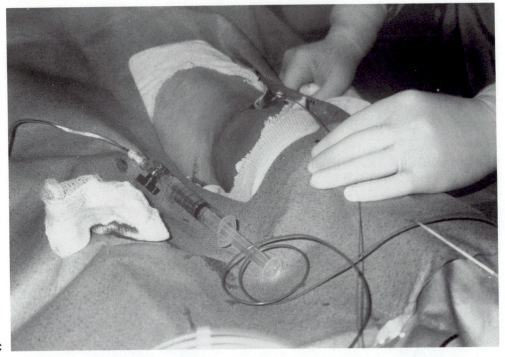

C

Figure 7–1. (*continued*) (**C**) The popliteal artery is punctured with the patient prone. (*Figure continues*)

foreshortening of the Wallstent during deployment. Due to this significant foreshortening, we were unable to integrate standard graft material with this stent in a unified delivery system. Thus, the procedure required placement of the graft and the stent separately. We accomplished this by achieving ipsilateral antegrade femoral access and retrograde popliteal artery access to facilitate initial delivery of the graft. Small platinum markers were sewn to each end of the graft and tethers consisting of 2-0 sutures were looped through the ends of the graft. Subsequently, the tethers were externally hooked with a wire and drawn through a 7 French guiding catheter previously advanced over a guide wire introduced from the popliteal sheath and maneuvered out the femoral sheath. The graft was then pulled through the femoral sheath into the superficial femoral artery. By externally manipulating the tethers on either end, the graft was positioned using the platinum markers as guides. A 6-mm–diameter 10-cm–long balloon catheter was then inflated along the length of the graft. Following balloon inflation as many Wallstents as necessary to line the graft were deployed from its distal to proximal end. The stent/graft was balloon-expanded to 6 mm, and the tethers were easily removed by pulling on one end of the loop.

Of the 18 patients composing the initial experience with these three techniques, the primary patency of endovascular stent/grafting for femoropopliteal occlusive disease was 57% at 15 months (mean). The secondary patency was 86% and usually required catheter-directed infusion of urokinase followed by angioplasty to rescue the graft. One patient with one-vessel tibial runoff occluded his graft 2 weeks after implantation. He subsequently required a surgical femoropopliteal *in situ* saphenous vein bypass; however, his foot perfusion did not improve despite patency of the bypass graft and peroneal artery runoff. Two weeks after bypass surgery he underwent

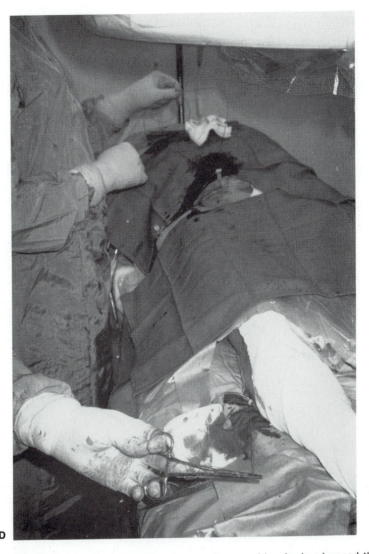

Figure 7–1. (*continued*) (**D**) With the patient supine, a guide wire is advanced through the popliteal access and maneuvered out the ipsilateral femoral artery sheath. (*Figure continues*)

below-knee amputation because of progressive ischemia of his left foot. He recovered uneventfully after surgery.

In our experience there were no technical failures resulting from an inability to recanalize an occlusion or successfully deploy the stent/graft device. There were two patients who consented to the procedure before angiography was performed but did not undergo percutaneous graft placement because of poor runoff.

To date, all but one of the failures has occurred in the rigid balloon-expandable stent group. Specifically, it appears that rigid stents placed in the region on the abductor canal may be extrinsically deformed due to the action of overlying muscles. In multiple failures the distal stent anchoring the prosthesis at the abductor canal region was obviously narrowed. Following regional thrombolysis the stent could be easily re-expanded by balloon angioplasty.

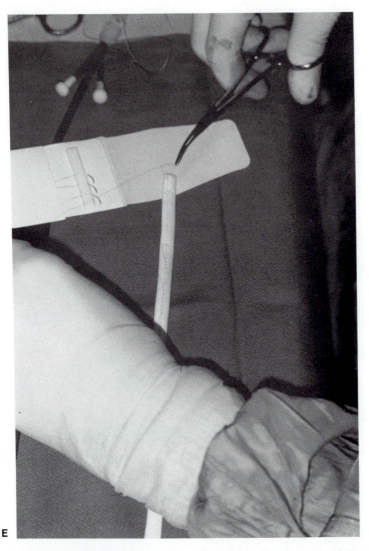

E

Figure 7–1. (*continued*) (**E**) Platinum markers are sutured to the ends of the graft to provide fluoroscopic landmarks. (*Figure continues*)

In all patients, irrespective of the stent technique, heparin was administered during the procedure and overnight, and oral warfarin was prescribed for 2 months.

Long-term evaluation of patients who have undergone endovascular treatment of diffuse femoropopliteal disease has failed to demonstrate durable patency, regardless of the type of device used. Restenosis following balloon angioplasty is due to the process of intimal hyperplasia, which is a manifestation of the healing process that causes renarrowing of the dilated vascular lumen. It has been demonstrated that the length of the treated arterial segment is directly proportional to the likelihood that intimal hyperplasia will result in a symptomatic renarrowing of the artery at some point along its treated segment.

Currently, due to the lack of effective endovascular means to address the restenosis phenomenon, femoropopliteal occlusive disease longer than 6 to 8 cm is usually treated by surgical bypass. The 5-year patency of above-knee bypass using PTFE is approximately 60%.[10] This is significantly better than the 5-year patency of long-

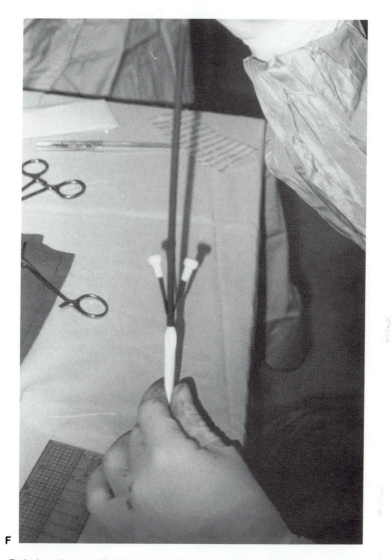

Figure 7–1. (*continued*) (**F**) The graft is compressed into a loading cannula, which is advanced into the femoral sheath before the graft is drawn into position by external tethers. (*Figure continues*)

segment femoropopliteal balloon angioplasty, which is less than 20%.[11] The theoretical basis for percutaneous intraluminal graft placement is to isolate the flow surface of the treated arterial segment by lining it with PTFE graft material. This material is microporous, but healing with endothelialization does not usually occur and intimal hyperplasia does not generally develop in the graft. It is commonly believed that most cases of PTFE bypass graft failure are due to pannus formation at the anastomoses. We hypothesize that endoluminal segmental graft placement would improve the durability of long-segment percutaneous femoral revascularization by restricting the formation of intimal hyperplasia to the anastomotic borders. If this is true, patency would be similar to angioplasty of focal lesions or surgical bypass. It is also possible that the patency of intraluminal grafts could be better than that of a similar surgical procedure, since arteriotomy and anastomotic suturing are not necessary.

There may be other possible advantages of percutaneous femoropopliteal graft placement. Customizing the length of the grafted segment may preserve collateral

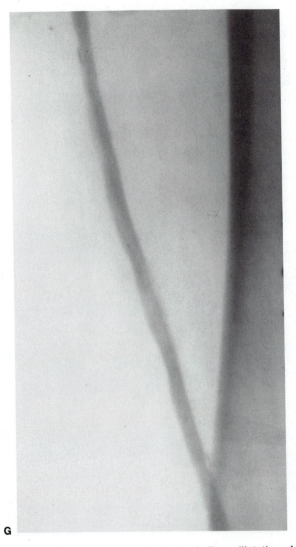

G

Figure 7–1. (*continued*) (**G**) An arteriogram following balloon dilatation of the 6-mm PTFE graft. (*Figure continues*)

vessels and render the patient less graft dependent. Similar to other endovascular procedures, percutaneous graft placement may postpone or eliminate the need for surgical bypass in some patients. Due to the significant 5- and 10-year mortality of patients with peripheral vascular disease secondary to underlying coronary or cerebral vascular disease, percutaneous graft placement may provide a suitable initial treatment when long-segment revascularization is required.

Although this discussion represents a general overview of the concept, the relative merits of the different techniques used in our experience warrant a brief examination.

1. Grafts with rigid balloon-expandable stents attached to each end are potentially easy to introduce and deploy. Limitations include relatively short graft lengths secondary to the current maximum commercially available balloon length of 10 cm, narrowing of the nonstented midgraft region due to elastic recoil of the artery, and difficulty maintaining the position of the coaxially crimped

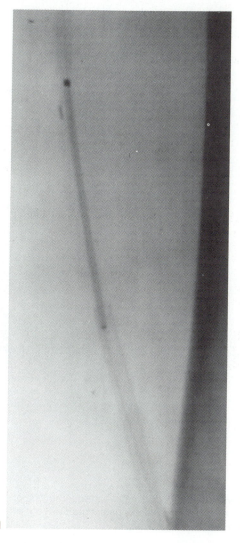

H

Figure 7–1. (*continued*) (**H**) Placement of a flexible self-expanding Wallstent within the graft. (*Figure continues*)

stent and graft on the balloon during introduction through the sheath due to friction. Perhaps the most profound concern, however, is the potential for crushing of the rigid stent after deployment. As a result of our experience in a number of patients and other recent anecdotal experience with patients treated with noncovered rigid stents in the region of the abductor canal, we believe that the use of these rigid stents in the femoral artery is not ideal. In our initial experience we did not note any kinking or twisting of the graft material during placement; however, this represents a potential problem requiring technical refinement. We did observe some compression of unsupported graft segments, presumably secondary to unopposed elastic recoil in the midportion of the graft. In the future we believe grafts will be supported throughout their length by flexible stents to eliminate the risk of deformation noted with rigid stents and to decrease the risk of elastic recoil as a cause of graft compression.

2. A graft supported along its entire length by a flexible nonforeshortening self-expandable stent is potentially simpler to place and reduces the risk of stent

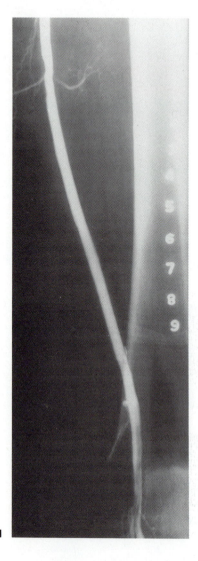

Figure 7–1. (*continued*) (**I**) A completion arteriogram demonstrating a smoothly contoured widely patent graft without evidence of residual arterial narrowing.

deformation and graft occlusion due to extrinsic trauma. Nonforeshortening stents possess the advantage of easy more accurate deployment at the target site. Stents that significantly foreshorten during expansion require a level of operator judgment and experience to allow precise placement.

Endovascular graft designs with thin support throughout the length of the graft may also minimize slack recoil, which may narrow an unsupported endoluminal graft. Current limitations of this technique include a relatively large delivery system (11 French); however, future development of ultrathin-walled graft material could eliminate this concern.

3. The pull-through technique using flexible foreshortening self-expandable stents allows placement of long graft segments through smaller sheaths because it does not require simultaneous stent placement. A current disadvantage of this technique is the requirement of popliteal artery access. This results in a relatively more complicated deployment technique requiring a significantly longer procedure time.

Although recent experience in the iliac artery suggests that primary recanalization and stent placement for chronic occlusions can be accomplished with a high technical success rate, a potential limitation of percutaneous intraluminal femoropopliteal graft placement is the inability to recanalize long-segment occlusions. Recent data, however, demonstrate relatively high technical success rates (85% to 91%) in recanalizing femoral artery occlusions.[12,13] Similarly, one report specifically addressed long-segment femoropopliteal occlusions and described a 76% technical success rate in recanalizing 71 arteries,[14] suggesting that the majority of occlusions can be successfully recanalized.

Other current limitations of the procedure include an inability to successfully address a diameter mismatch between the proximal femoral aspect of the graft and a smaller diseased popliteal artery, and the relatively poor outcome in patients with limited tibial runoff consisting of one vessel or less.

Our initial experience with 18 patients generally went well; hospitalization was short, and patient acceptance was good. Although technical success and short-term patency have been good in patients with flexible stents lining the entirety of the graft length, long-term patency is not yet known. Issues currently under study include the absolute need for stent placement within the midgraft segment; comparison of rigid balloon-expandable, flexible balloon-expandable, flexible foreshortening self-expandable, and flexible nonforeshortening self-expandable stents for graft fixation; and delivery system improvement. Clearly, the value of this technique will depend on its durability. This can only be established by years of dedicated follow-up carefully scrutinized in relation to traditional bypass surgery. Only after this is performed can the merits of this technique be truly validated and the procedure recommended on a wider scale.

REFERENCES

1. Murray RR Jr, Hewes RC, White RI Jr, et al. Long segment femoropopliteal stenosis: is angioplasty a boon or a bust? *Radiology.* 1987;162:473–476.
2. Becker GJ, Katzen BT, Dake MD. Noncoronary angioplasty: state of the art. *Radiology.* 1989;170:921–940.
3. Cragg AH, Gardiner GA, Smith TP. Vascular applications of laser. *Radiology.* 1989;172:925–935.
4. Huppert PE, Duda SH, Helbert U, et al. Comparison of pulsed laser-assisted angioplasty and balloon angioplasty in femoropopliteal artery occlusions. *Radiology.* 1992;184:363–367.
5. Nakawaga N, Cragg AH, Smith TP, et al. Peripheral atherectomy: experimental results with a new device. *JVIR.* 1990;1:127–132.
6. Katzen BT, Becker GJ, Benenati JF, et al. Long-term follow-up of directional atherectomy in the femoral and popliteal arteries. *JVIR.* 1992;3:38–39.
7. Sapoval MR, Long AL, Raynaud AC, et al. Femoropopliteal stent placement: long-term results. *Radiology.* 1992;184:833–839.
8. Moore WS, Quinones-Baldrich WJ. An argument against all-autogenous tissue for vascular bypasses below the inguinal ligament. *Adv Surg.* 1991;24:91–101.
9. Cragg AH, DeJong S, Barnhart W, et al. Preclinical evaluation of the Cragg stent. *Radiology.* 1992;185(P):162. Abstract.
10. Donaldson MC, Whittemore AD, Mannick JA. An argument in favor of all-autogenous tissue for vascular bypasses below the inguinal ligament. *Adv Surg.* 1991;24:69–90.
11. Capek P, McLean GK, Berkowitz HD. Femoropopliteal angioplasty: factors influencing long-term results. *Circulation.* 1991;83(suppl 1):70–80.

12. Morgenstern BR, Geetrajdman GI, Laffey KJ, et al. Total occlusions of the femoropopliteal artery: high technical success rate of conventional balloon angioplasty. *Radiology.* 1989;172:937–940.
13. Lammer J, Pilger E, Karnel F, et al. Laser angioplasty: results of a prospective multicenter study at 3-year follow-up. *Radiology.* 1992;178:335–337.
14. Bolia A, Miles KA, Brennan J, et al. Percutaneous transluminal angioplasty of occlusions of the femoral and popliteal arteries by subintimal dissection. *Cardiovasc Intervent Radiol.* 1990;13:357–363.

8

Angioscopic Technique for *In Situ* Bypass Grafting

Magruder C. Donaldson, MD

Widespread experience has proven *in situ* saphenous vein bypass to be a reliable technique for infrainguinal reconstruction.[1-3] The majority of causes of failure after *in situ* bypass are related to correctable errors in technique or operative management.[4] It is most important to ensure complete valve lysis and division of significant venous branches that may persist as large arteriovenous fistulas. The chosen vein should be at least 3 mm in outside diameter after gentle inflation and the vein should be free of areas of scar or wall thickening for optimal results. Areas of recanalization or luminal compromise are not always readily evident from outside inspection and manipulation. Because the method usually involves a long incision over the entire vein, wound healing problems can contribute to operative morbidity.[5] Completion imaging of the conduit, anastomosis, and runoff arteries helps eliminate many residual anatomic or technical problems that might have an impact on early and late patency. Operative arteriography is standard in many institutions, supplemented by other modalities, such as continuous wave ultrasound[6] and, more recently, duplex ultrasound. In addition, rapid development of endoscopic technology[7] has made angioscopy an alternative method for assisting in vein preparation, and completion imaging of the conduit and anastomoses.

Angioscopy has been perfected sufficiently to provide excellent visualization in most instances with relatively minimal logistical inconvenience. Despite the availability of a practical tool, the real value of the instrument as a supplement or substitute for established methods in vascular surgery remains unclear. In the case of *in situ* bypass, angioscopy could help eliminate technical causes of graft failure, and might even reduce the incidence of wound complications and postoperative length of hospital stay. On the other hand, these potential benefits may be outweighed by possible morbidity such as fluid overload and vein injury during angioscopy. This chapter reviews the techniques and results of angioscopically assisted *in situ* bypass to help assess the value of this method to the vascular surgeon.

TECHNIQUES OF ANGIOSCOPICALLY ASSISTED *IN SITU* BYPASS

Brigham & Women's Method

Over the last several years the vascular team at Brigham & Women's Hospital (Boston, Mass) has adapted a technique for angioscopically assisted *in situ* vein grafting.[8,9] The proximal femoral artery and saphenofemoral regions are exposed through a standard groin incision and the infrageniculate target artery and saphenous vein are exposed through a single distal incison. A large proximal branch at the saphenous bulb is used to insert a short self-sealing introducer with a side port 1 cm into the saphenous vein. A side branch near the distal end of the vein is used to secure a short 18- or 20-gauge Silastic catheter. The angioscopic flushing system is connected to the catheter and to the side port of the introducer by three-way stopcock after appropriate flushing with heparinized saline (1 U/mL) to remove air.

After full intravenous heparinization the saphenofemoral junction is occluded with a bulldog, and a 1.4-mm or 2.2-mm steerable angioscope (Olympus, Lake Success, NY) is positioned in the proximal vein via the introducer. The distal saphenous vein is ligated and a deflated 3 French embolectomy catheter is gently advanced to the groin through a second convenient side branch or a small transverse venotomy as heparinized crystalloid solution is flushed at low volume using a pump operated by foot pedal switch (Olympus) into the distal Silastic catheter to facilitate passage. If any obstruction to passage is encountered, a counterincision is made over the tip of the catheter to exclude the presence of a venous anomaly or abnormality. The deflated catheter is withdrawn and a modified Mills (Olympus) or Mehigan-Pilling (Pilling, Fort Washington, Pa) valvulotome with a long flexible shaft is advanced from the distal vein with the hook pointed toward the skin to minimize the chance of becoming caught on a side branch emerging lateral or deep to the main venous trunk (Fig. 8–1). The flushing system is switched by three-way stopcock to the side port of the introducer to allow proximal low-flow (50 mL/min) or high-flow (200 mL/min) irrigation under foot pedal control. With ambient light turned down, the valvulotome is withdrawn as the angioscope follows to allow valve lysis under direct vision (Fig. 8–2). The locations of branches identified by backbleeding are marked with skin staples over the transilluminated tissue. If increased inflow from branches obscures vision as the process moves distally, the irrigation can be switched to the distal catheter or an elastic tourniquet can be applied below the area being viewed. When the process reaches the end of the vein, the valvulotome is secured as the angioscope is withdrawn

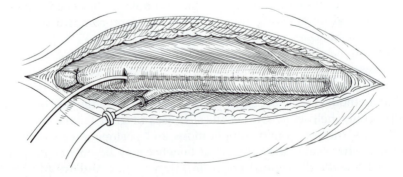

Figure 8–1. Ligated distal saphenous vein with an irrigating catheter via the side branch and the valvulotome being advanced until visualized by angioscope at the groin level.

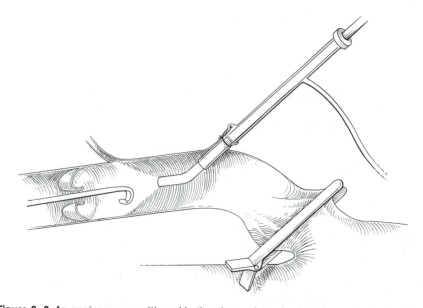

Figure 8–2. An angioscope positioned in the clamped proximal saphenous vein via introducer using the side port for irrigation as valvulotomy is visualized just distal to a vein branch.

to the groin, surveying the cut valves and rechecking branch locations. The angioscope, valvulotome, and irrigating catheters are removed and set aside.

The distal vein is divided and clamped and vein branches marked by staples are ligated via small longitudinal skin incisions. The proximal saphenous vein is detached from the femoral vein and the proximal and distal anastomoses are performed in standard fashion, taking care to remove the most proximal saphenous valve under direct vision and being certain that the introducer did not obscure presence of a second valve just distally. After establishing flow a sterile continuous wave Doppler ultrasound probe is used to insonate for residual arteriovenous fistulas[6] and completion angiography is performed to evaluate the graft, distal anastomosis, and runoff anatomy. In order to minimize trauma, particularly in tibial vessels, the angioscope is not routinely reintroduced to assess the distal anastomosis and runoff.

Alternative Methods

Other centers have found it useful to perform preoperative ultrasound scanning on the leg to map venous branches and anomalies. The marked branches can be divided prior to angioscopy, reducing flushing volume and improving visualization. Transverse skin incisions for branch ligation may be preferable, although longitudinal incisions may facilitate ligation of multiple adjacent branches via one wound. Rather than minimizing incisional side effects by using small counterincisions, a single long incision over the vein may facilitate safe passage of instruments and branch ligation. Other valvulotomes are available which feature removable or retractable cutting blades and can be passed up the vein with less chance of causing injury by becoming entangled in anomalous anatomy or side branches. A novel flushing valvulotome has been pioneered by a Swiss group.[10] Others[11–13] use the angioscope routinely to view the distal anastomosis and proximal runoff anatomy, with reduced need for completion angiography. There is some experience[14] with endovascular occlusion of side branches using coils deposited under fluoroscopic or angioscopic control, potentially avoiding all but small incisions over each end of the graft.

CLINICAL VALUE OF ANGIOSCOPY

Accuracy of Angioscopic Imaging

There is little question that modern angioscopy has opened a new window for improved imaging of a wide range of luminal abnormalities within grafts, anastomoses, and runoff arteries. Sales et al[15] demonstrated a high correlation between angioscopic and pathological findings in excised saphenous vein segments. Miller et al[16] found a 19% incidence of residual valve cusps and a 37% incidence of residual vein branches in a study of 155 *in situ* grafts. Studies by Baxter et al[11] and Miller et al[13] confirmed higher sensitivity for angioscopy than for operative angiography in detecting intraluminal defects. In a study of 20 *in situ* grafts, Gilbertson et al[12] found angioscopy to be substantially more sensitive than operative angiography and operative duplex ultrasound in detecting residual branches and valve cusps. Angioscopy revealed 66% of proven branches compared to 44% by angiography and only 12% by duplex scan. Sensitivity for residual valve cusps was 100% for angioscopy compared to 22% by angiography and 11% by duplex ultrasound. Furthermore, specificity of angioscopy in confirming an adequate distal anastomosis was 100%, whereas angiography and duplex scanning had false-positive rates of 20% and 10%, respectively, for identifying stenosis >30%.

Impact of Angioscopy on Outcome

It is difficult to prove that the added detail and resolution provided by modern angioscopy is of critical importance to improved results after bypass grafting. In some respects angioscopy may be too sensitive, revealing subtle abnormalities that have no clinical effect on graft natural history.[15] Significant findings such as retained valve leaflets are arguably rare enough[4,5] to make routine angioscopy to find them less fruitful. While Baxter et al[11] and Miller et al[13] found that findings detected by angioscopy led to a higher rate of graft correction at the time of surgery compared to angiography, there was no clear impact of this higher revision rate on the incidence of early graft occlusion. In the prospective randomized comparative study by Miller et al,[13] for example, 3.1% of the angioscopy group suffered graft failure within 30 days compared to 6.6% in the angiography group, an insignificant difference ($P = .11$).

In an effort to assess the impact of angioscopy on results of *in situ* bypass grafting, the vascular team at Brigham & Women's Hospital hypothesized that the angioscope might facilitate precise preparation of the *in situ* vein bypass with reduced operative morbidity and hospital stay and without incurring a negative impact on late graft patency.[17] During a 48-month period 59 consecutive patients requiring primary infrainguinal reconstruction to a target artery below the knee were randomized to one of two groups by a coin toss prior to surgery. Exclusion criteria included a need for secondary revision procedures, a history of prior inflow grafting, evidence of aneurysmal disease or a need for composite grafting. All patients underwent similar preoperative medical evaluation and received aspirin the night before surgery. Patients in the SCOPE group underwent angioscopically assisted *in situ* bypass as described above. Patients in the NO SCOPE group underwent standard *in situ* vein grafting, during which the entire vein was exposed through a single long incision, with ligation of

TABLE 8–1. PREOPERATIVE CHARACTERISTICS OF BRIGHAM & WOMEN'S HOSPITAL STUDY PATIENTS

Characteristic	SCOPE (*n* = 32)	NO SCOPE (*n* = 27)	All (*N* = 59)
Mean Age, y	71.0	71.2	71.1
Risk Factors, *n* (%)			
Diabetes	11 (34)	12 (44)	23 (39)
Smoking	12 (38)	12 (44)	24 (41)
Hypertension	19 (59)	18 (67)	37 (67)
Coronary disease	14 (44)	13 (48)	27 (46)
Indication, *n* (%)			
Claudication	11 (34)	5 (19)	16 (27)
Limb salvage	21 (66)	22 (82)	43 (73)
Rest pain	11 (34)	5 (19)	16 (27)
Ulcer	10 (31)[a]	11 (41)[a]	21 (36)
Gangrene	—	6 (22)[a]	6 (10)

[a] *P* < .003 SCOPE vs NO SCOPE.

vein branches and valvulotomy performed without intraluminal visualization using the short modified Mills valvulotome.[2] Patients from both groups received postoperative daily aspirin, were ambulated if possible on the first postoperative day, and had daily assessment of wound status and graft function. Following discharge, graft surveillance was accomplished by serial history and physical, ankle/brachial index, and color-flow duplex ultrasound scanning.

The preoperative characteristics of the two study groups are listed in Table 8–1. There were more patients with tissue necrosis in the NO SCOPE group (*P* < .003) and a somewhat higher frequency of claudicators in the SCOPE group (*P* = .07). Otherwise, the two groups were similar. Table 8–2 highlights the operative features, revealing a slight increase in operative time for the SCOPE group but no difference in fluid volume administered despite the average of 1131 mL related to the angioscope. Most grafts were infrapopliteal, with similar frequency of adjunctive procedures such as toe amputations in the two groups.

TABLE 8–2. INTRAOPERATIVE CHARACTERISTICS OF BRIGHAM & WOMEN'S HOSPITAL STUDY PATIENTS

Characteristic	SCOPE (*n* = 32)	NO SCOPE (*n* = 27)	All (*N* = 59)
Mean Operating Time, min	239[a]	206[a]	224
Vein Diameter, mm	3.6	3.3	3.5
Mean Operating Room Fluid, mL	2,640	2,238	2,436
Distal Anastomosis, *n* (%)			
Distal popliteal	15 (47)	10 (37)	25 (42)
Anterior tibial	6 (19)	3 (11)	9 (16)
Posterior tibial	6 (19)	5 (19)	11 (19)
Peroneal	3 (9)	7 (26)	10 (17)
Dorsalis pedis	2 (6)	2 (7)	4 (7)
Adjunctive Procedure, *n* (%)			
Toe amputation	2 (6)	2 (7)	4 (7)
Debridement	1 (3)	2 (7)	3 (5)

[a] *P* < .05 SCOPE vs NO SCOPE.

The postoperative outcome was similar for both groups (Table 8–3). Most remarkably, there was no difference in wound morbidity or early graft failure. There were no early complications such as fluid overload directly attributable to the angioscope. One early graft failure in the SCOPE group was related to valvulotome injury in a small vein, which occurred despite the use of the angioscope. There was not a likely preventive role for angioscopy in the other three failures, due to small vein caliber, distal embolization, and poor runoff. No retained valve leaflets or arteriovenous fistulas were recognized in either group. Overall and postoperative hospital lengths of stay were not influenced by use of the angioscope. Overall primary and secondary cumulative graft patencies were 62% and 85%, respectively, at 48 months and 13.6-month mean follow-up. There was no significant difference in patency between the two study groups, with primary patencies of 63% (SCOPE) and 61% (NO SCOPE) and secondary patencies of 79% (SCOPE) and 91% (NO SCOPE) ($P = .127$).

This relatively small randomized prospective study showed that angioscopy had neither a positive nor negative impact on the significant end points measured. The absence of an advantage in the SCOPE group may be more compelling considering the somewhat larger number of claudicators and the smaller number of open foot lesions compared to the NO SCOPE group. Although insignificant at follow-up to date, a difference in secondary patency rates favoring the NO SCOPE group may emerge as graft surveillance continues. Since angioscopy appears to provide no major benefit, the Brigham & Women's team has used it only for continued study purposes rather than routinely for in situ grafting. Alternatively, these results have been interpreted by others to confirm that there is no harm in the use of the angioscope and that its use should therefore be continued and expanded.

Maini et al[18] performed a prospective study with a hypothesis similar to that in the Brigham & Women's series, although with some significant differences in study methodology. Twenty-six grafts using routine preoperative vein mapping and angioscopic assistance were compared to a historical group of 24 standard in situ bypass grafts. There was a 6% incidence of limbs operated on for popliteal aneurysm and there were no claudicators nor urgently threatened limbs. The angioscopic technique

TABLE 8–3. POSTOPERATIVE MORBIDITY AND MORTALITY[a]

	SCOPE (n = 32)	NO SCOPE (n = 27)	All (N = 59)
Local Complications, n (%)			
Wound infection	1 (3)	1 (4)	2 (3)
Hematoma	2 (6)	—	2 (3)
Early graft failure	2 (6)	2 (7)	4 (7)
Systemic Complications, n (%)			
Myocardial infarction	1 (3)	1 (4)	2 (3)
Arrhythmia	—	1 (4)	1 (2)
Stroke	—	1 (4)	1 (2)
Pneumonia	—	1 (4)	1 (2)
Mean Length of Hospital Stay, Days (Range)			
Total	10.5 (4–27)	10.7 (4–23)	10.6 (4–27)
Postoperative	8.0 (2–25)	8.6 (2–21)	8.2 (2–25)
Mortality, n (%)	—	1 (4)	1 (2)

[a] No statistical difference between SCOPE and NO SCOPE groups.

was similar to that in the Brigham & Women's study. Results of this study demonstrated that the angioscopy group suffered significantly fewer wound complications than the historical group (4% and 38%, respectively). Postoperative ambulation averaged 1 day earlier and hospital discharge averaged 4.7 days earlier in the angioscope group. There appeared to be no immediate ill effects from angioscopy. However, cumulative primary graft patency at 12 months was 72% for the angioscope group compared to 95% for the comparison group.

The relatively high wound morbidity rate in the historical group is not unrealistic,[5] but the study design makes it difficult to attribute the improvement in the rate of wound complications conclusively to the angioscopically assisted technique. The dramatic difference in length of hospital stay may be the product of more factors than angioscopy alone and deserves further analysis, particularly in the present era of cost savings. The authors correctly caution about a possible detrimental impact of angioscopy on long-term patency, although differences may be explained in part by comparison of nonrandomized noncontemporary groups of patients.

CONCLUSION

Since early description of vascular endoscopy to assist in the treatment of mitral valve stenosis,[7] angioscopy has progressed through advances in modern fiber-optic technology to a truly spectacular level. Small-diameter angioscopes with high image resolution can be used to evaluate vessels and grafts following thrombectomy and endarterectomy, to assist in vein preparation during bypass, and to evaluate anastomotic and conduit adequacy. In applications involving the *in situ* vein bypass, the quality of visualization of valves and branches is uniformly good and often excellent with appropriate flushing strategies and coordination between the surgical and anesthesia teams to avoid undue fluid infusion. Angioscopy is the most sensitive method available for detecting intraluminal abnomalities, placing the surgeon's eye directly inside the vessel, using light rather than ultrasound or radiopaque contrast to illuminate structures such as valve leaflets.

It is remarkable that this device has not yet found an undisputed niche in the vascular armamentarium. One difficulty in the case of infrainguinal grafting is that the angioscope is competing with routines using older modalities such as continuous-wave ultrasound and operative angiography. Results of surgery using these methods have improved steadily, reducing the incentives to adopt new and unfamiliar technology, regardless of how spectacular or intriguing. Additional relative disincentive arises from real or potential concerns regarding cost, operating room logistics, and rapid obsolescence of evolving instrumentation. Most importantly, there are still no data that conclusively demonstrate a uniquely superior role for angioscopy in improving outcome after infrainguinal surgery.

Of all procedures with potential angioscopic applications, the *in situ* vein bypass offers unique opportunities for significant advances. Theoretically, angioscopy should be capable of increasing success and reducing morbidity by facilitating precise vein preparation and making bypass a minimally invasive procedure. Studies to date support the feasibility and operative safety of this application but fail to reach a strong consensus demonstrating superiority over traditional *in situ* techniques. The issue of a potential detrimental impact of angioscopy on long-term patency remains incompletely resolved. Angioscopically assisted techniques will remain valuable in some surgeons' hands as further study continues.

REFERENCES

1. Leather RP, Shah DM, Chang BB, et al. Resurrection of the in situ saphenous vein bypass: 1000 cases later. *Ann Surg.* 1988;208:435–442.
2. Donaldson MC, Mannick JA, Whittemore AD. Femoral-distal bypass with in situ greater saphenous vein: long-term results using the Mills valvulotome. *Ann Surg.* 1991;213:457–465.
3. Bergamini TM, Towne JB, Bandyk DF, et al. Experience with in situ saphenous vein bypasses during 1981 to 1989: determinant factors of long-term patency. *J Vasc Surg.* 1991;13:137–149.
4. Donaldson MC, Mannick JA, Whittemore AD. Causes of primary graft failure after in situ saphenous vein bypass grafting. *J Vasc Surg.* 1992;15:113–118.
5. Wengrovitz M, Atnip RG, Gifford RRM, et al. Wound complications of autogenous subcutaneous infrainguinal arterial bypass surgery: predisposing factors and management. *J Vasc Surg.* 1990;11:156–163.
6. Donaldson MC. Doppler detection of arteriovenous fistulas after in situ saphenous vein bypass. *Am J Surg.* 1988;155:263–265.
7. White GH, White RA, eds. *Angioscopy: Vascular and Coronary Applications.* Chicago: Year Book Medical Publishers, Inc; 1989.
8. Miller A, Stonebridge PA, Tsoukas AI, et al. Angioscopically directed valvulotomy: a new valvulotome and technique. *J Vasc Surg.* 1991;13:813–821.
9. Lamuraglia GM, Cambria RP, Brewster DC, et al. Angioscopy guided semiclosed technique for in situ bypass. *J Vasc Surg.* 1990;12:601–604.
10. Stierli P, Aeberhard P. Angioscopy-guided semiclosed technique for in situ bypass with a novel flushing valvulotome: early results. *J Vasc Surg.* 1992;15:564–568.
11. Baxter TB, Rizzo RJ, Flinn WR, et al. A comparative study of intraoperative angioscopy and completion arteriography following femorodistal bypass. *Arch Surg.* 1990;125:997–1002.
12. Gilbertson JJ, Walsh DB, Zwolak RW, et al. A blinded comparison of angiography, angioscopy, and duplex scanning in the intraoperative evaluation of in situ saphenous vein bypass grafts. *J Vasc Surg.* 1992;15:121–129.
13. Miller A, Marcaccio EJ, Tannenbaum GA, et al. Comparison of angioscopy and angiography for monitoring infrainguinal bypass vein grafts: results of a prospective randomized trial. *J Vasc Surg.* 1993;17:382–398.
14. Cikrit DF, Dalsing MC, Lalka SG, et al. Early results of endovascular-assisted in situ saphenous vein bypass grafting. *J Vasc Surg.* 1994;19:778–787.
15. Sales CM, Marin ML, Veith FJ, et al. Saphenous vein angioscopy: a valuable method to detect unsuspected venous disease. *J Vasc Surg.* 1993;18:198–204.
16. Miller A, Stonebridge PA, Jepsen SJ, et al. Continued experience with intraoperative angioscopy for monitoring infrainguinal bypass grafting. *Surgery.* 1991;109:286–293.
17. Clair DG, Golden MA, Mannick JA, et al. Randomized prospective study of angioscopically-assisted in situ saphenous vein grafting. *J Vasc Surg.* 1994;19:992–999.
18. Maini BS, Andrews L, Salimi T, et al. A modified, angioscopically assisted technique for in situ saphenous vein bypass: impact on patency, complications, and length of stay. *J Vasc Surg.* 1993;17:1041–1049.

III

Nonatherosclerotic Ischemia

9

Arteritides:

Current Status of
Diagnosis and Management

John William Joyce, MD

The arteritides are random infrequent occurrences that can challenge both diagnostic and therapeutic skills. These diseases usually affect several organ systems, producing multifaceted manifestations spread sequentially over several weeks or months, inhibiting early diagnosis. In many, a solitary organ dominates the clinical picture and a patient with arteritis may present in almost any medical or surgical discipline.

The generic term *arteritis* implies an arterial inflammatory response and could logically include reactions induced by infection, radiation, chemicals, drugs, or other mechanisms. The term is usually applied, however, to a diverse subset of diseases of immune or unknown etiology. These syndromes are preferably classified as the vasculitides, for venous involvement is common.

Classifications of the vasculitides are variable, inconstant, and evolving, often complex for erudition or simplified for practicality. They are based on various combinations of histological features, etiology, vessel size, and clinical syndromes. Each of these criteria may overlap in several entities, confounding classification and reflecting the slow evolution of knowledge and incomplete understanding of the basic etiological mechanisms. Vasculitis is characterized by acute or chronic inflammation or necrosis of the vessel wall, sometimes with associated thrombosis or intimal proliferation, and a late sclerotic stage. Recognized syndromes have common patterns of organ involvement, tempo, morbidity, mortality, and response to therapy. Systemic symptoms of fever, malaise, weight loss, and rheumatological, ocular, cutaneous, and central or peripheral neurological manifestations are common to many. Most are self-limiting, but intervention is essential to reduce morbidity and mortality, whether the disease is acute or indolent at presentation.

Understanding of the etiological mechanisms of the vasculitides is hindered by the low prevalence of the syndromes, and separating cause from effect can be problematic. Immune complex disease, cell-mediated immune responses, and hypersensitivity have been identified as basic mechanisms. Antigens, however, have been found in only a few entities, and triggering events are only occasionally noted clinically. These include drugs (hydralazine, sulfa, and procainamide), infection (hepatitis B and C, rickettsia, and streptococcus), inflammation (biliary cirrhosis and inflammatory bowel disease), and neoplasia. Responses noted in vasculitis are the activation of complement, production of immunoglobulins and cryoglobulins, and interactions of the endothelial cells with any of the leukocytes, macrophages, and platelets. Cytokines, arachidonic acid metabolites, growth factors, and both clotting and lytic factors contribute to the pathological process at the endothelial level. Several excellent contemporary reviews provide detailed information of the pathogenesis, classification, and clinical profiles of the vasculitic syndromes.[1-6] Just how much there is yet to learn will be apparent to the thoughtful reader.

The majority of the vasculitides are managed medically. However, significant stenoses, occlusions, aneurysms, and hemorrhagic and thrombosing events of major arteries and veins require surgical treatment. It is these syndromes that are reviewed here (Table 9–1). Interdisciplinary cooperation is often essential for the optimal management of these patients.

THE GIANT CELL ARTERITIDES

The two vasculitic syndromes that the surgeon will most frequently include in differential diagnosis or encounter are the giant cell arteritides: temporal and Takayasu arteritis. Major manifestations of both are occlusive and aneurysmal disease of the aorta

---

TABLE 9–1. A CLASSIFICATION OF VASCULITIS

Necrotizing Vasculitis
Polyarteritis nodosa[a]
Allergic granulomatosis (Churg–Strauss syndrome)
Overlap syndromes

Hypersensitivity Vasculitis
Hypersensitivity vasculitis
Henoch–Schönlein purpura
Serum sickness
Vasculitis with collagen disease
Vasculitis with infection
Vasculitis with malignancy
Vasculitis with cryoglobulinemia
Hypocomplementemic vasculitis

Giant Cell Arteritis
Temporal arteritis[a]
Takayasu arteritis[a]

Miscellaneous
Thromboangiitis obliterans[a]
Wegener's granulomatosis
Behçet's disease[a]
Kawasaki syndrome[a]
Relapsing polychondritis[a]

---
[a] Denotes large artery involvement.

and its branches, the domain of surgery. The histology of each is identical in the acute phase; systemic symptoms, laboratory tests, and angiographic findings are similar.

Several clinical features separate the two syndromes. Takayasu arteritis occurs predominantly in females less than 50 years of age, while the gender difference of temporal arteritis is less, and the disease is rare under age 50. Arterial lesions differ in extent, distribution, and frequency. Aortic involvement is almost universal in Takayasu arteritis; branch vessel lesions are frequent and often multiple, occurring near their aortic origin and sometimes beyond, rarely extending below the axilla or groin. Temporal arteritis has only a 10% incidence of extracranial arterial disease, most commonly stenotic or occlusive lesions of paired limb vessels at sites distal to their aortic takeoff. Lesions are seen on occasion below the axillae and knees but aortic disease is uncommon. Stenotic and occlusive lesions predominate in both syndromes, with about 10% incidence of aneurysm formation. Dissection of the aorta may occur with temporal arteritis.[6–10]

Surgical repair is often required for the lesions of Takayasu arteritis but is only rarely indicated for those of temporal arteritis. Of singular importance, steroid and immunosuppressive drugs can arrest or even improve the arterial complications when given in the acute phase of either disease.

TEMPORAL ARTERITIS

The name *temporal arteritis* does not adequately delineate this syndrome; other designations, such as Horton's disease or cranial, giant cell, or granulomatous arteritis, are also wanting or overlap with other diseases. I prefer the term *temporal arteritis* because of its common usage and historical origin. Male–female ratios were almost equal in early reports, but an increasing preponderance of women is now noted.[11] Most reviews come from white populations and northern climates. The incidence of the disease has been measured as 17.4 cases per 100,000 persons over age 50 annually, rising to almost 30 cases beyond age 70.[11] Diagnosis has been documented in patients under age 50, but is most common in the seventh and eighth decades. There are random reports of temporal arteritis in paired siblings.

Arterial Manifestations

Extracranial arterial involvement of the limb arteries can present as asymptomatic bruits or pulse deficits, claudication and, rarely, distal ischemia. Raynaud's phenomenon is sometimes noted. Arterial involvement typically begins in the second through fifth months of the disease; and while some patients initially present because of these symptoms, careful interrogation will define antecedent features of the disease. On occasion, a history of other symptoms cannot be elicited, and arteritis is defined by angiography and/or biopsy. On occasion, arterial deficits first appear during steroid taper, signaling incomplete suppression of disease activity; an elevated erythrocyte sedimentation rate (ESR) will be noted.[7]

Atherosclerosis causes most arterial problems in this age range. I advise angiography for any manifestation of occlusive or aneurysmal disease when other features of temporal arteritis are present or when findings evolve over a few weeks, suggesting arteritis.

Temporal arteritis of the limbs is characterized by a bilateral insidious progression from asymptomatic bruits to reduced or absent pulses, and then claudication over a few weeks. Collaterals develop and usually prevent ischemia, which occurs only with combined involvement of the superficial and profunda femoris, popliteal, and tibioperoneal trunk in a given patient. Paired limb involvement is invariably simultaneous: when symptoms are unilateral, bruits, reduced systolic pressures, or angiography identify contralateral disease. Lesions of the subclavian–axillobrachial system are the most common, followed by the profunda and superficial femoral arteries. Involvement of both upper and lower limbs together or staged over a few weeks is not infrequent. Focal lesions of the forearm, popliteal, and tibioperoneal arteries are noted on occasion. The development of bilateral limb arterial disease over a short period in those over 50 strongly suggests the disease and warrants arteriography.[7,12,13]

Other syndromes seen by the surgeon occur in temporal arteritis. Amaurosis fugax is noted in up to 10% and either transient ischemic attacks or cerebral infarction is seen in 7% of untreated patients.[14] Stenosis may be seen in the common carotid but is more common where the internal carotid or vertebral vessels enter the skull.[15-17] Intracranial arteritis is rare.[18] Myocardial infarction from arteritis can occur,[17] and we have confirmed superior mesenteric stenosis in a patient with abdominal angina. Aneurysms of the ascending, descending, and abdominal aortas are infrequent, but death from rupture or aortic dissection has been documented.[7,17] Renal artery stenosis thus far has been noted only in parenchymal branches, causing active urinary sediment and albuminuria.[7]

Angiographic Findings

Arteriography delineates classic lesions. Stenoses are usually bilateral, often multiple, and demonstrate long or short tapering segments. Poststenotic dilation is common. Total occlusion, when seen, is usually at the end of a tapered segment and collateral vessels are generous (Fig. 9–1). Most lesions are seen near the clavicle, but it is

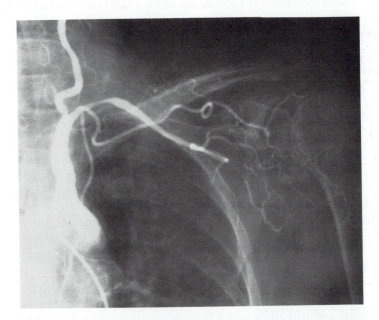

Figure 9–1. Focal stenosis of the left subclavian artery, complete occlusion of the axillary artery in a tapered stenosis, and collateral development. The right axillary artery showed a tapered stenosis. This 71-year-old woman presented with bilateral arm claudication, Raynaud's phenomenon, and a recent history of polymyalgia rheumatica. The ESR was 73 mm/h and a temporal artery biopsy was positive.

important to image the axillary artery where a dominant diagnostic lesion can be found (Fig. 9–2).[19]

Takayasu arteritis may cause identical lesions in the axillosubclavian system, in contrast to their usual location in the aortic root. Long tapered stenosis may also result from radiation fibrosis or the overuse of ergot. All three conditions can be easily differentiated from temporal arteritis by their historical features. Arteritis of the superficial femoral artery may be difficult to distinguish from atherosclerosis on occasion. This may be clarified by noting typical arteritic lesions in the adjacent profunda femoris or improvement of clinical and angiographic status after steroid therapy.

The Clinical Setting

Temporal arteritis usually begins insidiously with malaise and anorexia, followed by daily headache that can be focal or diffuse, sometimes intermittent, and often accompanied by scalp tenderness. These symptoms fade over weeks or overlap with fever, jaw claudication, and polymyalgia rheumatica. The latter is noted in one-third of patients and is characterized by significant pain and stiffness, with minimal tenderness, of the hip and shoulder girdles and neck. It may be most disabling and may persist for 1 year or more. Major eye symptoms occur in 15% to 20% of patients. These include central retinal artery or vein occlusion, extraocular muscle imbalance, amaurosis fugax, but most commonly ischemic optic neuritis causing partial or total blindness of one or both eyes. Ocular events occur after the second month of illness in most but have been documented as early as the third day of the illness. Extracranial arterial involvement occurs in about 10%, usually in the fifth through eighth months, but may be the presenting complaint. Forty percent of patients note inflamed temporal

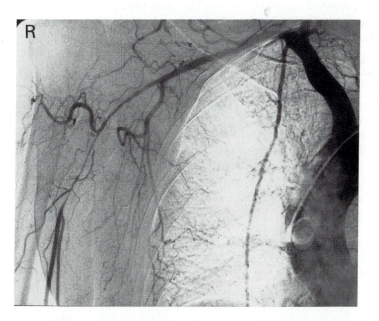

Figure 9–2. This 80-year-old man presented with bilateral arm claudication. The subclavian artery is not diagnostic, but the long tapered stenosis of the axillobrachial segment is diagnostic of arteritis. A similar lesion was present on the left side. A temporal artery biopsy was positive.

or occipital arteries in the early weeks, and these or fibrotic pulse vessels are found on examination in only half of proven cases.[7,11,20,21]

Temporal arteritis can be difficult to diagnose. Because the illness can mimic common transient problems and its phases can spread over several months, careful questioning of these aged patients or their families is often required in eliciting a complete history. Further, single components may dominate the presentation, such as severe headache or anemia, spiking fevers, and weight loss exceeding 15 pounds, all diverting extensive testing toward hematologic, neurogenic, malignant, or infectious processes. Definitive diagnosis remains essential, both to justify high-dose steroid therapy and because the morbidity of ocular complications and the disability and occasional death from vascular lesions can be prevented by adequate and timely steroid therapy.

Laboratory Findings

The ESR is elevated at a level of 40 to 140 mm/h in active temporal arteritis. A few patients present with a normal ESR and active disease, but the value becomes abnormal when anti-inflammatory drugs taken for fever or myalgias are discontinued. However, we and others have seen rare instances of a normal ESR with the disease active. Normocytic anemia of 11 g/dL is usual. Mild leukocytosis of 11,000 to 19,000 and moderate thrombocytopenia occur in many. Sight, nonspecific elevations of α_2-globulin, alkaline phosphatase, transaminase, and prothrombin time may be noted and may clear with therapy.

Temporal Artery Biopsy

The histological features of temporal arteritis are diagnostic and can be differentiated from the rare instance of necrotizing arteritis of the temporal vessels. Temporal artery bypass is an essential diagnostic tool in defining the presence or absence of arteritis in those with polymyalgia rheumatica and in the atypical cases of headache, anemia, obscure fever, and other unusual presentations. I require biopsy of patients with typical findings to justify committing the patient to steroid side effects, particularly osteoporosis, and to avoid late challenge of the diagnosis by others less familiar with the disease when steroid side effects push for rapid tapering.

Biopsy has been without morbidity in several hundred cases at Mayo Medical School (Rochester, Minn) and is done under local anesthesia. A specimen of 1 to 2 cm is adequate when the artery is frankly inflamed, but a 4- to 6-cm segment is taken when the clinical picture or observed artery is atypical. Because the disease is often focal and segmental with skipped areas, the longer specimens are examined microscopically at 3- to 5-mm intervals. Our diagnostic sensitivity is 92%, and of this, 14% is gained by biopsy of the contralateral artery when the first is negative. Biopsies are performed by designated surgeons familiar with the disease and the biopsy protocol.[22]

Medical Treatment

Temporal arteritis is unique in that the arterial complications can be prevented, improved, or cured by corticosteroid therapy. These agents were first used in 1949, and it became apparent that the initial or additional optic events could be prevented.[20,23] These observations established our practice of initiating treatment on the day of diagnosis, as visual loss can be unpredictable and sudden, followed by laboratory testing and biopsy. Steroids induce clinical improvement or restoration of pulses in 80% or more of patients with limb arteritis.[7,13] Stenotic lesions improve, documented on occasion by angiography but more often by Doppler pressures, and pulses and blood pressure normalize. Those with complete occlusion often improve, some by the development of collateral and others because of relief of stenosis in the same limb. Systemic symptoms and the ESR improve in the first week, often dramatically in 1 to 3 days. Arterial improvement may occur within 2 weeks, but more often is seen between the fourth and eighth weeks.[7]

The patient's symptoms, systolic pressures, and the ESR are monitored with each dosage change. Arterial occlusive disease can first be noted during steroid taper, and the ESR is not suppressed in these patients. Three instances of fatal aortic dissection occurred in patients without suppression of the ESR. Based on these observations, the steroid dosage and rate of taper are altered to keep the ESR normal. On occasion, initial or recurrent arterial events are first noted in the year following initial treatment. Monitoring the patient, limb pulses, and ESR quarterly for 1 year after therapy is prudent.[7]

Prednisone is the common choice for treatment; 60 mg in a single or divided daily dose is given for 1 week, then reduced to 45 mg/d if systemic symptoms and the ESR are suppressed. After 1 month of 45 mg/d, the dose is reduced by 5-mg increments at intervals of 2 to 3 weeks in those without extracranial arterial involvement and at 3- to 4-week intervals when arteritis is present. As noted, the findings and ESR are monitored at each dosage change, and the level is increased by 50% for 1 month if suppression is not complete. When the dosage reaches 10 mg/d, final reduction is by 1-mg increments. Recrudescence during treatment or subsequent recurrence occurs in 15% to 20% of patients.[7,24]

Patients with active visual or neurological symptoms are hospitalized and treated with intravenous steroids and heparin until symptoms stabilize. Antiplatelet agents are advocated by some for other forms of arteritis. However, sudden arterial thrombosis is not seen in treated temporal arteritis, and these agents are not indicated. At present, effective treatment programs to reduce osteoporosis during steroid therapy have not been documented. A controlled study of alternate-day steroid therapy, hoping to reduce osteoporosis, documented incomplete control of temporal arteritis at 1 month, but such a regimen is not advised.[25] Dapsone, cyclophosphamide, and azathioprine have been demonstrated to reduce steroid requirements, but each has additional side effects and the impact on osteoporosis has not been documented by controlled observations.[21] Further study is desirable. A program for tuberculosis prevention should be considered in patients with prior active disease. Both the patient and his or her family should be informed of the expected steroid side effects. A drug program of tuberculosis prophylaxis should be considered in patients with prior active disease. A no–added salt diet is advised, and both the patient and family are informed of expected steroid side effects.

Mortality

The incidence of death from temporal arteritis is small but not well defined. A population-based study of 42 patients noted a single death over a 25-year period. Autopsy documented acute aortitis with fatal dissection in a patient with inadequate steroid suppression.[11] Treated patients are said to have long-term survival similar to that of a matched population.[26] It is clear that deaths reported and appropriately studied are from major vascular events: usually aortic dissection or stroke and sometimes myocardial infarction.[7,15,17,24] In each of these studies, the majority of patients were untreated, and the others were either inadequately treated or in the first days of steroid suppression. These observations underscore the importance of early diagnosis, the efficacy of steroid therapy, and the value of ESR suppression as a guide to therapy.

The Role of Surgery

Reconstructive arterial surgery is not often needed. The significant improvement of stenoses with steroids, the development of shoulder collaterals in those with brachiocephalic occlusions, and the improvement of diseased profunda femoris arteries in those with femoropopliteal occlusions is such that few patients are handicapped enough to warrant repair. We have performed femoropopliteal or femorotibial saphenous vein bypass surgery in three patients with ischemic rest pain after the disease was suppressed. Each had femoropopliteal system occlusions accompanied by loss of an effective profunda femoris: two have been followed up and maintain patency at 5 and 8 years, respectively. Bilateral below-knee amputations were necessary for a patient whose claudication preceded the onset of temporal arteritis. Examination of the specimens showed extensive atherosclerosis and superimposed arteritis. A single patient with extensive axillobrachial arteritis had an ischemic finger pad ulcer following direct digital trauma and this healed spontaneously. Ischemic limb lesions and rest pain are rare with temporal arteritis.

A role for surgery can be predicted for those with aortic dissection, aneurysm of the aorta, symptomatic carotid disease,[16] and perhaps coronary involvement. All are, fortunately, uncommon. Failure of saphenous vein grafts placed in limbs when the arteritis has not been suppressed has been observed. It would seem essential that high-dose intravenous steroids be given perioperatively for any urgent surgery and that anastomoses be placed in adjacent healthy tissue when practical.

TAKAYASU ARTERITIS

Takayasu arteritis, of all the vasculitides, has the most extensive involvement of the aorta and its major branches. The lesions are multiple often complex combinations of occlusive and sometimes aneurysmal disease, both above and below the diaphragm, and surgical repair is required for many. It is also an uncommon arteritis with a reported incidence of only 2.6 cases per 1 million people per year.[9] The original description and subsequent studies that are a foundation for study come from Japan, but the disease is widespread and significant observations have been reported on natives of Mexico, India, Russia, Africa, Europe, and North America as well as other populations. Because of its infrequent ubiquitous occurrence, this condition has many names. It is now usually reported as nonspecific aortoarteritis or Takayasu artertis.

Eighty to ninety-five percent of these patients are female.[9,10,27] The age of onset varies from childhood through the sixties, with a peak incidence in the third and fourth decades. It has been traditional to describe two phases of the illness: an initial systemic period, followed months later by the appearance of the arterial deficits. It has, however, been clear for some years that the arterial lesions can develop during the acute systemic phase or that they may be the sole manifestations of the syndrome, without any identifiable antecedent illness. Because the systemic symptoms are not specific, a delay of several months from the onset of the disease to diagnosis is usual. On occasion, Takayasu arteritis has developed in defined cases of rheumatoid arthritis, scleroderma, ankylosing spondylitis, systemic lupus erythematosus, and inflammatory bowel disease. An association with tuberculosis is also frequently noted, but no causal relationship has been established, and these reports would seem to reflect the prevalence of tuberculosis in certain countries.

The Clinical Setting

The systemic phase is reported in 25% to 75% of patients and lasts a few weeks to several months. The most common symptoms are malaise, fever, night sweats, headache, and pleurisy. Myalgias, arthralgias, and synovitis are noted by 50% or more of patients; skin lesions such as rash, urticaria, or erythema nodosum are noted in about 15%.[9,10] The subsequent arterial involvement can cause claudication of the limbs, lightheadedness, posturally induced visual dimness, tunnel vision, amaurosis fugax, diplopia, hypertension, and on occasion stroke, myocardial infarction, or abdominal angina.

Laboratory Findings

Laboratory data are similar to those on temporal arteritis. A normochromic normocytic anemia is noted in 25% to 45%, leukocytosis in 10%, elevated α_2-globulin in 33%, and C-reactive protein in 25% of patients. ESR elevation in the range of 40 to 140 mm/h is found in 70% to 80% of patients with clinically active disease.[9,10,27] In contrast to temporal arteritis, however, the ESR normalizes in only one-half of the patients in apparent remission after treatment. Further, arterial biopsies taken at surgery can show active arteritis when the disease has been treated medically and the ESR is normal.[10,28] A better serologic marker of active disease is needed, both to direct drug therapies and to minimize the chance of graft failures reported when surgery is done during active arteritis.[9]

Arterial Manifestations

All patients with Takayasu arteritis have bruits and/or pulse deficits at the time of diagnosis, except for the occasional patient with only aneurysmal disease. Blood pressure can often be detected in involved limbs only by Doppler examination. The arterial lesions are predominantly branch vessel stenoses or occlusions, usually but not always at their aortic origin (Fig. 9–3), and irregularities of the aorta and vessel walls. Aneurysm or ectasia of the aorta, and sometimes of its branches, is noted in up to one-quarter of patients. Coarctation is present in the thoracic aorta in 15% to 25% and in the abdominal aorta in up to one-half of these studied.[9,10,27] The incidence of pulmonary artery stenosis is unknown, as this circulation is usually studied only when pulmonary hypertension is noted. When both the thoracic and abdominal aortas are studied, a typical distribution of lesions includes: thoracic aorta and its branches alone, 8% (type I); the abdominal aorta and its branches alone, 11% (type II); and both the abdominal and thoracic aortas and branches, 65% (type III).[29] Complete angiography is advised for all patients to detect aneurysms and occult occlusive disease. Limb runoff studies are added when clinical findings suggest disease distal to the truncal arteries (Fig. 9–4). Study of the coronary or pulmonary circulation is dictated by clinical findings.

Several clinical syndromes may result from the multiple lesions of Takayasu arteritis, and a given patient can demonstrate more than one. The most common are symptoms of orthostatic cerebral hypoperfusion, including dizziness and visual disturbance (Fig. 9–5), claudication of the arms and sometimes the legs (Figs. 9–6 and 9–7), and hypertension secondary to renal artery stenosis or aortic coarctation. There is a small incidence of stroke, coronary artery disease, aortic valve incompetence,

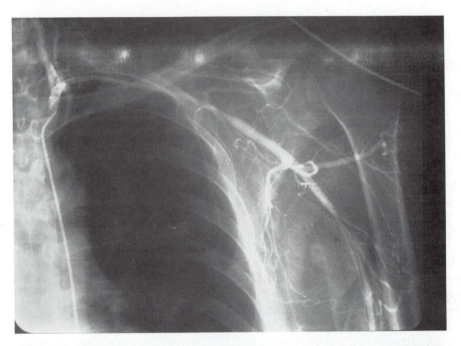

Figure 9–3. Subclavian, axillary, and brachial lesions in a 32-year-old woman during recurrence of Takayasu arteritis. Note the similarity to temporal arteritis. The patient initially presented with abdominal angina, which cleared with steroid therapy. She underwent bilateral renal artery saphenous bypass surgery following suppression of her recurrence.

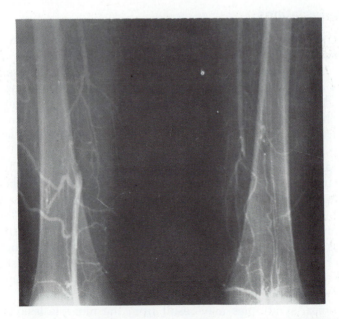

Figure 9–4. Bilateral superficial femoral artery occlusions in a 9-year-old boy. These lesions do not have features diagnostic of arteritis. He presented with bilateral claudication and his only other lesions were at the iliac level (see Fig 9–7). He experienced no systemic symptoms, and the ESR was never elevated. An iliac biopsy at the time of bypass surgery to increase left leg growth was positive, despite an antecedent course of steroids. He illustrates many of the diagnostic and therapeutic problems of Takayasu arteritis.

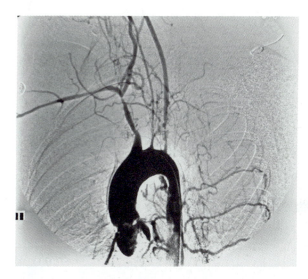

Figure 9–5. Tapered lesions of the brachiocephalic arteries typical of Takayasu arteritis. Note coarctation of the descending aorta (gradient, 44 mg Hg) and the collateral circulation. This female patient experiences visual blurring only with increased activity and left arm claudication. Surgery is planned following a course of steroid suppression.

and pulmonary hypertension. Congestive heart failure secondary to renovascular hypertension or thoracic coarctation may be seen late in the course of the disease.

Angiography

Retrograde angiography is accomplished with no mortality and rare morbidity in these youthful patients. An initial complete study is advised, as noted, to detect

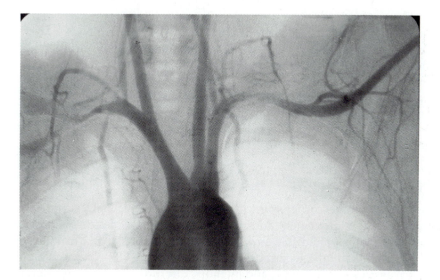

Figure 9–6. This 28-year-old woman presented with bilateral arm claudication and had experienced no systemic symptoms. The proximal subclavian lesions may be seen in either temporal or Takayasu arteritis. Note, however, early lesion of the left carotid artery near its origin. Such early irregularities are common in the aorta and its branch vessels with Takayasu arteritis. The patient's steroid management was erratic, and subsequently both common carotids were bypassed from the ascending aorta, following a full course of steroids and cyclophosphamide.

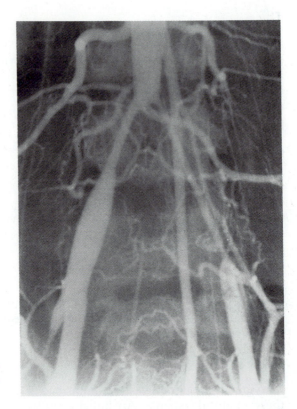

Figure 9–7. The same patient as Fig 9–4. Growth of the left leg was 1.5 inches less than that of the right. This was corrected after aortoiliac bypass.

occult lesions and to serve as a guide for surgical requirements and later medical follow-up. A representative incidence of the multiple lesions includes about 80% abdominal aorta and left subclavian and superior mesenteric arteries; 60% thoracic aorta and renal left common carotid, innominate, and celiac arteries; 40% right common carotid and vertebrals; and 25% axillobrachial system. Bilateral involvement is common but not universal in paired arteries.[9,10] Involvement of the internal carotid arteries is rare, and this facilitates bypass surgery of the brachiocephalic arteries when needed.

Medical Therapy

Corticosteroids are the cornerstones of therapy and effectively suppress systemic symptoms. While improvement and/or stability of stenotic lesions is observed, this is not as common or predictable as with temporal arteritis.[9,10,30] Treatment failure is seen in up to 40%, and the recurrence rate can approach 45%.[10] Immunosuppressive agents such as cyclophosphamide and methotrexate are combined with steroids when suppression is not obtained with steroids alone. Methotrexate has a lower incidence of significant side effects and is the current choice for a second agent.[31] Initial treatment averages 1 to 2 years, and recurrences occur for up to 5 years. Clearly, better understanding of the etiology of this disease and therefore more specific drug therapy are both needed. Long-term monitoring of the clinical course, serologic markers, and, when applicable, graft stability are essential.

The Role of Surgery

Inflammation of Takayasu arteritis is aggressive and, in contrast to atherosclerosis, produces multiple major lesions in months or a few short years. One-third to one-half of those affected will require surgical repair.[9,10] The indications are those learned from atherosclerosis, but operations are compounded by the problem of disease activity and the need for complex repairs of several vessels in combined or staged procedures, often through extensive incisions as thoracoabdominal or sternotomy with neck extensions. A high level of skill and experience is required of the surgical team.

The indications for surgery are well defined. These include significant hypertension from aortic coarctation, renal artery stenosis, and usually both; orthostatic cerebral hypoperfusion, amaurosis fugax, and cerebral ischemia; aneurysm; mesenteric angina and infarction; aortic value insufficiency; coronary artery disease (usually ostial); and limb bypass for ischemia, disabling claudication, and sometimes growth in young patients. Bypass and replacement grafts are commonly used, and patch grafts are sometimes appropriate. Endarterectomy is not favored by most surgeons. Grafts should be attached to unaffected or healed tissues. Grafts to the brachiocephalic vessels are best brought from the ascending aorta. Repair of multiple visceral and renal artery stenoses is demanding because thoracic or abdominal coarctation is commonly present and often extensive, requiring long thoracoabdominal grafts.[10,28,32,33]

Biopsies are taken when feasible, to assess disease activity and govern the direction of postoperative medical care. Catastrophic events such as aneurysm rupture, intestinal infarction, or increasing neurological events can occur when the arteritis is clearly active. We have treated such patients with intravenous steroids and proceeded with the indicated repair.

The concept of angioplasty for focal stenosis is attractive. Given the youth of these patients and the known finite durability of prosthetic and venous grafts, even the gain of a few years of effective patency would be of value. Several centers have reported high initial patency rates after dilation of ostial renal stenosis.[34] Recently, similar encouraging initial success has been obtained in stenosis of the thoracic and abdominal aortas measuring less than 4 cm.[35] Few reports have achieved 5-year follow-up, most being measured in months. It is to be hoped that angioplasty evolves as a selective successful addition for the care of these patients.

BEHÇET'S DISEASE

Behçet's disease is a clinical syndrome caused by cellular vasculitis of small and large blood vessels and veins. It is chronic and recurrent and characterized by three major manifestations: recurrent aphthous ulcers of the mouth and genitalia; uvitis and recurrent hypopyon; and a variety of skin lesions, including erythema nodosum, pustules, and hypersensitivity to needle punctures. Additional manifestations include synovitis, recurrent meningoencephalitis, inflammatory bowel disease, and an incidence of up to 25% of major arterial and venous problems. These manifestations are spread over several months and into a chronic recurring phase, with arterial and venous problems usually occurring in the second year of the disease or later. The diagnosis is established by the presence of two or three criteria with various combinations of minor criteria. With the exception of the aphthous oral lesions and ocular disease, there is no common agreement as to what constitutes major criteria. This disease has a prevalence of up to 1 in 1,000 in Mediterranean countries and Japan and of 1 in 25,000 persons in the United States. It is more common in men, and the usual age at presentation is in the fourth and fifth decades.[36-38]

The disease is fatal in 3% to 5% of patients; major arterial and venous diseases cause the bulk of these, followed by meningoencephalitis. Blindness is seen in up to 25% of patients with uvitis or hypopyon, and neurological involvement is most common in the brainstem, causing hemiplegia, paraplegia, and disturbances of the cranial nerves. Psychiatric syndromes often accompany neurological involvement. The ESR is elevated in up to 70% of patients and nonspecific elevations of α_2-globulin, C-reactive protein, and lymphocytes are noted. No single therapeutic agent has been demonstrated to be consistently effective in the manifestations of major organ systems, but steroids can suppress systemic symptoms and reduce the frequency of ocular attacks. In recent years chlorambucil has shown significant benefit in reducing the severity and frequency of both meningoencephalitis and ocular vasculitis.

Arterial and venous involvement has been noted in 6% to 25% of cases, and rupture of aneurysms, chiefly the aorta, is the leading cause of death. Almost any artery or vein can be involved, and venous lesions are more frequent than arterial ones. These consist of spontaneous thrombosis, most commonly of the superior and inferior vena cavae, with subclavian and femoral veins next in frequency; and almost any named vein, including the hepatic, renal, internal and external jugular, and the veins of the limbs, can be involved. It has been noted that recurrent phlebitis can occur in the face of warfarin therapy.

Aneurysms are more frequent than acute arterial occlusions. They most frequently affect the abdominal and thoracic aortas and the femoral and carotid arteries. They are also reported in all arteries of the upper and lower extremities and coronary, renal, and splenic arteries. The aneurysms tend to be irregular and saccular and are prone to rupture during acute exacerbations of the disease. Aneurysms of the pulmonary artery can cause recurrent hemoptysis that is eventually fatal. Acute arterial thrombosis is most common in the subclavian and pulmonary arteries and may occur in the common carotid artery, any of the vessels of the arms or legs, or the renal artery. An unusual, and useful, vascular manifestation of the syndrome is the development of an acute inflammatory reaction about 1 cm in size at the site of needle pricks or the development of a 2- to 4-cm superficial phlebitis at the site of simple needle puncture or indwelling catheters. This is now called the Behçetin phenomenon, and some include it as a major diagnostic criterion.

Arteriography is sometimes accompanied by significant hemorrhage or local thrombosis when the site of penetration is in an area of active disease. Standard surgical bypass procedures, attempting to place the grafts in adjacent healthy tissue, is the standard approach for aneurysms. Aneurysms occurring in paired arteries such as the forearm or tibioperoneal area can be ligated. The risk of anastomotic pseudoaneurysms is significant. Because of a favorable experience with chlorambucil, we have recently treated one patient in the active phase of the disease and suppressed his tendency toward pseudoaneurysm and anastomotic aneurysm formation in the superficial femoral artery. It can be anticipated that this therapy will have failures, like others before it, but its further use seems justified. The initial dosage is 0.1 mg/kg/d, continued for 1 year and then tapered over an additional 6 months. Ideally, arterial surgery is best attempted when the disease is in a quiescent phase, manifest by a normal sedimentation rate and control of the aphthous ulcerations (Fig. 9–8).

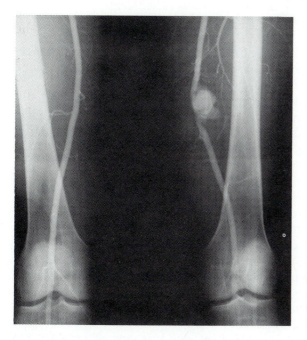

Figure 9–8. False aneurysm of a 33-year-old man with a 4-year history of Behçet's disease. Two saphenous vein bypass grafts each developed anastomotic aneurysms. No further aneurysms occurred during the 29 months after a 1-year course of chlorambucil. His monthly episodes of oral ulcers were also suppressed.

KAWASAKI DISEASE

Kawasaki disease (mucocutaneous lymph node syndrome) is a unique syndrome of infants, small children, and rarely those in their teens that occurs in epidemic fashion in Japan and endemically in Asia, Europe, and North America. It is characterized by an acute onset of high spiking fever with conjunctivitis; erythema of the trunk, sole, and palms; cervical adenopathy; and often cricopharyngeal edema. After a few days arthralgias, dryness of the lips, and desquamation of the skin occur. Laboratory changes are nonspecific and include mild anemia, neutrophilia, accelerated ESR, and thrombocytosis which can be quite marked. Meningitis, hepatitis, pleurisy, and diarrhea are uncommon features.

Approximately 1% to 2% of patients died in the acute or subacute phase from an intense necrotizing vasculitis of the small and medium arteries and veins identical to periarteritis nodosa histologically. This induces coronary artery ectasia and aneurysm in about 15% of people during the first month of disease but sometimes up to 4 years later. It can be recognized and followed by echocardiography, and death occurs from aneurysm thrombosis or rupture. Aspirin suppresses the acute symptoms of the disease. The addition of high-dose γ-globulin during the acute phase of the disease has significantly reduced the arteritis and coronary disease and is now standard therapy.

Aneurysmal disease of the abdominal aorta and also of the iliac, brachial, axillary renal, hepatic, and mesenteric arteries has been noted as late sequelae some years after the acute phase of the disease. When identified, standard surgical procedures of excision and grafting are effective. It is not yet clear whether the use of γ-globulin will reduce the incidence of late arterial aneurysm formation.[39–41]

RELAPSING POLYCHONDRITIS

Relapsing polychondritis is characterized by inflammatory degeneration of cartilage, chiefly of the ears, nose, larynx, and trachea, accompanied by arthritis. Its etiology is unknown; men and women are affected equally, and the age distribution is from 13 to 84 years, but most cases occur in the fifth and sixth decades. Malaise, fever, and elevation of the sedimentation rate occur in most patients. Episcleritis, conjunctivitis, and uvitis as well as audiovestibular damage are seen in one-quarter of the patients.

Approximately 15% of patients have an accompanying necrotizing arteritis of the small and medium-sized blood vessels, manifest as subcutaneous nodules, erythema nodosum, and panniculitis. However, syndromes similar to periarteritis nodosa occur with involvement of the kidneys and causing typical mononeuritis multiplex. In 5% to 8% of cases, arteritis of the aorta will result in aortic ring dilation with aortic incompetence, dissection of the ascending aorta, and aneurysm formation of the thoracic and abdominal aortas. On occasion, other forms of vasculitis overlap with polychondritis, and these include lupus erythematosus, Behçet's disease, and writers' syndrome.

The response of the systemic manifestations to steroids, aspirin, and dapsone is inconsistent. It is not clear whether later arteritis is prevented by any agent. Surgery is indicated for major valvular or aneurysm disease, and it is desirable to suppress the systemic process with steroids prior to repair (Fig. 9–9).[42,43]

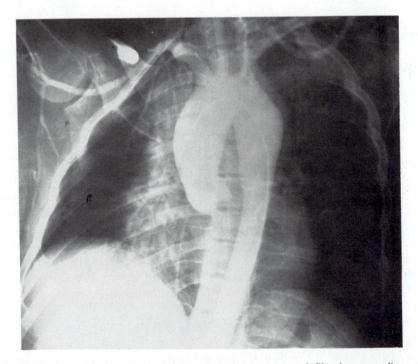

Figure 9–9. This aneurysm was noted on routine chest x-ray. A film 1 year earlier was normal when this 18-year-old girl presented with nose and ear lesions typical of relapsing polychondritis. She died 8 years after the onset of her illness following surgery for a false aneurysm of her original graft.

POLYARTERITIS NODOSA

Polyarteritis nodosa is a necrotizing arteritis that can affect any or all organ systems, and in a given patient there are usually several manifestations. Common patterns of presentation include the systemic illness presenting as unknown fever or weight loss, mononeuritis multiplex, glomerulitis, abdominal pain, acute hypertension, and arthralgias. Other findings can include skin rash, orchitis, stroke, and pulmonary infiltrates or pleurisy. Coronary, pericardial, and myocardial involvement is common at autopsy but is usually clinically silent. This disease is accompanied by an elevation of the sedimentation rate, modest anemia, and a moderate leukocytosis. The onset is usually insidious, with accumulating manifestation, but on occasion it is fulminant, with death in days or weeks.

Acute necrosis, with secondary thrombosis or late fibrosis, is a typical histological pattern, and lesions in different stages of evolution will be found in a given organ or artery. This disease can be seen throughout life from childhood on but is most common in the fourth through sixth decades, and males predominate.

Digital and microcirculatory disease of the extremities may manifest as finger pad infarction, livedoid vasculitis of the distal limbs that may ulcerate, and Raynaud's phenomenon. Medium-sized blood vessels in the gastrointestinal and renal circulations may occlude or more commonly become aneurysmal. Multiple aneurysms of the secondary and tertiary branches of the visceral, renal, hepatic, and lumbar arteries are characteristic of the syndrome on angiography. Vessel occlusion can result in acute cholecystitis, appendicitis, and more commonly perforation of the gut with gastrointestinal hemorrhage. Aneurysmal disease can cause intra-abdominal hemorrhage and shock, and ischemic bowel obstruction is sometimes seen following visceral vessel occlusions. Of importance, intra-abdominal and renal aneurysms have been noted to regress under appropriate steroid or immunosuppressive therapy. Asymptomatic aneurysms can be watched, but if regression does not occur, elective surgery is advised. Second-look surgery is often imperative in patients with bowel ischemia or recurrent hemorrhage.[44-46]

REFERENCES

1. Cheng Ng S, Kono DH, Paulus HE. Upper extremity manifestations of systemic vascular disorders. In: Machledge HI, ed. *Vascular Disorders of the Upper Extremity.* Mount Kisco, NY: Futura Publishing Co; 1989;305–401.
2. Churg A, Churg J, eds. *Systemic Vasculitides.* New York: Igaku-Shoin; 1991.
3. Conn DL. Vasculitic syndromes. In: Conn DL, ed. *Vasculitic Syndromes. Rheumatic Disease Clinics of North America.* Philadelphia: WB Saunders Co; 1990.
4. Calabrese LH, Clough JD. Systemic vasculitis. In: Young JR, Graor RA, Olin JW, et al, eds. *Peripheral Vascular Diseases.* St Louis, Mo: Mosby–Year Book; 1991;339–360.
5. Pariser KM, Wolff SM. The clinical spectrum of vasculitis. In: Loscalzo J, Creager MA, Dzau VJ, eds. *Vascular Medicine.* Boston: Little, Brown; 1992;1011–1048.
6. Fauci AS, Haynes BF, Katz P. The spectrum of vasculitis: clinical, pathologic, immunologic, and therapeutic considerations. *Ann Intern Med.* 1978;89:660–676.
7. Klein RG, Hunder GG, Stanson AW, et al. Large artery involvement in giant cell (temporal) arteritis. *Ann Intern Med.* 1975;83:806–812.
8. Shelhamer JH, Volkman DJ, Parrillo JE, et al. Takayasu's arteritis and its therapy. *Ann Intern Med.* 1985;103:121–126.
9. Hall S, Barr W, Lie JT, et al. Takayasu arteritis: a study of 32 North American patients. *Medicine.* 1985;64:89–99.

10. Kerr GS, Hallahan CW, Giordano JT, et al. Takayasu arteritis. *Ann Intern Med.* 1994;120:919–929.

11. Huston KA, Hunder GG, Lie JT, et al. Temporal arteritis: a 25-year epidemiologic, clinical and pathologic study. *Ann Intern Med.* 1978;88:162–167.

12. Hamrin B, Jonsson N, Landberg T. Involvement of large vessels in polymyalgia arteritica. *Lancet.* 1965;1:1193–1196.

13. Walz-Leblanc BAE, Ameli FM, Keystone EC. Giant cell arteritis presenting as limb claudication. Report and review of the literature. *J Rheumatol.* 1991;18:470–472.

14. Caselli RJ, Hunder GG, Whisnant JP. Neurologic disease in biopsy-proven giant cell (temporal) arteritis. *Neurology.* 1988;38:352–359.

15. Wilkinson IMS, Russel RWR. Arteritis of the head and neck in giant cell arteritis: a pathologic study to show the pattern of arterial involvement. *Arch Neurol.* 1972;27:378–391.

16. Fortner GS, Thiele BL. Giant cell arteritis involving the carotid artery. *Surgery.* 1984;95:759–762.

17. Save-Soderbergh J, Malmvall BE, Andersson R, et al. Giant cell arteritis as a cause of death: report of nine cases. *JAMA.* 1986;255:493–496.

18. Enzmann D, Scott WR. Intracranial involvement of giant cell arteritis. *Neurology.* 1977;27:794–797.

19. Stanson AW, Klein RG, Hunder GG. Extracranial angiographic findings in giant cell (temporal) arteritis. *Am J Roentgenol.* 1976;127:957–963.

20. Hollenhorst RW, Brown JR, Wagener HP, et al. Neurologic aspects of temporal arteritis. *Neurology.* 1960;10:490–498.

21. Hunder GG. Giant cell (temporal) arteritis. In: Conn DL, ed. *Vasculitic Syndromes. Rheumatic Disease Clinics of North America.* Philadelphia: WB Saunders Co; 1990;399–409.

22. Hall S, Hunder GG. Is temporal artery biopsy prudent? *Mayo Clin Proc.* 1984;59:793–796.

23. Birkhead NC, Wagener HP, Shick RM. Treatment of temporal arteritis with corticosteroids: results in fifty-five cases in which the lesion was proved at biopsy. *JAMA.* 1957;163:821–827.

24. Fauchald P, Rygvold O, Oystese B. Temporal arteritis and polymyalgia rheumatica: clinical and biopsy findings. *Ann Intern Med.* 1972;77:845–852.

25. Hunder GG, Sheps SG, Allen GL, et al. Daily and alternate-day corticosteroid regimens in treatment of giant cell arteritis: comparison in a prospective study. *Ann Intern Med.* 1975;82:613–618.

26. Andersson R, Malmvall BE, Bengtsson BA. Long-term survival in giant cell arteritis including temporal arteritis and polymyalgia rheumatica. A follow-up study of 90 patients treated with corticosteroids. *Acta Med Scand.* 1986;220:361–364.

27. Lupi-Herrera E, Sanchex-Torres G, Marcushamer J, et al. Takayasu's arteritis. Clinical study of 107 cases. Am Heart J. 1977;93:94–103.

28. Kieffer E, Piquois A, Bertal A, et al. Reconstructive surgery of the renal arteries in Takayasu's disease. *Ann Vasc Surg.* 1990;4:156–165.

29. Nakao K, Ikeda M, Kimata SI. Takayasu's arteritis: clinical report of eighty-four cases and immunologic studies of seven cases. *Circulation.* 1967;35:1141–1155.

30. Fraga A, Mintz G, Valle L, et al. Takayasu's arteritis: frequency of systemic manifestations (study of 22 patients) and favorable response to maintenance steroid therapy with adrenocorticosteroids (12) patients. *Arthritis Rheum.* 1972;15:617–624.

31. Hoffman GS, Leavitt RY, Kerr GS, et al. Treatment of glucocorticoid-resistant or relapsing Takayasu arteritis with methotrexate. *Arthritis Rheum.* 1994;37:578–582.

32. Kieffer E, Natali J. Supraortic trunk lesions in Takayasu's arteritis. In: Bergan JJ, Yao JST, eds. *Cerebrovascular Insufficiency.* New York: Grune & Stratton Inc; 1983;395–415.

33. Pokrovsky AV. Nonspecific aortoarteritis. In: Rutherford RB, ed. *Vacular Surgery.* 3rd ed. Philadelphia: WB Saunders Co; 1989;217–237.

34. Sharma S, Rajani M, Kaul U, et al. Initial experience with percutaneous transluminal angioplasty in the management of Takayasu's arteritis. *Br J Radiol.* 1990;63:517–522.

35. Tyagi S, Kaul UA, Nair M, et al. Balloon angioplasty of the aorta in Takayasu's arteritis: initial and long-term results. *Am Heart J.* 1992; 124:876–882.

36. Shimizu T, Erlich GE, Inaba G, et al. Behçet disease (Behçet syndrome). *Semin Arthritis Rheum.* 1979;8:223–260.

37. Durham JR, Yao JST. Aneurysms and Behçet's disease. In: *Aneurysms: New Findings and Treatments*. Norwalk, CT: Appleton & Lange; 1994;367–378.
38. O'Duffy JD, Kokmen E. *Behçet's Disease: Basic and Clinical Aspects*. New York: Marcel Dekker; 1991.
39. Yanagawa H, Kawasaki T, Shigematsu I. Nationwide survey of Kawasaki disease in Japan. *Pediatrics*. 1987;80:58–62.
40. Amano S, Hazama F, Hamashimi Y. Pathology of Kawasaki disease: II. Distribution and incidence of the vascular lesions. *Jpn Circ J*. 1987;43:741–748.
41. Newburger JW, Takahasi M, Burns JC, et al. The treatment of Kawasaki syndrome with intravenous gammaglobulin. *N Engl J Med*. 1986;315:341–347.
42. Michet CJ, McKenna CH, Luthra HS, et al. Relapsing polychondritis: survival and predictive role of early disease manifestations. *Ann Intern Med*. 1986;104:74–78.
43. Esdaile J, Hawkins D, Gold P, et al. Vascular involvement in relapsing polychondritis. *Can Med Assoc J*. 1977;116:1019–1022.
44. Cohen RD, Conn DL, Ilstrup DM. Clinical features, prognosis, and response to treatment in polyarteritis. *Mayo Clin Proc*. 1980;55:146–155.
45. McCauley RL, Johnston MR, Fauci AS. Surgical aspects of systemic and necrotizing vasculitis. *Surgery*. 1985;97:104–110.
46. Sellke FW, Williams GB, Donovan DL, et al. Management of intra-abdominal aneurysms associated with periarteritis. *J Vasc Surg*. 1986;4:294–298.

10

The Antiphospholipid Syndrome
and Peripheral Arterial Occlusion

Richard M. Green, MD, and Cynthia K. Shortell, MD

The antiphospholipid syndrome (APS) includes a number of clinical entities associated with a hypercoagulable state in which the antiphospholipid antibodies either
are markers or are in some way implicated in the thrombotic process. APS either may
result in spontaneous thrombotic events that require treatment or may have an adverse
effect on arterial reconstructions for other occlusive processes.

DEFINITIONS

APS is a syndrome originally described in patients with systemic lupus erythematosis
(SLE) and other systemic collagen vascular disorders characterized by the presence
of acquired antiphospholipid antibodies, including anticardiolipin and the "lupus
anticoagulant." These antibodies bind negatively charged or neutral phospholipids
and circulate as polyclonal immunoglobulins. The lupus anticoagulant can exist independently of any collagen vascular disease. Clinical manifestations include venous and
arterial thromboses, recurrent fetal loss, thrombocytopenia, and/or neuropsychiatric
disorders.[1,2] This syndrome occurs in a primary form when no other disease is present
or as a secondary phenomenon. Secondary APS occurs in association with autoimmune diseases, various infections including acquired immunodeficiency syndrome
(AIDS), malignant neoplasms, and drugs such as chlorpromazine.[3] Since its original
description, the umbrella of APS has expanded to include a large variety of thrombotic
conditions.[4] Those features that are relevant in the consideration of peripheral arterial
occlusion are discussed.

MECHANISM OF THROMBOTIC ARTERIAL OCCLUSION IN APS

The hemostatic–antithrombotic systems normally operate to provide hemostasis at
the site of an injury and to prevent thrombosis. In the diseased state the same mechanisms may result in thrombosis. The factors involved in this process can be divided
into two categories: (1) those effecting platelet activation and (2) those inhibiting

fibrin deposition. The former are derived mostly from the endothelium and include prostacyclin, endothelium-derived relaxing factor (EDRF), or nitric oxide and ADPase. The latter include antithrombin III; protein C and its cofactor, protein S; tissue pathway inhibitor (TFPI); and the fibrinolytic system.[5]

Rudolf Virchow postulated in 1856 that the three components of vascular thrombosis were vessel wall abnormalities, diminished blood flow, and increased coagulability of the blood.[6] This triad remains valid today, even though arterial and venous thromboses have some distinguishing pathogenetic elements. Stasis, or reduced blood flow, is the most important factor in the pathogenesis of venous thrombosis. The venous thrombus itself is composed of fibrin and red blood cells, with relatively few platelets. Changes in the vessel wall are not readily apparent. In contrast, an arterial thrombus consists mainly of platelets, with very little fibrin and red blood cells. Abnormalities in the arterial wall, usually due to atherosclerotic plaques, supersede hypercoagulability in the pathogenesis of an arterial thrombus.[4] These distinctions help explain why venous thrombosis is far more common than arterial occlusion in patients with the inherited hypercoagulable states, that is, antithrombin III, protein C or S deficiency, and fibrinolytic abnormalities.

Antithrombin III is a protein synthesized in the liver and excreted in the urine and functions as a direct antagonist of thrombin. Deficiency states may be primary or secondary, as with severe liver failure or the nephrotic syndrome. Protein C increases fibrinolytic activity and inhibits the formation of thrombin.[7] Protein S is a cofactor that is necessary for protein C to exert its antithrombin effect.[8] Arterial occlusions can occur in these hypercoagulable patients, especially those with protein S deficiency. Two series have been reported in which patients under 45 years of age found to be heterozygous for protein S deficiency presented with arterial thrombosis with no other risk factors for atherosclerosis.[9,10] Finally, arterial thromboemboli may originate in the venous system and travel through a patent foramen ovale. In a series of patients under the age of 55 with ischemic stroke, the incidence of a patent foramen ovale was 40% as compared to a 10% prevalence in a control group without stroke.[11] Aside from these cases of clinical overlap, arterial thrombosis is usually the result of abnormalities of the vessel wall and/or the platelets, and venous thrombosis is the result of abnormal coagulation.

The autoantibodies associated with APS have been established as a causative factor in arterial thrombosis only in patients with SLE. All other associations remain controversial, since many patients followed up for long periods have antiphospholipid antibodies without subsequent thrombosis. Likewise, the mechanism of arterial thrombosis in patients with APS is unknown. In a study comparing patients with arterial manifestations of APS with a time-matched cohort of patients with atherosclerotic arterial disease, it was found that the patients with APS tended to be young female nonsmokers who had a higher than expected incidence of upper extremity arterial involvement, cerebrovascular disease with varying angiographic patterns, and unexplained bypass graft failure.[12] Eliminating the patients with SLE from this study may well change the conclusions, and therefore no solid evidence exists that the APS autoantibodies are themselves thrombogenic. Prospective longitudinal studies in patients with the antiphospholipid antibodies are required to determine the actual risk of thrombosis.

Although direct clinical evidence is lacking, there are experimental data indicating that patients with APS are hypercoagulable. For instance, urinary metabolites of both platelet-derived thromboxane A_2 and vascular-derived prostacyclin demonstrate an increase in thromboxane A_2 in patients with APS.[13] Also, the common association of thrombocytopenia suggests that platelet activation and consumption are occurring in areas of thrombus formation. Alternatively, the thrombocytopenia may be the result of platelet destruction as the antiphospholipid antibodies bind to the phospholipids on the platelet membrane and the complex is destroyed by the reticuloendothelial system.[14] Finally, immunoglobulin fractions from patients with APS often react with endothelial cells and may have an adverse effect on the antithrombotic capabilities of the endothelium.[15] Inhibition of the thrombomodulin-dependent protein C activation,[16] inhibition of prostacyclin release,[17] induction of procoagulant tissue factor expression,[18] and von Willebrand factor release[12] have all been documented. Despite these interesting observations, no specific biochemical or platelet abnormality has been irrefutably associated with antiphospholipid antibodies, which may only be markers of a thrombotic tendency rather than the cause.[3]

DIAGNOSIS OF APS

The diagnosis of APS should be suspected in any patient with an unusual presentation of venous or arterial thrombosis. This would include young patients, those with a family history of thrombosis, those with associated medical problems (particularly autoimmune diseases), those with thromboses in unusual sites, those with no known risk factors for atherosclerosis, those resistant to conventional anticoagulant therapy, those with a history of spontaneous abortion, and those with an unexplained early occlusion of an arterial reconstruction (Table 10–1). Thromboses can occur in any artery, but most arteries report the highest involvement in the cerebral and extremity vessels.

Since the work-up is quite expensive, clinical judgment is important and a shotgun approach should not be used. Search for an underlying systemic disorder is important in establishing a cause and a possible solution for the hypercoagulable state. A partial thromboplastin time (PTT), prothrombin time (PT), and platelet count should be routinely obtained. The PTT and, less frequently, the PTs may be elevated. This is not associated with an increased risk for hemorrhage unless thrombocytopenia is also present.[9] The antibodies produce an elevation in the PTT because they interfere with the phospholipid-dependent coagulation factors. Testing for the hereditary deficiency syndromes, such as antithrombin III and proteins C and S, should be done when clinically indicated, especially in patients with venous thrombosis. Investigations in patients with arterial thrombosis should begin identifying possible platelet or vascular abnormalities. The different approaches to arterial and venous thromboses are merely guidelines, since the distinctions between the two are not absolute.

TABLE 10–1. CLINICAL CLUES IN THE DIAGNOSIS OF ANTIPHOSPHOLIPID SYNDROME

Young patients
Familial history of thrombosis
Autoimmune disorders
Thromboses in unusual sites
Absent risk factors for atherosclerosis
Resistance to anticoagulants
History of spontaneous abortion
Unexplained early failure of arterial reconstruction

TABLE 10–2. DEMOGRAPHIC DIFFERENCES BETWEEN THE POPULATIONS OF PATIENTS WITH ATHEROSCLEROSIS AND ANTIPHOSPHOLIPID SYNDROME

Characteristic	Atherosclerosis (n = 1,078)	Antiphospholipid Syndrome (n = 19)	P Value
Age (y)	63.6 ± 0.4	46.2 ± 3.3	<.0001
% Female	411 (38%)	13 (68%)	<.02
Cigarette smokers	700 (65%)	1 (5%)	<.0001
Upper/lower extremity involvement	13 (1%)	8/18 (44%)*	<.0001

* One patient had disease involving carotid artery only, without extremity lesions.
Adapted from Shortell CK, Ouriel K, Green RM, et al. Vascular disease in the antiphospholipid syndrome: a comparison with the patient population with atherosclerosis. *J Vasc Surg.* 1992;15:158–166.

Since clinical hematology laboratories evaluate bleeding rather than thrombotic tendencies, the detection of the thrombotic state is difficult. Furthermore, although experimental evidence suggests that increased levels of circulating coagulation factors are thrombogenic, a causal relationship among thrombosis and thrombocytosis, a shortened bleeding time, PTT or PT, or increased amounts of individual clotting factors has not been established.[19] Increased plasma levels of fibrinogen and factor VIII have been found to be markers for risk of stroke and myocardial infarction, but no causal relationship with thrombogenesis has been established.[20,21] As clinical experience grows with the more sensitive indicators of thrombin generation, such as radioimmunoassays for plasma fibrinopeptide A, prothrombin fragments F_1 and F_2, and the thrombin–antithrombin complex, the true relationship between the APS antibodies and the coagulation system will be better defined.[22]

THE RELATIONSHIP OF APS TO THE VASCULAR SURGEON

Vascular surgeons are likely to encounter patients with APS in two settings. A patient may present for treatment with an arterial or venous occlusion, or APS may have an adverse effect on a reconstruction. There are some important demographic differences between the atherosclerotic patient population that normally visits a vascular surgeon and the population with APS. These differences are described in Table 10–2. They show a preponderance of young women in the APS group, which makes sense since the most common autoantibody identified is the lupus anticoagulant.

TABLE 10–3. SCREENING FOR THE HYPERCOAGULABLE STATE IN THE VASCULAR SURGICAL PATIENT

Platelet count
Prothrombin time
Partial thromboplastin time
Antithrombin III
Protein C
Protein S
Anticardiolipin antibody
Lupus anticoagulant
Heparin-induced platelet aggregation

TABLE 10–4. INCIDENCE OF HYPERCOAGULABLE STATES IN VASCULAR SURGICAL POPULATIONS[a]

Laboratory Abnormality	Boston, Mass[24]	Rochester, NY[12]
Anticardiolipin antibody	0/42	16/19
Lupus anticoagulant	18/42	10/19
Platelet count <150,000	NR	3/19
Prolonged PTT	NR	8/19
Antithrombin III deficiency	3/42	NM
Protein C deficiency	11/42	NM
Protein S deficiency	4/42	NM
Heparin-induced platelet activation	5/42	NM

[a]NR indicates not reported; PTT, partial thromboplastin time; NM, not measured routinely.

The possibility that the APS and the hypercoagulable state may have an adverse effect on the results of arterial reconstruction was first suggested by Donaldson et al.[23] They identified 27 *in situ* vein grafts that failed within the first 30 postoperative days. Nine of these failures (33%) were probably due to a hypercoagulable state. This preliminary study led to a screening program designed to identify the significance of these syndromes in a vascular surgical practice. One hundred fifty-eight patients underwent preoperative screening as listed in Table 10–3 and abnormalities were detected in 15 patients (9%).[24] There were 5 patients with lupus anticoagulant autoantibodies, 4 with heparin-induced platelet activation, 4 with protein C deficiency, 2 with antithrombin III deficiency, and 1 with protein S deficiency. A variety of arterial procedures were performed on 137 of the 158 patients and postoperative thromboses occurred in 11 of these patients (8%). There were 5 infrainguinal graft occlusions, 2 myocardial infarctions, 3 strokes, and 1 deep venous thrombosis. Three of the 14 patients (21%) previously identified as hypercoagulable sustained graft thrombosis as compared to a 2% incidence of graft thrombosis in the patients with normal coagulation tests. These results were confirmed after a review of 9 patients with APS undergoing 12 peripheral arterial operations at the University of Rochester (NY).[12] The mean graft patency in the group of patients who underwent lower extremity bypass, either aortoiliac or femoropopliteal, was only 5.5 months. Technical errors and inadequate

TABLE 10–5. TREATMENT OF THE HYPERCOAGULABLE SYNDROMES IN THE VASCULAR SURGICAL PATIENT

Syndrome	Treatment
Antithrombin III deficiency	Intravenous heparin and fresh-frozen plasma; concentrate effective in hip surgery, role in peripheral arterial reconstruction unclear
Protein C or S deficiency	Perioperative heparin and long-term warfarin
Antiphospholipid (lupus anticoagulant or anticardiolipin antibody)	Warfarin until antibody levels are no longer detectable; heparin and aspirin in the perioperative period; steroids and cyclophosphamide (Cytoxan) controversial but may be effective against underlying autoimmune process
Unexplained graft failure with no hematologic abnormalities	Chronic warfarin therapy, although no convincing data exist

RIGHT FOOT   **LEFT FOOT**

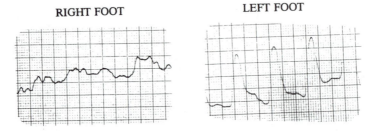

Figure 10–1. Digital photoplethysmography in a patient with ischemic toes and a lupus anticoagulant. The wave forms are flattened, suggestive of digital artery emboli. The wave forms in each toe are flattened on the right foot. The left side is normal, as seen in this representative sampling.

inflow/outflow were ruled out as causes of failure in each of these patients at the time of revision. These poor results compare to an early occlusion rate of only 3% in a time-matched cohort of patients undergoing similar operations but without APS. The specific entities in the patients with graft occlusions are listed in Table 10–4. Both series underestimate the true incidence of these abnormalities because of incomplete screening. Nonetheless, these data suggest that APS has an adverse effect on the results of arterial reconstruction.

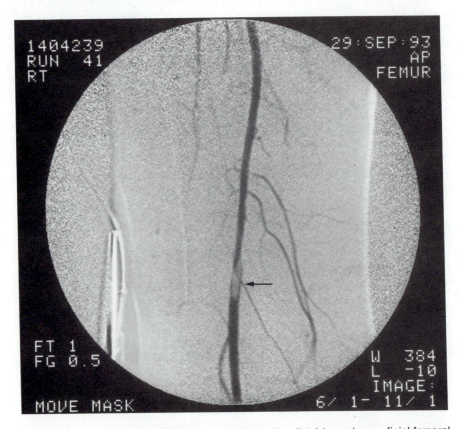

Figure 10–2. An arteriogram showing a thrombus in the distal (arrow) superficial femoral artery.

TREATMENT OF ARTERIAL THROMBOSIS IN ASSOCIATION WITH APS

The treatment of arterial or graft occlusions in association with APS should be directed at reducing the thrombotic potential. Patients with deficiency syndromes are treated with both anticoagulants and replacement therapy. Antithrombin III deficiency should be treated with intravenous heparin and fresh-frozen plasma in the perioperative period.[25] Exogenous antithrombin III is available and is effective in reducing venous thrombosis following joint replacement.[26] Administration of antithrombin III concentrate at the time of arterial reconstruction and chronic therapy with warfarin have not been proven effective. Patients with protein C or S deficiency are managed with perioperative heparin and long-term warfarin therapy.

The presence of autoantibodies complicates therapy since reduced levels would seem desirable, even though direct evidence of the thrombotic potential of these antibodies is not available. There is evidence that patients with APS and either arterial or venous thrombosis should be treated with warfarin until antiphospholipid antibody levels are no longer detectable.[27] The role of prophylactic warfarin in patients with antibody but no thrombosis is controversial.[28] Since the incidence of subsequent thrombosis is around 25%, this risk must be balanced against the risk of complications from the anticoagulation. Our bias is to treat patients with antiphospholipid antibodies with warfarin prior to a thrombotic episode, since we have observed two untreated

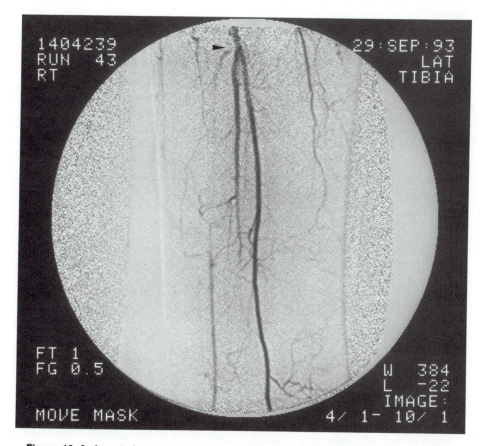

Figure 10–3. An arteriogram showing a proximal occlusion of the anterior (arrowhead) and posterior tibial arteries and a patent posterior tibial artery.

patients with APS and spontaneous retinal artery thrombosis.[12] The use of parenteral steroids and immunosuppressive agents is controversial.[29] APS patients undergoing arterial reconstruction should be treated with both antiplatelet and anticoagulant therapies. Occasionally, a patient presents with an early bypass graft failure with no explanation. No technical errors are identified and no inflow or outflow lesions are present. Hematologic work-up is normal. This patient is probably hypercoagulable and should be treated with warfarin after graft revision or replacement. These principles are outlined in Table 10–5.

A REPRESENTATIVE CASE REPORT OF ARTERIAL OCCLUSION IN A PATIENT WITH APS

A.K. is a 54-year-old white female with a history of SLE, recurrent deep venous thromboses, and diabetes mellitus. This patient was maintained on 20 mg/d prednisone. The patient presented with ischemic toes on her right foot. Digital photoplethysmography (Fig. 10–1) showed flattening of the wave forms in all five toes. The femoral pulse was normal and the popliteal and pedal pulses were present but weak. The ankle/brachial index was 0.85 on the affected side and 1.16 on the other leg. Segmental pressure measurements indicated a stenosis or occlusion in the distal superficial femo-

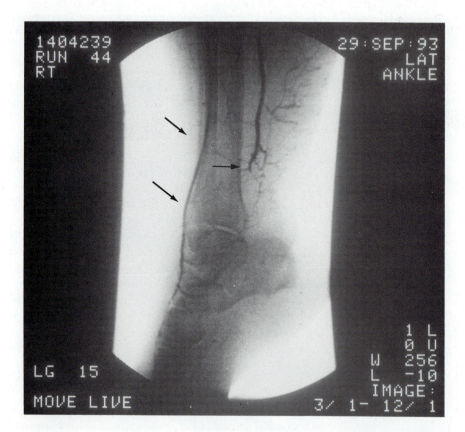

Figure 10–4. An arteriogram showing reconstitution of the anterior tibial artery (ATA) and a distal occlusion of the posterior tibial artery (PTA). The anterior artery reconstitutes the ATA and the PTA occludes abruptly at the ankle.

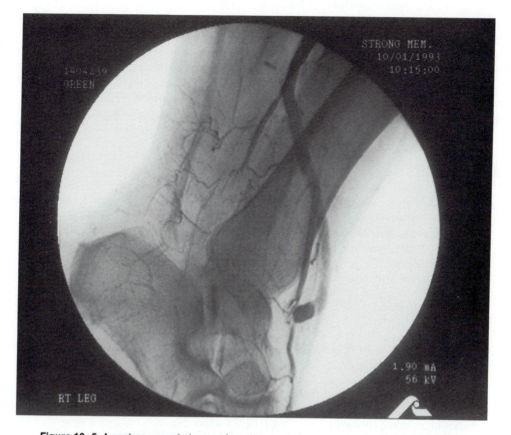

Figure 10–5. A saphenous vein bypass from the posterior tibial artery to the dorsalis pedis artery restored flow to the foot.

ral artery. Hematologic work-up demonstrated an elevated PTT and a high lupus anticoagulant titer. An arteriogram was performed which showed a thrombus in the distal superficial femoral artery (Fig. 10–2), occlusion of the proximal anterior tibial artery (Fig. 10–3), and a distal occlusion of the posterior tibial artery with reconstitution of the anterior tibial artery (Fig. 10–4). The patient was treated with aspirin and intravenous heparin. At the time of operation, the dorsalis pedis artery was explored and was found to be a very small vessel, as suggested on the digital film of the foot (Fig. 10–5). The lateral plantar artery was then identified and was patent. The popliteal artery was explored and an old thrombus was extracted with a balloon catheter. The posterior tibial vessel could not be thrombectomized, and a short graft was created between the distal posterior tibial artery and the lateral plantar artery using a segment of saphenous vein. The heparin and aspirin were continued in the perioperative period. The patient had an uneventful recovery with healing of her toes. She is currently being maintained on warfarin.

CONCLUSION

APS is a syndrome that must be recognized by those treating patients with vascular disease. Although the antibodies themselves may not be the cause of the thrombosis, these patients are hypercoagulable. Venous thrombosis is the most common problem encountered, but arterial occlusions do occur. These arterial lesions are often in a younger patient population without the usual atherosclerotic risk factors. The vascular surgeon will see most patients with APS when a reconstruction fails for unknown causes. When any of these patients requires reconstruction, both anticoagulant and antiplatelet therapies are indicated. Chronic warfarin therapy is required postoperatively as long as antibody levels are present, which is lifelong for most patients.

REFERENCES

1. Bowie EJW, Thompson JH, Pascuzzi CA, et al. Thrombosis in systemic lupus despite circulating anticoagulants. *J Lab Clin Med.* 1963;62:416–430.
2. Love PE, Santoro SA. Antiphospholipid antibodies: anticardiolipin and the lupus anticoagulant in systemic lupus erythematosus (SLE) and in non-SLE disorders. *Ann Intern Med.* 1990;112:682–698.
3. Schafer AI. The hypercoagulable states. *Ann Intern Med.* 1985;102:814–828.
4. Asherson RA, Cervera R. The antiphospholipid syndrome: a syndrome in evolution. *Ann Rheum Dis.* 1992;51:147–150.
5. Schafer AI, Kroll MH. Nonatheromatous arterial thrombosis. *Annu Rev Med.* 1993; 44:155–170.
6. Virchow R. *Gesammelte Abhandlungen zur Wissenschaftlichen Medizineschem.* Frankfurt, Germany: Meidinger Sohn; 1856.
7. Broekmans AW, Veltkamp JJ, Bertina RM. Congenital protein C deficiency and venous thromboembolism: a study of three Dutch families. *N Engl J Med.* 1983;309:340–344.
8. Comp PC, Esmon CT. Recurrent venous thromboembolism in patients with a partial deficiency of protein S. *N Engl J Med.* 1984;311:1525–1528.
9. Allaart CF, Aronson DC, Ruys T, et al. Hereditary protein S deficiency in young adults with arterial occlusive disease. *Thromb Haemostasis.* 1990;64:206–210.
10. Wiesel ML, Borg JY, Grunebaum L, et al. Influence of protein S deficiency on the arterial thrombosis risk. *Presse Med.* 1991;20:1023–1027.
11. Lechat P, Mas JL, Lascault G, et al. Prevalence of patent foramen ovale in patients with stroke. *N Engl J Med.* 1988;318:1148–1152.
12. Shortell CK, Ouriel K, Green RM, et al. Vascular disease in the antiphospholipid syndrome: a comparison with the patient population with atherosclerosis. *J Vasc Surg.* 1992;15:158–166.
13. Lellouche F, Martinuzzo J, Markiewicz W, et al. Imbalance of thromboxane/prostacyclin biosynthesis in patients with lupus anticoagulant. *Blood.* 1991;78:2894–2899.
14. Harris EN, Asherson RA, Hughes GRV. Antiphospholipid antibodies. *Clin Rheum Dis.* 1985;11:591–609.
15. McCrae KR, DeMichele A, Samuels P, et al. Detection of endothelial cell-reactive immunoglobulin in patients with lupus anticoagulant. *Br J Haematol.* 1991;79:595–605.
16. Cariou R, Tobelem G, Bellucci S, et al. Effect of lupus anticoagulant on antithrombogenic properties of endothelial cells—inhibition of thrombomodulin-dependent protein C activation. *Thromb Haemostasis.* 1988;60:54–58.
17. Watson KV, Schorer AE. Lupus anticoagulant inhibition of in vitro prostacyclin release is associated with a thrombosis-prone subset of patients. *Am J Med.* 1991;90:47–53.
18. Tannenbaum SH, Finko R, Cines DB. Antibody and immune complexes induce tissue factor production by human endothelial cells. *J Immunol.* 1986;137:1532–1538.
19. Ratnoff OD. The role of haemostatic mechanisms. *Clin Haematol.* 1981;10:261–281.
20. Wilhelmsen L, Svardsudd K, Korsan-Bengtsen K, et al. Fibrinogen as a risk factor for stroke and myocardial infarction. *N Engl J Med.* 1984;311:501–550.
21. Meade TW, North WRS, Chakrabarti R. Hemostatic function and cardiovascular death: early results of a prospective study. *Lancet.* 1980;1:1050–1054.
22. Lowe GDO. Laboratory evaluation of hypercoagulability. *Clin Haematol.* 1981;10:407–442.

23. Donaldson MC, Weinberg DS, Belkin M, et al. Screening for hypercoagulable states in vascular surgical practice: a preliminary study. *J Vasc Surg.* 1990;11:825–831.
24. Whittemore AD, Donaldson MC, Mannick JA. Detection and treatment of hypercoagulable states: can they improve infrainguinal bypass results? In: Veith FJ, ed. *Current Critical Problems in Vascular Surgery,* vol. 3. St. Louis, MO: Quality Medical Publishing, 1991;81–85.
25. Towne JB, Bernhard VM, Hussey C, et al. Antithrombin III deficiency—a cause of unexplained thrombosis in vascular surgery. *Surgery.* 1981;89:735–742.
26. Francis CW. Antithrombin III: clinical trials. In: *Research Initiatives in Vascular Disease.* Bethesda, Md: National Heart, Lung and Blood Institute–National Institutes of Health; 1990;41–44.
27. Elias M, Eldor A. Thromboembolism in patients with the "lupus"-type circulating anticoagulant. *Arch Intern Med.* 1984;144:510–551.
28. Asherson RA, Chan JHK, Harris EN, et al. Anticardiolipin antibody, recurrent thrombosis, and warfarin withdrawal. *Ann Rheum Dis.* 1985;44:823–825.
29. Ahn SS, Kalunian K, Rosove M, et al. Postoperative thrombotic complications in patients with the lupus anticoagulant: increased risk after vascular procedures. *J Vasc Surg.* 1988;7:749–756.

11

Popliteal Artery Pathology

Walter J. McCarthy, MD, and Richard R. Keen, MD

Arterial pathology of the popliteal space is sufficiently unique to warrant detailed consideration. Although the conditions for discussion are different in their mechanism and treatment, grouping them in a single chapter allows easy reference when such pathology is encountered. Abnormalities of the arterial wall are presented with details of popliteal aneurysm management and the entity of cystic adventitial disease. Conditions arising because of the popliteal artery's intimate relationship to the knee joint and musculature include popliteal entrapment and the management of popliteal injury associated with knee dislocation. Finally, some comments on popliteal artery exposure emphasizing the less familiar posterior approach are useful for popliteal exposure in selected cases.

POPLITEAL ANEURYSM

Popliteal aneurysms have challenged surgeons since antiquity. The first reported surgical intervention was by Antyllus in the second century AD, with ligation above and below the aneurysm sac. Paré espoused proximal ligation only, as did John Hunter. Hunter's technique of proximal ligation was utilized for more than a century and was reported to result in approximately 10% limb loss. In 1888 Rudolph Matas first performed the technique of endoaneurysmorrhaphy, successfully reducing the aneurysm size while maintaining flow. This method reportedly reduced limb loss to about 5%.[1]

Popliteal aneurysms are the second most common arterial aneurysm after those involving the abdominal aorta. They compose about 70% of aneurysms peripheral to the aorta.[2] Almost all popliteal aneurysms are atherosclerotic, reflected by 231 of 233 in a recent series by Wychulis et al.[3] Approximately one-half of popliteal aneurysms are bilateral, with a range reported between 38% and 58%. One must always suspect and examine for other arterial aneurysms once a popliteal aneurysm is located, and about one-half of patients will have an abdominal aortic aneurysm concurrently.

Retrospective surgical series usually report that more than one-half of their patients have had symptomatic popliteal aneurysms. Evans et al[4] noted thrombosis in 36%, distal emboli in 25%, and frank popliteal aneurysm rupture in 7% of patients from an atypical retrospective review. This distinction is worthwhile, as patients presenting with thrombosis are considerably more likely to have amputation as a final outcome. Gifford and associates[5] found that 8 of 24 limbs operated on for ischemia ended with eventual amputation. Other symptoms related to this pathology include individuals with large popliteal aneurysms who occasionally present complaining of leg swelling from popliteal vein compression or even with frank deep venous thrombosis. In addition, occasionally large aneurysms cause neurological compression resulting in calf pain.

The exact definition of a popliteal aneurysm must be based on comparison with the normal adjacent artery. Generally, aneurysms are defined as those vessels greater than 2 cm in diameter or 1.5 times the diameter of the normal adjacent superficial femoral artery.

The natural history of popliteal aneurysms is to eventually thrombose or embolize into the distal arterial circulation. For this reason most authors recommend surgical correction once the diagnosis has been established in a reasonable-risk patient. This seemingly sound advice is occasionally questioned[6] and recently Hands and Collin[7] have proposed observation for asymptomatic aneurysms because of graft failure and resulting limb loss in some cases. They reported amputation after elective repair in 3 of 11 limbs with asymptomatic popliteal aneurysms. These results are in contrast to much higher success rates in other series.[8] Thus, the recommendation to proceed with repair of asymptomatic aneurysms is predicted on the assumption of good locally achievable results.

The surgical approach to popliteal aneurysms is almost always by way of the medial exposure. Popliteal aneurysms without involvement of the superficial femoral artery are usually managed by aneurysm ligation and a saphenous vein interposition graft. The saphenous vein is anastomosed either end to side or end to end to the distal superficial femoral artery and the below-knee popliteal artery. After bypass the popliteal artery is ligated above and below the knee to isolate the artery. Actual surgical removal of the popliteal aneurysm is usually not necessary unless the aneurysm is large enough to cause nerve or bypass graft compression. In some cases subcutaneous graft tunneling, following lessons learned from the *in situ* technique, allow grafting around a large ligated popliteal aneurysm.

Angiographic evaluation of patients with popliteal aneurysm often provides successful anatomic visualization to about the knee level and then dilution of contrast within the aneurysm and no below-knee popliteal or tibial visualization (Fig. 11–1). The surgeon should not despair at these findings and will almost always find vessels for a distal anastomosis by using intraoperative angiography and exploration. Should the popliteal artery be occluded, femoral-to-tibia bypass grafting will provide useful revascularization. Recently, the use of thrombolytic therapy has been reported to be successful related to popliteal aneurysm management.[1] The technique seems most appropriate for patients who have moderate, not severe, ischemia at the time of presentation, that is, patients who will tolerate 12 to 24 hours of observation during the thrombolytic process. Successful thrombolysis may open recently thrombosed popliteal and tibial vessels, allowing a more successful standard surgical repair (Fig. 11–2).

Surgical results and long-term graft patency depend on the anatomy at surgical intervention. Shortell et al[8] recently reviewed a 25-year experience in Rochester, NY, and emphasized this point. One-year graft patency comparing emergency versus elective surgery was 69% versus 100%. Stratification by runoff showed a 3-year patency with good runoff of 89% compared to 30% if the runoff was poor. These findings validate the general recommendations that popliteal aneurysms should be repaired

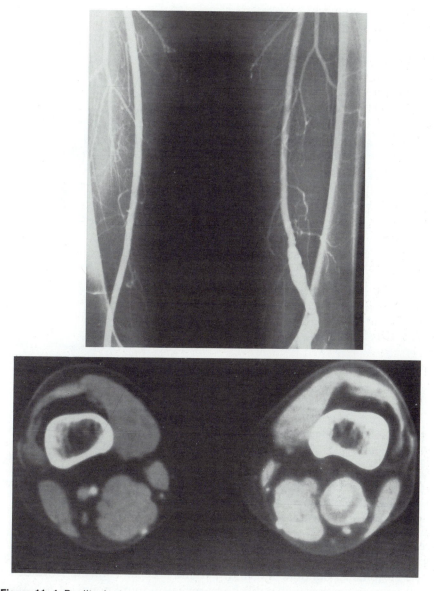

Figure 11–1. Popliteal artery aneurysms that appear small on arteriography are frequently lined with laminated thrombus, as demonstrated here by CT scan.

once they are diagnosed and before they thrombose or embolize, destroying the distal circulation.

ADVENTITIAL CYSTIC DISEASE

Adventitial cystic disease of the popliteal artery is a very unusual condition; approximately 200 cases have been reviewed in the world literature. The first of these was reported by Hierton and Lindberg[9] in 1957. The conduct of this case, operated on in Stockholm, Sweden, in 1953, was described by the author as "proceeding with a

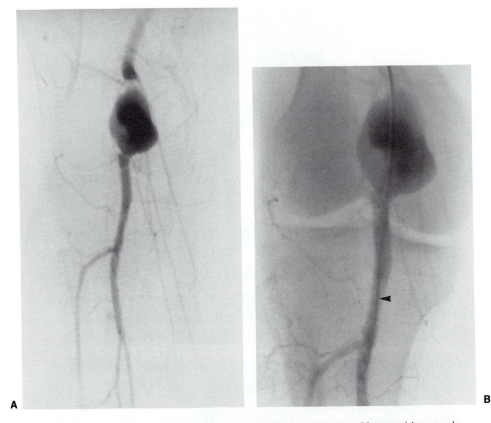

Figure 11–2. (A) Arteriography reveals a popliteal aneurysm in a 56-year-old man who presented with right foot rest pain and a pulsatile mass in his right popliteal fossa. The right leg arteries were not imaged beyond the level of the midleg, suggesting distal embolization of thrombus. **(B)** Placement of an infusion catheter distal to the aneurysm (arrowhead) permitted the infusion of urokinase to the occluded distal arteries. (*Figure continues*)

transverse incision in an apparently thickened artery and releasing two thimbles full of raspberry jelly–like material."[10] Charles Rob, then a professor of surgery at St Mary's Hospital in London, England, became familiar with the work of Hierton and Lindberg and together they published a review of four known cases in the *British Journal of Surgery* in 1957.[10,11] Beginning in 1969 the Division of Vascular Surgery at Northwestern University Medical School (Chicago, Ill) began to record incidental cases involving adventitial cystic disease from around the world. This resulted in a paper by Flanigan et al,[10] published in 1979, which summarized 115 cases collected by distributing newsletters on this topic worldwide in 1975 and 1976. Surgeons were asked to communicate their findings and observations related to the management of adventitial cystic disease.

Adventitial cystic disease affects young patients, primarily men, who typically present with claudication in their third decade. Symptoms may be quite pronounced if arterial occlusion has occurred or may fluctuate with changes in symptoms. Along with these symptomatic changes, occasionally the ankle brachial index may actually be seen to fluctuate on repeated office examination. Ishikawa et al[12] noticed that forceful dorsiflexion of the ankle often causes pulse loss when this condition is present. Eastcott[10,13] observed the presence of a posterior popliteal murmur related to stenosis. After physical examination, evaluation by duplex scanning is recommended and either

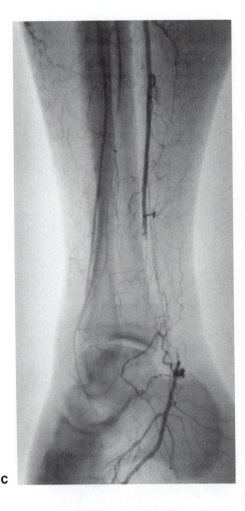

C

Figure 11–2. (*continued*) (**C**) After 48 hours in thrombolytic therapy the rest pain had resolved. Repeat arteriography demonstrated lysis of the clot in the posterior tibial artery at the ankle.

computed tomography (CT) scan or magnetic resonance imaging is excellent as a second diagnostic modality. Once the diagnosis has been confirmed, angiography should be undertaken to plan surgical repair. At angiography a half-moon–shaped near-occlusion of the popliteal artery caused by cystic compression has been termed "the scimitar sign" after an ancient curved sword (Fig. 11–3).

Treatment of popliteal compression by an adventitial cyst is generally best obtained by surgical exposure. Alternative proposals have included blind needle aspiration, performed in 1965, followed more recently by CT-guided aspiration techniques. Aspiration could theoretically be curative but is usually technically difficult. Percutaneous transluminal angioplasty (PTLA) seems intuitively wrong and has been demonstrated to fail in this application. PTLA and CT-guided aspiration leave the adventitial cyst unrelieved and are quite susceptible to fluid reaccumulation. Operative approaches may best be divided into arterial resection and nonresection techniques. In the review by Flanigan et al[10] of 115 cases, the exact operative technique could be ascertained for 98. Of these, 42 underwent arterial resection, with 30 having vein graft interposition. Seven patients had synthetic material placed, 2 had arterial homografts, and 3 had end-to-end anastomosis as their repair. The 56 nonresectable cases involved cystic incision or in some cases excision with patch angioplasty of a weakened arterial wall. Of these 98 patients, although follow-up was obviously sketchy, only 1 was reported to have undergone leg amputation and 2 patients were found to claudi-

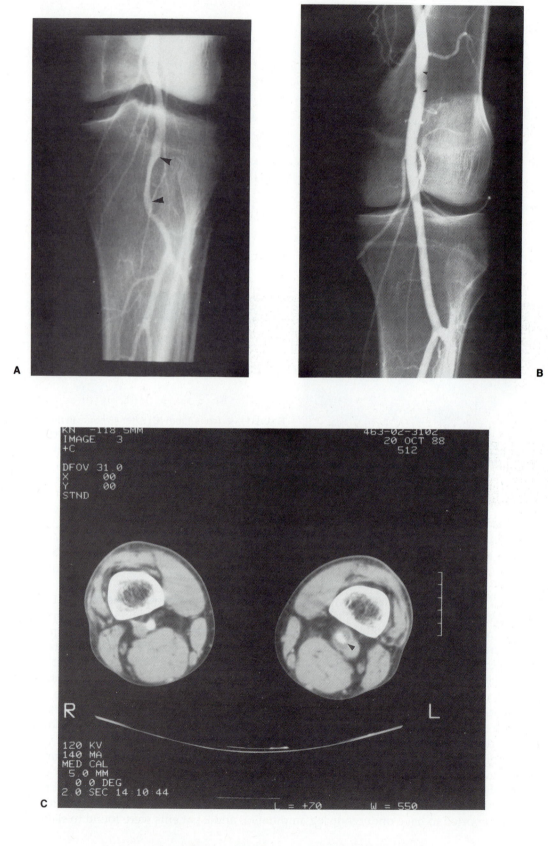

cate. Approximately 10% of the patients with cyst resection alone required reoperation because of cyst fluid reaccumulation.

A recent useful adjunct to standard treatment has been the lysis of occluding thrombus by urokinase. Samson and Willis[14] reported a patient presenting with sudden onset of claudication, an adventitial cyst, and popliteal artery thrombosis. After lytic therapy the characteristic scimitar sign replaced an arterial blockage and standard surgical treatment resulted in normal leg function.

The etiology of adventitial cystic disease is still open to speculation. Workable theories include a posttraumatic condition, expansion of an embryonic rest of cells, or formation of a ganglia related to the knee joint or tendon sheaths. The concept of a ganglion is perhaps the most attractive, because occasionally during dissection a distinct communication can be seen between the knee joint and the affected arterial segment. DeLaurentis et al[15] have described the material within the adventitial cyst as acid mucopolysaccharide and hyaluronic acid radicals.

POPLITEAL VASCULAR INJURY

Popliteal vascular injuries are both common and significant. Injuries of the popliteal artery account for one-quarter of all extremity arterial injuries significant enough to require repair with an interposition graft.[16] In recent series the rate of limb loss for all civilian extremity arterial injuries has been as low as 3%. However, popliteal artery injuries are associated with limb loss rates as high as 12%[17] to 22%.[18] It has been shown that 50% of all extremity vascular injuries that require amputation involve the popliteal artery.[16]

Unique anatomic features of the popliteal region make it extremely susceptible to limb-threatening trauma and explain why popliteal vascular injuries carry such an inordinately high risk of limb loss.[19] First, the presence of a single axial artery in the popliteal region makes any arterial injury in this location more likely to completely interrupt arterial flow to the leg. Injuries in the thigh, where both the superficial and profunda femoral arteries exist, or the leg, where the three tibial vessels perfuse the distal extremity, are less likely to completely interrupt lower leg perfusion. The perigenicular and gastrocnemius arteries, which serve as the collateral supply around the knee, are small and easily compromised by any associated skeletal or soft tissue trauma. These features makes the popliteal region especially susceptible to ischemia after penetrating trauma.

The popliteal artery begins at the adductor magnus tendon and ends at the bifurcation into the posterior tibial and peroneal arteries. The tibioperoneal trunk is usually considered a portion of the popliteal artery for discussion purposes. Blunt trauma is responsible for approximately 70% of all civilian popliteal arterial injuries.[17]

Figure 11–3. (A) The scimitar sign and intraluminal contrast filling the popliteal artery lumen in the shape of the named saber (arrowhead) suggest adventitial cystic disease of the popliteal artery. **(B)** Arteriography is not always diagnostic in adventitial cystic disease of the popliteal artery (arrowheads). **(C)** In this case CT scan demonstrated adventitial cystic disease (arrowhead). **(B** and **C** reprinted with permission from Rizzo FJ, Flinn WR, Yao JST, et al. Computed tomography for the evaluation of arterial disease in the popliteal fossa. J Vasc Surg. 1990;11:112–119.)

The popliteal artery is unusually susceptible to skeletal injuries because it is tethered to the distal femoral shaft by the adductor magnus tendon and to the tibia by the tendonous arch of the soleus muscle. Consequently, knee dislocations—the most common type of severe blunt trauma observed in this region—distal femur fractures, and proximal tibial–fibular fractures can all result in direct injury, stretching, or entrapment[20] of these arteries. Arterial injuries occur in 23% to 32% of knee dislocations[21] but arterial injuries accompany only 2% of tibial–fibular fractures and less than 1% of femoral fractures.[22]

Complex skeletal, nerve, or soft tissue injuries will render some limbs sustaining popliteal artery injuries unsalvageable. Both associated fractures and shock are associated with increased rates of limb loss in injuries to the popliteal vessels.[23] However, prompt recognition and repair of popliteal artery injuries has been demonstrated to improve limb salvage in these patients. The critical variable in optimizing limb salvage after popliteal injury is minimizing the length of time of severe limb ischemia.[18,23] In the series reported by Downs and MacDonald[18] no patient among 19 with severe ischemia revascularized in less than 6 hours required amputation, while 13 of 39 patients (33%) treated after 6 hours of ischemia sustained limb loss.

Careful physical examination appears sensitive in detecting limb-threatening ischemia after popliteal artery injury. Treiman et al[21] found that 23 of 29 patients with knee dislocations and an abnormal ipsilateral pedal pulse had a popliteal artery injury on arteriography. Eighty-six additional patients with normal pedal pulses underwent arteriography, and while no arteriographic abnormalities were found in 77 patients, 5 patients had arterial spasm and 4 had intimal flaps. None of these 86 patients with normal pulses, managed without operation, sustained an adverse outcome.

Routine arteriography in all cases of posterior knee dislocation remains a useful protocol but has been challenged not only by this recent series[21] but also by several others, which claimed that physical examination was adequate in determining which patients required popliteal arteriography. Dennis et al[24] reviewed 37 patients with posterior knee dislocation secondary to blunt trauma and found that the information from arteriography did not alter management in any case. Seven patients with arteriographic findings of isolated intimal defects or vasospasm were managed without operation or anticoagulation with no adverse outcomes.[24] The presence of normal pulses found after reduction of a knee dislocation, when limb ischemia existed prior to reduction, does not negate the need for arteriography to diagnose a popliteal artery injury that requires operative treatment.[25]

The operative approach for popliteal vascular trauma may be by either a medial or posterior approach. Straightforward isolated popliteal artery injuries, such as those secondary to a posterior knee dislocation which do not require orthopedic fixation, can be safely repaired by a posterior approach. More complex injuries, such as combined popliteal artery and vein injuries or popliteal vascular injuries with associated fractures, are more safely addressed from a medial approach. When in doubt, a medial approach is recommended.

Sfeir et al[23] reported a series of popliteal vascular injuries from the recent Lebanon War in which 44% of patients had an associated fracture. The high frequency of combined orthopedic and arterial injuries poses a potential dilemma regarding the order in which vascular and orthopedic repairs should be performed. Sfeir and colleagues[23] concluded that because of the critical role that an ischemia time of less than 6 hours has on outcome, arterial repair should be performed as soon as possible and prior to orthopedic repair. The amputation rate for 90 patients repaired in less than 6 hours was 7% (6 patients), significantly lower than the amputation rate of 33% (8 of 24 patients) who were revascularized later than 6 hours following injury ($P = .014$). Small vessel thrombosis, which often occurs following prolonged ischemia, can result in a patent bypass, but a distal limb that continues to be severely ischemic is eventually amputated. In cases of a flail extremity, a temporary arterial shunt may be placed while orthopedic stabilization is undertaken.[17,26]

Popliteal venous injuries are uncommon in blunt trauma but occur in combination with arterial injuries in up to 50% of cases of penetrating injury to the popliteal region. Isolated popliteal venous injuries are infrequent, and only 8 of 178 patients (4%) in the series by Sfeir et al[23] sustained isolated popliteal vein injuries. Repair of the popliteal vein, which should follow popliteal artery repair, will improve runoff and decrease the incidence of compartmental hypertension. The venous outflow through the saphenous system of the injured extremity can be crucial to limb salvage in the immediate postoperative period. In all cases of combined popliteal artery and vein injury, the donor saphenous vein should be harvested from the contralateral extremity. A significant size discrepancy between an injured popliteal vein and the donor saphenous vein can be resolved by constructing a paneled vein graft for the venous repair. Interestingly, an associated venous injury does not necessarily result in a higher extremity amputation rate.[17,23]

Systemic heparin administered at the time of proximal clamp placement, completion arteriography (Fig. 11–4), and the liberal use of four-compartment fasciotomy have been associated with improved limb salvage rates in popliteal artery injuries.[27] Mannitol and dextran may also be important adjuncts in the management of this

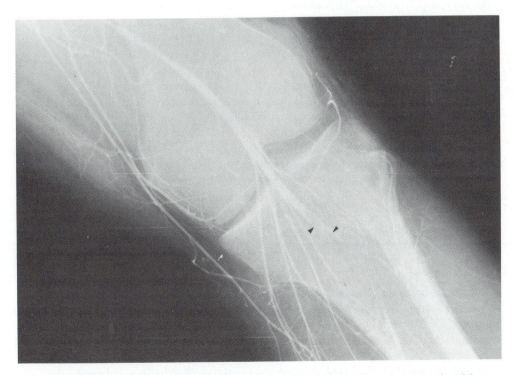

Figure 11–4. Completion arteriography detected distal into arterial thrombus (arrowheads) following vein graft repair of a more proximal popliteal artery gunshot wound. Distal thrombus formation can be a frequent finding in cases in which proximal arterial control must be achieved prior to systemic anticoagulation with heparin.

problem. Shah et al[26] reported no amputations and only two fasciotomies in 16 patients with popliteal artery injuries treated with mannitol, as opposed to 9 patients requiring fasciotomy of 14 patients who did not receive mannitol.[28] Sfeir et al[23] also observed a positive but not statistically significant effect of dextran on limb salvage, in which none of the patients receiving dextran required amputation.

POPLITEAL ENTRAPMENT

Popliteal artery entrapment syndrome is an unusual cause of claudication and limb ischemia. Although popliteal artery entrapment is a congenital anomaly, presentation before the third decade is unusual. This infrequent syndrome can be due to either abnormal muscle development in the popliteal region or an abnormal course of the popliteal artery. Most commonly, it is characterized by altered spatial relationships between the medial head of the gastrocnemius muscle and the popliteal artery, leading to compression of the popliteal artery between the muscle belly and the medial femoral condyle whenever the muscle contracts.

Popliteal entrapment was first described in 1879 by a medical student, T. P. A. Stuart,[29] who discovered the abnormality while dissecting the limb of 64-year-old man with a popliteal aneurysm who had developed distal gangrene. Stuart observed that the popliteal artery remained medial to the medial head of the gastrocnemius muscle, instead of passing between its two heads as it traversed the popliteal fossa. He recognized that the origin of the medial head of the muscle was much more proximal than was usually found.[29] This finding provided a clue to the etiology of this particular type of popliteal artery entrapment. An excessively proximal origin of the medial head of the gastrocnemius muscle could prevent the popliteal artery at the adductor hiatus from coursing between the two heads of the gastrocnemius muscle.

More than 300 cases of popliteal artery entrapment have been reported.[30,31] Five major types of popliteal artery entrapment are recognized.[32-36] (Type I) The medial head of the gastrocnemius muscle is in its normal location, or its origin is too proximal (type Ia), and as a result the popliteal artery is deviated medially. (Type II) The medial head of the gastrocnemius originates too lateral and the artery descends in a relatively straight location to the popliteal fossa without excessive medial deviation. (Type III) An accessory slip of muscle originates from the lateral aspect of the medial head, transversing from craniolateral to caudomedial. This muscle bundle or fibrous band serves to compress the artery against the medial femoral condyle. In this scenario the popliteal artery can actually go between different sections of the medial head of the gastrocnemius muscle. (Type IV) The deeper popliteus muscle or fibrous bands can compress the artery against the medial femoral condyle. This band may or may not be medial to the medial head of the gastrocnemius. (Type V) The popliteal vein can also be entrapped with the popliteal artery.[34-36] An acquired form of popliteal artery entrapment has also been described.[37]

Variations in the popliteal fossa anatomy that characterize popliteal artery entrapment can be explained by errors in the migration of the medial head of the gastrocnemius muscle or errors in development of the popliteal artery.[38,39] At 7 weeks' gestation development of the gastrocnemius muscle originates at the calcaneus, and it migrates cephalad to attach to the lateral femoral epicondyle.[40] At the same time, the deep popliteal artery, the termination of the sciatic artery, which lies anterior to the popliteus muscle, regresses. The new superficial popliteal artery, which evolves into the adult popliteal artery, arises posterior to the popliteus muscle. At the same time that the deep popliteal artery regresses and the superficial popliteal artery develops, the medial head of the gastrocnemius muscle migrates from the lateral to the medial femoral epicondyle across the superior aspect of the popliteal fossa.

Types I, Ia, II, III, and V of popliteal artery entrapment can be explained by variations in the migration and attachment of the medial head of the gastrocnemius muscle (Table 11–1). Type I popliteal artery entrapment, in which the medial head of the gastrocnemius muscle is in its normal anatomic position, but the artery is deviated medially, can be explained by the premature development of the superficial popliteal artery or by the late migration of the medial head of the gastrocnemius muscle. Type V popliteal artery entrapment, in which both the artery and the vein are compressed, is unusual because the popliteal vein normally develops much later than the popliteal artery or the gastrocnemius muscle. Delayed migration of the medial head of the gastrocnemius muscle could also explain type V variation.[34–36] Type Ia can be explained by too cephalad an attachment; type II, by too lateral an attachment; and type III, by delayed migration of the medial head of gastrocnemius relative to superficial popliteal artery formation. Failure of the deep popliteal artery to regress and of the superficial popliteal artery to develop explains compression of the popliteal artery by the popliteus muscle (type IV).

Popliteal artery entrapment should be suspected in young men presenting with calf claudication. Specific diagnostic maneuvers that can be used to facilitate the diagnosis of popliteal artery entrapment involve contraction of the gastrocnemius muscle. The loss of pedal pulses or compression by duplex scan can be observed with active plantar flexion or with passive dorsiflexion of the ankle. Both maneuvers stretch and compress the popliteal artery against the medial femoral condyle in the popliteal fossa if popliteal artery entrapment exists. In suspected cases of popliteal artery entrapment, a lower extremity arteriogram of both extremities should be performed in both the neutral position and with active plantar flexion (Fig. 11–5). Arteriographic findings can include popliteal artery occlusion, stenosis, aneurysm, or a normal-appearing artery. The popliteal artery can be in its normal anatomic location or it can be deviated medially. In cases of distal vessel occlusion suggesting thrombotic emboli from the

TABLE 11–1. POPLITEAL ARTERY ENTRAPMENT

Type	Medial Head Gastrocnemius (MHG)	Popliteal Artery (PA)	Etiology (Proposed)
I	Normal location	Medial deviation	MHG: Delayed migration from lateral to medial relative to formation of PA
Ia	Origin too cephalad	Medial deviation	MHG: Continued cephalad migration
II	Origin too lateral	Normal location	MHG: Failure to migrate from lateral to medial
III	Accessory bundle; broad attachment	Normal location; pierces muscle	MHG: Delayed migration from lateral to medial
IV	Normal location	Anterior to popliteus muscle	PA: Failure of DPA to regress and of SPA to develop into PA
V	Normal location	Medial division along with popliteal vein	MHG: Delayed migration from lateral to medial

DPA indicates deep popliteal artery; SPA, superficial popliteal artery.
Adapted from Inshua et al,[32] Gibson et al,[20] Donayre,[39] and Bardeen.[40]

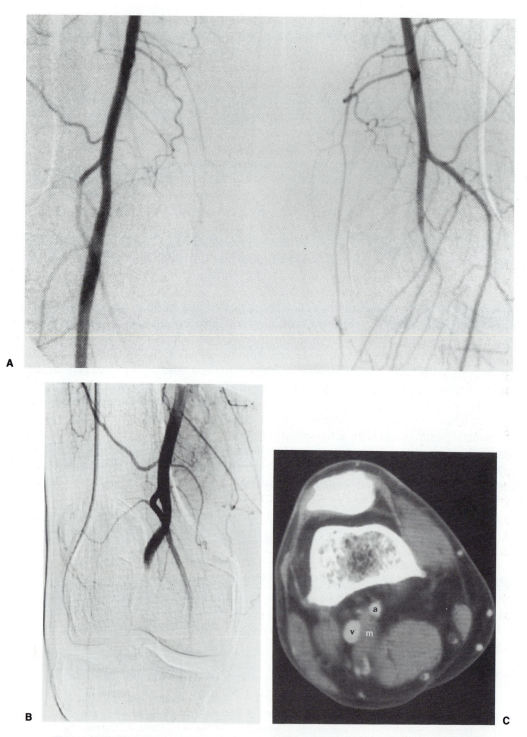

Figure 11–5. (A) Arteriography in the neutral position in a 37-year-old man who presented with left calf claudication and an asymptomatic right leg reveals left popliteal artery occlusion. The patent right popliteal artery is imaged in its normal location. **(B)** Planar flexion causes complete occlusion of the right popliteal artery. **(C)** CT scan confirms type II popliteal artery entrapment. The medial head of the gastrocnemius muscle (m) has failed to migrate and is lateral. The right popliteal artery (a) and vein (v) are in their normal locations.

area of the popliteal entrapment, thrombolytic therapy can be considered prior to definitive operation intervention. Evaluation of both extremities is emphasized because of the high incidence of asymptomatic popliteal entrapment at the time the symptomatic limb is evaluated. Both unilateral and bilateral popliteal artery entrapment can occur, with bilateral entrapment being found in appoximately 25% of cases.[33]

Contrast-enhanced CT scans of the popliteal fossa should be performed in suspected cases of popliteal entrapment, as this will often localize the type of muscular anomaly responsible for the syndrome.[41–43] These muscular or fibrous abnormalities are usually well imaged on CT scan. Magnetic resonance imaging is extremely useful in detailing popliteal fossa pathology but does not appear to have any specific advantages over CT scan in evaluating popliteal artery entrapment.

In many cases of bilateral popliteal entrapment, an asymptomatic leg is discovered along with a symptomatic extremity for which the patient sought medical treatment. There are several options for the care of these patients. For the patient who presents with extensive chronic distal thrombosis necessitating an extensive revascularization, the asymptomatic leg may logically be repaired first in order to prevent further complications to this otherwise undiseased arterial system. Once the asymptomatic leg has been treated to prevent arterial complication of the uncompromised extremity, the arterial repair can be undertaken for the symptomatic leg. Staging of these operations may be recommended. Patients with bilateral popliteal artery entrapment and no arterial occlusion may have both extremities released during the same anesthetic. The long-term outcome for patients with popliteal artery entrapment has been studied by di Marzo et al.[31] Simple myotomy in 18 limbs was associated with a patency rate of 94% with a mean follow up of 48 months.

Surgical Exposure for Popliteal Entrapment

Popliteal artery entrapment syndrome is best exposed using a posterior surgical approach. The primary disadvantage of a medial approach is difficulty in identifying the fibromuscular abnormality responsible for the arterial compression. The posterior approach provides the necessary exposure for defining and treating the underlying pathological lesion and is also adequate for arterial bypass should one be necessary. An exception in which the posterior approach may not be preferred is cases with popliteal artery or tibial arterial thrombosis requiring a distal tibial bypass.

The saphenous vein is readily harvested from the medial thigh incision when utilizing a posterior approach, and we have not encountered difficulty in harvesting the vein when arterial reconstructions are performed in the popliteal fossa. The lesser saphenous vein is also easily harvested if its use is required.

The popliteal fossa is approached through an S-shaped incision, with the medial aspect of the incision beginning on the posterior medial thigh to facilitate saphenous vein harvest from the thigh. The incision extends 5 cm below the knee. The deep fascia is incised to reveal the medial cutaneous sural nerve and the lesser saphenous vein, which can be traced cephalad to its termination in the popliteal vein within the popliteal fossa. The lesser saphenous vein should not be sacrificed because it is sometimes of adequate caliber to be used as a bypass or patch. The popliteal artery should be identified and then traced along its entire course within the popliteal fossa. Once the gastrocnemius muscle pathology is identified, it should be transected. Resecting a portion of the muscle is not associated with any disability and should be performed in cases in which the muscle appears to be hypertrophied. If the artery is normal, no further treatment is needed. To test the adequacy of the fibromuscular release, the ankle should be plantar and dorsiflexed while palpating the space between the posterior aspect of the medial femoral condyle and the popliteal artery. This will ensure that there is no residual compression. A short-segment arterial bypass can be fashioned through this posterior approach in the standard manner if needed.

CONCLUSION

Few anatomic regions present as much varied arterial pathology as the popliteal space. The common theme uniting adventitial cystic disease and popliteal entrapment is that patients often present with claudication symptoms at a very young age. To overlook or ignore these symptoms will often lead to permanent arterial damage after thrombosis and possibly a lifelong disability. Popliteal injuries from blunt or penetrating trauma are as challenging as they are treacherous and require prompt intervention, as there is often insufficient collateral flow to sustain the distal extremity. Popliteal aneurysms are easily managed with early surgical intervention, but if unrecognized until severe ischemia develops, they are profoundly limb threatening. Taken together, these conditions indeed provide a fascinating challenge for the surgeon.

Acknowledgment
Research for this chapter was sponsored in part by the Agency for Health Care Policy and Research grant RO1 HS07184-02.

REFERENCES

1. Giddings AEB. Influence of thrombolytic therapy in the management of popliteal aneurysms. In Yao JST, Pearce WH, eds. *Aneurysms: New Findings and Treatments.* Norwalk, Conn: Appleton & Lange; 1994;493–508.
2. Gaylis H. Popliteal arterial aneurysms. A review and analysis of 55 cases. *S Afr Med J.* 1974;48:75–80.
3. Wychulis AR, Spihell JA Jr, Wallace RB. Popliteal aneurysm. *Surgery.* 1970;68:942–952.
4. Evans WE, Conley JE, Bernhard V. Popliteal aneurysms. *Surgery.* 1971;70:762–767.
5. Gifford RW, Hines EA, Janes JM. An analysis and follow-up study of 100 popliteal aneurysms. *Surgery.* 1953;33:284–293.
6. Quraishy MS, Giddings AEB. Treatment of asymptomatic popliteal aneurysm: protection at a price. *Br J Surg.* 1992;79:731–732.
7. Hands LJ, Collin J. Infra-inguinal aneurysms: outcome for patient and limb. *Br J Surg.* 1991;78:996–998.
8. Shortell CK, DeWeese JA, Ouriel K, et al. Popliteal artery aneurysms: a 25-year surgical experience. *J Vasc Surg.* 1991;14:771–779.
9. Hierton T, Lindberg K. Cystic adventitial degeneration of the popliteal artery. *Acta Chir Scand.* 1957;44:348.
10. Flanigan DP, Burnham SJ, Goodreau JJ, et al. Summary of cases of adventitial cystic disease of the popliteal artery. *Ann Surg.* 1979;189:165–175.
11. Hierton T, Lindberg K, Rob C. Cystic degeneration of the popliteal artery. *Br J Surg.* 1957;44:438.
12. Ishikawa K, Mishima Y, Kobayashi S. Cystic adventitial disease of the popliteal artery. *Angiology.* 1961;12:357.
13. Eastcott HHG. Cystic degeneration of the popliteal artery. *Br Med J.* 1972;1:111.
14. Samson RH, Willis PD. Popliteal artery occlusion caused by cystic adventitial disease: successful treatment by nonresectional cystotomy. *J Vasc Surg.* 1990;12:591–593.
15. DeLaurentis DA, Wolferth CC Jr, Wolf FM. Mucinous adventitial cysts of the popliteal artery in an 11 year old girl. *Surgery.* 1973;74:456.

16. Keen RR, Meyer JP, Durham JR, et al. Autogenous vein graft repair of injured extremity arteries: early and late results with 134 consecutive patients. *J Vasc Surg.* 1991;13:664–668.
17. Peck JJ, Eastman AB, Bergan JJ, et al. Popliteal vascular trauma, a community experience. *Arch Surg.* 1990;125:1339–1344.
18. Downs AR, MacDonald P. Popliteal artery injuries: civilian experience with sixty-three patients during a twenty-four year period (1960 through 1984). *J Vasc Surg.* 1986;4:55–62.
19. Snyder WH III. Popliteal and shank arterial injury. *Surg Clin North Am.* 1988;68:787–807.
20. Hall RF Jr, Gonzales M. Fracture of the proximal part of the tibia and fibula associated with an entrapped popliteal artery. *J Bone J Surg.* 1986;68-A:941–943.
21. Treiman GS, Yellin AE, Weaver FA, et al. Examination of the patient with a knee dislocation. *Arch Surg.* 1992;127:1056–1063.
22. Howe HR Jr, Poole GV Jr, Hansen KJ, et al. Salvage of lower limb extremities following combined orthopedic and vascular trauma: a predictive salvage index. *Am Surg.* 1987;53:205–208.
23. Sfeir RE, Khoury GS, Haddah FF, et al. Injury to the popliteal vessels: the Lebanese War experience. *World J Surg.* 1992;16:1156–1159.
24. Dennis JW, Jagger C, Butcher JL, et al. Reassessing the role of arteriograms in the management of posterior knee dislocations. *J Trauma.* 1993;35:692–697.
25. Kendall RW, Taylor DC, Salvian AJ, et al. The role of arteriography in assessing vascular injuries associated with dislocations of the knee. *J Trauma.* 1993;35:875–878.
26. Shah DM, Naraynsingh V, Leather RP, et al. Advances in the management of acute popliteal vascular blunt injuries. *J Trauma.* 1985;25:793–797.
27. Lim LT, Michuda MS, Flanigan DP, et al. Popliteal artery trauma: 31 consecutive cases without amputation. *Arch Surg.* 1980;115:1307–1313.
28. Shah PM, Wapnir I, Babu S, et al. Compartmental syndrome in combined arterial and venous injury of the lower extremity. *Am J Surg.* 1989;158:136–139.
29. Stuart TPA. Note on a variation in the course of the popliteal artery. In: Barker WF, ed. *Clio Chiurgical, The Arteries.* Austin, Tex: RG Landes Co; 1992;473.
30. Persky JM, Kempczinski RF, Fowl RJ. Entrapment of the popliteal artery. *Surg. Gynecol Obstet.* 1991;173:84–90.
31. di Marzo L, Cavallaro A, Sciacca V, et al. Surgical treatment of popliteal artery entrapment syndrome: a ten year experience. *Eur J Vasc Surg.* 1991;5:59.
32. Inshua JA, Young JR, Humphries AW. Popliteal artery entrapment syndrome. *Arch Surg.* 1970;101:771–775.
33. Whelan TJ Jr. Popliteal artery entrapment. In: Ernst CB, Stanley JC, eds. *Current Therapy in Vascular Surgery.* 2nd ed. Philadelphia: BC Decker; 1991;779–783.
34. Rich NM, Collins GJ Jr, McDonald PT, et al. Popliteal vascular entrapment: its increasing interest. *Arch Surg.* 1979;114:1377–1384.
35. Rich NM, Hughes CW. Popliteal artery and vein entrapment. *Am J Surg.* 1967:113:696.
36. Rich NM. Popliteal entrapment and adventitial cystic disease. *Surg Clin North Am.* 1982;62:449–465.
37. Baker WH, Stanley RJ. Acquired popliteal entrapment syndrome. *Arch Surg.* 1972;106:780.
38. Gibson MHL, Mills JG, Johnson GE, et al. Popliteal entrapment syndrome. *Ann Surg.* 1977;185:341–348.
39. Donayre CE. Entrapment syndromes. In: White RA, Hollier LH, eds. *Vascular Surgery: Basic Science and Clinical Correlation.* Philadelphia: JB Lippincott Co; 1994;207–215.
40. Bardeen CR. Development and variation of the nerves and the musculature of the inferior extremity and the neighboring regions of the trunk in man. *Am J Anat.* 1907;6:259–390.
41. Williams LR, Flinn WR, McCarthy WJ, et al. Popliteal artery entrapment: diagnosis by computed tomography. *J Vasc Surg.* 1986;3:360–363.
42. Rizzo RJ, Flinn WR, Yao JST, et al. Computed tomography for the evaluation of arterial disease in the popliteal fossa. *J Vasc Surg.* 1990;11:112–119.
43. Muller N, Morris DC, Nichols DM. Popliteal artery entrapment demonstrated by CT. *Radiology.* 1984;151:157–158.

12

Management of Heparin-Induced Ischemia

John G. Adams, Jr, MD, and Donald Silver, MD

The omniuse of heparin, especially in patients with cardiovascular disorders, requires that cardiovascular surgeons be familiar with the potential complications of heparin therapy. One complication, heparin-induced thrombocytopenia syndrome, with its high morbidity and mortality, occurs in 0.9% to 31% (average, 2% to 4%) of patients receiving heparin. This chapter reviews the history, pathophysiology, clinical spectrum, diagnosis, and management of heparin-induced thrombocytopenia syndrome.

HISTORY

In 1941 Copely and Robb reported that heparin, *in vitro* and *in vivo*, reduced platelet counts in dog and mice venous blood (mice *in vivo* only) and concluded that ". . . heparin has disintegrating effects upon platelets."[1] In 1948, Copely demonstrated platelet emboli in rabbits and hamsters following an injection of heparin[2] and Fidlar and Jaques demonstrated a ". . . swift disappearance and return of platelets from the general circulation. . ." in dogs and humans.[3] Gollub and Ulin in 1962 suggested that the acute reversible thrombocytopenia found after intravenous administration of heparin might be secondary to "transient sequestration" of the platelets.[4] This transient rapidly reversible heparin-induced thrombocytopenia has no clinical sequelae and may represent only in *in vitro* effect of heparin.[5,6]

In 1958 Weismann and Tobin reported 10 cases (6 deaths) of arterial embolism in patients receiving heparin.[7] The emboli were ". . . pale, soft, salmon-colored. . ." and were composed of ". . . fibrin, platelets and leukocytes; red cells were rare." No platelet counts were recorded. They suggested that the embolizations ". . . were precipitated by some unknown local effect of systemic heparinization." Roberts and associates in 1964 reported 11 cases (16 embolectomies and 4 deaths) of arterial embolism in patients receiving heparin. The emboli were ". . . of a light color, seemingly made up primarily of fibrin and platelets. . .". They speculated about the development of an "antiheparin factor."[8] In 1973 Rhodes and associates reported on 2 patients with thromboembolism in whom heparin-induced thrombocytopenia had developed.[9]

Their platelet aggregation and complement fixation studies established a heparin-dependent antibody as the cause for the thrombocytopenia. In recent years heparin-induced thrombocytopenia syndrome has been recognized with increased frequency, with 28 references to this syndrome listed in the 1993 *Index Medicus*.

CLINICAL SPECTRUM

Immune heparin-induced thrombocytopenia occurs in 0.9% to 31% of patients receiving heparin. The triad of events that occur in patients with heparin-induced thrombocytopenia syndrome include thrombocytopenia, resistance to anticoagulation with heparin, and new or progressive thromboembolic events—mostly arterial but occasionally venous. Hemorrhage is a rare occurrence. There are no known patient characteristics that help the clinician identify the patient at risk for developing heparin-associated antiplatelet antibodies. The development of the antibodies is independent of patient age, sex, blood type, amount of heparin received, type of heparin given, or route of heparin administration. Newborns are at risk for becoming sensitized by heparin. The manifestations of heparin-induced thrombocytopenia syndrome in infants are similar to those in adults. Heparin-induced thrombocytopenia has been described in patients who have received pork, beef, and low-molecular-weight heparins. In the past a higher percentage of patients receiving beef heparin was sensitized than those receiving pork heparin. However, there is currently little, if any, difference between the sensitization rates by beef or pork heparin. The development of the antibodies is not related to the amount of heparin received by the patient. The antibodies have been detected in patients receiving therapeutic amounts of heparin, prophylactic amounts, and even the minuscule amounts used in "flushes" to maintain indwelling catheter patency. We have noted the development of antibodies in patients receiving as little as 1 U of heparin per hour. The small amount of heparin released from heparin-coated catheters is capable of sustaining the thrombocytopenia that occurs in patients with heparin-associated antiplatelet antibodies.[10]

Low-molecular-weight heparin has been reported to be both useful and detrimental in the management of patients with this syndrome. We have found that plasma from patients who aggregate platelets in the presence of unfractionated heparin frequently also aggregates platelets in the presence of low-molecular-weight heparins. We recommend that patients with known heparin antibodies be tested for the cross-reactivity of the antibodies before receiving a low-molecular-weight heparin.[11]

The thromboembolic complications of heparin-induced thrombocytopenia syndrome are virtually always preceded by a falling platelet count and/or thrombocytopenia. The interval between the initiation of the use of heparin and the onset of thrombocytopenia is between 4 and 15 days (mean, 8 days) for patients receiving heparin for the first time. The nadir of the platelet counts occurs between the second and ninth days (mean, 5 days) for those who have previously received heparin.[12] We have observed the occurrence of thrombocytopenia during the first day of heparin re-exposure in previously sensitized patients. The duration of the presence of the heparin-associated antibodies varies from a few days to more than 13 years.

Patients with heparin-associated antiplatelet antibodies are at risk for the development of limb- and/or life-threatening thromboembolic, rarely hemorrhagic, complications when exposed to any form of heparin. Lower limb (and occasionally upper limb) ischemia from aortic, iliac, and/or femoral artery thrombosis is not uncommon. Myocardial infarction, pulmonary embolism, bowel infarction, cerebral thrombosis, graft thrombosis, deep venous thrombosis, and primary pulmonary embolism have been reported. Any new thromboembolic event in a patient receiving heparin should promote a search for heparin-associated antiplatelet antibodies.

The mortality and morbidity of the heparin-induced thrombocytopenia syndrome (when recognized and treated late) have been as high as 23% and 61%, respectively.[13] Laster and associates noted a decrease in mortality and morbidity to 12% and 25%, respectively, when they detected the heparin-induced thrombocytopenia syndrome early and initiated early management.[13,14] There are no signs or symptoms that allow the clinician to predict which patient will develop thromboembolic complications. Therefore, laboratory monitoring with platelet counts of all patients receiving heparin is recommended to detect this process before complications arise.

PATHOPHYSIOLOGY

It is accepted that patients with the immune form of heparin-induced thrombocytopenia have heparin-associated antiplatelet antibodies which, in the presence of heparin, cause platelet activation and aggregation. The antibodies are usually of the immunoglobulin G (IgG), occasionally of the IgM, and rarely of the IgA classes. Although complement is deposited on platelets in the presence of the antibodies and heparin, complement activation does not have an important role in the activation or aggregation of platelets.[15] Bone marrow studies in patients with heparin-induced thrombocytopenia have revealed the presence of normal megakaryocytes. The thrombocytopenia is related to the peripheral consumption and/or destruction of platelets. This association is supported by the elevated plasma levels of β-thromboglobulin and platelet factor IV that occur during heparin-induced thrombocytopenia.

The sequence of the complexing of the heparin-associated antibody and the platelet has been under intense study. Studies have suggested that circulating heparin combines with the many (up to approximately 5,000 on an inactivated platelet) platelet heparin receptors.[15-17] Antiheparin IgG then binds with heparin, forming an immune complex. It has also been suggested that the IgG and heparin combine in the plasma and then attach to the platelet. The heparin–IgG immune complex interacts with the platelet Fc receptors, resulting in platelet activation and aggregation. Recent studies in our laboratory indicate that the antibody is specific for heparin. These studies confirm that the Fc component of the antibody is required to produce platelet aggregation.

It has been demonstrated that the antibody, perhaps by interacting with the available heparan sulfate, can interact with endothelial cells and cause expression of tissue factor.[18] This altering of the endothelium not only may contribute to thrombosis but would also cause the endothelium to be ineffective in inhibiting thrombosis. This activation of platelets and the alteration of endothelium cause patients receiving heparin to be at risk for thrombosis and, to a much lesser degree, hemorrhage. Platelet aggregation is thought to play a major role in the thrombus formation, which occurs usually in major arteries (eg, aorta, iliac, and femoral) and occasionally in major veins (eg, femoral and iliac).

LABORATORY DIAGNOSIS

Heparin-induced thrombocytopenia should be suspected when any patient receiving heparin develops thrombocytopenia, a resistance to heparin anticoagulation, or new or extending thromboembolic events. Laboratory confirmation is based on platelet activation in the presence of the patient's heparin-associated antiplatelet antibodies and heparin.

The thrombocytopenia is usually progressive and sustained and will not remit until the patient's exposure to heparin ceases. Any patient receiving heparin who demonstrates a progressive decline in platelet count or a platelet count of less than 100,000/mm^3 (less than 70,000/mm^3 in the newborn) may have heparin-induced thrombocytopenia. The average platelet count nadir is 68,000/mm^3 [19]; however, platelet counts as low as 5,000/mm^3 have been reported.[12] Cessation of heparin therapy is associated with substantial increases in the platelet count in most patients, usually within 48 hours.

Laboratory evidence of disseminated intravascular coagulation is usually lacking. In addition to eliminating intravascular coagulation as a cause of the thrombocytopenia, an attempt should be made to ensure that the low platelet count is not associated with other thrombocytopathies (eg, post-transfusion thrombocytopenia, infectious thrombocytopenia, idiopathic thrombocytopenic purpura, and other drug-induced thrombocytopenias).

The increased resistance to heparin anticoagulation is usually documented by a decreasing partial thromboplastin time (PTT) during a constant infusion of heparin. Substantial increases of the amount of heparin infused are usually required to maintain a constant PTT.

Platelet aggregation studies have been used most frequently to detect the presence of heparin-associated antiplatelet antibodies. The aggregation test consists of mixing normal donor platelet-rich plasma with the plasma containing the suspected antibody and with heparin. (1.0 and 100 U/mL) in the aggregometer cuvettes.[9,19–21] Platelet aggregation is assessed in the test samples and control samples (normal donor platelet-rich plasma and normal donor plasma). It should be noted that aggregation testing may be falsely negative if the patient is receiving heparin at the time of testing. If the aggregation test remains negative at 96 hours following cessation of heparin, the patient has a very low probability of having heparin-associated antiplatelet antibodies. Platelet aggregation testing is relatively simple, inexpensive, and rapidly completed. Although the sensitivity of platelet aggregation testing has been questioned by some authors,[22,23] it has been shown by others to be highly sensitive and specific for the detection of heparin-associated antiplatelet antibodies.[12,24]

The carbon 14 serotonin assay is a modification of the heparin-dependent platelet aggregation test. The test measures carbon 14 sertotonin release from washed donor platelets in the presence of heat-treated patient serum. The test utilizes a low heparin concentration (0.1 to 1.0 U/mL) and a high heparin concentration (100 U/mL) and is considered positive if serotonin release occurs at the lower concentration but not at the higher concentration. This test has been proposed as being more sensitive and specific for the detection of heparin-associated antiplatelet antibodies than platelet aggregation.[14,25] However, the test is not widely used and its value has not been validated.

β-Thromboglobulin (BTG) is released by platelets during degranulation[26] and has been shown to be a sensitive marker for the presence of heparin-associated antiplatelet antibodies. In a recent series sera from 169 patients with heparin-induced thrombocytopenia syndrome (confirmed by clinical presentation combined with platelet aggregation testing) were assayed for BTG; all patients with heparin-induced thrombocytopenia syndrome had significantly elevated levels of BTG compared to controls.[13]

Platelets from patients with heparin-induced thrombocytopenia syndrome have been found to have increased levels of platelet-associated IgG and complement.[18,27,28]

However, increases in platelet-associated IgG are found in many other disorders (eg, idiopathic thrombocytopenic purpura), which result in thrombocytopenia and are therefore not specific for heparin-induced thrombocytopenia syndrome.[29] Because of this lack of specificity, a modification of the platelet-associated IgG test has been described in which fluorescein-labeled or enzyme-linked anti-immunoglobulin probes are used to assess the heparin-dependent binding of IgG to platelets.[30–34] The roles of these tests in establishing the presence of heparin-associated antiplatelet antibodies require further evaluation.

MANAGEMENT

Heparin-induced thrombocytopenia syndrome has been associated with a 61% morbidity and a 23% mortality if detected and treated late. The rates decline to 22.5% and 12%, respectively, when the process is detected and treated early.[12,13] It is important that this entity be recognized before thromboembolic complications occur. Therefore, daily platelet-count monitoring is recommended for all patients receiving heparin.

When heparin-induced thrombocytopenia is suspected, all sources of heparin exposure (including heparin-coated catheters, parenteral flushes, etc.) must be eliminated. Cessation of heparin administration usually results in rapid resolution (2 to 3 days) of the thrombocytopenia and markedly reduces the risk of thromboembolism. Complications of heparin-induced thrombocytopenia syndrome often include thromboembolic obstructions of major arteries with secondary ischemia. Management of these arterial (occasionally venous) obstructions consists of cessation of heparin administration, platelet function inhibition, alternate forms of anticoagulation, thrombolytic therapy, and/or revascularization surgery.

Platelet function inhibitors are adminstered to patients with heparin-induced thrombocytopenia syndrome to inhibit platelet activation and aggregation. Aspirin is the platelet inhibitor most commonly used; it significantly decreases the thromboembolic complications in patients re-exposed to heparin.[35,36] Dipyridamole, an inhibitor of platelet activation, has also been used in the management of heparin-induced thrombocytopenia syndrome (usually in combination with aspirin); however, there are few data to support its use. Low-molecular weight dextran has been reported to reduce heparin-induced platelet aggregation and may be of benefit in the treatment of these patients, although no conclusive data are available. The efficacy of ticlopidine in the treatment of heparin-induced thrombocytopenia syndrome has not been studied. Iloprost, a prostacyclin derivative, has proven successful in inhibiting platelet activation in patients with heparin-induced thrombocytopenia syndrome who require additional exposure to heparin. The administration of iloprost has been accompanied by hypotensive effects.[37,38] Iloprost is not currently available in the United States.

Several agents have been used to treat patients with heparin-induced thrombocytopenia syndrome who require continued anticoagulation. Warfarin is the most frequently used alternative. Ancrod, a defibrinogenating agent prepared from pit viper venom, has been used successfully for short-term anticoagulation in patients with heparin-induced thrombocytopenia syndrome.[39] Anticoagulation is achieved by blocking the final stage of the coagulation cascade and by preventing platelet aggregation.[40] Ancrod is not currently available in the United States. A heparinoid, Org 10172 (Organon, Oss, The Netherlands), has been used for interval anticoagulation with favorable results in a few patients with heparin-induced thrombocytopenia syndrome.[41-45] It also is not available for routine clinical use. Low-molecular-weight heparins have also been adminstered to patients with heparin-associated antiplatelet antibodies with varying results.[46-52] In a recent study plasma samples from patients with heparin-induced thrombocytopenia syndrome were found to have a cross-reactivity rate of approximately 20% with Org 10172, 26% with Fragmin (Kabi-Vitrum, Stockholm, Sweden) (a low-molecular-weight heparin), and 61% with Mono-Embolex NM (Sandoz Pharmaceuticals, East Hanover, NJ) (a low-molecular-weight heparin) when evaluated with platelet aggregometry.[11] It is recommended that heparinoids and low-molecular-weight heparins be tested for possible cross-reactivity with the patient's heparin-associated antiplatelet antibodies prior to administration of these agents to the patient.

Patients with heparin-induced thrombocytopenia syndrome who develop ischemic complications frequently require lytic and/or surgical intervention. Thrombolytic therapy with or without adjunctive endovascular procedures has been successfully utilized in the management of thromboses of major vessels in these patients.[53-57] Thrombolytic therapy has been used successfully to treat critical ischemia of the lower extremity,[53,55] pulmonary artery and coronary artery saphenous vein graft thromboses,[56] and multiple pulmonary emboli.[57] An additional report of iliofemoral venous thrombosis and critical ischemia of the opposite extremity was unsuccessfully treated with lytic therapy.[55] Because of the major contraindications involved with the administration of lytic agents (eg, active internal bleeding, recent cerebrovascular accident, intracranial pathology, recent major surgery/trauma, active peptic ulcer disease, and uncontrollable hypertension), many patients with heparin-induced thrombocytopenia syndrome are not candidates for thrombolytic therapy. We have found that the heparin-induced "white clots" are more resistant to lysis with thrombolytic agents than are comparable "red clots."

In a recent series of 231 patients with heparin-induced thrombocytopenia syndrome, 50 patients (22%) developed thromboembolic ischemic complications requiring surgical intervention.[13] In the early part of the series, 35% (22/62) of the patients required a surgical procedure for thromboembolic ischemic complications; in the later part of the series, when early detection and treatment of heparin-induced thrombocytopenia syndrome were emphasized, only 17% (28/169) of the patients required a surgical procedure. Thromboembolectomy of the abdominal aorta or the iliofemoral arteries was the most common procedure performed for ischemic complications (33/50). Additional procedures consisted of amputations (9/50), exploratory laparotomies for mesenteric ischemia and/or gastrointestinal hemorrhage (5/50), mediastinal exploration for hemorrhage following median sternotomy for cardiac surgery (2/50), and evacuation of an extremity hematoma (1/50). It should be noted that despite the overall decrease in morbidity and mortality in patients with heparin-induced thrombocytopenia syndrome who are detected and treated early, there continues to be a high mortality rate (55%) when a patient has an ischemic complication.[13] In a patient who requires surgical intervention for thromboembolic-induced ischemia, (1) the administration of heparin should cease, (2) flow should be restored quickly with a thromboembolectomy, (3) dextran or saline solution flushes should be used liberally, (4) the patient should be pretreated with platelet inhibitors and an alternate anticoagulant (usually warfarin) if indicated, and (5) re-exposure to heparin must be limited[40] (see below). If heparin is continued in a patient with the heparin-associated antiplatelet antibodies, the recurrence rate for thromboembolic complications is high (approaching 100%).[19]

HEPARIN RE-EXPOSURE

Patients with heparin-associated antiplatelet antibodies may require diagnostic or therapeutic procedures necessitating re-exposure to heparin. Elective procedures should be postponed until platelet aggregation testing fails to demonstrate the presence of the antibody. At that time heparin can be safely administered in the standard fashion with a low risk of immediate thromboembolic complications. In the postprocedural period the platelet count should be followed daily. A falling platelet count or a new thromboembolic event should raise concern about the redevelopment of heparin-associated antiplatelet antibodies.

Patients who have heparin-associated antiplatelet antibodies and who receive additional heparin during surgery, angiography, hemodialysis, etc, without being "pretreated" with platelet inhibitors have been shown to have a 75% thromboembolic complication rate.[36] Conversely, similar patients receiving heparin during peripheral vascular and cardiovascular procedures who were pretreated with platelet inhibitors (most often aspirin) had no complications.[35,36] A recent series reported on 9 patients with heparin-associated antiplatelet antibodies who were given aspirin (325 mg twice daily) and/or dipyridamole (200 to 300 mg/d) and were subsequently re-exposed to 5,000 to 12,000 U of heparin during 11 vascular procedures without thromboembolic or hemorrhagic complications.[36] Others have found that iloprost offered protection to patients with heparin-associated antiplatelet antibodies during heparin re-exposure.[37]

In summary, patients with known heparin-associated antiplatelet antibodies can safely tolerate limited re-exposures to heparin if their platelet function is inhibited prior to the re-exposure. We currently administer aspirin preoperatively, use a limited amount of heparin intraoperatively or during the study, and continue aspirin postoperatively/poststudy. If anticoagulation will be required postoperatively, warfarin therapy is usually initiated preoperatively.

REFERENCES

1. Copely AL, Robb TP. The effect of heparin on the platelet count in dogs and mice. *Am J Physiol.* 1941;133:248. Abstract.
2. Copely AL. Embolization of platelet agglutination thrombi in the hamster's pouch produced by heparin. *Fed Proc.* 1948;7:22–23.
3. Fidlar E, Jaques LB. The effect of commercial heparin on the platelet count. *J Lab Clin Med.* 1949;33:1410–1423.
4. Gollub S, Ulin AW. Heparin-induced thrombocytopenia in man. *J Lab Clin Med.* 1962;59:430–435.
5. Davey MG, Lander H. Effect of injected heparin on platelet levels in man. *J Clin Pathol.* 1968;21:55–59.
6. Salzman EW, Rosenberg RD. Effect of heparin and heparin fractions on platelet aggregation. *J Clin Invest.* 1980;65:64–73.
7. Weismann RE, Tobin RW. Arterial embolism occurring during systemic heparin therapy. *Arch Surg.* 1958;76:219–227.
8. Roberts B, Rosato FE, Rosato EF. Heparin—a cause of arterial emboli? *Surgery.* 1964; 55:803–808.
9. Rhodes GR, Dixon RH, Silver D. Heparin-induced thrombocytopenia with thrombotic and hemorrhagic manifestations. *Surg Gynecol Obstet.* 1973;136:409–416.
10. Laster JL, Silver D. Heparin coated catheters and heparin-induced thrombocytopenia. *J Vasc Surg.* 1988;7:667–672.

11. Kikta MJ, Keller MP, Humphrey PW, et al. Can low molecular weight heparins and heparinoids be safely given to patients with heparin-induced thrombocytopenia syndrome? *Surgery*. 1993;114:705–710.

12. Silver D, Kapsch DN, Tsoi EK. Heparin-induced thrombocytopenia, thrombosis, and hemorrhage. *Ann Surg*. 1983;198:301–306.

13. Laster JL, Cikrit D, Walker N, et al. The heparin-induced thrombocytopenia syndrome: an update. *Surgery*. 1987;102:763–770.

14. Sheridan D, Carter C, Kelton JG. A diagnostic test for heparin-induced thrombocytopenia. *Blood*. 1986;67:27–30.

15. Chong BH, Castaldi PA, Berndt MC. Heparin-induced thrombocytopenia: effects of rabbit IgG, and its Fab and Fc fragments on antibody–heparin–platelet interaction. *Thromb Res*. 1989;55:291–295.

16. Kelton JG, Sheridan D, Santos A, et al. Heparin-induced thrombocytopenia: laboratory studies. *Blood*. 1988;72:925–930.

17. Horne MK, Chao ES. Heparin binding to resting and activated platelets. *Blood*. 1989;74:238–243.

18. Cines DB, Kaywin P, Bina M, et al. Heparin-associated thrombocytopenia. *N Engl J Med*. 1980;303:788–795.

19. Kapsch D, Silver D. Heparin-induced thrombocytopenia with thrombosis and hemorrhage. *Arch Surg*. 1981;116:1423–1427.

20. Babcock RB, Dumper CW, Scharfman WB. Heparin-induced immune thrombocytopenia. *N Engl J Med*. 1976;295:237–241.

21. Fratantoni JC, Pollet R, Gralnick HR. Heparin-induced thrombocytopenia: confirmation of diagnosis with in vitro methods. *Blood*. 1975;45:395–401.

22. Kelton JG, Sheridan D, Brain H, et al. Clinical usefulness of testing for a heparin-dependent platelet-aggregating factor in patients with suspected heparin-associated thrombocytopenia. *J Lab Clin Med*. 1984;103:606–612.

23. Greinacher A, Michels, I, Kiefel V, et al. A rapid and sensitive test for diagnosing heparin-associated thrombocytopenia. *Thromb Haemostasis*. 1991;66:734–736.

24. Kapsch DN, Adelstein EH, Rhodes GR, et al. Heparin-induced thrombocytopenia, thrombosis, and hemorrhage. *Surgery*. 1979;86:148–155.

25. Warkentin TE, Kelton JG. Heparin and platelets. *Hematol Oncol Clin North Am*. 1990; 4:243–264. Review.

26. Moore S, Pepper DS, Cash JD. The isolation and characterization of platelet specific β-globulin (beta-thromboglobulin) and the detection of antiurokinase and antiplasmin from thrombin-aggregated washed human platelets. *Biochim Biophys Acta*. 1975;379:360–369.

27. Kelton JG, Powers PJ. Heparin-associated thrombocytopenia: an immune disorder. In: Lundblad RL, Brown WV, Mann KG, et al, eds. *Chemistry and Biology of Heparin*. New York: Elsevier/North Holland Inc; 1980;365–375.

28. Stead RB, Schafer AI, Rosenberg RD, et al. Heterogeneity of heparin lots associated with thrombocytopenia and thromboembolism. *Am J Med*. 1984;77:185–188.

29. Kelton JG, Powers P, Carter CJ. A prospective study of the usefulness of the measurement of platelet-associated IgG for the diagnosis of idiopathic thrombocytopenic purpura. *Blood*. 1982;60:1050–1053.

30. Follea G, Hamandjian I, Trzeciak MC, et al. Pentosan polysulphate associated thrombocytopenia. *Thromb Res*. 1986;42:413–418.

31. Howe SE, Lynch DM. An enzyme-linked immunosorbent assay for the evaluation of thrombocytopenia induced by heparin. *J Lab Clin Med*. 1985;105:554–559.

32. Silberman S, Kovarik P. Heparin-induced thrombocytopenia: use of indirect immunofluorescence. *Ann Clin Lab Sci*. 1987;17:106–110.

33. Wolf H, Glassl H, Nowack H, et al. Identification of binding site for heparin and other polysulfated glycosaminoglycans on human thrombocytes. *Int Arch Allergy Appl Immunol*. 1986;80:231–238.

34. Wolf H, Nowack H, Wick G. Detection of antibodies interacting with glycosaminoglycan polysulfate in patients treated with heparin or other polysulfated glycosaminoglycans. *Int Arch Allergy Appl Immunol*. 1983;70:157–163.

35. Walls JT, Curtis JJ, Silver D, et al. Heparin-induced thrombocytopenia in open heart surgical patients: sequelae of late recognition. *Ann Thorac Surg.* 1992;53:787–791.
36. Laster J, Elfrink R, Silver D. Reexposure to heparin of patients with heparin-associated antibodies. *J Vasc Surg.* 1989;9:677–682.
37. Kappa JR, Cottrell ED, Berkowitz HD, et al. Carotid endarterectomy in patients with heparin-induced platelet activation: comparative efficacy of aspirin and iloprost (ZK36374). *J Vasc Surg.* 1987;5:693–701.
38. Kappa JR, Fisher CA, Berkowitz HD, et al. Heparin-induced platelet activation in sixteen surgical patients: diagnosis and management. *J Vasc Surg.* 1987;5:101–109.
39. Cole CW, Bormanis J. Ancrod: a practical alternative to heparin. *J Vasc Surg.* 1988;8:59–63.
40. Sobel M. Heparin-induced thrombocytopenia. *Perspect Vasc Surg.* 1992;5:1–30.
41. Chong BH, Ismail F, Cade J, et al. Heparin-induced thrombocytopenia: studies with a new low molecular weight heparinoid, Org 10172, *Blood.* 1989;73;1592–1596.
42. Harenberg J, Zimmermann R, Schwartz F, et al. Treatment of heparin-induced thrombocytopenia with thrombosis by new heparinoid. *Lancet.* 1983;1:986–987. Letter.
43. Rowlings PA, Mansberg R, Rozenberg MC, et al. The use of a low molecular weight heparinoid (Org 10172) for extracorporeal procedures in patients with heparin dependent thrombocytopenia and thrombosis. *Aust N Z J Med.* 1991;21:52–54.
44. Ortel TL, Gockerman JP, Califf RM, et al. Parenteral anticoagulation with the heparinoid Lomoparan (Org 10172) in patients with heparin induced thrombocytopenia and thrombosis. *Thromb Haemostasis.* 1992;67:292–296.
45. Greinacher A, Drost W, Michels I, et al. Heparin-associated thrombocytopenia: successful therapy with the heparinoid Org 10172 in a patient showing cross-reaction to LMW heparins. *Ann Hematol.* 1992;64:40–2.
46. Vitoux JF, Mathieu JF, Roncato M, et al. Heparin-associated thrombocytopenia treatment with a low molecular weight heparin. *Thromb Haemostasis.* 1986;55:37–39.
47. Roussi JH, Houbouyan LL, Goguel AF. Use of low-molecular-weight heparin in heparin-induced thrombocytopenia with thrombotic complications. *Lancet.* 1984;1:1183. Letter.
48. Horellou MH, Conard J, Lecrubier C, et al. Persistent heparin induced thrombocytopenia despite therapy with low molecular weight heparin. *Thromb Haemostasis.* 1984;51:134. Letter.
49. Leroy J, Leclerc MH, Delahousse B, et al. Treatment of heparin-associated thrombocytopenia and thrombosis with low molecular weight heparin (CY 216). *Semin Thromb Haemostasis.* 1985;11:326–329.
50. Robitaille D, Leclerc JR, Laberg R, et al. Cardiopulmonary bypass with a low-molecular-weight heparin fraction (enoxaparin) in a patient with a history of heparin-associated thrombocytopenia. *J Thorac Cardiovasc Surg.* 1992;103:597–599.
51. van Besien K, Hoffman R, Golichowski A. Pregnancy associated with lupus anticoagulant and heparin induced thrombocytopenia: management with a low molecular weight heparinoid. *Thromb Res.* 1991;62:23–29.
52. Goualt-Heilmann M, Huet Y, Adnot S, et al. Low molecular weight heparin fractions as an alternative therapy in heparin-induced thrombocytopenia. *Haemostasis.* 1987;17:134–140.
53. Fiessinger JN, Aiach M, Roncato M, et al. Critical ischemia during heparin-induced thrombocytopenia. Treatment by intra-arterial streptokinase. *Thromb Res.* 1984;33:235–238.
54. Clifton GD, Smith MD. Thrombolytic therapy in heparin-associated thrombocytopenia with thrombosis. *Clin Pharm.* 1986;5:597–601.
55. AbuRahma AF, Boland JP, Witsberger T. Diagnostic and therapeutic strategies of white clot syndrome. *Am J Surg.* 1991;162:175–179.
56. Dieck JA, Rizo-Patron C, Unisa A, et al. A new manifestation and treatment alternative for heparin-induced thrombosis. *Chest.* 1990;98:1524–1526.
57. Cohen JI, Cooper MR, Greenber CS. Streptokinase therapy of pulmonary emboli with heparin-associated thrombocytopenia. *Arch Intern Med.* 1985;145:1725–1726.

IV

Surgical Treatment of Upper Extremity Ischemia

13

Occupational Injuries

Spencer W. Galt, MD, and James S.T. Yao, MD, PhD

Occupational injury to the upper extremity includes those injuries resulting from repetitive and forceful use of the hands and arms, known collectively as cumulative trauma disorders[1] (CTDs), and those resulting from exposure involving a single accident in the workplace. According to the US Bureau of Labor Statistics, the incidence of CTD has increased steadily in recent years, accounting for 20 work-related repetitive motion disorders per 100,000 workers in 1989. Furthermore, CTDs have accounted for more than 50% of all occupational illnesses reported in the United States.[2] Most CTDs involve the musculoskeletal system, but a significant number of workers suffer arterial injury to the upper extremity sufficient to cause hand and arm ischemia. Occupation-associated arterial injuries include hand–arm vibration syndrome, hypothenar hammer syndrome, acro-osteolysis, thoracic outlet compression to the subclavian–axillary artery, and hand ischemia related to athletic activities.

HAND–ARM VIBRATION SYNDROME

Hand–arm vibration syndrome (HAVS) is a constellation of symptoms induced by long-term occupational exposure to vibration. HAVS consists of (1) Raynaud's phenomenon, (2) peripheral neuropathies, and (3) musculoskeletal injuries.[3] The vasospastic component of HAVS has been variably referred to as vibration white finger, Raynaud's phenomenon of occupational origin, and traumatic vasospastic disease. Regardless of the terminology, the common presenting vascular symptoms are of Raynaud's phenomenon, owing to the prolonged use of vibrating mechanical tools.

Raynaud's disease–like symptoms in Italian miners using pneumatic tools were first reported by Loriga in 1911.[4] In the United States Hamilton[5] established the definitive linkage. In 1918 she reported on limestone cutters and carvers using pneumatic tools in Bedford, Ind, who had a prevalence of Raynaud's phenomenon of 80%. Despite a subsequent plethora of studies over the intervening years reaffirming the association, the National Institute for Occupational Safety and Health estimated 64 years later, in 1982, that 1.2 million Americans may have had significant exposure to high-frequency vibration, and as many as 89% of selected populations may be affected.[6] The association of HAVS and handheld tools, such as pneumatic hammers, drills, grinders, and chain saws is well known. However, the injury is not restricted to a few types of tools, but occurs in a variety of situations in which the hands of workers are subjected to significant vibration exposure.[7] Table 13–1 lists the types of tools that commonly cause HAVS.

Publications concerning HAVS have been sparse in the United States, but epidemiological studies from northern Europe and Japan illustrate the magnitude of the problem. The prevalence of HAVS has been reported to be from 7% to 84% in workers exposed to vibration injury in various industries.[8–16] The variability of occurrence undoubtedly relates to differences in individual susceptibility to HAVS and to the fact that clinical manifestations rarely occur until the worker has been exposed for at least 2,000 hours.[17] Initial symptoms of HAVS are numbness and tingling, consistent with compression neuropathy. Confusion with carpal tunnel syndrome may occur, or the two may coexist.[3] Continued vibration exposure, typically over years, results in attacks of blanching of one or more of the vibration-exposed fingers, commonly precipitated by cold. Vasospastic symptoms usually last about 1 hour and are terminated with a reactive hyperemia and considerable pain. Further exposure to vibration may induce a blue–black cyanotic appearance to the affected fingers. All digits of both hands may eventually become involved, although the thumbs are usually spared.[18] Despite the severity of the vasculopathy, only about 1% of the cases will progress to ulceration or gangrene. In order to grade the attacks as objectively as possible, various staging systems have been proposed. Most commonly used is the the Stockholm Hand–Arm Vibration Syndrome Grading scale (Table 13–2). The Stockholm scale has been recommended by the National Institute for Occupational Safety and Health for the basis of worker protection, including mandatory and fully compensated work removal for stage 2 sensorineural or peripheral vascular symptoms.[19]

The pathophysiology of HAVS remains obscure. Experimental and observational studies have lent support to multiple theories, but none has been proven. Obviously, the vibrating tool causes a repetitive trauma, which may have both local and systemic effects. Olsen[20] suggested that hyper-reactivity of a centrally mediated sympathetic reflex mechanism during cooling is responsible for the pronounced vasospasm. Further support for centrally mediated effects has been reported by Harada et al[21] and Miyashita et al,[17] who have demonstrated increased secretion of catecholamines and thyroid hormones, but this has not been a consistent finding by all investigators.[22] Numerous reports have focused on local phenomena. Gemne et al[23] have suggested

TABLE 13–1. TOOLS ASSOCIATED WITH HAND–ARM VIBRATION SYNDROME

Pneumatic tools
  Riveting
  Caulking
  Drilling
  Clinching and flanging
Rotary burring tools
Pneumatic hammers
Chain saws
Grinders
  Pedestal
  Handheld
Chipping hammers
Concrete vibro-thickener
Concrete leveling vibro-tables

TABLE 13–2. THE STOCKHOLM HAND–ARM VIBRATION SYNDROME GRADING SCALE

Vascular Assessment			Sensorineural Assessment	
Stage	Grade	Description	Stage	Symptoms
0		No attacks	0SN	Exposed to vibration but no symptoms
1	Mild	Occasional attacks affecting the tips of one or more fingers	1SN	Intermittent numbness, with or without tingling
2	Moderate	Occasional attacks affecting the distal and middle (rarely also proximal) phalanges of one or more fingers	2SN	Intermittent or persistent numbness, reducing sensory perception
3	Severe	Frequent attacks affecting *all* phalanges of most fingers	3SN	Intermittent or persistent numbness, reducing discrimination and/or manipulative dexterity
4	Very severe	As in stage 3, with trophic skin change in the fingertips		

Reprinted with permission from the International Standards Organization (ISO). *Guidelines for the Measurement and the Assessment of Human Exposure to Hand-transmitted Vibration.* Publication 5349. Geneva, Switzerland: ISO; 1986.

that patients with HAVS have increased peripheral resistance independent of the sympathetic nervous system. Other authors have reported that vibration-exposed vessels are highly responsive to vasoconstrictive stimuli,[24] possibly through perturbation of pacinian corpuscles[25] or peripheral damage to sympathetic nerves, allowing an increased vasoconstrictive reflex.[26] Hematologic abnormalities have been implicated as well. Vibration has been reported to increase platelet activation with the release of vasoconstrictive and mitogenic factors.[27,28] Alterations in blood viscosity and red blood cell deformity may also result from vibration exposure.[29] Undoubtedly, HAVS is a combination of local effects on the vessels and peripheral nerves, over which a central sympathetic effect may be superimposed.

The diagnosis of the vasospastic component of the HAVS is made from a history of the chronic use of vibrating tools and classic Raynaud's symptoms. Objective diagnostic tests may be useful in documenting vasospasm and digital vessel occlusion, but none is specific for HAVS. Cold provocation tests, which rely on either the delayed recovery of digital temperature[30,31] or abnormal diminution of finger systolic pressure detected by laser Doppler,[32] may aid in diagnosis. In advanced cases with digital artery occlusion, transcutaneous Doppler ultrasound[33] or B-mode scanning[34] is useful. Of 80 chippers evaluated at the Northwestern University (Chicago, Ill) Blood Flow Laboratory, 25% had a significant reduction in systolic pressure in one or more digits.[35] In six of these patients, arteriography demonstrated occlusion of the digital arteries (Fig. 13–1).

Treatment of the vasospastic component of HAVS consists of the symptomatic treatment of Raynaud's phenomenon; no specific therapy for HAVS exists. Most important, use of vibrating tools should be discontinued. In early stages of the disease, reversal of symptoms is possible, although this may take years. In advanced cases symptoms are typically irreversible, and may even progress despite cessation of vibra-

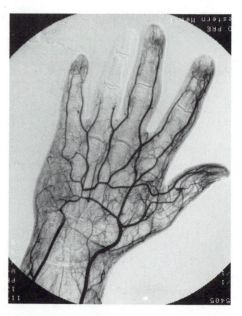

Figure 13–1. Arteriogram of a chipper exposed to arm vibration. There is complete occlusion of the digital arteries of the fourth finger.

tory injury. Patients should be advised to abstain from smoking, and avoidance of caffeine may be helpful. Ergotamine preparations and β-adrenergic blocking agents should be avoided, as should cold exposure. Biofeedback, therapeutic or aquatic exercises, heat treatment, and massage may provide some relief of symptoms.[36] Pharmacological therapy includes that for Raynaud's phenomenon, although a few trials have addressed HAVS specifically. Nifedipine and diltiazem have demonstrated effectiveness[36–38] for some patients. Other potentially useful agents include α-receptor blockers (prozosin) and prostacyclin analogs (iloprost). Prevention remains more effective than cure, however. Antivibration gloves should be used when exposure is unavoidable. Hand-grip force should be minimized on tools, and tools should be operated at reduced speeds when possible.[39] Antivibration measures, including education, worker counseling, periodic examination of exposed workers, avoidance of continued exposure, and adherence of factories to acceptable standards as suggested by the National Institute for Occupational Safety and Health in 1989, should be encouraged.[19]

HYPOTHENAR HAMMER SYNDROME

The hypothenar hammer syndrome is a traumatic arterial injury of the ulnar artery caused by the repetitive use of the palm of the hand as a blunt instrument to push, pound, or twist. It also may result from the use of vibratory tools, independent of HAVS.[40] Raynaud's phenomenon, aneurysm formation with digital embolization, or ulnar artery thrombosis may result.

The ulnar artery is the main supply of the superficial palmar arch, from which the digital vessels are usually based. The ulnar artery enters the hand through Guyton's canal (Fig. 13–2), which is a groove bounded by the hook of the hamate and the pisiform on its ulnar aspect. The floor of the canal is formed by the pisohamate ligament, an extension of the transverse carpal ligament. Just distal to the pisiform, the ulnar artery lies quite superficially, covered here only by the skin, subcutaneous

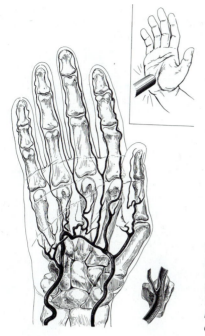

Figure 13–2. Mechanism of ulnar artery injury in hypothenar hammer syndrome. The ulnar artery is vulnerable to injury because of its superficial location and close proximity to the hamate bone. (*Reprinted with permission from Yao JST. Occupational vascular problems. In: Rutherford RB, ed. Vascular Surgery. 3rd ed. Philadelphia: WB Saunders Co; 1989;1:900.*)

tissue, and the palmaris brevis muscle. It is in this 2-cm subcutaneous segment that the ulnar artery is vulnerable to blunt trauma. Distally, it courses through the superficial palmar fascia to a more protected position.

In 1934 Von Rosen[41] provided the first descriptive report of this condition, and only since 1948 has it been recognized as an occupational disease.[42] Patients with the hypothenar hammer syndrome may present with symptoms of Raynaud's phenomenon, although the traditional triphasic color (white–blue–red) changes and thumb involvement are uncommon.[43] Embolization to digital arteries may occur form an ulnar aneurysm, or the ulnar artery may thrombose. The type of arterial injury will depend on the nature of the damage to the vessel. Intimal damage often results in thrombotic occlusion, whereas injury to the media causes aneurysm formation (Fig. 13–3). Physical examination may reveal a prominent callus over the hypothenar eminence, coldness or mottling of the involved fingertip, and atrophic ulceration. A positive Allen's test, indicating ulnar artery occlusion, is common. In the series of patients described by Conn and colleagues,[44] the ring finger was the one most commonly involved. Occasionally, an aneurysm can be found as a pulsatile mass in the palm. The diagnosis is made by a consistent history and presenting symptoms and may be confirmed by noninvasive testing. B-mode scan is of particular value in detecting ulnar aneurysms. Arteriography is helpful in the diagnosis and planning of treatment. It will define the type of vascular lesion (spasm, aneurysm, or occlusion) and may demonstrate a characteristic "corkscrew" pattern.[45] Not infrequently, an incomplete superficial palmar arch is seen in the asymptomatic hand.

Treatment of hypothenar hammer syndrome should be guided by symptoms, noninvasive studies, and arteriographic findings. All patients should be encouraged to avoid use of the hand as a blunt instrument and to acquire the appropriate tools and padded gloves. Supportive therapy of ulnar artery occlusion is often sufficient. Interposition vein grafting rarely may be appropriate,[46] particularly in patients with an incomplete superficial palmar arch. Recently, we have used thrombolytic therapy

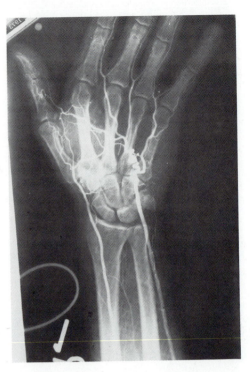

Figure 13–3. Aneurysm of the ulnar artery in a patient with hypothenar hammer syndrome. (*Reprinted with permission from Yao JST. Occupational vascular problems. In: Rutherford RB, ed.* Vascular Surgery. *3rd ed. Philadelphia: WB Saunders Co; 1989;1:901.*)

(urokinase infusion) to treat a patient with thrombosis of the ulnar artery. An underlying thrombosed aneurysm was uncovered after 24 hours of infusion (Figs. 13–4 and 13–5). Aneurysm of the ulnar artery should be resected to eliminate the source of embolization. If good collateral flow is demonstrated with a complete superficial palmar arch, excision and ligation may be performed; otherwise, end-to-end ulnar artery anastomosis or interposition vein grafting is necessary.[47–49]

OCCUPATIONAL ACRO-OSTEOLYSIS

Occupational acro-osteolysis is a syndrome of osteolysis of the distal phalanges of the hand, Raynaud's phenomenon, and scleroderma-like skin induration first described by Wilson and colleagues[50] in workers exposed to the manufacturing and polymerization of polyvinyl chloride. The dominant presenting symptoms are those of Raynaud's phenomenon. Diagnosis is made by obtaining the proper occupational history and a consistent physical examination and by excluding other causes of Raynaud's phenomenon. Although the syndrome is well recognized, its prevalence of 1% in chronically exposed workers[50,51] suggests an idiosyncratic response in a minority of individuals, and a potential genetic defect has been indentified.[52] Few reports of angiography in this syndrome have been published to document digital artery injury.[53–55] The findings include multiple arterial stenoses and occlusions of the digital arteries, along with areas of hypervascularity adjacent to the areas of bony resorption. The reason for the hypervascularity is not clear, but it may be related to the stasis of contrast in digital pulp arteries, secondary to shortening and retraction of the fingers. The digits may be clubbed, a finding that has been associated with hypervascularity of the fingertips. There is suggestion that cessation of exposure may allow the symptoms to abate.[56]

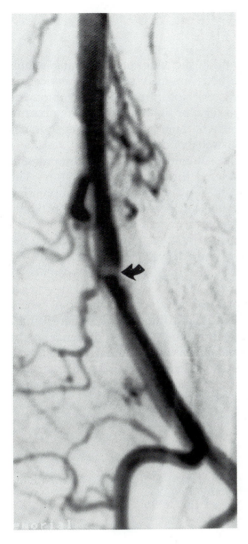

Figure 13–4. Occlusion (*arrow*) of the ulnar artery in a patient with hypothenar hammer syndrome.

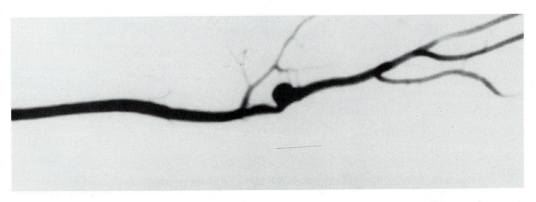

Figure 13–5. In the same patient as in Fig 13–4, an ulnar artery aneurysm was discovered after 24 hours of urokinase therapy.

THORACIC OUTLET COMPRESSION TO THE SUBCLAVIAN–AXILLARY ARTERY

Thoracic outlet compression due to overhead working activities or exaggerated shoulder motion is well known. The presence of a bony anomaly such as a cervical rib or anomalous first rib may be the causative factor. Not infrequently, symptomatic compression of the axillary artery, subclavian artery, or their branches may occur in any athlete, particularly a professional athlete, who engages in vigorous shoulder motions in the extremes of position. Reports of basebal pitchers, swimmers, kayakers, tennis players, oarsmen, and weight lifters who suffered symptomatic compression of the axillary and subclavian arteries are scattered throughout the literature. The increasing number of athletes diagnosed with these various causes of compression over the past several years probably results from an increased recognition of the problem, rather than a true increase in prevalence.

In the absence of cervical bands or ribs, arterial compression around the thoracic outlet and the shoulder may occur in four discrete locations (Fig. 13–6). Proximally, after exiting the thorax, the subclavian artery passes just posterior to the anterior scalene muscle, which may compress the artery if the scalene muscle is hypertrophic. The next site at which compression may occur is the point where the subclavian artery courses between the clavicle and the first rib, where it may become scissored between them. The axillary artery then courses posterior to the pectoralis minor, where it may be compressed against the thorax, particularly if the pectoralis minor is hypertrophic and the shoulder is abducted and externally rotated to the extreme. The suprascapular, subscapular, and posterior humeral

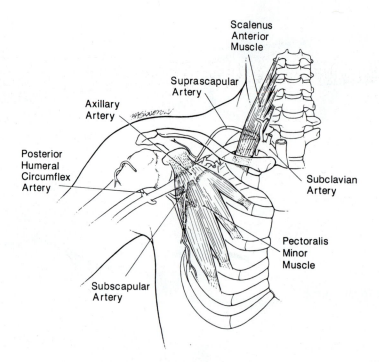

Figure 13–6. Anatomy of the subclavian and axillary arteries, demonstrating potential sites of compression around the thoracic outlet and shoulder. (*Reprinted with permission from McCarthy WJ, Yao JST, Schafer MF, et al. Upper extremity arterial injury in athletes. J Vasc Surg. 1989;9:321.*[60])

circumflex arteries may be compressed or become aneurysmal[57] (Figs. 13–7 and 13–8). In this same position the head of the humerus rotates anteriorly, which may cause the axillary artery to pull across it in a bowstring fashion, the fourth site of compression.[58] Hypertrophy of the humeral head has been described in athletes,[59] and this may contribute to the mechanism of compression.

Professional athletes suffering from compression may present with claudication-like symptoms, distal embolization, or thrombosis. Claudication-like symptoms manifest initially as early arm fatigue in an otherwise well-conditioned athlete. Baseball pitchers suffer a measurable loss of pitching velocity and are unable to pitch more than one to three innings.[60] Forearm pain, throwing arm heaviness, and hand coldness may also occur. Arterial injury in professional baseball pitchers includes thrombosis of the subclavian or axillary artery (Fig. 13–8)[58,61] and aneurysm of the circumflex artery with digital embolization. Rarely, retrograde propagation of the thrombus may result in a right hemispheric stroke, and this has been reported in a professional baseball pitcher.[62]

Evaluation of such symptoms requires close communication with an orthopedic sports specialist. Clearly, upper extremity symptoms in athletes are common, most of them resulting from musculoskeletal conditions. A careful history, including the motion and position that elicit the pain, is necessary. Localization of the pain is of obvious importance. Pulses should be palpated in the neutral, abduction-external rotation, and specific playing positions, along with auscultation for bruits. Noninvasive evaluation, including duplex scanning of the axillosubclavian segment in the various postures, is also useful. Arteriography remains the definitive technique, and

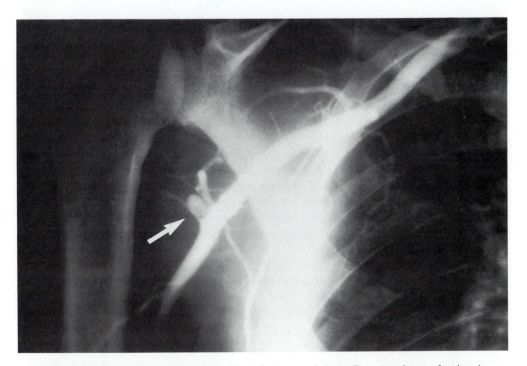

Figure 13–7. Aneurysm (*arrow*) of the posterior humeral circumflex artery in a professional baseball player. (*Reprinted with permission from Benjamin ME, Yao JST. Aneurysms of secondary and tertiary branches of major arteries. In: Yao JST, Pearce WH, eds. Aneurysms: New Findings and Treatments. Norwalk, Conn: Appleton & Lange; 1994;511.*)

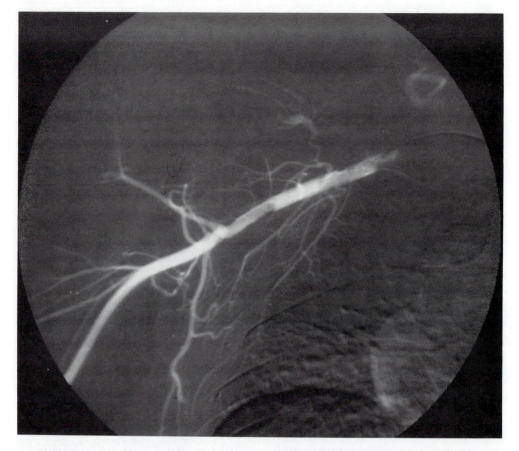

Figure 13–8. Partially occluding thrombus of the axillary artery in a professional baseball player.

also must be performed in the extremes of position. However, it is important to remember that some degree of detectable compression may be apparent in about 50% of individuals who are asymptomatic,[58] and therefore careful consideration of alternative diagnoses is recommended.

Treatment must be individualized and largely depends on the extent of arterial injury. For compression without signs of arterial injury, cessation of the aggravating activity is probably the most effective treatment, although this is likely to be considered unacceptable to the professional athlete. Alteration of the pitching motion has been effective in a number of the professional pitchers seen at Northwestern University. If not, division of the offending muscle and tendon or bony abnormality may be necessary. Aneurysm requires resection and bypass grafting along with decompression. We have chosen to use the saphenous vein graft, with good results. For a short stenotic artery, patch angioplasty may suffice. Thrombolytic therapy may also play a role for athletes with distal embolization or thrombosis with noncritical ischemia, but definitive treatment of the underlying cause will be necessary. Treatment of humerus head compression without arterial injury remains uncertain, and further experience is needed to establish the proper surgical approach in these patients.[63]

HAND ISCHEMIA IN ATHLETES

Hand ischemia in athletes may result from either distal emolization of a source around the thoracic outlet or, more commonly, repetitive local trauma to the hand with subsequent occlusion of the radial, ulnar, or digital arteries. Hand ischemia from repetitive blunt trauma in the athlete is analogous to the hypothenar hammer syndrome, but the distribution of digital artery disease may be different, depending on the sport.[60]

Any sport in which repetitive blunt trauma to the hand occurs may lead to ischemia. Most commonly, it is seen in baseball catchers[60] and handball players[64] but has also been reported in karate experts; frisbee, lacrosse, and volleyball players[65]; and a bare-handed softball player.[66] Patients usually present with symptoms of chronic hand complaints, including cold hypersensitivity, finger numbness, finger coolness, and blanching. Baseball catchers often first seek medical attention in the off-season, when engaged in outdoor activity in the cool autumn or winter. Occasionally, the athlete will present with severe post-traumatic hand ischemia, complaining of severe finger and palm pain.[60]

The diagnosis is established by history and physical examination and may be substantiated with upper extremity noninvasive tests. Segmental brachial, radial, and ulnar artery pressures are measured, as are digital systolic pressures and the competency of the palmar arch by the Doppler technique. Cold sensitivity may be assessed with thermistors on the fingertips.[33] Arteriography is reserved for those patients with severe and continuous painful ischemia.

Considering the speed of the baseball and the force exerted on the hand with impact, arterial injury in professional catchers may be more frequent than has been suspected. Lowrey et al[67] have reported decreased digital perfusion to the index finger of the glove hand of 13 of 22 minor league catchers studied. In a series of 10 catchers studied at Northwestern University, 40% had evidence of digital artery occlusion.[35] As one might suspect, the cumulative effect of the trauma is important. Sugawara et al[68] reported that injury to the digital arteries is uncommon in junior high school players, with an increased prevalence in high school and college players. Buckhout[64] has estimated that players with greater than 200 hours of accumulated handball playing time are at greater risk.

Treatment of hand ischemia is most often nonoperative. In a recent series at Northwestern University,[60] no patient required surgical intervention. In two patients with acute severe ischemia, intra-arterial vasodilator therapy during arteriography relieved spasm, followed by dextran and heparin administration. Patients with chronic complaints should be advised to avoid cold exposure and increase the padding in the glove of the affected hand. If a palmar artery aneurysm is detected, resection is recommended.

REFERENCES

1. Rempel DM, Harrison RJ, Barn Hart S. Work-related cumulative trauma disorders of the upper extremity. *JAMA.* 1992;267(6):838–842.
2. *Bureau of Labor Statistics Reports on Survey of Occupational Injuries and Illnesses in 1977–1989.* Washington, DC: Bureau of Labor Statistics, US Department of Labor; 1990.
3. Boyle JC, Smith NJ, Burke FD. Vibration white finger. *J Hand Surg (British).* 1988;13B:171.
4. Loriga G. Ill lavoro con i martelli pneumatic boll. *Ipsett.* 1911;2:35.

5. Hamilton A. A study of spastic anemia in the hands of stonecutters: an effect of the airhammer on the hands of stonecutters. *Ind Acc Hygiene Ser.* 1918;236/19.

6. National Institute for Occupational Safety and Health. *Vibration White Finger Disease in US Workers Using Pneumatic Chipping and Grinding Hand Tools. I: Epidemiology.* Washington, DC: US Department of Health and Human Services; 1982;82:118.

7. Griffen MJ. *Vibration Injuries of the Hand and Arm: Their Occurrence and the Evaluation of Standards and Limits.* London, England: Her Majesty's Stationery Office; 1980.

8. Harkonen H, Riihimaki H, Tola S, et al. Symptoms of vibration syndrome and radiographic findings in the wrists of lumberjacks. *Br J Ind Med.* 1984;41:133.

9. Futatsaka M, Ueno T. Vibration exposure and vibration-induced white finger due to chain saw operation. *J Occup Med.* 1985;27:257

10. Brubaker RL, MacKenzie CJ, Hutton SG. Vibration induced white finger among selected underground rock drillers in British Columbia. *Scand J Work Environ Health.* 1986;12:296.

11. Dandell R, Engstrom K. Vibration from riveting tools in the frequency range of 6 Hz–10 MHz and Raynaud's phenomenon. *Scand J Work Environ Health.* 1986;12:338.

12. Yu ZS, Chao H, Qiao L, et al. Epidemiologic survey of vibration syndrome among riveters, chippers, and grinders in the railway system of the People's Republic of China. *Scand J Work Environ Health.* 1986;12:289.

13. Nilsson T, Burstrom L, Hagberg M. Risk assessment of vibration exposure and white fingers among platers. *Int Arch Occup Environ Health.* 1989;61:473.

14. Hedlund U. Raynaud's phenomenon of fingers and toes of miners exposed to local and whole-body vibration and cold. *Int Arch Occup Environ Health.* 1989;61:457.

15. Dimberg L, Oden A. White finger symptoms: a cross sectional study. *Aviat Space Environ Med.* 1991;62:879.

16. Letz R, Cherniak MG, Gerr F, et al. A cross sectional epidemiological survey of shipyard workers exposed to hand–arm vibration. *Br J Ind Med.* 1992;49:53.

17. Miyashita K, Shiomi S, Itoh N, et al. Epidemiological study of vibration syndrome is response to total hand-tool operating time. *Br J Ind Med* 1983;40:92.

18. Taylor W. Vibration white finger in the workplace. *J Soc Occup Med.* 1982;32:159.

19. National Institute for Occupational Safety and Health. *Occupational Exposure to Hand–Arm Vibration. Criteria for a Recommneded Standard 1989.* Washington, DC: US Department of Health and Human Services; 1989;89-106.

20. Olsen N. Hyperactivity of the central nervous system in vibration induced white finger. *Kurume Med J.* 1990;37:S109.

21. Harada N, Nakamoto M, Kohno H, et al. Hormonal response to cold exposure in subjects with vibration syndrome. *Kurume Med J.* 1990;37:S45.

22. Bovenzi M. Vibration white finger, digital blood pressure and some biochemical findings on workers operating vibrating tools in the engine manufacturing industry. *Am J Ind Med.* 1988;14:575.

23. Gemne G, Pyykko I, Starck J, et al. Circulatory reaction to heat and cold in vibration-induced white finger with and without sympathetic blockade—an experimental study. *Scand J Work Environ Health.* 1986;12:371.

24. Futatsaka M, Pyykko I, Farkkila M, et al. Blood pressure, flow and peripheral resistance of digital artery in vibration syndrome. *Br J Ind Med.* 1983;40:434.

25. Pyykko I, Hyvarinen J, Farkkila M. Studies on the etiological mechanism of the vasospastic component of the vibration syndrome. In: Brammer AJ, Taylor W, eds. *Vibration Effects of the Hand and Arm in Industry.* New York: John Wiley & Sons; 1982;13–25.

26. Ho ST, Yu HS. Ultrastructural changes of the peripheral nerve induced by vibration: an experimental study. *Br J Ind Med.* 1989;46:157.

27. Ikehata K, Kawauchi S, Kohno F, et al. Increased platelet function and von Willebrand factor in vibration syndrome. *Tokushima J Exp Med.* 1980;27:23.

28. Biondi ML, Marasini B. Abnormal platelet aggregation in patients with Raynaud's phenomenon. *J Clin Pathol.* 1989;42:716.

29. Belch JF, McLaren M, Chopra M, et al. Blood coagulation and rheology in patients with vibration white finger disease. Proceedings of a symposium on the assessment and associ-

ated problems of vibration white finger; October 19, 1988; New Cross Hospital, Wolverhampton, England.

30. Kurumatani N, Iki M, Hirata K, et al. Usefulness of fingertip skin temperature for examining peripheral circulatory disturbances of vibrating tool operators. *Scand J Work Environ Health.* 1986;12:245.

31. Bovenzi M. Finger thermometry in the assessment of subjects with vibration induced white finger. *Scand J Work Environ Health.* 1987;13:348.

32. Allen JA, Doherty CC, McGrann S. Objective testing for vasospasm in the hand–arm vibration syndrome. *Br J Ind Med.* 1992;49:688.

33. Baxter BT, Blackburn DR, Payne K, et al. Noninvasive evaluation of the upper extremity. *Surg Clin North Am.* 1990;70:1.

34. Payne KM, Blackburn DR, Peterson LK, et al. B-mode imaging of the arteries of the hand and upper extremity. *Bruit.* 1986;10:168.

35. Bartel P, Blackburn DR, Peterson LK, et al. The value of non-invasive tests in occupational trauma of the hands and fingers. *Bruit.* 1984;8:15.

36. Matoba T, Kuwahara H. Treatments for hand–arm vibration disease in Japan. *Kurume Med J.* 1990;37:S123.

37. Harada N. The effect of nifedipine (Aldalat) on vibration syndrome. *J Jpn Coll Angiol.* 1986;26:403.

38. Nilsson H, Jonason T, Leppert J, et al. The effect of the calcium channel blocker nifedipine on cold induced digital vasospasm. *Acta Med Scand.* 1987;221:53.

39. Wasserman D. The control aspects of occupational hand–arm vibration. *Appl Ind Hygiene.* 1989;4:F22.

40. Kaji H, Honma H, Usui M, et al. Hypothenar hammer syndrome in workers occupationally exposed to vibrating tools. *J Hand Surg (British).* 1993;18B:761.

41. Von Rosen S. Einfall von thrombose in der Arteria ulnaris nach einwirkung von stumpfer gewalt. *Acta Chir Scand.* 1934;73:500.

42. Short DW. Occupational aneurysm of the palmar arch. *Lancet.* 1948;2:217.

43. Pineda CJ, Weisman MH, Bookstein JJ, et al. Hypothenar hammer syndrome: form of reversible Raynaud's phenomenon. *Am J Med.* 1985;79:561.

44. Conn J, Bergan JJ, Bell JL. Hypothenar hammer syndrome: post-traumatic digital ischemia. *Surgery.* 1970;68:1122.

45. Hammond DC, Matloub HS, Yousif NJ, et al. The corkscrew sign in hypothenar hammer syndrome. *J Hand Surg (British).* 1993;18B:767.

46. Melhoff TL, Wood MB. Ulnar artery thrombosis and the role of interposition vein grafting: patency and microsurgical technique. *J Hand Surg (American).* 1991;16(2):274.

47. Vayssairat M, Debure C, Cormier J, et al. Hypothenar hammer syndrome: seventeen cases with long-term follow-up. *J Vasc Surg.* 1987;5:835.

48. Harris EJ, Taylor LM, Edwards JM, et al. Surgical treatment of distal ulnar artery aneurysms. *Am J Surg.* 1990;159(5):527.

49. Rothkopf DM, Bryan DJ, Cuadros CL, et al. Surgical management of ulnar artery aneurysms. *J Hand Surg (American).* 1990;15(6):891.

50. Wilson R, McCormick W, Tatton C, et al. Occupational acro-osteolysis. *JAMA.* 1967;210:577.

51. LaPlanche A, Claval-Chapelon F, Contassot JC, et al. Exposure to vinyl chloride monomer: results of a cohort study after seven year follow up. *Br J Ind Med.* 1992;45(2):134.

52. Black C, Pereira S, McWhirter A, et al. Genetic susceptibility to scleroderma-like syndrome in symptomatic and asymptomatic workers exposed to vinyl chloride. *J Rheum.* 1986;13(6):1059.

53. Veltman G. Raynaud's syndrome in vinyl chloride disease. In: Heidrich H, ed. *Raynaud's Phenomenon.* Berlin, Germany: TM-Verlag; 1979;211–216.

54. Falappa P, Magnavita N, Bergamarchi A, et al. Angiographic study of the digital arteries in workers exposed to vinyl chloride. *Br J Ind Med.* 1982;39:169.

55. Bookstein JJ. Arteriography. In: Poznanski AK, ed. *The Hand in Radiologic Diagnosis with Gamuts and Pattern Profiles.* 2nd ed. Philadelphia: WB Saunders Co; 1984;97–112.

56. Freudiger H, Bounameaux H, Garcia J. Acroosteolysis and Raynaud's phenomenon after vinyl chloride exposure. *Vasa.* 1988;17:216.

57. Nuber GW, McCarthy WJ, Yao JST, et al. Arterial abnormalities of the shoulder in athletes. *Am J Sports Med*. 1990;18(5):514.

58. Rohrer MJ, Cardullo PA, Pappas AM, et al. Axillary artery compression and thrombosis in throwing athletes. *J Vasc Surg*. 1990;11:761.

59. Jones HH, Priest JD, Hayes WC, et al. Humeral hypertrophy in response to exercise. *J Bone J Surg*. 1977;59A:204.

60. McCarthy WJ, Yao JST, Schafer MF, et al. Upper extremity arterial injury in athletes. *J Vasc Surg*. 1989;9:317.

61. Tullos HS, Erwin WD, Woods GW, et al. Unusual lesions of the pitching arm. *Clin Orthop*. 1972;88:169.

62. Fields WS, Lemak NA, Ben-Menachem Y. Thoracic outlet syndrome: a review and reference to stroke in a major league pitcher. *AJNR*. 1986;7:73.

63. Durham JR, Yao JST, Pearce WH, et al. Arterial injuries in the thoracic outlet syndrome. Presented at Society for Vascular Surgery Annual Meeting; June 7, 1994; Seattle, Wash.

64. Buckhout BC, Warner MA. Digital perfusion of handball players: effect of repeated ball impact on structures of the hand. *Am J Sports Med*. 1980;8:206.

65. Ho PK, Dellon AL, Wilgis EFS. True aneurysms of the hand resulting from athletic injury: report of two cases. *Am J Sports Med*. 1985;13:136.

66. Kaplan EB, Zeide MS. Aneurysms of the ulnar artery: a case report. *Bull Hosp J Dis*. 1972;33:197.

67. Lowrey CW, Chadwick RO, Waltman EN. Digital vessel trauma from repetitive impact in baseball catchers. *J Hand Surg (American)*. 1976;1:236.

68. Sugawara M, Ogino T, Minami A, et al. Digital ischemia in baseball players. *Am J Sports Med*. 1986;14:329.

14

Hand and Finger Ischemia in Patients with Connective Tissue Disorders

Robert B. McLafferty, MD, Lloyd M. Taylor, Jr, MD, and John M. Porter, MD

Diverse disease processes affecting the small arteries of the hand may produce ischemic symptoms ranging from mild episodic skin color changes to severe rest pain, ulceration, and gangrene. The true frequency with which various diseases produce hand ischemia is difficult to determine because of inconsistent referral patterns at various medical centers. It appears clearly established, however, that connective tissue disorders (CTDs) are responsible for a significant proportion of severe hand and finger ischemia in our population. Since 1974, we in the Division of Vascular Surgery at Oregon Health Sciences University (Portland) have prospectively evaluated and followed up more than 1,000 patients with symptomatic hand ischemia. Patients with CTDs represent approximately 30% of this population. Some patients who initially presented with hand ischemia and no associated diagnosis subsequently have been found to have a CTD. This chapter reviews the history, clinical presentation, epidemiology, pathophysiology, differential diagnosis, and treatment of hand ischemia, with special emphasis on CTDs.

HISTORY

In 1862 Maurice Raynaud described a group of patients with digital vasospastic attacks.[1] Because most of his patients had normal wrist pulses, he theorized that the episodic digital ischemia was caused by vasospasm resulting from overactivity of the sympathetic nervous system. At the turn of the century, Hutchinson recognized that episodic digital ischemia was frequently associated with other conditions, such as arteriosclerosis, scleroderma, and heart failure.[2] He coined the term *Raynaud's phenomenon* for episodes of finger ischemic color changes common to multiple diseases. In 1932 Allen and Brown published a clinical approach to episodic finger ischemia still used by many clinicians.[3] They proposed characterizing digital vasospastic attacks as Raynaud's disease (a benign idiopathic condition) or Raynaud's phenomenon (a symptom complex occurring in association with one or more of a variety of associated disorders). They further proposed that if no associated disorder developed within 2 years of the onset of symptoms, primary Raynaud's disease could be diagnosed with confidence. Many investigators since Allen and Brown's influential publication have reported their observations using this classification.[4–6] At our institution we have chosen to classify patients presenting with intermittent digital ischemic symptoms as having Raynaud's syndrome (RS) recognizing that they have an increased lifelong risk for the development of a CTD or other associated disorder.

CLINICAL PRESENTATION

Raynaud's Syndrome

Classic RS attacks consist of episodes of intense pallor when the fingers are cooled followed by cyanosis and rubor upon rewarming. This is frequently accompanied by numbness and discomfort, but severe pain is rare. Vasospastic attacks are occasionally induced by emotional stress. Full recovery generally takes 15 to 45 minutes after resolution of the precipitating event. Variations in classic sequential tricolor attacks are observed in many patients with RS. Patients may present with only cold hands and no color changes yet by vascular laboratory or angiography have identical pathology to those with classic tricolor changes. Typically, both hands are affected, with sparing of the thumbs. The majority of patients have mild symptoms in the hands. The feet are also affected in about 50% of patients, whereas only 10% of patients have symptoms in the feet alone.

Rest Pain, Ulceration, and Gangrene

Ischemic rest pain, finger ulceration, and finger gangrene are obviously symptoms of severe ischemia, which are frequently associated with intermittent digital vasospastic attacks. Fixed digital ischemia always indicates the presence of an underlying disease associated with significant small artery occlusion in the hand. In addition to severe pain in the affected digits, which are extremely sensitive to touch, chronic deformative changes in the fingernails, swelling, rubor, and infection (particularly under the nails) are frequent findings. Patients with a prior history of stable mild RS may, on occasion, present with painful digital ulceration.[7] Conversely, patients may experience the abrupt onset of severe digital ischemia as the first symptom and go on to develop chronic RS following resolution of the acute symptoms.[8–10]

EPIDEMIOLOGY

In damp cool climates, including the Pacific Northwestern United States, England, and Denmark, approximately 20% to 25% of all people between the ages of 18 and 45 years are affected by varying degrees of RS. Most patients with RS are women under 30 years of age. The prevalence of RS in patients with a CTD is extremely high. It is estimated that 80% or more of patients with CTDs are afflicted with RS.[11–13] Epidemiological research has more often focused on determining the prevalence of associated diseases, including CTDs in patients with RS.

An early series from the Mayo Clinic (Rochester, Minn) found that of 204 patients with RS, 57 (28%) had an associated systemic disease, frequently scleroderma or arthritis.[14] Blain, Coller, and Carver at the University of Michigan in 1950 reported that 119 (50%) of 238 patients with RS had an associated disease process, using the criteria of Allen and Brown.[15] More than 100 patients had been followed up longer than 5 years, and of these, 69% remained unchanged or improved, 6% had moderate disease progression, and 25% had severe disease progression. In 1962 de Takats and Fowler challenged the 2-year limit for diagnosis of primary Raynaud's disease.[6] It became clinically apparent that many years could elapse between the onset of RS and the development of a CTD. Clearly, the 2 years specified by Allen and Brown was not long enough. A publication from our laboratory in 1976 indicated that 59 (81%) of 73 patients with RS had an associated disease.[16] However, subsequent data have demonstrated a lower percentage of associated diseases (46%), clearly reflecting changes in referral patterns.[17] As our interest in RS became known, we began to receive patients with milder symptoms. An important study by Priollet, Vayssairat, and Housset in 1987 classified 240 patients with RS.[18] Seventy patients (29%) had no associated disease and 26 patients (11%) had one or more abnormal immunologic tests without meeting American Rheumatism Association criteria. The remaining 144 (60%) patients were diagnosed with a CTD. Those patients suspected of having primary RS and those suspected of having an associated CTD were followed for a mean of 4.7 years. Forty-nine of the 70 patients originally diagnosed with primary RS were available, one of whom became reclassified as having a suspected CTD. Twenty-four of the 26 patients originally having a serologic abnormality without a diagnosis of CTD were available, 14 of whom went on to receive a firm diagnosis of CTD. This led to the conclusion that patients initially presenting with one or more specific CTD laboratory abnormalities are at increased risk for developing an associated CTD over the long term and should be followed up carefully. Conversely, patients with no findings at initial evaluation can be reliably diagnosed as having primary RS.

The prevalence of RS caused by associated disorders unrelated to CTD has not been fully established. Large artery causes include atherosclerosis, proximal or distal aneurysmal disease, and trauma.[7,19,20] Small artery causes include hypersensitivity angiitis, Buerger's disease, cold injury (frostbite), and chronic vibration disorder.[21–24] Hematologic abnormalities, cancer, and disorders of thyroid function have also been implicated.[25–29] Velayos et al reported a nearly equal proportion of patients having a non–CTD-associated disease (38%) as compared to those with a CTD (42%).[30] A more recent study by Mills et al found 27% of patients to have a CTD, 19% to have other associated diseases, and 54% showing no evidence of either.[31] Edwards and Porter reported classification of 635 patients with RS. They determined 27% to have an associated CTD, 19% to have a non–CTD-associated disease, and 54% without an associated disease.[17] More recent data from Porter et al on 911 patients are illustrated in Table 14–1.[32]

PATHOPHYSIOLOGY

The pathophysiology responsible for Raynaud's syndrome can be divided into two distinct mechanisms: obstructive and vasospastic.[7,33,34] Both mechanisms are capable of producing ischemia sufficient to incite a Raynaud's attack. Some patients exhibit signs, symptoms, and vascular laboratory findings consistent with both mechanisms, suggesting a continuum of disease rather than two separate entities.

TABLE 14–1. ASSOCIATED DISEASES

	No. of Patients	Total
Connective Tissue Disorders (CTDs)		290 (32%)
Scleroderma	108	
Systemic lupus erythematosus	21	
Rheumatoid arthritis	17	
Sjögren's disease	21	
Mixed CTD	17	
Undifferentiated CTD	34	
Miscellaneous/unknown CTD	72	
Other Associated Diseases		223 (24%)
Atherosclerosis	51	
Cancer	10	
Buerger's disease	16	
Frostbite/cold exposure	31	
Carpal tunnel syndrome	26	
Hypothyroidism	13	
Vibration exposure	15	
Erythromelalgia	9	
Hypersensitivity angiitis	21	
Hematologic abnormalities	15	
Trauma	16	
Absence of Associated Disease	398	398 (44%)
TOTAL		911

Vasospastic Mechanisms

In spite of 100 years of research, the basic underlying molecular mechanisms causing vasospastic RS are unknown. At room temperature patients with vasospastic RS have normal resting digital artery pressures. A Raynaud's attack takes place when the constrictive force of the arterial wall exceeds the intraluminal distending pressure, causing blood flow to cease. The fact that complete closure of digital arteries occurs during a Raynaud's attack was first observed by Lewis.[4,35] Subsequent studies with plethysmography and angiography have shown complete digital artery closure after a cold challenge despite previously normal digital artery pressure and the absence of significant arterial obstruction.[36–38] Once the critical closing pressure was reached, digital artery pressure remained in the range of only 5 mm Hg.[35] Krahenbuhl and associates[36] discovered that patients with vasospastic RS had moderate decreases in digital artery pressure until a critical temperature of 28°C was reached, when finger artery pressure suddenly became unmeasurable (Fig. 14–1). Coffman and Cohen demonstrated after detailed studies of patients with RS that decreases in digital flow after cooling could be overcome by blocking sympathetic reactivity with reserpine.[33,39] These findings suggested increased adrenergic neuroeffector activity contributing to the pathophysiology of RS.

Other observations suggest that the defect causing abnormal vasospasm is a local rather than systemic phenomenon. One theory implicating a local defect in the arterial wall is alteration in α-adrenergic receptors.[40] Keenan and Porter discovered a significantly higher level of α_2-adrenoceptors in circulating platelets of patients with vasospastic RS compared to patients with obstructive RS as well as normal controls.[41] Although α-adrenoceptors in vascular smooth muscle have not been quantitated in

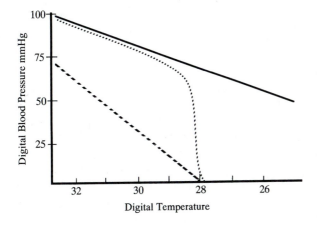

Figure 14–1. The response of digital blood pressure to cold exposure in normal controls (solid line), patients with Raynaud's syndrome (dotted line), and patients with obstructive Raynaud's syndrome (dashed line). (*From Edwards JM, Porter JM. Evaluation of upper extremity ischemia. In: Bernstein EF, ed. Noninvasive Vascular Diagnosis. 4th ed. St Louis, Mo: Mosby–Year Book Inc; 1993;631.*)

digital arteries, numerous experimental and clinical studies support the theory of altered receptors in patients with vasospastic RS.

Many other local and systemic abnormalities have been hypothesized to contribute to vasospastic RS. Deficiencies, excesses, and abnormalities in β-adrenoceptors, endothelin, serotonin receptors, and calcitonin gene-related peptide have all been proposed as contributing to digital hyperreactivity upon cold exposure.[42–46] In addition, alterations in blood viscosity, abnormal serum proteins, and altered shear stress have been implicated in vasospastic RS.[24–28]

Obstructive Mechanisms

In the presence of decreased intraluminal pressure from fixed arterial obstruction, a normal vasoconstrictive response to cold or emotional stimuli results in digital artery closure. Research by Hirai has shown with the use of plethysmography and digital artery blood pressure that mild arterial obstruction is not associated with RS.[47] The onset of a Raynaud's attack requires that both digital arteries in a single digit be obstructed, a situation producing significantly decreased digital pressure.

The mechanisms causing obstruction of small arteries of the hands of patients with CTDs are unknown. The presumed explanation is an antigen–antibody reaction causing transmural necrotizing vasculitis.[29,46] Interestingly, arteries other than in the distal upper extremity are affected less frequently by autoimmune arteritis, with the exception of a few with consistent organ system involvement. Different CTDs have been observed to cause varying amounts of digital artery obstruction. Patients diagnosed with Sjögren's syndrome, progressive systemic sclerosis, or undifferentiated connective tissue disease typically have more diffuse arterial obliteration and hence greater ischemic symptoms than those diagnosed with mixed connective tissue disease, rheumatoid arthritis, or systemic lupus erythematosus.

Distal ischemic symptoms in the upper extremity associated with RS may also be caused by proximal large artery disease.[48] Digital artery obstruction can be caused by emboli from proximal lesions such as subclavian aneurysms. Severe stenosis in proximal arteries can cause a reduction in digital artery blood pressure, leading to Raynaud's attacks in response to cold or emotional stimuli. The most frequent cause of large artery obstruction is atherosclerosis. A variety of other conditions may also affect the large arteries, including Takayasu's disease, giant cell arteritis, thoracic outlet syndrome, radiation arteritis, fibromuscular dysplasia, and trauma.[48–53] In addition, the heart can be a source of embolization, causing large and small artery occlusion.[54,55]

DIFFERENTIAL DIAGNOSIS

Special emphasis should be directed to the pulse examination and blood pressures in both arms. In most instances the diagnosis of RS can be made prior to the vascular laboratory determination of an obstructive versus vasospastic pattern. Our initial patient evaluation also includes a radiograph of the hand to detect the presence of tuft resorption, calcinosis, or arthritis, as well as a basic immunologic screen including a complete blood cell count, chemistry profile, erythrocyte sedimentation rate, antinuclear antibody, and rheumatoid factor. In addition, the vascular laboratory can provide critical adjuvant information to objectively diagnose large artery and/or small artery disease of the upper extremity.

Segmental Pressure Measurement

The first objective step in localizing large artery occlusive disease of the upper extremity is segmental arm measurements with a multiple-cuff system. Using Doppler arterial detection at the wrist, significant decreases in segmental arm pressures can be determined as indexed to the contralateral arm pressure or lower extremity pressure in the case of bilateral upper extremity disease.

Digital Pressures and Wave Forms

The primary tests to differentiate vasospastic from obstructive Raynaud's syndrome are digital blood pressures and analysis of photoplethysmographic (PPG) wave forms. A normal systolic brachial-to-finger pressure gradient ranges from 10 to 20 mm Hg. Significant palmar or digital artery obstruction is present when a brachial-to-finger ratio is greater than 20 mm Hg, more than 20 mm Hg exists between any two fingers, or an absolute finger blood pressure is less than 70 mm Hg.[56] The test is performed by attaching a PPG probe to the test finger with double-sided tape and placing a 2-cm cuff around the proximal phalanx. The cuff is then inflated and the pressure is recorded when the wave form disappears. The specific finding of a peaked pulse on the digital arterial wave form has been associated with RS.[57,58] Representative tracings of normal, vasospastic (peaked pulse), and obstructive wave forms are shown in Figure 14–2. It is important to note that normal arterial wave forms can be present in digits with only one artery occluded or with occlusion distal to the cuff.

Measurement of digital pressures should be performed to determine whether digital ischemia is caused by palmar or proximal digital artery obstruction. If obstruction of one or more digital arteries exists in conjunction with normal arm pressure, upper extremity duplex scanning may be indicated to look for a subclavian aneurysm or other sources of emboli, particularly if symptoms are present only in one hand.[59]

Duplex Scanning

Using the appropriate duplex probe, Doppler signals can be obtained from the aortic arch to the radial and ulnar arteries. The subclavian artery should be viewed from several approaches (eg, infraclavicular fossa, supraclavicular fossa, and sternal notch) to rule out the presence of a subclavian aneurysm. Step-by-step scanning of arterial

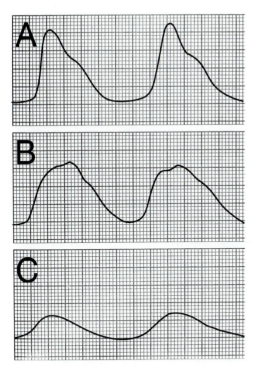

Figure 14–2. (**A**) A normal PPG wave form, (**B**) a peaked pulse associated with vasospastic Raynaud's syndrome, and (**C**) an obstructive digital PPG wave form. (*From Edwards JM, Porter JM. Evaluation of upper extremity ischemia. In: Bernstein EF, ed.* Noninvasive Vascular Diagnosis. *4th ed. St Louis, Mo: Mosby–Year Book Inc; 1993;636.*)

segments, searching for increased velocity and spectral broadening, may indicate the presence of a significant stenosis.

Cold Challenge Testing

Changes in digital pressure after exposure to cold are typically quite different in vasospastic and obstructive Raynaud's patients. As shown in Figure 14–1, normal individuals have less than a 20% drop in digital artery pressure in response to cold.[60,61] Abrupt arterial closure occurs in patients with primary vasospasm when a critical temperature threshold is reached. Digits with obstructive disease show a hypothermic pressure decrease paralleling normal at lower starting pressures.

Fingertip temperature recovery time after immersion in ice water was the first temperature-related vascular laboratory test.[62] Many patients with RS and normal individuals exhibit similar resting digital temperatures and temperature drops after exposure to ice water. Differences occur in the time required for Raynaud's patients to recover to the previous baseline temperature. Typically, Raynaud's patients take more than 20 minutes to recover, as opposed to 5 to 10 minutes in normal individuals (Fig. 14–3). Despite its excellent specificity (100%), this test is no longer widely used due to poor sensitivity (59%).

In 1977 Nielsen and Lassen described a test to determine digital blood pressure in response to 5 minutes of digital occlusive hypothermia.[37] The test requires a temperature-controlled double-inlet cuff around the second finger (test finger) and a single-inlet cuff around the fourth finger (reference finger). Mercury-in-Silastic strain gauges are then placed around the two fingertips and the cuffs are inflated for 5 minutes. The test finger is sequentially perfused with water at 30°C, 15°C, and 10°C during each test. As the cuff pressure is slowly released after each 5-minute period, the strain gauge on the tip of each finger measures the return of pulsatile flow. A

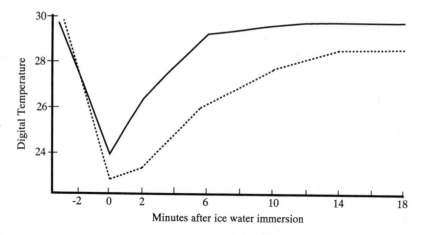

Figure 14–3. Recovery of finger temperature after immersion in ice water. Patients with Raynaud's syndrome (dotted line) have a prolonged recovery compared to normal controls (solid line). (*From Edwards JM, Porter JM. Evaluation of upper extremity ischemia. In: Bernstein EF, ed.* Noninvasive Vascular Diagnosis. *4th ed. St Louis, Mo: Mosby–Year Book Inc; 1993;637.*)

positive test is present when the pressure in the test finger detects 20% below that of the reference finger (Fig. 14–4). The Medimatic model SP2 strain gauge plethysmograph with digital cooling system (Medsonics, Mountain View, Calif) in use in our vascular laboratory is shown in Figure 14–5.

Our vascular laboratory found this test to be 87% specific and 90% sensitive, with an overall accuracy of 92% compared to clinical diagnosis in 100 patients.[63] This test will objectively diagnose most patients afflicted with cold-induced RS even though the magnitude of the pressure drop has not been conclusively shown to correspond with the severity of symptoms. Therefore, we are not convinced that this test is reliable in measuring a response to treatment.

Arteriography

In patients who exhibit moderate to severe ischemic symptoms of the hands, arteriography may be required. We recommend arteriography in patients with diminished arm pulses and/or unilateral hand symptoms. In patients with normal pulses to the wrist, obstructive wave forms in all fingers, and serologic abnormalities typical for CTD, arteriography is unlikely to change the course of treatment. An example of hand arteriography illustrating marked arterial obstruction in a patient with CTD is shown in Figure 14–6.

TREATMENT

The treatment for patients with RS caused by CTD is palliative. Since the majority of patients with RS have mild to moderate symptoms secondary to vasospasm alone, simple preventative measures provide significant relief of symptoms in most patients. Patients with CTD have an increased risk for developing more virulent hand ischemia due to palmar and/or digital artery obstruction. In evaluating more than 900 patients with RS at our institution, we encountered 100 patients with finger ulceration or gangrene.[31,64] More than half of these patients had a CTD, of which the majority

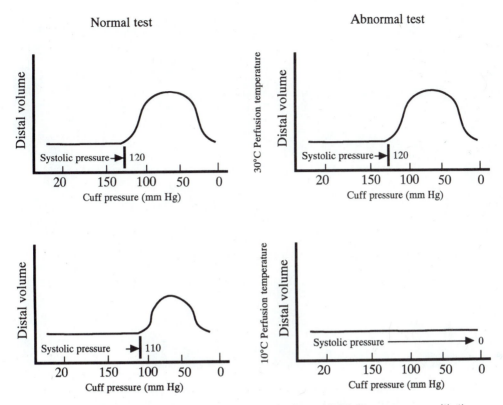

Figure 14–4. A normal test (**left**) and an abnormal test (**right**) for vasospasm with the digital hypothermic challenge test. (*From Edwards JM, Porter JM. Evaluation of upper extremity ischemia. In: Bernstein EF, ed.* Noninvasive Vascular Diagnosis. *4th ed. St Louis, Mo: Mosby–Year Book Inc; 1993;638.*)

had scleroderma or the CREST variant (chondrocalcinosis, RS, esophageal motility disturbance, sclerodactyly, and telangiectasias).

Regardless of the severity of RS, all patients are empirically counseled to cease smoking. Studies have shown significant decreases in arterial blood flow in the hand and increased precapillary sphincter tone in response to smoking.[65–68] In addition, finger temperatures have been shown to drop after cigarette smoking, and temperature recovery after ice bath immersion is longer in smokers.[69] In our opinion the physician should act as a resource guide to stop-smoking programs and continually be supportive when patients relapse.

Patients should actively minimize cold exposure to their hands.[68] Helpful measures include keeping all rooms at a comfortable temperature, using an electric blanket when sleeping, washing vegetables in tepid water, and protecting hands with potholders when removing food from the freezer. Patients should keep an extra pair of gloves near the front door for quick trips outside. For patients with severe cold-induced vasospasm, electrically heated gloves are now available.[70] Certain drugs may also predispose patients to frequent Raynaud's attacks. The use of oral contraceptives,[71] ergotamine preparations,[72] and β-adrenergic blockers in some studies[73] has been shown to exacerbate RS and should be supplanted with alternative treatments.

Pharmacological Therapy

Certain medications may alleviate symptoms in patients with severe vasospastic RS. Patients with concomitant obstructive RS may also benefit. Currently, there are no

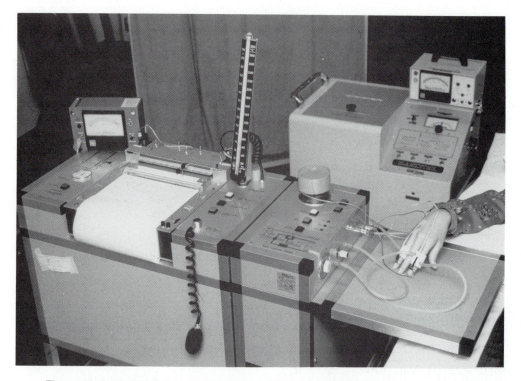

Figure 14–5. Medimatic model SP2 strain gauge plethysmograph with digital cooling system. Note digital cuffs on the second and fourth fingers. (*From Edwards JM, Porter JM. Evaluation of upper extremity ischemia. In: Bernstein EF, ed.* Noninvasive Vascular Diagnosis. *4th ed. St Louis, Mo: Mosby–Year Book Inc; 1993;637.*)

vascular laboratory tests that correlate with improvements in symptoms after drug therapy. Uncontrollable factors such as environmental temperature and the patient's emotional state greatly hamper the development of such a test. Drug therapy therefore has relied on anecdotal reports of efficacy. Patients with vasospastic RS are more likely to respond to drug therapy than are those with obstructive RS. Many patients require treatment only during the winter months.

In recent years calcium channel blockers have been the first-line pharmacological therapy.[74,75] The most potent vasodilator in this group is nifedipine, which has produced anecdotal improvement in 50% to 60% of patients with RS. Side effects include dizziness, headaches, and ankle swelling, which unfortunately cause problems in 50% of patients with RS. Currently, we recommend taking 30 mg of the extended-release form at bedtime, which appears to minimize the untoward effects.

Prostaglandins (PGs) have been used to treat patients with ischemic digital ulceration.[76] Both PGE_1 and PGI_2 are potent vasodilators and inhibitors of platelet aggregation. Clifford et al[77,78] and Pardy et al[79] had encouraging initial results with infusion therapy. In a randomized double-blind trial by Mohrland et al in 1985, patients with RS and no digital ulceration showed no significant benefit of treatment with PGE_1.[80] Iloprost, a stable derivative of PGI_2, was demonstrated in a randomized double-blind trial to be superior to nifedipine in the treatment of ischemic digital ulcers.[81] Patients experienced rapid healing of digital ulcers, a reduction in the occurrence of new lesions, and a decrease in the duration and severity of Raynaud's attacks over a 16-week period.

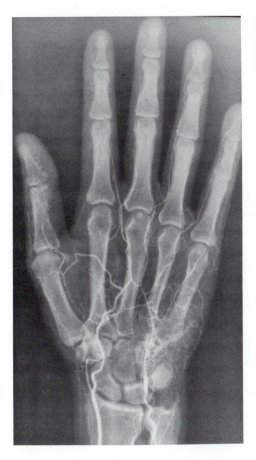

Figure 14–6. Hand arteriogram showing diffuse arterial obstruction in a patient with CTD.

A variety of new drugs and other unconventional treatments have been used in the treatment of RS. The hemorrheologic agent pentoxiphylline is thought to increase the rate of healing in ischemic ulcers.[82] Currently, we recommend 400 mg three times per day until complete healing of ulceration occurs. A selective serotonin-2 receptor blocker called ketanserin has been reported as useful in the treatment of obstructive RS but is not available in the United States.[83] Stanozolol, an anabolic steroid capable of stimulating impaired fibrinolytic activity, has shown improvement in preliminary uncontrolled trials in patients with ischemic digital ulcers associated with progressive systemic sclerosis.[83] Initial studies of angiotensin-converting enzyme inhibitors have shown some promising results, but large multicenter trials are needed.[84] The competitive antagonism of α-mediated noradrenalin receptors by thymoxamine has shown some anecdotal improvements in small series of patients.[85] Other therapies, such as omega-3 fatty acids (fish oil) and plasmapheresis, have been tried with varied results.[86,87]

Surgical Therapy

Over the past 30 years patients with vasospastic or obstructive RS have been treated with cervicothoracic sympathectomy.[88,89] Response rates to sympathectomy have varied widely in different series. Typically, dramatic improvement is observed for several months followed by a quick return of symptoms. No studies have shown superiority over conventional drug therapy for palliation.

In recent years sympathectomy has been applied locally to digital arteries by stripping the adventitia, dividing the terminal sympathetic nerve branches with microscopic assistance.[90] No controlled clinical trials exist comparing this mode of therapy to other forms of treatment. In addition, this procedure does not address the underlying arterial obstruction and has no effect on the inherent local factors thought to cause vasospastic RS. A small number of patients have undergone microsurgical arterial reconstruction of the palmar and digital arteries. This procedure is not indicated for the majority of patients in whom diffuse obstructive arterial disease is present.

Supportive Therapy

Sympathectomy and vasodilator infusion therapy have been reported to heal up to 85% of digital ischemic ulcers.[78–80,89,90] We found in our current series of 100 consecutive patients with digital ischemic ulcers that complete healing could be accomplished in 88% of patients with conservative wound care alone.[65] Patients undergo a treatment program that includes twice-daily gentle soap and water scrubs followed by a protective bandage. Frequent outpatient visits may be required to debride any necrotic tissue in order to facilitate healing. Close inspection should be made with regard to infection and a low threshold should exist for treatment. Cultures should be taken and appropriate antibiotics prescribed. Close attention to infection under the fingernail is warranted, with removal necessary if infection is present. Occasionally, patients require admission to the hospital for intravenous antibiotics and more aggressive wound care. Finger amputation is only rarely necessary. A finger with an ischemic ulcer is shown in Figure 14–7 before and after 4 weeks of conservative therapy.

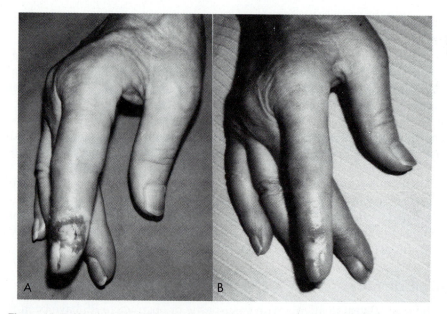

Figure 14–7. (A) Ischemic digital ulcer in a patient with CTD. **(B)** Complete healing was obtained after conservative wound care. (*From Edwards JM, Porter JM. Raynaud's syndrome. In: Sabiston DC, ed.* Textbook of Surgery. *Philadelphia, Pa: WB Saunders Co; 1991;1646.*)

CONCLUSION

Ischemic hand symptoms in patients diagnosed with a CTD range from Raynaud's syndrome to rest pain, ulcer, and gangrene. Epidemiological studies show that approximately 30% of patients with ischemic symptoms of the hand have an associated CTD. Multiple digital and palmar arteries are obliterated by thrombosis secondary to a transmural necrotizing vasculitis. The differential diagnosis primarily relies on screening blood chemistries and vascular laboratory testing. Treatment is palliative and predominantly involves preventive and pharmacological measures to alleviate symptoms. Premature finger amputation should be avoided in patients with finger ulcers and a CTD, since the majority will heal with aggressive wound care.

Acknowledgment
The work presented in this chapter was supported by grant RR00334 of the General Clinical Research Centers Branch, Division of Research Resources, National Institutes of Health.

REFERENCES

1. Raynaud M. On local asphyxia and symmetrical gangrene of the extremities. In *Selected Monographs.* London, England: New Sydenham Society; 1888.
2. Hutchinson J. Raynaud's phenomena. *Med Press Circular* 1901;128:403–405.
3. Allen E, Brown G. Raynaud's disease: a critical review of minimal requisites for diagnosis. *Am J Med Sci.* 1932;83:187–200.
4. Lewis T, Pickering GW. Observations upon maladies in which the blood supply to the digits ceases intermittently or permanently and upon bilateral gangrene of the digits: observations relevant to so-called "Raynaud's disease." *Clin Sci.* 1934;1:327–366.
5. Gifford RW Jr, Hines EA Jr. Raynaud's disease among women and girls. *Circulation.* 1957;16:1012–1021.
6. de Takats G, Fowler EF. Raynaud's phenomenon. *JAMA.* 1962;179:1–8.
7. Porter JM, Rivers SP, Anderson CJ, et al. Evaluation and management of patients with Raynaud's syndrome. *Am J Surg.* 1981;142:183–189.
8. Baur GM, Porter JM, Bardana EJ Jr, et al. Rapid onset of hand ischemia of unknown etiology. *Ann Surg.* 1977;186:184–189.
9. Mills JL, Friedman EI, Taylor LM Jr, et al. Upper extremity ischemia caused by small artery disease. *Ann Surg.* 1987;154:123.
10. Taylor LM Jr, Baur GM, Porter JM. Finger gangrene caused by small artery occlusive disease. *Ann Surg.* 1981;193:453–461.
11. Dodds AJ, O'Reilly MJG, Yates CJP, et al. Hemorrheological response to plasma exchange in Raynaud's syndrome. *Br Med J.* 1979;2:1186.
12. Edwards JM, Porter JM. Long-term outcome of Raynaud's syndrome. In Yao JST, Pearce WH, eds. *Long-Term Results in Vascular Surgery.* Norwalk, Conn: Appleton & Lange; 1993; 345–352.
13. Strandness DE Jr. Episodic digital ischemia. In: Strandness DE Jr, ed. *Peripheral Arterial Disease: A Physiologic Approach.* Boston, Mass: Little, Brown & Co; 1969;265.
14. Allen E, Brown G. Raynaud's disease: a clinical study of 147 cases. JAMA 1932;99:1472–1478.
15. Blain A III, Coller FA, Carver GB. Raynaud's disease: a study of criteria for prognosis. *Surgery.* 1951;29:387–397.
16. Porter JM, Bardana EJ, Baur GM, et al. The clinical significance of Raynaud's syndrome. *Surgery.* 1976;80:756–764.

17. Edwards JM, Porter JM. Associated diseases in patients with Raynaud's syndrome. In: Corkle E, Nicolaides A, Porter JM, eds. *Program in the Investigation and Management of Raynaud's Phenomenon*. London, England: Med-Orion Publishing; 1990;61–69.

18. Priollet P, Vayssairat M, Housset E. How to classify Raynaud's phenomenon: long-term follow-up study of 73 cases. *Am J Med*. 1987;83:494–498.

19. James EC, Khun NT, Fedde CW. Upper limb ischemia resulting from arterial thromboembolism. *Am J Surg*. 1979;137:739.

20. Porter JM, Taylor LM Jr, Friedman EI. Indications for cervical and first rib excisions. In: Greenhalgh RM, ed. *Indications in Vascular Surgery*. Orlando, Fla: Grune & Stratton, Inc; 1987;215.

21. Porter JM, Taylor LM, Harris EJ. Nonatherosclerotic vascular disease. In: Moore WS, ed. *Vascular Surgery, a Comprehensive Review*. 4th ed. Philadelphia, Pa: WB Saunders Co; 1993;108–146.

22. Mills JL, Porter JM. Buerger's disease (thromboangiitis obliterans). *Ann Vasc Surg*. 1992;5:570–572.

23. Urschel JD. Frostbite: predisposing factors and predictors of poor outcome. *J Trauma*. 1990;30:340–342.

24. Harris EJ, Edwards JM, Taylor LM, et al. Vibration arterial trauma. In: Flanigan DP, ed. *Civilian Vascular Trauma*. Philadelphia, Pa: Lea & Febiger; 1992;306–315.

25. Powell KR. Raynaud's phenomena preceding acute lymphocytic leukemia. *J Pediatr*. 1973;82:539.

26. Rudolph RI. Vasculitis associated with hairy-cell leukemia. *Arch Dermatol*. 1980;116:1077.

27. O'Donnell JR, Keaveney TV, O'Donnell LG. Digital arteritis as a presenting feature of malignant disease. *Ir J Med Sci*. 1980;149:326.

28. Taylor LM Jr, Hauty MG, Edwards JM, et al. Digital ischemia as a manifestation of malignancy. *Ann Surg*. 1987;206:62–68.

29. Blunt RJ, Porter JM. Raynaud's syndrome. *Semin Arthritis Rheum*. 1981;10:282–308.

30. Velayos E, Roginson H, Porciuncula F, et al. Clinical correlation analysis of 137 patients with Raynaud's phenomenon. *Am J Med Sci*. 1970;262:347–356.

31. Mills JL, Friedman EI, Taylor LM Jr, et al. Upper extremity ischemia caused by small artery disease. *Ann Surg*. 1987;206:521–528.

32. Porter JM, et al. Unpublished data. 1994.

33. Coffman JB, Cohen AS. Total and capillary fingertip blood flow in Raynaud's phenomenon. *N Engl J Med*. 1971;285:259.

34. Zweifler AJ, Trinkaus P. Occlusive digital artery disease in patients with Raynaud's phenomenon. *Am J Med*. 1984;77:995–1001.

35. Lewis T, Kerr WJ. Experiments relating to the peripheral mechanism involved in spasmodic arrest of the circulation in the fingers, a variety of Raynaud's disease. *Heart*. 1929;15:7–101.

36. Krahenbuhl B, Nielsen SL, Lassen NA. Closure of digital arteries in high vascular tone states as demonstrated by measurement of systolic blood pressure in the finger. *Scand J Clin Lab Invest*. 1977;37:71.

37. Nielson SL, Lassen NA. Measurement of digital blood pressure after local cooling. *J Appl Physiol*. 1977;43:907–910.

38. Rosch J, Porter JM, Gralino BJ. Cryodynamic hand angiography in the diagnosis and management of Raynaud's syndrome. *Circulation*. 1977;55:807–814.

39. Coffman JD. Total and nutritional blood flow in the finger. *Clin Sci*. 1972;42:243–250.

40. Edwards JM, Phinney ES, Taylor LM Jr, et al. Alpha-2 adrenoreceptor differences in vasospastic and obstructive Raynaud's syndrome. *J Vasc Surg*. 1987;5:38–45.

41. Keenan EJ, Porter JM. Alpha-2 adrenergic receptors in platelets from patients with Raynaud's syndrome. *Surgery*. 1983;94:204–209.

42. Brotzu G, Falchi S, Mannu B, et al. The importance of presynaptic beta receptors in Raynaud's disease. *J Vasc Surg*. 1989;9:767–771.

43. Zamora MR, O'Brien RF, Rutherford RB, et al. Serum endothelin-1 concentrations and cold provocation in primary Raynaud's phenomenon. *Lancet*. 1990;336:1144–1147.

44. Halpern A, Kuhn PH, Shaftel HE, et al. Raynaud's disease, Raynaud's phenomenon, and serotonin. *Angiology*. 1960;11:151–167.

45. Bunker CB, Terenghi G, Springall DR, et al. Deficiency of calcitonin gene-related peptide in Raynaud's phenomenon. *Lancet.* 1990;336(8730):1530–1533.
46. Dale WA. Occlusive arterial lesions of the wrist and hand. *J Tenn Med Assoc.* 1964;57:402–406.
47. Hirai M. Cold sensitivity of the hand in arterial occlusive disease. *Surgery.* 1979;85:140.
48. Williams SJ. Chronic upper extremity ischemia: current concepts in management. *Surg Clin North Am.* 1986;66:355.
49. Fauci AS, Haynes BF, Katz P. The spectrum of vasculitis: clinical, pathologic, immunologic, and therapeutic considerations. *Ann Intern Med.* 1978;89:660.
50. Rob CG, Standeven A. Arterial occlusion complicating thoracic outlet compression syndrome. *Br Med J.* 1958;7:709–712.
51. Butler MS, Lane RHS, Webster JHH. Irradiation injury to large arteries. *Br J Surg.* 1980;67:341–343.
52. Edwards JM, Antonious JI, Porter JM. Critical hand ischemia caused by forearm fibromuscular displasia. *J Vasc Surg.* 1985;2459–2463.
53. Borman KR, Snyder WH II, Weigelt JA. Civilian arterial trauma of the upper extremity: an 11 year experience in 267 patients. *Am J Surg.* 1985;148:796.
54. Abbott WM, Maloney RD, McCabe CC, et al. Arterial embolism: a 44 year perspective. *Am J Surg.* 1982;143:460.
55. Forgarty TJ, Daily PO, Shumway NE, et al. Experience with balloon catheter technic for arterial embolectomy. *Am J Surg.* 1971;122:231.
56. Edwards JM, Porter JM. Evaluation of upper extremity ischemia. In: Bernstein EF, ed. *Noninvasive Vascular Diagnosis.* 4th ed. St Louis, Mo: Mosby–Year Book Inc; 1993;630–640.
57. Holmgren K, Baur GM, Porter JM. The role of digital photoplethysmography in the evaluation of Raynaud's syndrome. *Bruit.* 1981;5:19.
58. Sumner DS, Strandness DE. An abnormal finger pulse associated with cold sensitivity. *Ann Surg.* 1972;175:294.
59. Alexander S, Cummings C, Figg-Hoblyn L, et al. Usefulness of digital peaked pulse for diagnosis of Raynaud's syndrome. *J Vasc Technol.* 1988;12:71–75.
60. Carter SA. The effect of cooling on toe systolic pressures in subjects with and without Raynaud's syndrome in the lower extremities. *Clin Physiol.* 1991;11:253–261.
61. Carter SA, Dean E, Kroeger EA. Apparent finger systolic pressures during cooling in patients with Raynaud's syndrome. *Circulation.* 1988;77(5):988–996.
62. Porter JM, Snider RL, Bardana EJ, et al. The diagnosis and treatment of Raynaud's phenomenon. *Surgery.* 1975;77:11–23.
63. Gates KH, Tyburczy JA, Zupan T, et al. The noninvasive quantification of digital vasospasm. *Bruit.* 1984;8:34–37.
64. Porter JM. Upper extremity ischemia: role of the vascular surgeon in Raynaud's syndrome and finger gangrene. In: Veith FJ, ed. *Critical Problems in Vascular Surgery.* New York, NY: Appleton-Century-Crofts; 1982;277–295.
65. Holmberg JT, Thulesius O, Gjores JE. Effect of nicotine on isolated human blood vessels. *Acta Chir Scand.* 1975;465(suppl):71–73.
66. Ludbrook J, Vincent AH, Walsh JA. The effects of sham smoking and tobacco on hand blood flow. *Aust J Exp Biol Med Sci.* 1974;52:285.
67. Matsubara I, Sano T. Effect of cigarette smoking in human precapillary sphinctors. *Br J Pharmacol.* 1974;45:13.
68. Lennihan R Jr, Porter JM, Sumner DS. When your patient has Raynaud's syndrome. *Patient Care.* 1983;17:70–102.
69. Hansteen V. Medical treatment in Raynaud's disease. *Acta Chir Scand.* 1975;465(Suppl): 87–91.
70. Kempson GE, Coggon D, Acheson ED. Electrically heated gloves for intermittent digital ischemia. *Br Med J.* 1983;286:268.
71. Eastcott HHG. Raynaud's and the oral contraceptive pill. *Br Med J.* 1976;2:447.
72. Graham MR. Methylsergide for prevention of headaches: experience in five hundred patients over five years. *N Engl J Med.* 1964;270–67.
73. Frolich ED, Tarayi RC, Dutson MP. Peripheral arterial insufficiency as a complication of beta-adrenergic blocking therapy. *JAMA.* 1969;208:2471.

74. Gjorup T, Kelbaek H, Hartling OJ, et al. Controlled double-blind trial of the clinical effect of nifedipine in the treatment of idiopathic Raynaud's phenomenon. *Am Heart J.* 1986;111:742–745.

75. Porter JM, Friedman EI, Mills JL Jr. Raynaud's syndrome: current concepts and treatment. *Med Tribune Ther.* May 19, 1988;23–25.

76. Szczeklik A, Cryglewski RJ, Nizankowski R, et al. Prastacyclin therapy in peripheral arterial disease. *Thromb Res.* 1980;19:191.

77. Clifford PC, Martin MFR, Dieppe PA, et al. Prostaglandin E1 infusion for small vessel arterial ischaemia. *J Cardiovasc Surg.* 1983;24:503–508.

78. Clifford PC, Martin MFR, Sheddon EJ, et al. Treatment of vasospastic disease with prostaglandin E1. *Br Med J.* 1980;281:1031–1040.

79. Pardy BJ, Lewis JD, Eastcott HHG. Preliminary experience with prostaglandins E_1 and I_2 in peripheral vascular disease. *Surgery.* 1980;88:826.

80. Mohrland JS, Porter JM, Smith EA, et al. A multiclinic, placebo-controlled, double-blind study of prostaglandin E1 in Raynaud's syndrome. *Ann Rheum Dis.* 1985;44:754–760.

81. Rademaker M, Cooke ED, Almond NE, et al. Comparison of intravenous infusions of Iloprost and oral nifedipine in the treatment of Raynaud's phenomena in patients with systemic sclerosis: a double blind randomized study. *Br Med J.* 1989;298:561.

82. Roath S. Management of Raynaud's phenomena, focus on newer treatments. *Drugs.* 1989;37:700–712.

83. Jayson MIV. Ketanserin and stanozolol in Raynaud's syndrome. In: Coke ED, Nicolaides AN, Porter JM, eds. *Raynaud's Syndrome.* Los Angeles, Calif: Med-Orion Publishing; 1991;177–182.

84. Rustin MHA, Almond NE, Beachem JA, et al. The effect of captopril on cutaneous blood flow in patients with Raynaud's phenomena. *Br J Dermatol.* 1987;117:751.

85. Grigg MJ, Nicolaides AN, Papadakis K, et al. The efficacy of thymoxamine in primary Raynaud's phenomena. *Eur J Vasc Surg.* 1989;3:309.

86. Edwards JM, Porter JM. Update on Raynaud's syndrome. *Semin Vasc Surg.* 1990;3:227–235.

87. O'Reilly MJG, Dodds AJ, Roberts VC, et al. Plasma exchange in Raynaud's phenomena—its assessment by Doppler ultrasound velocimetry. *Br J Surg.* 1979;66:712.

88. Kirtley JA, Riddell DH, Stoney WS, et al. Cervicothoracic sympathectomy in neurovascular abnormalities of the upper extremities: experiences in 76 patients with 104 sympathectomies. *Ann Surg.* 1967;165:869–879.

89. Machleder HI, Wheeler E, Barber WF. Treatment of upper extremity ischemia by cervicodorsal sympathectomy. *Vasc Surg.* 1979;13:399–404.

90. Flatt AE. Digital artery sympathectomy. *J Hand Surg.* 1980;5:550.

15

Long-Term Results of
Arterial Reconstruction of the
Upper Extremity

Jan Brunkwall, MD, PhD, and
Sven-Erik Bergentz, MD, PhD

HISTORICAL REMARKS

Stenosis or occlusion of the innominate artery or the proximal part of the left subclavian artery often produces cerebral symptoms but may also give rise to upper extremity ischemia. The first suggestion of this was made by Harrison as early as 1829.[1] The first description of the condition with stenosis or occlusions of the aortic arch branches was made by Savory in 1856,[2] followed by Broadbent in 1875,[3] but the condition with aortitis leading to stenosis or occlusions became more well known after the 1908 report by Takayasu, for whom the disease is named.[4]

The first case of surgical correction of an aortic arch branch occlusion was reported in 1951 by Shimizu and Sano, who made a bypass between the aortic arch and the common carotid artery.[5] In a patient with innominate artery occlusion from atherosclerosis, Davis performed in 1956 a thromboendarterectomy, which resulted in a weak pulse in the carotid artery but no pulse in the right arm.[6] De Bakey was, in 1958, the first to report on two arterial reconstructions of the upper extremity, performed in 1956 and 1957, due to chronic upper extremity ischemia.[7] He performed a thoracotomy and used a bifurcated graft from the aorta to the right common carotid and subclavian arteries in one case and a thrombendarterectomy of the left subclavian artery in the other. In 1962 Crawford et al described thrombendarterectomy for stenotic lesions of the upper extremity,[8] and in 1964 Parrot described the carotid–subclavian transposition procedure for subclavian steal syndrome.[9] In 1967 Dietrich et al introduced the carotid–subclavian bypass procedure using the extrathoracic approach.[10] These methods were widely used until 1980, when Mathias et al[11] and Bachman and Kim[12] suggested that transluminal angioplasty could also be used for the treatment of lesions of the subclavian or innominate artery, a procedure which has since gained widespread popularity.[13]

CAUSES OF THE VASCULAR LESIONS

Upper extremity ischemia can be divided into three groups: (1) chronic ischemia from atherosclerosis or inflammatory disease, (2) emboli, and (3) trauma. Embolism and chronic ischemia account for equal numbers of arterial operations in the upper extremity at Malmö (Sweden) General Hospital.[14] Trauma (with increasing number of iatrogenic type) also plays an important role. An example of this is the brachial artery injury due to cardiac catheterization. Iatrogenic occlusions of the brachial artery are frequently left untreated due to the mild symptomatology in otherwise sick patients.

As few data are available on the long-term results of treatment for trauma and embolism, this chapter focuses mainly on chronic upper limb ischemia. Most of the patients with upper extremity ischemia have a proximal stenosis or occlusion localized to the subclavian, innominate, or, less often, axillary artery as the cause of their symptoms. This in turn is often due to atherosclerosis, even though Takayasu's nonspecific transmural arteritis is occasionally found, especially in younger females, affecting the aortic arch and its branches. Takayasu's disease can often be divided into two phases, the first being characterized by an active inflammation, for which the treatment is nonsurgical. In the second phase there may be stenosis or occlusion, for which surgical therapy is sometimes indicated.

Giant cell arteritis[15,16] may be seen in middle-aged women and is more distally located, as is thromboangitis obliterans (Buerger's disease), giving rise to rest pain and gangrene. Buerger's disease is seen in middle-aged males who are heavy smokers. Secondary Raynaud's syndrome[17] is often associated with collagenosis, which may give rise to upper extremity ischemia and more often peripheral gangrene than effort fatigue.

Radiation injury developing several years after radiation has three regions of predominance: the iliac, carotid, and subclavian and axillary arteries.[18] The typical picture of radiation injury is that of a premature and severe atherosclerosis localized to areas usually saved from this condition, and appearing many years after radiation therapy.[18] When affecting the subclavian and axillary arteries, it may cause upper extremity ischemia.[19]

Intake of ergotamine to reduce attacks of migraine may sometimes cause chronic upper extremity ischemia, although more often it results in acute ischemia.[20]

AGE, SEX, AND ANATOMICAL DISTRIBUTION

Most reported series on surgery or percutaneous angioplasty of the aortic arch branches include patients with both cerebral and upper extremity symptoms, and very few deal only with upper extremity ischemia. Some of the results reported in the following therefore deal with both types of symptomatology.

Arterial reconstructions for upper limb ischemia are much less frequent than for lower limb ischemia and constitute in reported series only 1% to 4% of the total numbers of reconstructions.[14,21-24] The left subclavian artery is affected about twice as often as the right one (including the innominate artery), and so far there has been no explanation for this discrepancy. In reported series with upper extremity ischemia only, as well as upper extremity ischemia and cerebral symptoms, the left-right ratio is 2.2 for operated cases, whereas for those undergoing percutaneous transluminal angioplasty (PTA) (only combined series) the predominance of the left side is even more prominent, with a ratio of 4.1. One possible explanation for this might be that it is easier to gain access with the PTA catheter to the left artery than to the right one.

Of the 2,124 patients who underwent surgery for upper limb ischemia with or without cerebral symptoms (1,813 patients), the male-female ratio was 1.25. For those 404 of 570 patients (only combined symptoms) treated with PTA, the ratio was 1.6. For patients operated on for upper limb ischemia only, the pooled data result in a male-female ratio of 0.9. Thus, the sex distribution is comparable to recent data from patients undergoing reconstruction for aortoiliac occlusive disease in which females are more frequently represented than in femorocrural occlusive disease.[25,26]

The median age of patients reported with upper extremity ischemia was 55 years (range, 17 to 88 years), which is also comparable with that of patients undergoing surgery for aortoiliac disease.

Risk factors for patients with upper extremity ischemia are similar to those seen in patients operated on for lower limb ischemia with proximal disease. Seventy-five percent to 93% are smokers and about half of these are being treated for hypertension.[8,22,27–29] About one-third have had previous vascular operations, but diabetes is not over-represented as in patients operated on with infrainguinal bypass.[30–32] Diabetes is also over-represented in younger patients undergoing various types of vascular reconstructions.[33–35]

SYMPTOMS

In the case of proximal lesions in which both the vessels to the brain and the arm are involved, the patient may suffer from ischemia from both territories. Cerebral symptoms may include transient ischemic attacks, minor stroke, amaurosis fugax, drop attacks, diplopia, vertigo, and ataxia. A special form of vascular lesion may result in a subclavian steal syndrome first described in 1961 by Reivich[36] and Fisher.[37] Occlusion of the innominate artery or the subclavian artery proximal to the verebral artery may lead to reversed flow in the vertebral artery and from there to the subclavian artery.[38] The finding can be seen by angiography but clinical symptoms are less frequent,[22] although it has been suggested that patients with subclavian steal syndrome have an increased risk of developing transient ischemia attacks.[39]

The collateral circulation around the shoulder to the arm is very good, the demand on blood flow to the upper extremity is less than on that to the lower, and therefore the ischemia symptoms from the upper extremity are less frequent and less pronounced. In addition, there are seldom any multiple stenoses or occlusions as in the lower extremity, and therefore amputations due to upper extremity ischemia are rare. Symptoms most often include effort fatigue, especially when the arm is used in the above-shoulder position. Rest pain and gangrene are sometimes seen after an acute arterial occlusion, but are in most cases temporarily due to development of good collateral circulation.

Repeated microemboli with occlusions in the small arteries in the hand and fingers cause severe pain and may result in a substantial tissue loss. Microembolism may be the indication for surgical correction in as much as 35% of the patients,[14,22,40–43] and this condition should therefore lead to angiography, which may reveal the underlying cause, such as an aneurysm or an atheromatous plaque. Microembolization may also, as in other territories, be a concomitant phenomenon to occlusion of the subclavian artery.

DIAGNOSIS

Blood pressure in each arm will be different in the case of a significant proximal arterial stenosis or occlusion. The Doppler device could be of use when the pressure is not heard with an ordinary stethoscope. It is not uncommon that even patients without any symptoms have different arm blood pressures, and thus the bare presence of different arm pressures should not lead to any further investigation in preparation for surgical correction. In patients with microembolism, a murmur at the level of the subclavian artery may give a suspicion of an aneurysm or a stenosis. Subclavian aneurysms are atherosclerotic, traumatic, or poststenotic[44] and are usually seen on an arteriogram, even though they have a mural thrombus.

Arteriography is the method of choice for anatomical description of the lesion. When combined with a plexus anesthesia, more information about the spasm-prone distal bed can be retrieved, and in the case of microembolism, distal occlusions may be visualized.

TREATMENT OPTIONS

Principally, there are three ways of treating proximal upper extremity stenosis or occlusions. The oldest is the intrathoracic approach, which, to a large extent, is replaced by the extrathoracic approach (Fig. 15–1). During the last 10 to 15 years the use of percutaneous angioplasty has increased (Fig. 15–2).

Intrathoracic Alternatives

By a sternum split there is easy access to all the aortic branches and then it is possible either to perform a thrombendarterectomy of the subclavian or innominate arteries or to make a bypass from the aorta. A side clamp is placed on aorta when performing the aortic anastomosis. The intrathoracic approach is mandatory only when there are occlusions of all major branches from the aortic arch. When one of the branches has a stenosis and the others are occluded, it is sometimes possible to percutaneously dilate the stenosis of the donor artery prior to an extrathoracic bypass procedure.

Extrathoracic Alternatives

Most of the proximal arterial occlusions or stenoses may be treated via an extrathoracic approach. In such cases several options are available. Theoretically, the most favorable technique is to ligate the subclavian artery distal to the occlusion or stenosis, divide the subclavian artery, and then transpose the distal end to the common carotid artery on the ipsilateral side (Fig. 15–1.) This method can be used when the occlusion is distal to the origin of the vertebral artery. When the lesion is located proximal to the vertebral artery, it is preferable to use a carotid–subclavian bypass. We prefer Dacron, which is easy to handle and gives good long-term results. In occlusion of the innominate artery, a carotid–carotid bypass, preferably with Dacron, between the common carotid arteries is performed. A fourth option is to do a thrombendarterectomy with or without a patch of the subclavian artery from the supra- or infraclavicular fossa, but this is technically more demanding.

A femoroaxillary bypass is possible to perform in cases with occlusion of all major aortic arch branches, but the durability of such bypass is limited and it is therefore used mostly in very high-risk patients.

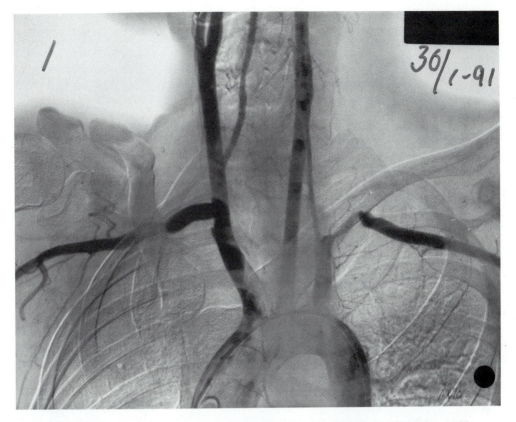

Figure 15–1. Angiogram of the aortic arch in a 28-year-old male with a nonspecific arteritis showing a patent carotid–subclavian transposition performed 3 years earlier due to effort fatigue caused by occlusion of the *right* subclavian artery. On the left side he has an asymptomatic subclavian artery stenosis.

Transluminal Angioplasty

Using a femoral approach, it is possible to dilate a stenosis of the subclavian artery. On the right side it might be hard to pass a guidewire and in such cases a brachial approach may facilitate. Occlusions of the subclavian arteries are more difficult to dilate. Stenting may be necessary due to the otherwise inferior long-term results (discussed below). Stenosis of the innominate artery can also be dilated, using an occluding balloon in the common carotid artery to prevent embolization to the brain.

RESULTS

As the number of treated patients is so low at each institution, there are no prospective studies comparing various therapeutic options. Thus, one is restricted to retrospective and nonrandomized studies in order to analyze the outcome. On the other hand, there are numerous reports on surgical and angioplastic procedures, making deductions relatively reliable.

Mortality

Mortality after surgery for upper extremity ischemia is quite favorable in comparison with surgery for lower limb ischemia (Fig. 15–3). The intrathoracic approach, including

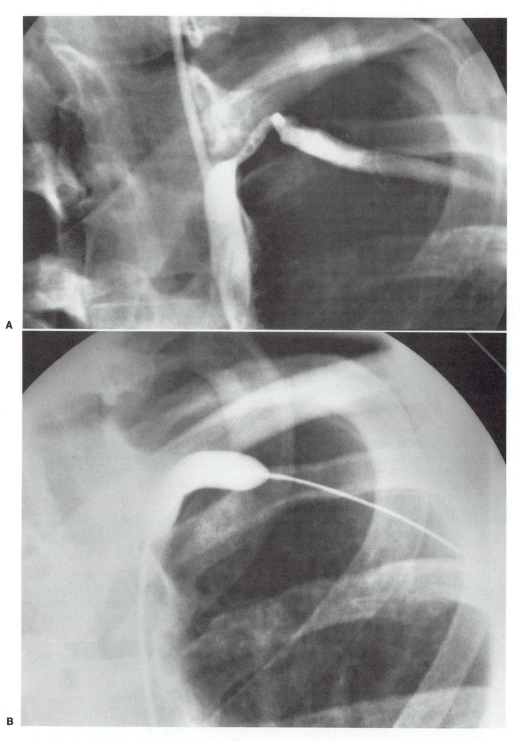

Figure 15–2. The same patient as in Fig 15–1. (**A**) He had developed effort fatigue in the *left* arm due to a severe stenosis of the left subclavian artery, which (**B**) was treated with transluminal angioplasty. (*Figure continues*)

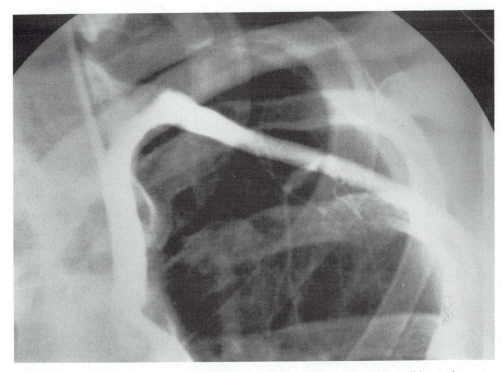

C

Figure 15–2. (*continued*) (**C**) A residual stenosis remained but the patient did not give any symptoms.

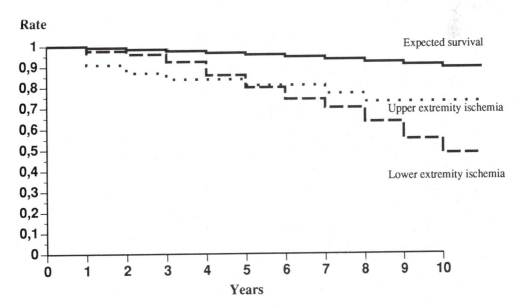

Figure 15–3. Kaplan–Meier curve showing the expected survival rate of the normal population, compared with that from the group operated on for chronic upper extremity ischemia in Malmö, Sweden (mean age, 58 years), and the group reported by Hertzer, which was operated on for lower extremity ischemia (mean age, 57 years).

both thrombendarterectomy and bypass surgery, bears the highest mortality, in the range of 3% to 15% after 1 month.[28,45–48]

The extrathoracic approach means a minor trauma and bears a 1-month mortality rate of less than 4%, with a median of 1%.[49–53] This has become the method of choice, bearing in mind that there are cases with bilateral occlusions when one must choose an intrathoracic approach. Using the extrathoracic approach, there does not seem to be any difference in mortality between the various methods (carotid–subclavian–brachial bypass, carotid–subclavian transposition, or axilloaxillary bypass).

Long-Term Survival Rates

Long-term survival for patients with upper extremity ischemia with or without cerebral symptoms is reported to be in the range of 89% to 100%, with a mean of 94% after 1 year (Table 15–1).[1–20,22–95] The mean 5-year survival rate is 85% and the mean 10-year survival, 65%. In studies in which the procedures have been performed for upper extremity ischemia only, the median 5-year survival rate is 84%[22,24,54,55] and the 10-year survival rate, 73%.[22] Thus, there seem to be comparable survival rates for patients with upper extremity ischemia with or without cerebral symptoms.

Patency

Patency is often reported only as the primary patency, probably due to the good results. Pooled data from all types of arterial reconstructions reveal a 1-month patency rate in patient groups with upper extremity and/or cerebral ischemia of 97%, a mean 1-year patency of 92%, a 5-year patency of 96%, and a 10-year patency of 84%[22,56,57] (Table 15–2). Patients being operated on for upper extremity ischemia only have a primary 1-month patency of 93%, a 1-year patency of 90%, a 5-year patency of 77%,[22,55] and a 10-year patency of 80%.[22]

These mortality and patency rates can be compared with those of acute ischemia due to embolism or thrombosis. In the Swedish vascular registry (Swedvasc), are 394 embolectomies and 44 thrombectomies of the upper limb are registered, with a survival rate of 77% after 1 year and 65% after 5 years, and no difference between embolectomy and thrombectomy. These numbers are statistically significantly lower than those for chronic upper limb ischemia (using the log-rank test). Even though the group with acute ischemia is 20 years older, the difference in survival rate between the groups is still significant when corrected for the difference in age. The patency rates for embolectomies, at 1 year 98% and at 2 years 96%, are not statistically different from those of chronic upper limb ischemia. Thrombectomies, on the other hand, have patency rates of 91% and 88%, respectively, significantly lower than in chronic upper limb ischemia.

TABLE 15–1. SURVIVAL AFTER SURGICALLY TREATED PROXIMAL ARTERIAL STENOSIS OR OCCLUSIONS OF THE UPPER EXTREMITY

Time	No. Alive	Survival (%)	References
1 month	2,034/2,078	98	1–20, 22–95
1 year	853/903	94	10, 22, 28, 29, 38, 46, 50, 52, 55, 56, 67, 76, 78, 79–81
5 years	1,070/1,262	85	10, 22, 24, 28, 29, 46, 47, 49, 50, 52–55, 67, 69, 70, 72, 76, 78, 79
10 years	387/592	65	29, 46, 56, 57, 69, 70, 76, 79

TABLE 15–2. PATENCY AFTER SURGICALLY TREATED PROXIMAL ARTERIAL STENOSIS OR OCCLUSIONS OF THE UPPER EXTREMITY

Time	Patent Reconstructions	Patency (%)	References
1 month	1,579/1,652	96	1–20, 22, 23, 25, 26, 29–44, 46, 48–68, 70, 71, 74–80, 82–96
1 year	1,054/1,143	92	10, 14, 22, 29, 38, 46–48, 50–56, 58, 67, 75, 76, 78–80, 95, 96
5 years	160/166	96	22, 29, 46, 47, 49–53, 55, 56, 58, 67, 76, 79, 96
10 years	191/227	84	22, 56, 57, 67

Thus, there does not seem to be any difference in patency after embolectomy for acute upper limb ischemia and reconstructions for chronic upper limb ischemia. On the other hand, the patients with acute upper limb ischemia are older and have a lower survival rate, which is similar for those with acute ischemia of the lower limb.

There have been few comparisons between the various operative methods used for upper limb arterial reconstructions, all in a retrospective fashion. AbuRahma et al compared polytetrafluoroethylene (PTFE) grafts used for carotid–subclavian bypass (28 patients) or axilloaxillary bypass (31 patients) in patients with stenotic or occlusive lesions giving cerebral as well as upper limb ischemic symptoms.[58] They found a 94% 10-year primary patency rate for the carotid–subclavian bypass group versus 66% for the axilloaxillary group ($P < .05$). No difference in mortality or morbidity was found.

Kretschmer et al compared, in patients with both cerebral and upper limb symptoms, carotid–subclavian transposition (32 patients) with carotid–subclavian bypass (19 patients: 4 with veins grafts and 15 with Dacron grafts).[53] They found a better patency rate in the transposition group, 100% versus 80% at 15 to 72 months, but no difference in the survival rate. Sandmann et al made a similar comparison between 20 patients undergoing various bypass procedures and 59 operated on with carotid–subclavian transposition, and found no difference in patency and survival at 4 years.[45] Sterpetti et al also made a comparison between carotid–subclavian transposition (16 patients) and bypass surgery (30 patients: 4 with vein grafts and 26 with Dacron or PTFE grafts) for subclavian occlusions.[51] At 4 years there was 100% patency in the former group and 86% in the latter.

Cherry et al reported their experience with the transthoracic approach to the innominate artery with endarterectomy in 10 patients and bypass grafting in 16 patients, and found no difference in patency at 5 years.[27]

Gerety et al used endarterectomy in 14 patients, Dacron bypass in 8, and a vein bypass in 12 patients with subclavian stenosis or occlusion.[59] They found five occlusions in the vein group but none in the other two groups. Gross et al used vein grafts in 48 patients with various causes of upper extremity ischemia and had eight failures within 1 year.[21]

Weimann compared the transthoracic approach (44 patients) with the extrathoracic approach (81 cases) in patients with cerebral as well as upper limb ischemic symptoms.[57] They found an 89% patency rate in the transthoracic group and 82% in the extrathoracic group at 10 years.

Thus, there seem to be comparable patency rates with the various methods used. In subclavian artery occlusion carotid–subclavian transposition seems to give the best

TABLE 15–3. SURVIVAL AFTER TRANSLUMINAL ANGIOPLASTY OF PROXIMAL UPPER EXTREMITY STENOSIS OR OCCLUSIONS

Time	No. Alive	Survival (%)	References
1 month	373/373	100	13, 63–66, 82–91
1 year	210/214	98	62–64, 82, 83, 85, 87, 90
3 years	109/142	77	62

result and reconstruction with vein graft the worst, as seen from two studies[60,61] and our own experience. For more distally located anastomoses, though, autogenous vein seems superior to prosthetic material.[55]

TRANSLUMINAL ANGIOPLASTY

There are no reports with long-term follow-up on patients being treated with PTA for upper extremity ischemia only, so this review is based on patient groups with combined symptoms.

Mortality

There is almost no mortality reported after PTA, and even after 1 year the median survival rate is close to 100%. At 3 years the survival rate is 98%[62] (Table 15–3).

Patency

Patency is less favorable. In patients with *occlusions* the primary success rate varies between 15% and 88%.[63–65] In two reports in which the 1-year patency is mentioned, it was 50% and 80%, respectively.[63,65]

Stenotic lesions are more easily dilated and also have a better patency than occluded vessels. The primary patency rate at 1 month is 89%; at 1-year, 91%; and at 5-years, 82% (Table 15–4). There are no reports on longer follow-up.

Farina et al made a comparison between extrathoracic bypass and transposition surgery (15 patients) from one center in the United States and angioplasty of the subclavian artery (21 patients) from an Italian center.[96] They found no difference in patency at 1 month, but after 5 years the PTA group had a patency of 54% and the surgery group 86%.

In summary, it appears that stenotic lesions of the subclavian and innominate arteries can be treated with angioplasty with 1-month and 1-year patency rates similar to those accomplished by surgery, but long-term data are scarce and do not favor angioplasty. The patency rate after 5 years (82%) in the angioplasty group is statistically

TABLE 15–4. PATENCY AFTER TRANSLUMINAL ANGIOPLASTY OF PROXIMAL UPPER EXTREMITY STENOSIS OR OCCLUSIONS

Time	Patent Reconstructions	Patency (%)	References
1 month	507/570	89	13, 62–66, 82–92, 94, 96
1 year	326/359	91	63–65, 82, 83, 85, 87, 92, 94, 96
5 years	82/101	82	89, 92, 96

significantly different from that of the surgery group (96%) ($P <$ .001). The survival rate, though, is in favor of angioplasty, with 98% survival at 1 year and 94% for the surgery group ($P <$ .05). Occlusions seem to be better treated with surgical procedures than with angioplasty, many of which fail due to technical difficulties in penetrating the lesion and with early reocclusions.[65] This seems to be particularly evident in lesions due to inflammatory vascular disease, in which a stent may be necessary to keep the artery patent (Fig. 15–4).

As the presented data are based on retrospective reports, a prospective randomized trial is needed to scientifically clarify which procedure has the best survival and patency rates.

CONCLUSION

Arterial reconstructions for upper extremity ischemia constitute 1% to 4% of all arterial interventions. Due to this low number, there are no randomized trials comparing either various types of surgery or surgery and transluminal angioplasty. Surgical interventions are more common on the left side than on the right (ratio, 2.2/1) and females are slightly over-represented when operations are performed for upper limb

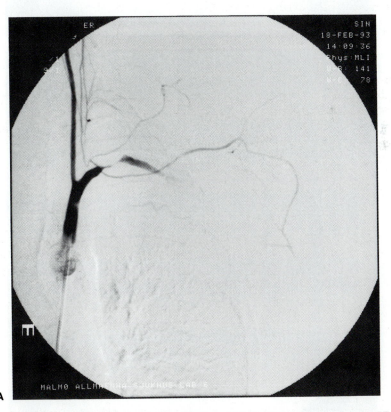

Figure 15–4. The same patient as in Figs 15–1 and 15–2. (**A**) Two years after the PTA he developed a very tight restenosis of the left subclavian artery, (**B**) which was redilated, but due to a poor result (**C**) a Wallstent was placed which kept the artery patent. This patient is without any arm symptoms 1 year later. (*Figure continues*)

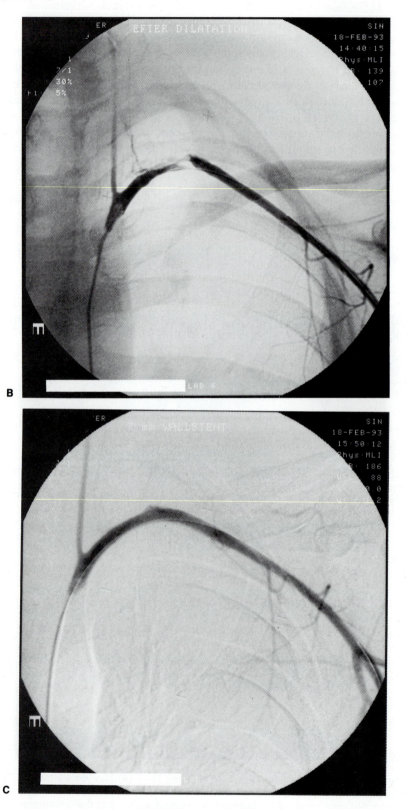

Figure 15–4. (*continued*)

ischemia only, whereas when cerebral symptoms are included, there is a male predominance.

Survival rates after surgery for upper limb and/or cerebral ischemia are: at 1 month, 98%; 1 year, 94%; 5 years, 85%; and 10 years, 65% (pooled data). Patency rates for carotid–subclavian bypass or transposition are: 1 month, 93%; 1 year, 90%; and 10 years, 80%. Carotid–subclavian transposition procedures have better patency rates than carotid–subclavian vein bypasses.

The survival rates after angioplastic procedures for lesions of the subclavian or innominate artery, causing upper limb and/or cerebral ischemia, are: at 1 month, 100%; 1 year, 98%; and 3 years, still 98%. Patency rates for angioplastic treatment of stenotic lesions are reported to be: at 1 month, 89%; 1 year, 91%; and 5 years, 82%. Occluded arteries are more difficult to treat and to keep patent by angioplasty procedures.

Survival and patency rates after arterial reconstructions for upper limb ischemia are favorable when compared with those for lower limb ischemia. Survival rates after treatment for chronic upper limb ischemia compare favorably with those of embolic and thrombotic occlusions.

Acknowledgment
We are deeply thankful to Dr Thomas Troeng of the Steering Committee of Swedvasc for preparing the data on survival and patency in acute upper extremity ischemia.

REFERENCES

1. Harrison P. In: Hodges, Smith, eds. *The Surgical Anatomy of the Arteries of the Human Body.* Dublin, Ireland: 1829.
2. Savory WS. Case of a young woman in whom the main arteries of both upper extremities and of the left side of the neck were throughout completely obliterated. *Med–Chir Trans.* 1856;39:205.
3. Broadbent WH. Absence of pulsation in both radial arteries, vessels being full of blood. *Trans Clin Soc, London* 1875;8:165–168.
4. Takayasu M. Case of queer changes in central blood vessels of retina. *Acta Soc Ophthalmol Jpn.* 1908;12:554.
5. Shimizu K, Sano K. Pulseless disease. *J Neuropathol Clin Neurol.* 1951;1:37–47.
6. Davis JB, Grove WJ, Julian OC. Thrombic occlusion of branches of aortic arch. Martorell's syndrome: report of case treated surgically. *Ann Surg.* 1956;144:124–126.
7. De Bakey ME, Morris GC Jr, Jordan GL Jr, et al. Segmental thrombo-obliterative disease of branches of aortic arch. Successful surgical treatment. *JAMA.* 1958;166(9):998–1003.
8. Crawford ES, De Bakey ME, Morris GC Jr, et al. Thrombo-obliterative disease of the great vessels arising from the aortic arch. *J Thorac Cardiovasc Surg.* 1962;43:38.
9. Parrot JD. The subclavian steal syndrome. *Arch Surg.* 1964;88:661–665.
10. Dietrich EB, Garrett HE, Ameriso J, et al. Occlusive disease of the common carotid and subclavian arteries treated by carotid–subclavian bypass. Analysis of 125 cases. *Am J Surg.* 1967;114:800–808.
11. Mathias K, Staiger J, Thron A, et al. Perkutane Katheterangioplastik der Arteria subclavia. *Dtsch Med Wochenschr.* 1980;105:16–18.
12. Bachman DM, Kim RM. Transluminal dilatation for subclavian steal syndrome. *AJR.* 1980;135:995–996.
13. Motarjeme A, Keifer JW, Zuska AJ. Percutaneous transluminal angioplasty of the brachiocephalic arteries. *AJNR.* 1982;3:169–174.
14. Bergqvist D, Ericsson BF, Konrad P, et al. Arterial surgery of the upper extremity. *World J Surg.* 1983;7:786–791.

15. Rivers SP, Baur GM, Inahara T, et al. Arm ischemia secondary to giant cell arteritis. *Am J Surg.* 1982;143:554–558.

16. Halpin DP, Moran KT, Jewell ER. Arm ischemia secondary to giant cell arteritis. *Ann Vasc Surg.* 1988;2(4):381–384.

17. Porter JM, Bardana ES Jr, Baur GM, et al. The clinical significance of Raynaud's syndrome. *Surgery.* 1976;80:756.

18. Bergentz S-E, Bergqvist D. *Iatrogenic Vascular Injuries.* Berlin, Germany: Springer-Verlag; 1989.

19. Heidenberg WJ, Lupovitch A, Tarr N. "Pulseless disease" complicating Hodgkin's disease. A case apparently caused by radiotherapy. *JAMA.* 1966;195:194–197.

20. Mumme A, Ernst R, Brandt J, et al. Extremitätenbedrohende Ischämie bei Ergotismus. Erfolgreiche Behandlung durch intraarterielle Gabe von Nifedipin. *Dtsch Med Wochenschr.* 1991;116:137–140.

21. Gross WS, Flanigan DP, Kraft RO, et al. Chronic upper extremity arterial insufficiency. Etiology, manifestations, and operative management. *Arch Surg.* 1978;113:419–423.

22. Brunkwall J, Bergqvist D, Bergentz S-E. Long-term results of arterial reconstruction of the upper extremity. *Eur J Vasc Surg.* 1994;8:47–51.

23. Perrault L, Lassonde J, Laurendeau F. Chirurgie artérielle du membre supérieur. *Ann Chir.* 1991;45(9):765–769.

24. Welling RE, Cranley JJ, Krause RJ, et al. Obliterative arterial disease of the upper extremity. *Arch Surg.* 1981;116:1593–1596.

25. Cronenwett JL, Davis JT, Gooch JB, et al. Aortoiliac occlusive disease in women. *Surgery.* 1980;88(6):775–784.

26. Brewster DC, Darling RC, Optimal methods of aortoiliac reconstruction. *Surgery.* 1978;84(6):739–748.

27. Cherry KJ Jr, McCullough JL, Hallett JW Jr, et al. Technical principles of direct innominate artery revascularization: a comparison of endarterectomy and bypass grafts. *J Vasc Surg.* 1989;9:718–724.

28. Cormier F, Ward A, Cormier J-M, et al. Long-term results of aortoinnominate and aortocarotid polytetrafluoroethylene bypass grafting for atherosclerotic lesions. *J Vasc Surg.* 1989;10:135–142.

29. Rosenthal D, Ellison RG Jr, Clark MD, et al. Axilloaxillary bypass: is it worthwhile? *J Cardiovasc Surg.* 1988;29:191–195.

30. Veith FJ, Gupta SK, Ascer E, et al. Six-year prospective multicenter randomized comparison of autologous saphenous vein and expanded polytetrafluoroethylene grafts in infrainguinal arterial reconstructions. *J Vasc Surg.* 1986;3:104–114.

31. Harris PL, How TV, Jones DR. Prospectively randomized clinical trial to compare in situ and reversed saphenous vein grafts for femoropopliteal bypass. *Br J Surg.* 1987;74:252–255.

32. Taylor LM Jr, Edwards JM, Porter JM. Present status of reversed vein bypass grafting: five-year results of a modern series. *J Vasc Surg.* 1990;11:193–206.

33. De Bakey ME, Crawford ES, Garrett E, et al. Occlusive disease of the lower extremities in patients 16–37 years of age. *Ann Surg.* 1964;159(6):873–890.

34. Pairolero PC, Joyce JW, Skinner CR, et al. Lower limb ischemia in young adults: prognostic implications. *J Vasc Surg.* 1984;1:459–464.

35. Brunkwall J, Weibull H, Bergqvist D, et al. Arterial surgery and angioplasty in patients under 40 years of age: a retrospective study. *Med Principles Pract.* 1989;1:37–43.

36. Reivich M, Holling HE, Roberts B, et al. Reversal of blood flow through the vertebral artery and its effect on cerebral circulation. *N Engl J Med.* 1961;265:878.

37. Fisher CM. New vascular syndrome—"subclavian steal." *N Engl J Med.* 1961;265:912.

38. Lawson JD, Petracek MR, Buckspan GS, et al. Subclavian steal: review of the clinical manifestations. *South Med J.* 1979;72(11): 1369–1373.

39. Moran KT, Zide RS, Persson AV, et al. Natural history of subclavian steal syndrome. *Am Surg.* 1988;54:643–644.

40. Holleman JH Jr, Hardy JD, Williamson JW, et al. Arterial surgery for arm ischemia. *Ann Surg.* 1980;191(6):727–737.

41. Bryan AJ, Hicks E, Lewis MH. Unilateral digital ischaemia secondary to embolisation from subclavian atheroma. *Ann R Coll Surg Engl.* 1989;71:140–142.

42. Banis JC, Rich N, Whelan TJ. Ischaemia of the upper extremity due to non-cardiac emboli. *Am J Surg.* 1977;134:131–139.

43. Sachatello CR, Ernst CB, Griffin WO. The acutely ischaemic upper extremity: selective management. *Surgery.* 1974;76:1002–1009.

44. Pairolero PC, Walls JT, Payne WS, et al. Subclavian–axillary artery aneurysms. *Surgery.* 1981;90(4):757–763.

45. Sandmann W, Kniemeyer HW, Jaeschock R, et al. The role of subclavian–carotid transposition in surgery for supra-aortic occlusive disease. *J Vasc Surg.* 1987;5:53–58.

46. Vogt DP, Hertzer NR, O'Hara PJ, et al. Brachiocephalic arterial reconstruction. *Ann Surg.* 1982;196(5):541–552.

47. Liljeqvist L, Ekeström S, Nordhus O. Intrathoracic approach for subclavian and innominate artery reconstruction. *Scand J Thorac Cardiovasc Surg.* 1979;13:309–314.

48. Van Damme H, Caudron D, Defraigne JO, et al. Brachiocephalic arterial reconstruction. *Acta Chir Belg.* 1992;92:37–45.

49. Luosto R, Ketonen P, Harjola P-T, et al. Extrathoracic approach for reconstruction of subclavian and vertebral arteries. *Scand J Thorac Cardiovasc Surg.* 1980;14:227–231.

50. Moore WS, Malone JM, Goldstone J. Extrathoracic repair of branch occlusions of the aortic arch. *Am J Surg.* 1976:132;249–257.

51. Sterpetti AV, Schultz RD, Farina C, et al. Subclavian artery revascularization: a comparison between carotid–subclavian artery bypass and subclavian–carotid transposition. *Surgery.* 1989;106:624–632.

52. Livesay JJ, Atkinson JB, Baker JD, et al. Late results of extra-anatomic bypass. *Arch Surg.* 1979;114:1260–1267.

53. Kretschmer G, Teleky B, Marosi L, et al. Obliteration of the proximal subclavian artery: to bypass or to anastomose. *J Cardiovasc Surg.* 1991;32:334–339.

54. Harris RW, Andros G, Dulawa LB, et al. Large-vessel arterial occlusive disease in symptomatic upper extremity. *Arch Surg.* 1984;119:1277–1282.

55. Mesh CL, McCarthy WJ, Pearce WH, et al. Upper extremity bypass grafting. A 15-year experience. *Arch Surg.* 1993;128:795–802.

56. Reul GJ, Jacobs MJ, Gregoric ID, et al. Innominate artery occlusive disease: surgical approach and long-term results. *J Vasc Surg.* 1991;14(3):405–412.

57. Weimann S. Extrathorakale versus transthorakale Methoden zur operativen Korrektur von Stenosen und Verschlüssen der Aortenbogenäste: ein Vergleich. *Wien Klin Wochenschr.* 1989;101(21):740–743.

58. AbuRahma AF, Robinson PA, Khan MZ, et al. Brachiocephalic revascularization: a comparison between carotid–subclavian artery bypass and axilloaxillary artery bypass. *Surgery.* 1992;112:84–91.

59. Gerety RL, Andrus CH, May AG, et al. Surgical treatment of occlusive subclavian artery disease. *Circulation.* 1981;64(suppl II):228–230.

60. Criado FJ. Extrathoracic management of aortic arch syndrome. Proffered review. *Br J Surg.* 1982;69(suppl):45–51.

61. Ziomek S, Quinones-Baldrich WJ, Busuttil RW, et al. The superiority of synthetic arterial grafts over autologous veins in carotid–subclavian bypass. *J Vasc Surg.* 1986;3:140–145.

62. Millaire A, Trinca M, Marache P, et al. Subclavian angioplasty: immediate and late results in 50 patients. *Cathet Cardiovasc Diagn.* 1993;29:8–17.

63. Düber C, Klose KJ, Kopp H, et al. Percutaneous transluminal angioplasty for occlusion of the subclavian artery: short- and long-term results. *Cardiovasc Intervent Radiol.* 1992;15:205–210.

64. Hebrang A, Maskovic J, Tomac B. Percutaneous transluminal angioplasty of the subclavian arteries: long-term results in 52 patients. *AJR.* 1991;156:1091–1094.

65. Mathias KD, Lüth I, Haarmann P, Percutaneous transluminal angioplasty of proximal subclavian artery occlusions. *Cardiovasc Intervent Radiol.* 1993;16:214–218.

66. Bogey WM, Demasi RJ, Tripp MD, et al. Percutaneous transluminal angioplasty for subclavian artery stenosis. *Am Surg.* 1994;60:103–106.

67. Branchereau A, Magnan PE, Espinoza H, et al. Subclavian artery stenosis: hemodynamic aspects and surgical outcome. *J Cardiovasc Surg.* 1991;32:604–612.
68. Brandl R, Jauch K-W, Bae JS. Früh- und Spätergebnisse nach Subclaviatransposition. *Chirurg.* 1990;61:171–177.
69. Carlson RE, Ehrenfeld WK, Stoney RJ, et al. Innominate artery endarterectomy. A 16-year experience. *Arch Surg.* 1977;112:1389–1393.
70. Crawford ES, Stowe CL, Powers RW Jr. Occlusion of the innominate, common carotid, and subclavian arteries: long-term results of surgical treatment. *Surgery.* 1983;94(5):781–791.
71. DePalma RG, Broadbent RV. Management of occlusive disease of the subclavian and innominate arteries. *Am J Surg.* 1981;142:197–202.
72. Eisenhardt HJ, Zehle A, Pichlmaier H. Indikationsstellung und operationstechnisches Vorgehen bei chronischen Verschlüssen des Truncus brachiocephalicus und der A. subclavia im Abschnitt I. *Langenbecks Arch Chir.* 1980;351:161–169.
73. Ekeström S, Liljeqvist L, Nordhus O. Surgical management of obliterative disease of the brachiocephalic trunk. Experience from 24 cases. *Scand J Thorac Cardiovasc Surg.* 1983;17:305–309.
74. Garrett HE, Morris GC, Howell JF, et al. Revascularization of upper extremity with autogenous vein bypass graft. *Arch Surg.* 1965;91:751–757.
75. Katz SG, Kohl RD. Direct revascularization for the treatment of forearm and hand ischemia. *Am J Surg.* 1993;165:312–316.
76. Perler BA, Williams GM. Carotid–subclavian bypass—a decade of experience. *J Vasc Surg.* 1990;12:716–723.
77. Rapp JH, Reilly LM, Goldstone J, et al. Ischemia of the upper extremity: significance of proximal arterial disease. *Am J Surg.* 1986;152:122–126.
78. Rostad H, Hall KV. Arterial occlusive disease of the upper extremity. *Scand J Thorac Cardiovasc Surg.* 1980;14:223–226.
79. Schroeder T, Buchardt Hansen HJ. Arterial reconstrution of the brachiocephalic trunk and the subclavian arteries. 10 years' experience with a follow-up study. *Acta Chir Scand.* 1980;502:122–130.
80. Shifrin EG, Anner H, Levy P, et al. Extrathoracic approach in surgical treatment of subclavian steal. *Isr J Med Sci.* 1986;22:567–571.
81. Zelenock GB, Cronenwett JL, Graham LM, et al. Bracheocephalic arterial occlusion and stenoses. *Arch Surg.* 1985;120:370–376.
82. Mathias K, Bockenheimer S, von Reutern G, et al. Katheterdilatation hirnversorgender Arterien. *Radiologe.* 1983;23:208–214.
83. Gordon RL, Haskell L, Hirsch M, et al. Transluminal dilatation of the subclavian artery. *Cardiovasc Intervent Radiol.* 1985;8:14–19.
84. Vitek JJ, Keller FS, Duvall ER, et al. Brachiocephalic artery dilation by percutaneous transluminal angioplasty. *Radiology.* 1986;158:779–785.
85. Wilms G, Baert A, Dewaele D, et al. Percutaneous transluminal angioplasty of the subclavian artery: early and late results. *Cardiovasc Intervent Radiol.* 1987;10:123–128.
86. Gershony G, Basta L, Hagan AD. Correction of subclavian artery stenosis by percutaneous angioplasty. *Cathet Cardiovasc Diagn.* 1990;21:165–169.
87. Insall RL, Lambert D, Chamberlain J, et al. Percutaneous transluminal angioplasty of the innominate, subclavian, and axillary arteries. *Eur J Vasc Surg.* 1990;4:591–595.
88. Kumar S, Mandalam KR, Rao VRK, et al. Percutaneous transluminal angioplasty in nonspecific aortoarteritis (Takayasu's disease): experience of 16 cases. *Cardiovasc Intervent Radiol.* 1990;12:321–325.
89. Kachel R, Basche S, Heerklotz I, et al. Percutaneous transluminal angioplasty (PTA) of supra-aortic arteries especially the internal carotid artery. *Neuroradiology.* 1991;33:191–194.
90. Tesdal IK, Jaschke W, Haueisen H, et al. Perkutane transluminale Angioplastie (PTA) der armversorgenden Arterien bei brachialer und zerebraler Ischämie. *Fortschr Roentgenstr.* 1991;155(4):363–369.
91. Sharma S, Kaul U, Rajani M. Identifying high-risk patients for percutaneous transluminal angioplasty of subclavian and innominate arteries. *Acta Radiol.* 1991;32:381–385.

92. Selby JB Jr, Matsumoto AH, Tegtmeyer CJ, et al. Balloon angioplasty above the aortic arch: immediate and long-term results. *AJR*. 1993;160:631–635.
93. Arlart IP. Ballonkatheterdilatation in der Behandlung des Subclavian-Steal-Syndroms. *Fortschr Roentgenstr*. 1988;149(3):263–266.
94. Qi Jianpin, Zeitler E. Katheterdilatation der arteriellen Stenosen supraaortaler Gefässe und Spätergebnisse. *Fortschr Roentgenstr*. 1991;155(4):357–362.
95. McCarthy WJ, Flinn WR, Yao JST, et al. Result of bypass grafting for upper limb ischemia. *J Vasc Surg*. 1986;3:741–746.
96. Farina C, Mingoli A, Schultz RD, et al. Percutaneous transluminal angioplasty versus surgery for subclavian artery occlusive disease. *Am J Surg*. 1989;158:511–514.

16

Endoscopic Thoracic
Sympathectomy

W.P. Hederman, MD, MCh, FRCS (Ireland)

HISTORY

The procedure of sympathectomy has had a long, checkered, and frequently contentious history. Initially, it was used in various conditions in the lower limb, mainly vascular.

The first account of sympathectomy of the upper limb appears to be in 1928, when Royle described a sympathetic trunk section for Raynaud's disease.[1]

Adson and Brown in 1929 resected the stellate and second dorsal ganglia for Raynaud's disease.[2] In 1935 Adson et al went on to describe cervical sympathectomy in the management of hyperhydrosis.[3] Also in 1935, Telford described what became the classic anterior supraclavicular approach to upper limb sympathectomy.[4]

Smithwick in 1937 described the posterior approach, resecting the inner ends of the second and third ribs.[5] Sir Hedley Atkins in 1949 described the axillary route, claiming better access to more of the chain.[6] Over the subsequent years these three operative approaches or variations thereof have been used for a variety of vascular conditions in the upper limb, frequently with disappointing long-term results after apparent initial improvement. In primary Raynaud's disease most cases revert to their preoperative condition after several months, and in collagen diseases such as scleroderma the effect is extremely transitory. Causalgia, in very carefully selected cases, can be helped by sympathectomy, but the results are variable.

There is, however, one condition for which sympathectomy is almost universally and permanently successful: hyperhydrosis, or excessive sweating from the palms of the hands or the armpits. Unfortunately, many surgeons in the past have been reluctant to undertake sympathectomy for a condition such as hyperhydrosis, which is neither life nor limb threatening, since each of the three traditional approaches—the anterior, the posterior, and the axillary—is associated with a definite incidence of morbidity and complications and requires fairly specialized surgical skills. For example, the axillary approach can only be performed on one side at a time and is frequently so painful in the postoperative period that some patients refuse to have the second side operated on.

However, I have rarely encountered a more grateful group of patients than those whose clammy hands have previously made their lives a misery, interfering with their social and professional activities, especially those whose work involved handling delicate or slippery materials or frequently meeting members of the public. Charles Dickens gave a beautiful description of the condition in the character of Uriah Heep in *David Copperfield*: "His damp cold hand felt so like a frog in mine that I was tempted to drop it and run away. He took out his pocket handkerchief, and began wiping the palms of his hands."

Therefore, when Kux in 1978 described his endoscopic approach to the upper dorsal sympathetic chain, a new era began for these patients.[7] We took up his idea and, using a standard laparoscope inserted into the pleural cavity through the anterior part of the axilla, found we had an excellent view of the upper dorsal sympathetic chain. Kux used a two-stage procedure, first inducing a pneumothorax under local anesthesia and subsequently excising portions of the sympathetic chain through a thoracoscope using grasping forceps and scissors. We used a unipolar diathermy probe and simple electrocoagulation under general anesthesia with a double-lumen endotracheal tube, and found it simple, straightforward, and easy to learn.[8] Patients had very little postoperative discomfort and virtually no complications.

PATIENT SELECTION

At Mater Misericordicue Hospital, Dublin, Ireland, our main indication for this procedure is palmar hyperhydrosis which is interfering significantly with the patient's lifestyle. It is important to exclude patients with more generalized sweating, either from systemic conditions or from psychological instability, and a careful assessment must be made. In practice we find that we reject almost two-thirds of the patients referred to us for consideration, either because they are not severe enough or sufficiently localized or they appear to have an underlying emotional instability or a medical condition.

Routine chest x-ray is carried out to exclude the possibility of apical pleural adhesions. Thyroid function studies and other routine preoperative tests are carried out.

Patients must be warned about a certain postoperative incidence of compensatory sweating from the trunk or the head.

TECHNIQUE

We use general anesthesia with a double-lumen endotracheal tube. The patient is placed supine with his arms abducted to a right angle on arm boards.

The tip of the surgeon's index finger identifies a suitably wide intercostal space in the anterior axilla immediately behind the pectoralis major muscle (this is usually the fourth space) (Fig. 16–1). A Verres needle is then introduced into the pleural cavity through a small stab incision, after the ipsilateral portion of the endotracheal tube has been detached from the anesthetic machine. About 0.5 L of carbon dioxide is insufflated carefully while checking that the pressure in the gas line does not go above 10 cm of water and also that the pressure varies with respiration.

The Verres needle is then removed and a standard laparoscope is introduced through a cannula at the same site. We use the smallest cannula that will take our standard telescope in order to avoid pressure on intercostal nerves. The mediastinum

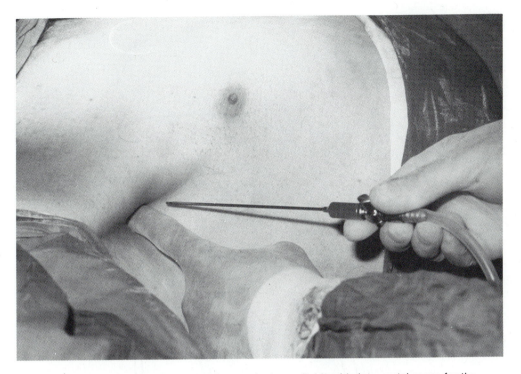

Figure 16–1. The surgeon's index finger selects a suitably wide intercostal space for the introduction of the Verres needle, and subsequently the telescope.

is inspected and in most cases the sympathetic chain can be identified under the pleura running vertically over the necks of the upper ribs just lateral to the bulge of the costovertebral junction, which glistens in the light.

Other anatomical features to be identified are the superior vena cava and the azygos vein on the right side and the subclavian artery and arch of the aorta on the left side and the phrenic and vagus nerves on each side.

Next, it is important to identify accurately the position of the second dorsal sympathetic ganglion. The highest rib that one sees easily is usually the second, and the ganglion lies on or just below its neck. It is equally important to note the presence of a characteristically yellow pad of fat at the apex of the pleural cavity, which covers the stellate ganglion and hides it completely from view and out of harm's way.

At this stage we introduce a second small cannula in the front of the chest, in the midclavicular line about the third intercostal space. An insulated unipolar diathermy probe with a slightly bent tip is introduced through this cannula and can be used to depress the apex of the lung to get a better view, and further carbon dioxide gas is introduced if necessary (Fig. 16–2).

If the sympathetic chain is not readily visible on inspection, it can be identified by palpating with the tip of the diathermy probe, stroking it along the neck of the second or third rib as one would do with one's index finger in an open sympathectomy. The chain can be seen and felt slipping out from under the tip of the probe during this maneuver (Fig. 16–3).

Using diathermy, the pleura is incised vertically over the second ganglion and down to just above the third ganglion. The second ganglion is then divided and coagulated right down onto the underlying rib until it presents a charred appearance.

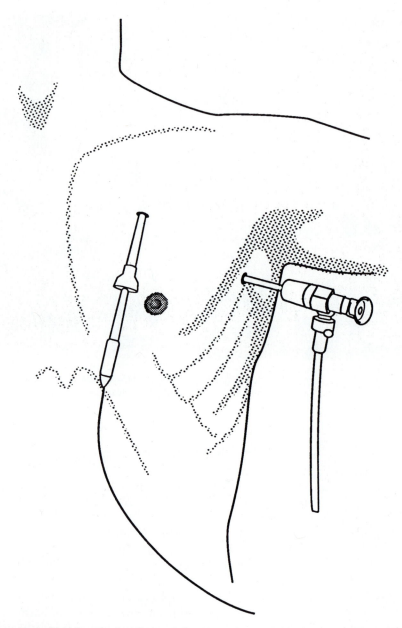

Figure 16–2. Showing the locations of the two cannulae with the telescope and the diathermy probe.

We also apply diathermy to the portions of the chain immediately above and below the ganglion and we then carry the incision in the pleura laterally for 1 in or so along the surface of the second and third ribs to deal with the possible presence of the nerve of Kuntz.[9] This nerve may occur in about 10% of cases and is not always visible. It may carry sympathetic fibers and cause recurrence of symptoms if not destroyed (Fig. 16–4.)

When coagulation on the first side is complete, the lung is re-expanded by reconnecting the appropriate side of the endotracheal tube to the anesthetic machine, disconnecting the carbon dioxide, removing the diathermy probe, and observing the reinflation of the apex of the lung through the scope. The operation is then repeated

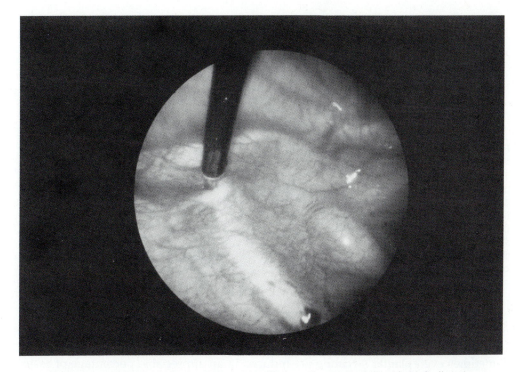

Figure 16–3. The sympathetic chain is identified on the neck of the third left rib being displaced by the blunt tip of the diathermy probe as it is stroked laterally along the rib.

on the other side without delay. No chest drains are used, but a routine postoperative chest x-ray is taken. There is usually a small apical pneumothorax which can be safely ignored.

Light or mild flimsy pleural adhesions can be divided with endoscopy diathermy scissors without difficulty. It is sometimes necessary to retract the apex of the lung to one side, using a simple metal probe inserted through a small stab incision lower in the axilla. However, very dense adhesions over the area of the sympathetic chain can render the operation impossible, because even if one carefully dissects off the lung from the mediastinum, the resultant "battleground" makes identification of the chain very difficult indeed.

In recent years we have limited the extent of our sympathectomy to the second dorsal ganglion and the adjoining portions of the chain, as described above, in all cases. Initially, like most other workers, we dealt with the second, third, fourth, and sometimes the fifth dorsal ganglia, especially if the skin of the axilla was involved. We found, however, on long-term review that up, to 64% of the patients continued to experience compensatory hyperhydrosis from around the waist, the back of the chest, or the head. The vast majority of patients said that this was infinitely preferable to the preoperative palmar sweating, but nevertheless we felt that we should try to reduce its severity and incidence. We discovered that Hyndman and Wolkin in 1942 had shown that only the second dorsal ganglion needed to be removed for complete sympathectomy of the upper limb,[10] and this was confirmed by O'Riordan et al in 1993.[11]

Since limiting the extent of the sympathectomy, the incidence of compensatory hyperhydrosis has been reduced to about 25% and, subjectively, seems to be less severe, while not reducing the success rate of the procedure as far as hand sweating

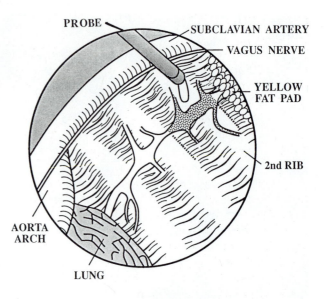

Figure 16–4. The diathermy probe (**top**) points to the second left dorsal ganglion. The stippled area indicates the extent of electrocoagulation. The dotted lines along the upper edges of the second and third ribs represent the lines of division of the pleura to divide a possible nerve of Kuntz.

is concerned. The curious factor that emerges from our own cases and those of others who are practicing this more limited sympathectomy is that axillary sweating and sometimes even plantar sweating are reduced in an appreciable percentage of cases. Why? Of course, the anatomy of the sympathetic nervous system is immensely variable, as has been shown in many anatomical studies over the years.

We have seen a much lower incidence of gustatory sweating than that in some other series: only 3%. This may be because the Irish do not eat very hot or spicy foods.

Those patients who continue to have excessive sweating from the axillae can be treated by local excision of the sweat glands. Plantar sweating is managed by localized phenol injection of the lumbar sympathetic chain.

RESULTS

We have reviewed 300 cases of palmar hyperhydrosis treated by sympathectomy from 1980 to 1992. There was an immediate success rate of 98%. Six of the early cases had to be reoperated on and were then successful. No doubt this was due to our initial timidity with the diathermy. On long-term follow-up, 5% of patients have developed some further sweating from one hand or the other. Four percent regard their compensatory hyperhydrosis as more distressing than their initial symptoms.

We feel that there are very few other indications for sympathectomy in the upper limb because of the early return of symptoms in vascular conditions. In 6 cases of causalgia, 3 have had very good results and the other 3 have shown some improvement. Twenty-four elderly patients with arterial disease unsuitable for reconstruction improved to varying degrees after the procedure.

We do not regard Raynaud's syndrome as an indication for sympathectomy unless there is severe ulceration not responding to conservative measures, such as 5-day intravenous infusion of low-molecular-weight dextran. We have operated on 10 such cases and the ulceration has healed following operation, but the patients continue to require observation and treatment.

COMPLICATIONS

We have had no permanent cases of Horner's syndrome, and just 3 transient ones. We have had bleeding in 1 case which required control with a clip and 2 cases of pneumothorax requiring underwater chest drainage.

This low complication rate compares with several other recently reported series and confirms the safety of the procedure and is in marked contrast to reports of complications in series of open operations in which permanent Horner's syndrome, brachial plexus or phrenic nerve injuries, or even subclavian artery injuries have all been reported.

One of the outstanding features of the procedure is the relative lack of postoperative pain or discomfort and the ability to discharge the patient from the hospital the day following the operation. Operating time is also short: usually 20 to 30 minutes for both sides. We have no difficulty with operating on both sides during the same admission. Continuous blood gas studies have shown no significant alterations during the procedure.

Cosmetically, the scars following endoscopic thoracic sympathectomy are far more acceptable to the patient than those after the open surgical procedures. This is important, since a high percentage of our patients are young and female.

This procedure has now gained wide acceptance in Europe and in the Far East, where hyperhydrosis seems to occur more frequently than in the West.

With the increasing expertise in the use of endoscopes and the increased sophistication of instrumentation, we feel that the thoracoscopic approach is currently ideal for patients requiring sympathectomy of the upper limb.

REFERENCES

1. Royle ND. Sympathetic trunk section: a new operation for Raynaud's disease and spastic paralysis of the upper limb. *Med J Aust*. 1928;2:436–439.
2. Adson AW, Brown GE. Raynaud's disease of the upper extremity; successful treatment by resection of sympathetic cervicothoracic and 2nd thoracic ganglia and intervening trunk. *JAMA*. 1929;92:444–447.
3. Adson AW, Craig WM, Brown GE. Essential hyperhidrosis cured by sympathetic ganglionectomy and trunk resection. *Arch Surg*. 1935;31:794–798.
4. Telford ED. The technique of sympathectomy. *Br J Surg*. 1935;23:448–450.
5. Smithwick R. The value of sympathectomy in the treatment of vascular diseases. *N Engl J Med*. 1937;216:141–150.
6. Atkins HJB. Peraxillary approach to the stellate and upper thoracic sympathetic ganglia. *Lancet*. 1949;2:1152–1154.
7. Kux M. Thoracic endoscopic sympathectomy in palmar and axillary hyperhidrosis. *Arch Surg*. 1978;113:264–266.
8. Malone PS, Duignan JP, Hederman WP. Transthoracic electrocoagulation (TTEC): a new and simple approach to upper limb sympathectomy. *Ir Med J*. 1982;75:20–21.
9. Kuntz A. Distribution of the sympathetic rami to the brachial plexus. *Arch Surg*. 1927;15:871–877.
10. Hyndman OR, Wolkin J. Sympathectomy of the upper extremity. Evidence that only the second dorsal ganglion need be removed for complete sympathectomy. *Arch Surg*. 1942;45:145–155.
11. O'Riordan DS, Maher M, Waldron DJ, et al. Limiting the anatomical extent of upper thoracic sympathectomy for primary palmar hyperhidrosis. *Surg Gynecol Obstet*. 1993;176:151–154.

17

Arterial Complications of Thoracic Outlet Syndrome

Edouard Kieffer, MD, Carlo Ruotolo, MD,
Fabien Koskas, MD, and Amine Bahnini, MD

Arterial complications of thoracic outlet syndrome (TOS) are observed far less frequently than neurological or even venous manifestations. In a recent review of the English-speaking literature, Sanders and Craig[1] found only 218 reported cases of arterial complications of TOS managed surgically. According to the largest series in the literature, arterial complications account for less than 5% of operations performed for TOS.[1] Their prognostic implications, however, may be extremely severe. Pathological changes of the subclavian artery (SA), mainly aneurysmal in nature, are the result of longstanding arterial compression leading to intimal alterations, mural thrombosis, and severe thromboembolic complications jeopardizing the viability of the upper extremity. The variety of clinical presentations can sometimes be misleading, so that one does not even think to request an arteriography. Unlike neurological complications, surgical decompression of the thoracic outlet, although necessary, is not sufficient, and proximal as well as distal arterial lesions must also be treated, sometimes with technical difficulties. As a consequence of diagnostic delay, advanced cases may be associated with severe functional impairment or even loss of integrity of the upper extremity, despite adequate surgical treatment. This chapter reviews the clinical and surgical aspects of these complications, based on a review of the recent literature and our experience with 60 surgically treated cases, 38 of which have already been reported.[2]

ANATOMIC LESIONS

An intermittent positional arterial compression is commonly observed in most cases of TOS, including the majority of those with purely neurological symptoms. This is also present in up to 50% to 60% of normal adults, especially those who are young or athletic.[3,4] However, in this subset of normal individuals, permanent arterial damage has never been reported. The mechanism of severe arterial lesions is always a significant, permanent, and longstanding compression. This accounts for (1) the nature of the compression itself, mainly secondary to bony abnormalities of the thoracic outlet, and (2) the long delay before arterial lesions develop and symptoms appear. Patients having arterial complications are an average of 10 years older than those experiencing neurological or venous symptoms. Accordingly, in Short's series of arterial complications of cervical ribs,[5] the mean ages of patients with and without thromboembolic complications were 44 and 24 years, respectively.

Although the compression may involve any of the three consecutive narrowings of the thoracic outlet, it primarily affects the costoscalene passage and, less frequently, the costoclavicular passage. The SA compression occurs anteroposteriorly in the former and cephalad to caudad in the latter. Arterial complications due to compression in the retropectoral passage have been reported very rarely.[6]

Elements of Compression

Congenital bony abnormalities are the most frequent causative factors. Cervical ribs are present in 0.5% to 1.0% of normal individuals. Among them, only 5% to 10% have clinical symptoms, usually of neurological origin.[3] Cervical ribs are by far the most common congenital bony abnormalities in almost all series of patients with arterial complications of TOS.

The arterial consequences of complete versus incomplete cervical ribs have been emphasized by several investigators.[5,7–9] Complete long cervical ribs are articulated or fused to a tubercle on the upper aspect of the first thoracic rib, just behind the distal insertion of the anterior scalene muscle (ASM). If a large spatulated anterior end of the cervical rib is present, the resulting arterial compression may be accentuated. Incomplete short cervical ribs do not directly reach the first thoracic rib, although they are commonly associated with a fibrous band that follows the same trajectory as a complete cervical rib. Incomplete cervical ribs, when symptomatic, usually cause nerve compression, whereas complete cervical ribs appear as the main causative factor of arterial compression and complications. Accordingly, in Short's report[5] arterial complications were observed in 15 of 21 cases with complete cervical ribs and in none of 7 cases with incomplete cervical ribs. Aneurysms were frequently observed when the cervical rib was lateral, articulating with the first rib at the lateral border of the ASM. Complications were much less frequent when the cervical rib was medial, articulating with the first thoracic rib just behind the ASM. These complications may also develop as a result of an incomplete cervical rib or an elongated C7 transverse process, but this occurs much less frequently.[2] In both situations the bony abnormality is usually prolonged by a fibrous band inserted on the first thoracic rib just behind the tubercle of the ASM.

Congenital abnormalities of the first thoracic rib are less common than those of the cervical ribs, as they are found in 0.07% to 0.5% of the normal population.[10–12] However, when present, they seem to be an even more frequent cause of arterial complications than cervical ribs.[13] Mercier et al[10] reported three arterial complications among 8 patients with first rib abnormalities and only five arterial complications among 31 patients with cervical ribs. Although first-rib abnormalities are rarely more prevalent than cervical ribs, they are reported in virtually all large series of arterial complications of TOS. Very few series do not mention such abnormalities as a causative factor. The most common abnormality is agenesis of the anterior part of the first rib. In these cases the posterior part of the rib may be articulated with or fused to the second rib in the same manner that a complete cervical rib articulates with a normal first thoracic rib. In other cases the anterior end of the partially agenetic first rib may be free and pulled upward by the ASM that inserts on it. Synostosis of the first two ribs,[8] bifidity,[14] or an abnormal tubercle of the first rib[15–17] is less frequently encountered.

Although they are mainly responsible for neurological symptoms, isolated congenital bands,[3] as well as hypertrophic ASM, have been described in a small number of patients with arterial complications of TOS.[15,18–21.] In the collected series by Sanders and Craig of 218 patients treated for arterial complications of TOS, only 19 (9%) had no bony abnormalities.[1]

Acquired bony abnormalities affecting mainly the clavicle and, less frequently, the first thoracic rib are even less common.[22] Malunion of a fractured clavicle is more likely to cause arterial problems than a hypertrophic callus. Anecdotal cases of hypertrophic callus[17] or exostosis[23] of the first thoracic rib, as well as cases of sequelae of osteomyelitis of the clavicle,[15,24] have also been reported.

Whatever its cause, location, and mechanism, arterial compression is usually intermittent at onset. Later, it becomes permanent as a result of a variety of physiological, pathological, or traumatic factors. The most important of these factors is the physiological dropping of the shoulder girdle, which usually takes place during the third decade of life, especially in women. Whiplash cervical injuries or athletic trauma[19,25] may also precipitate arterial compression by causing trauma and subsequent fibrosis of the scalene muscles.

Arterial Lesions

The initial consequence of a tight longstanding compression of the SA in the costoclavicular passage of the thoracic outlet is localized stenosis. Even after many years this lesion is probably entirely reversible by surgical decompression. However, with the passage of time and mechanical trauma caused by shoulder motion, the arterial wall becomes thick and fibrotic, and inflammatory changes of the adventitia fix the artery to the surrounding structures. In most cases poststenotic dilatation develops and is a characteristic complication of arterial compression in the thoracic outlet caused by the fragility of the SA in young persons. The most common mechanism for this dilatation, at least in compressions in the costoscalene passage, is poststenotic turbulence,[5] which is secondary not only to the presence of tight stenosis but also to angulation in the frontal plane. Indeed, the bony abnormality usually pushes the artery upward in the lower cervical region, resulting in acute angulation before it reaches the axillary region. The resulting vibrations affect the fragile arterial wall, distending and rupturing components of the media, thus giving rise to circumferential dilatation of the artery (Fig. 17–1).[26–29] Localized jet lesions may be present in very tight stenoses and account for the rare occurrence of saccular aneurysms. Similarly, repeated trauma from the moving clavicle may be responsible for a localized lesion of the upper aspect of the SA when compression takes place in the costoclavicular passage.

These arterial lesions may have different consequences, among which thromboembolic complications are the most common and potentially the most dangerous (Fig. 17–1). Distal ischemia secondary to proximal tight stenosis without any thromboembolic complication is rarely observed.[2,30] To our knowledge rupture of a poststenotic aneurysm, although theoretically possible, has never been reported. Similarly, poststenotic aneurysms rarely develop to such an extent as to compress the adjacent venous or nervous structures.

Thromboembolic complications are the real threat of these lesions. An intimal lesion may occur either at the site of compression and stenosis of the SA or in the poststenotic dilatation, often at the site of impact of the poststenotic jet (Fig. 17–2).

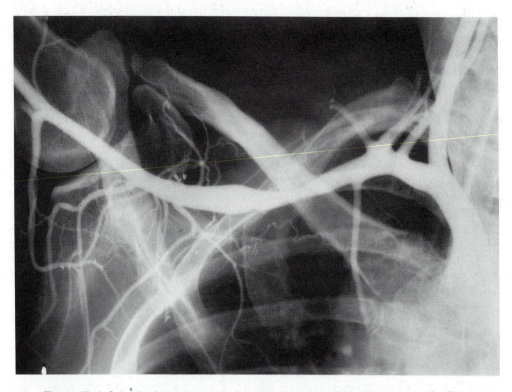

Figure 17–1. Selective innominate arteriography demonstrating mild poststenotic dilatation of the subclavian artery in a patient with an anomalous first rib.

Distal microembolization of platelet aggregates formed on this intimal lesion is now commonly considered to be the usual mechanism of Raynaud's syndrome and of digital necrosis with normal distal pulses occurring as a complication of TOS. These microemboli are especially frequent in the thumb and the index finger, probably as a result of the straightforward pathway through the radial artery as opposed to that of the ulnar artery. The formation of a mural thrombus is even more ominous.[31] Although mechanical factors are usually predominant, they may be accelerated by hematologic or hormonal disturbances, including the use of contraceptive pills.[10,20] Ischemic consequences of the resulting macroembolization vary according to the site and extent of distal occlusion. An isolated proximal embolus often has less serious consequences than more distal emboli, owing to the greater possibilities of collateral circulation. If the SA abnormality is not corrected early, emboli will occur repeatedly, with progressive obliteration of the distal arterial bed and aggravation of ischemia. In some cases effective treatment may be impossible and major irreversible ischemia will follow. Thrombotic occlusion of the SA is rarely encountered, but when it does occur, occlusion usually remains initially limited to the subclavian and axillary arteries, while good collateral circulation develops (Fig. 17–3). In these cases distal ischemia is usually mild or even absent. When it occurs after many episodes of distal embolization, ischemia is usually severe and may even be irreversible because of difficulties in clearing the distal arterial bed. Retrograde embolization to the cerebral arteries, although rare, is a serious potential complication.[19,32–34] Reported cases have always been associated with mural thrombosis of the subclavian artery and with previous upper extremity embolic complications. In case of proximal extension of thrombosis, the mechanism of cerebral embolization is easy to understand. When the thrombus

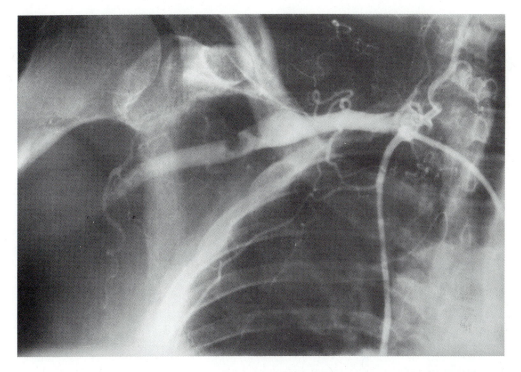

Figure 17–2. Selective subclavian arteriography demonstrating aneurysm of the subclavian artery with mural thrombus in a patient with an anomalous first rib.

involves only the poststenotic arterial segment, then the mechanism probably is complete positional occlusion of the subclavian artery, followed by fragmentation of the proximal part of the thrombus, turbulence above the occlusion, and retrograde embolization in the proximal SA.

CLINICAL SYMPTOMS

Diagnosis is rarely made at an early stage, before the appearance of thromboembolic complications. Three different clinical situations may result in an early diagnosis: (1) a pulsatile supraclavicular mass revealing an asymptomatic subclavian aneurysm[35,36]; (2) isolated neurological symptoms associated with a cervical rib or any bony abnormality of the thoracic outlet, a situation that, in our opinion, warrants arteriography or an ultrasound study; and (3) an incidental finding on arteriography performed for a symptomatic lesion of the opposite upper extremity.[16]

In many cases the disease remains undiagnosed until thromboembolic complications occur. The most frequent early symptoms are due to embolic occlusions of the digital arteries of the palmar arch. Raynaud's syndrome or its equivalents, including episodic pallor and/or cyanosis, paresthesia, coldness, pain, and cold sensitivity of the hands and digits, are commonly found at this stage of disease. They must be recognized as vascular symptoms and their source must be properly managed before further showers of microemboli or a larger embolus result in ischemic lesions of the fingertips or even frank gangrene of part or all of one or more digits.[37] In the presence of such distal vascular findings, the diagnosis of arterioarterial embolism is favored by (1) late age of onset; (2) predominant distribution in the radial artery bed of the

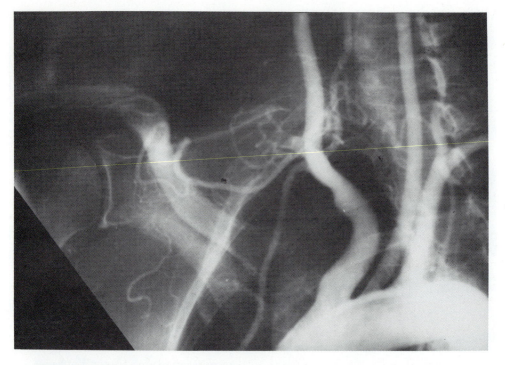

Figure 17–3. Arch aortography demonstrating occlusion of the subclavian artery in a patient with a cervical rib. Note extensive collateral circulation to the upper extremity.

hands and digits; (3) absence of other etiology, such as collagen vascular disease, occupational arterial trauma, or Buerger's disease; and (4) strictly unilateral nature, clearly indicating their secondary origin.[8,15] In some series of the literature, TOS is not even mentioned as a cause of Raynaud's syndrome,[38] whereas it seems to be associated with 5% of all Raynaud's syndromes and digital gangrene[37] and up to 25% of unilateral Raynaud's syndromes.[39] Although digital gangrene should always suggest distal arterial occlusion, Raynaud's syndrome or its equivalent may sometimes raise diagnostic problems. This happens when, despite recognition of TOS, symptoms are attributed to sympathetic irritation because of nerve compression rather than to arterial complications, which may be overlooked.[8] Another misleading clinical situation is encountered when a cervical rib is associated in the same patient with Raynaud's syndrome of different origin.[40]

Microembolization may last months or even years before major embolic complications occur. Acute ischemia owing to proximal embolism is the most frequent complication. A proximal arterial source accounts for 25% to 50% of all upper extremity emboli,[41] and complications of TOS are the most common. This source must be suspected in the presence of any proximal embolus in the upper extremity, especially when a cardiac source is not found. A major error would be to proceed to a standard isolated embolectomy.[2,5,18,21,42] This first episode of embolization usually has a favorable outcome, even if not treated surgically. The resulting ischemia may become subacute or chronic or even completely disappear owing to the development of collateral circulation. However, sooner or later, recurrent embolization will occur if its cause has not been eradicated through proper management. In these cases ischemia becomes severe and does not regress spontaneously, and surgical management becomes extremely difficult because of multiple emboli of different ages located at various levels in the extremity. Outcome may be unfavorable in more advanced cases, with major amputations becoming necessary. Subacute or chronic ischemia is usually associated with proximal segmental occlusion with good collateral circulation. In a few cases, usually with isolated SA occlusion, ischemia does not develop, and it may be difficult to establish the differential diagnosis with chronic occlusions due to trauma, cardiogenic embolism, or even Takayasu's arteritis.

Retrograde embolization in the cerebral circulation is, fortunately, rare. For obvious anatomic reasons, the right hemisphere is almost always affected, with left hemiplegia being the most common symptom. The constant association with thromboembolic complications affecting the right upper extremity should allow prompt recognition of the syndrome. Any delay in treatment should be avoided, since it entails a high risk of recurrence, with the possibility of leaving a young individual with both upper extremities compromised, due to arterial ischemia on the right and hemiplegia from right cerebral embolism on the left.[33]

DIAGNOSIS

A high index of suspicion of TOS is of crucial importance when faced with a patient with ischemic upper extremity. A clinical history of a fractured clavicle or first rib, with late complications of hypertrophic callus and/or malunion, may suggest diagnosis. More frequently, the presence of a cervical rib may be known for some time from a previous chest roentgenogram. Symptoms secondary to associated nerve compression are present in only one-third of the cases.

The diagnosis may be established by physical examination. A pulsatile mass in the supraclavicular area is often palpable but does not usually correspond to the SA aneurysm itself. A more precise examination usually shows that the palpable abnormality is the bony abnormality, pushing the artery upward. Arterial dilatation is slightly more distal, behind the clavicle. A bruit may be heard over the SA, occasionally only in extreme positions of the upper extremity. These positions may also diminish or even abolish the distal pulses. Although these findings have some value in these clinical circumstances, they are not specific, because they are often present in normal persons.

Anteroposterior and oblique cervical spine and upper thoracic roentgenograms are most important, since a bony abnormality is nearly always present. As previously mentioned, the most frequent is a cervical rib, usually long, complete, and fused or articulated to the first rib. Agenesis of the anterior part of the first thoracic rib is less commonly found. Still rarer are other congenital abnormalities of the first rib or acquired abnormalities of the clavicle or the first rib. The absence of a bony abnormality, however, should not rule out the diagnosis of arterial complications of TOS, since a few cases have been described with only muscular or fibrous elements of compression.

Noninvasive techniques have been used for more than two decades to investigate these patients. Doppler examination may be useful in describing and quantifying the postural changes in arterial circulation of the upper extremity. It may also localize the arterial occlusion and assess the collateral circulation. B-mode ultrasonography is useful in establishing the diagnosis of poststenotic dilatation (Fig. 17–4) and mural thrombus. It may also be used to follow asymptomatic arterial dilatation associated with the cervical rib which does not yet require surgical treatment, in order to avoid repeated arteriography.

Arteriography should visualize the entire upper extremity, from the aortic arch to the digital arteries. The usual technique is catheterization through the femoral artery and selective injection in the proximal SA. Diagnosis of arterial complications of the TOS is not always easy.[42] Subtraction techniques are useful. A fusiform aneurysm is usually obvious, especially if located distal to permanent arterial stenosis (Fig. 17–5). An irregular lining or filling defect strongly suggests the presence of mural thrombus (Fig. 17–6). Although arteriography is seldom entirely normal, some features may be difficult to recognize. A mural thrombus may obliterate part of the aneurysmal sac. In symptomatic patients even the smallest poststenotic dilatation is a strong clue to diagnosis, and in these patients a mural thrombus will often be found at the time of operation. The SA stenosis is not always obvious on the anteroposterior view, because compression in the costoscalene passage takes place in the same plane. Dynamic views help define the exact site of compression. Arteriography is also helpful in demonstrating distal arterial occlusions and the development of collateral circulation (Fig. 17–7). In the presence of Raynaud's syndrome or digital gangrene due to occlusive disease of the distal arteries, magnification films, including those obtained after intra-arterial injection of a vasodilator, may help in the differentiation between local lesions and emboli.[43]

In a small number of patients with cervical ribs or other bony abnormalities and symptoms of thromboembolic disease in the upper extremity, the SA may appear grossly normal or only slightly dilated on arteriography (Fig. 17–8). In these rare situations we strongly advocate surgical exploration as an integral part of the diagnostic work-up. Intraoperative arterial palpation is unreliable and may be dangerous, since it entails the risk of mobilizing the thrombus with further distal embolization. We

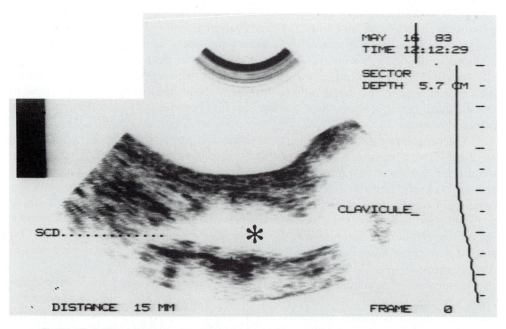

Figure 17–4. Ultrasonogram demonstrating poststenotic dilatation of the subclavian artery without mural thrombus.

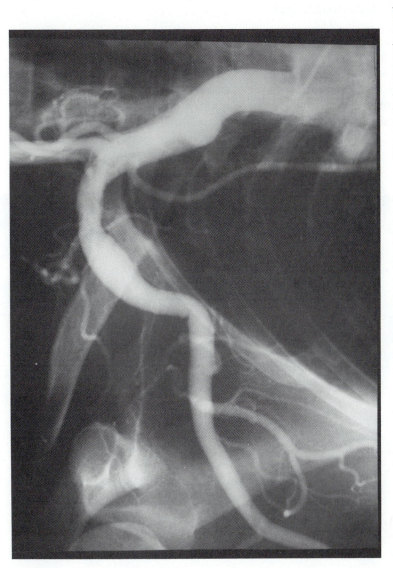

Figure 17–5. Selective innominate arteriography demonstrating uncomplicated fusiform aneurysm of the subclavian artery in a patient with a cervical rib.

believe that an exploratory longitudinal arteriotomy is best in these cases. This seemingly aggressive attitude is the only way to rule out with certainty a small intimal lesion that must be treated if recurrent emboli are to be avoided.[8,14,15,20,44] If the arterial intima appears normal, it is very simple to close the artery using a continuous suture, tailored to correct the poststenotic dilatation.

SURGICAL MANAGEMENT

The treatment of arterial complications of TOS is surgical. Surgery often must be performed on an emergency or semiemergency basis, not only in the presence of acute or subacute ischemia of the upper extremity but also every time a mural thrombus has been recognized, since severe embolic complications are unpredictable and may rapidly become difficult to manage.[9] The three anatomic components of the disease process—namely, arterial compression, subclavian–axillary arterial lesions, and, less consistently, distal emboli—must be treated simultaneously.

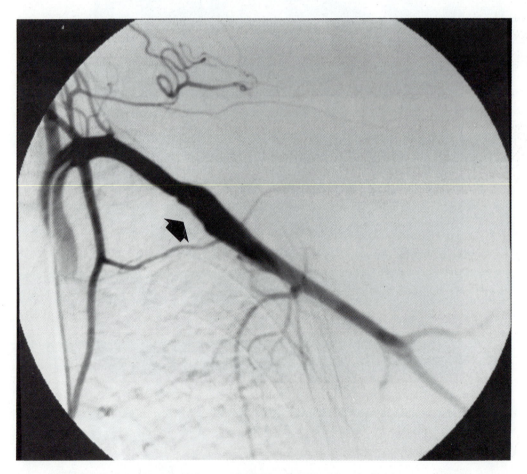

Figure 17–6. Selective subclavian arteriography demonstrating fusiform aneurysm of the subclavian artery with mural thrombus (arrow) in a patient with a cervical rib.

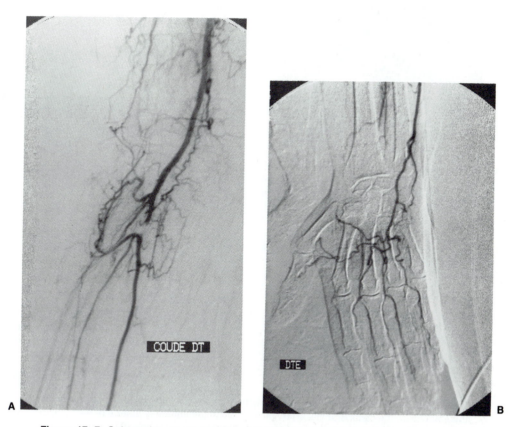

Figure 17–7. Subtraction arteriography of the upper extremity demonstrating embolic occlusion of the brachial artery bifurcation (**A**), palmar arches, and digital arteries (**B**).

Surgical Approach

The ideal surgical approach should allow simultaneous thoracic outlet decompression, treatment of the subclavian–axillary arterial lesions, and upper dorsal sympathectomy when indicated. The whole upper extremity should be accessible to the surgeon in order to allow for distal embolectomy when necessary.

The *transaxillary* approach is largely used for isolated rib resection in the presence of neurological symptoms. A concomitant upper dorsal sympathectomy may be easily added. However, this approach does not offer a satisfactory exposure of the subclavian–axillary artery and is therefore contraindicated in the management of arterial complications. Although a few surgeons have used it in isolated cases, Van Dongen[45] is the only author to advocate its routine in the treatment of arterial complications of TOS. The same objections apply to the anterolateral thoracic approach. In addition, a thoracic incision represents an unnecessary surgical approach, even in young or middle-aged patients.

The *transclavicular* approach allows for wide exposure of the supraclavicular and axillary regions. One of two techniques may be used. Although temporary transection of the middle part of the clavicle followed by osteosynthesis seems logical, it may lead to orthopedic complications such as malunion and/or hypertrophic callus of the

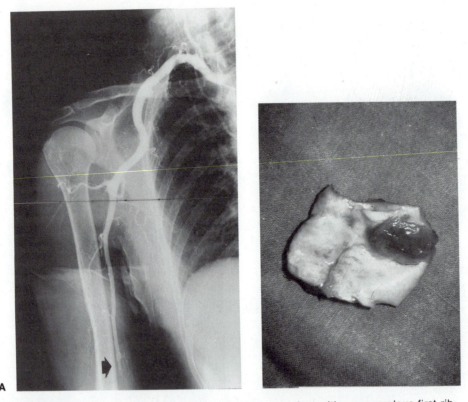

Figure 17–8. Selective subclavian arteriography in a patient with an anomalous first rib and embolus to the distal brachial artery (arrow). Despite minimal dilatation of the subclavian artery (**A**), a mural thrombus was found at the time of operation (**B**).

clavicle, with or without infection.[10,16] Resection of the middle part or medial two-thirds of the clavicle is simpler and has a low incidence of cosmetic and functional impairment.[15,20] However, since the same surgical procedures can be performed without dividing the clavicle, using a supraclavicular approach, the only indications for clavicular resection are the rare cases of arterial complications due to malunion and/or hypertrophic callus of the clavicle.

The *supraclavicular* approach offers complete exposure of the SA, cervical rib, and muscular or fibrous bands.[7,9,15,42] Using this approach, resection of the normal first rib is simple and safe, provided that the SA and the brachial plexus are entirely dissected and the entire upper extremity is prepared and draped so that it may be raised when resection of the anterior part of the rib is undertaken. Complete resection of the posterior part of the first rib is easily achieved, and it is straightforward to detect and treat any type of associated muscular or fibrous abnormality. Difficulties may arise in the presence of arterial lesions extending to the axillary artery. In these cases additional exposure is obtained through a deltopectoral or infraclavicular incision, leaving the clavicle undisturbed.[9]

Thoracic Outlet Decompression

Complete resection of a cervical rib or abnormal first rib is obviously necessary. Regardless of whether there are associated neurological symptoms, it seems logical to add routine resection of the normal first rib to preclude late occurrence of neurological manifestations or even recurrence of arterial compression.[2,16,35,36,46] Clavicular resection should be performed in cases of malunion and/or hypertrophic callus complicating a fractured clavicle. In any case resection of the bony abnormality must be accompanied by removal of any abnormal muscular or fibrous element. Scalenectomy seems definitely preferable to scalenotomy, since the scalene muscles may reattach themselves to the bed of the resected cervical or first rib and be responsible for recurrent arterial or nerve compression.

Proximal Arterial Reconstruction

Arterial reconstruction is necessary in the presence of an arterial aneurysm and/or mural thrombosis, with or without distal thromboembolic complications. However, mild poststenotic dilatation without clinical or radiological evidence of mural thrombus warrants discussion. Many surgeons still consider this entity an indication to conservative management because of its anticipated regression after isolated arterial decompression.[1,7,10,36,44,47] We believe that it does not always represent a benign condition and dictates at least surgical exploration. The presence of intimal arterial disease and/or mural thrombus is difficult to rule out unless an exploratory arteriotomy is performed. Very few cases of actual regression of the dilatation after isolated arterial decompression have been reported.[30] Severe arterial complications have been reported after these conservative procedures.[14,46,48,49] Although the initial arterial lesions have not always been described precisely, these cases constitute a strong argument in favor of direct arterial reconstruction in the presence of a seemingly benign poststenotic dilatation.

Surgical techniques must be tailored to the arterial lesions. Resection is required in the presence of a subclavian–axillary aneurysm. An excessive arterial length is usually obtained after resecting the cervical and first thoracic ribs. This allows for end-to-end anastomosis in most cases. In the presence of a lengthy arterial dilatation, a short segment of graft may have to be interposed in order to bridge the arterial defect. The preferred graft material is autogenous saphenous vein. When unavailable, we favor the use of an arterial autograft[42] rather than a Dacron or polytetrafluoroethylene (PTFE) graft.

A mild fusiform poststenotic dilatation should be opened longitudinally over its entire length and closed with a continuous tailoring suture after an intimal lesion has been ruled out or treated either by intimectomy or limited segmental resection. Although this technique appears easy and appealing, it may sometimes be difficult to perform. The use of an indwelling stent may be necessary for suitable aneurysmorrhaphy. Proximal or distal transection of the artery may also be useful when dealing with arterial lesions extending behind the clavicle. This allows visualization of the entire diseased artery through the supra- or infraclavicular incision. After the aneurysmorrhaphy has been performed, the artery is placed in its normal position and an end-to-end anastomosis is performed. A limited arterial resection may be added if excessive arterial length is present.

In rare cases an isolated intimal fibrous plaque without any associated arterial dilatation may be treated by intimectomy with or without patch angioplasty closure of the artery. In case of complete occlusion of the subclavian artery, a carotid–axillary bypass can be performed without resection of the arterial lesion. Associated decompression of the thoracic outlet should be added to prevent late neurological or vascular compression.

Management of Distal Embolic Occlusions

Distal embolic occlusions often introduce major difficulties in the surgical management of these patients. They are usually multiple and diffuse with emboli of different ages.

Some occlusions are recent and easily cleared by thromboembolectomy; others are older, adherent to the arterial wall, and inaccessible to direct or indirect embolectomy. In such cases unsuccessful surgical attempts at disobliteration may result in extensive thrombosis. In the presence of a seemingly old and well-compensated distal embolic occlusion, direct surgical treatment should be avoided. In most of these cases, upper dorsal sympathectomy is probably all that is required.

If distal arterial occlusion involves the proximal arteries, is apparently of recent onset, and results in severe distal ischemia, an attempt at direct revascularization is appropriate.[2,16] It may be possible to perform embolectomy by introducing the Fogarty balloon catheter through the distal SA at the site of proximal reconstruction. Distal passage of the catheter through the entire upper extremity is often difficult or impossible. Selective catheterization of the radial and ulnar arteries may also be difficult, and a separate approach to the brachial artery bifurcation is usually necessary. An intraoperative arteriogram is advisable in most cases. Although persisting occlusion of the forearm or hand arteries classically requires a direct approach to the radial and/ or ulnar arteries at the wrist and selective embolectomy of the palmar arches, intra-arterial infusion of thrombolytic agents is probably a better alternative in most cases.[50] In the presence of chronic brachial occlusion complicated by proximal recent embolus, it may be sufficient to revascularize the deep brachial artery,[2,14,16] which plays the same physiological collateral role in the upper extermity as does the deep femoral artery in the lower extremity, provided that the periarticular arterial network of the elbow is patent.

If embolectomy is impossible, ineffective, or incomplete, a distal bypass using autogenous vein may be performed in an attempt to revascularize one of the forearm arteries, usually the interosseous artery.

Difficulty in clearing the distal arterial bed accounts for the incomplete revascularization of the forearm and the hand in the most advanced cases. A significant number of major amputations are still reported, often after multiple surgical attempts to revascularize the upper extremity.[15,20,42] Distal amputations are mentioned in most large series and some patients, although they have a viable upper limb, will suffer disabling ischemic sequelae such as Raynaud's syndrome, Volkmann's contracture, claudication, or fatigability of the forearm. These results are in sharp contrast with those obtained in the absence of distal embolization, when clinical and anatomic results are consistently good if the initial surgical management has been appropriate.

PERSONAL EXPERIENCE AND RESULTS

From January 1973 to December 1993, 483 surgical decompressions of TOS have been performed in the Department of Vascular Surgery of Pitié-Salpétrière University Hospital, Paris, France. A total of 60 upper extremities with arterial complications were treated in 57 patients, accounting for 12% of the entire series. There were 45 female and 12 male patients, with a mean age of 40.3 years (ranges, 17 to 78 years).

Congenital bony abnormalities were almost constant. Thirty-two cases were associated with a cervical rib, including 23 complete cervical ribs, articulating with or fused to the first thoracic rib, and nine incomplete cervical ribs prolonged by a fibrous band. An abnormality of the first rib was present in 14 cases, including 11 ageneses of the anterior part and three hypertrophies of the anterior part with synostosis to the second rib. An elongated C7 transverse process was present in 2 patients. Malunion of the clavicle was present in 2 patients, the origin being congential in 1 case and secondary to a pathological fracture due to bone metastasis in the other. In 10 cases there was no bony abnormality but tight fibrous bands and/or hypertrophic scalene muscles. An arterial aneurysm distal to the site of an arterial compression was present in 46 cases. Among these aneurysms, 16 were uncomplicated, 25 had been the source of distal (11) or proximal (14) emboli, and 5 were completely occluded. In 1 case the aneurysm had developed distal to an aberrant right subclavian artery. The arterial diameter was normal in the remaining 14 cases. Among these, 8 cases had an atheromatous plaque at the site of compression, with intimal ulceration, and distal emboli. In the other 6 cases the subclavian artery was completely occluded.

Only 3 patients were asymptomatic and the diagnosis was made in the presence of a pulsatile supraclavicular mass. The majority of patients had arterial symptoms, either isolated (35 patients) or associated with neurological symptoms (7 patients) or venous symptoms (1 patient). The remaining 12 patients had isolated neurological symptoms. A total of 43 upper extremities presented with arterial symptoms. In 30 cases ischemia was associated with abolition of distal, brachial, and sometimes axillary pulses. Among these, 12 had chronic and 18 had acute ischemia jeopardizing the viability of the affected upper extremity and requiring emergency treatment. Distal pulses were present in 30 cases, including 5 cases with digital gangrene of one or several fingers and 8 cases with isolated intermittent vasomotor symptoms. Twelve cases presented with neurological symptoms, isolated with 6 cases and associated with arterial symptoms in the others. Bilateral selective subclavian angiograms visualizing the entire upper extremity were performed in all but 2 patients operated on an emergency basis.

Since the late 1970s all patients have had Doppler ultrasound studies and B-mode sonograms in order to detect the presence of a subclavian mural thrombosis and/or occlusion of the digital arteries.

One female patient had already undergone in another center partial resection of a cervical rib with Fogarty catheter embolectomy of the upper extremity and a repeat Fogarty catheter embolectomy, 3 and 1 year(s), respectively, before she was admitted with acute ischemia of the upper extremity. Both previous operations had misdiagnosed the presence of a subclavian aneurysm as the source of distal emboli. Four other patients had undergone elsewhere isolated Fogarty catheter embolectomy of the upper limb, 5 months and 23, 8, and 6 days, respectively, before surgical treatment of the proximal SA lesion was performed in our center.

All patients underwent surgical treatment with direct arterial reconstruction. Among the 60 cases in our series, resection of the inner half of the clavicle was the surgical approach in only 6, including the 2 patients with malunion of the clavicle. In the remaining 54 cases a supraclavicular incision was used to approach the thoracic outlet. Treatment of the proximal arterial lesion required an associated deltopectoral or inflaclavicular approach in 31 cases and a transaxillary approach in 3 cases. Bony abnormalities were resected whenever present. Among the 32 cases associated with a cervical rib 11 had an isolated resection of the cervical rib early in our experience, whereas 21 more recent cases had an associated cervical and first rib resection. An abnormal first rib was resected in 14 cases. A normal first rib was also resected in 10 cases of isolated fibrous and/or muscular compression and in 2 cases of an elongated C7 transverse process. In the 2 cases with malunion of the clavicle, surgical decompression of the throacic outlet was obtained by partial cleidectomy.

Surgical treatment of the proximal arterial lesion was usually not technically demanding. Resection of the diseased arterial segment followed by end-to-end anastomosis, whenever possible, was our technique of choice. Twenty-four subclavian arteries lesions were thus treated. In 19 cases the length of the arterial lesion did not allow a direct end-to-end anastomosis and required an interposition graft. The choice of graft material has evolved during the two-decade time frame of our series. One Dacron graft and 11 saphenous vein grafts were used early in our experience, whereas more recently seven femoral artery autografts were harvested for upper extremity arterial reconstruction and replaced by either a PTFE (6 cases) or saphenous vein graft (1 case). The rationale for this policy was that in case of degenerative changes of the venous or prosthetic grafts, repeat surgery would be more difficult and dangerous at the level of the thoracic outlet than at the level of the proximal superficial femoral artery.

In 5 cases of complete subclavian occlusion without associated arterial dilatation, a subclavian–axillary (3 cases) or carotid–axillary (2 cases) bypass graft was performed, without resection of the arterial lesion. Due to the length of the graft needed, a saphenous vein was used in all 5 cases. One patient with associated tight stenosis of the axillary artery had resection of an SA aneurysm and a carotid–axillary venous bypass graft. In the patient with an aberrant right SA, treatment consisted of resection of the aberrant artery through a cervical approach, including its retroesophageal portion, followed by carotid–axillary bypass using a femoral artery autograft replaced by a saphenous vein graft. Transposition of the right vertebral artery to the common carotid artery was also associated. In nine uncomplicated poststenotic dilatations a longitudinal arteriotomy was followed by aneurysmorrhaphy closure using a continuous modeling suture, after significant intimal lesion had been eliminated.

Management of distal thromboembolic complications was by far more challenging. A Fogarty balloon catheter embolectomy was attempted in 12 cases, most often through one or several distal arteriotomies. In an attempt to achieve older clot lysis, in 2 recent cases Fogarty catheter embolectomy was followed by intra-arterial thrombolytic therapy, with infusion of 100,000 U of urokinase into the distal bed. Due to the severity of ischemia and the difficulty in clearing the distal bed from old emboli, venous bypass to the interosseous artery was performed in 4 cases. An upper dorsal sympathectomy was associated in 23 cases.

There were no postoperative deaths or major amputations. Advanced gangrene of one digit required distal amputation in only 1 case. In the other 4 cases of digital gangrene, proximal revascularization combined with upper dorsal sympathectomy allowed spontaneous healing of the pulpar necrosis. One case of left chylothorax was successfully managed by chest tube drainage and parenteral hyperalimentation. Early reoperation was required in 3 patients with arterial proximal reconstruction. The causes were bleeding, occlusion of a bypass vein graft requiring thrombectomy, and an infected supraclavicular hematoma in 1 case each. The saphenous vein graft could be preserved in all 3 patients. In another patient early reocclusion of the brachial artery required a repeat Fogarty catheter thrombectomy. Chest x-rays showed phrenic nerve palsy in 6 patients, only 1 of whom had clinical complaints.

Early clinical results were excellent in 51 cases, with complete absence of ischemic symptoms. Besides the 1 patient with distal amputation, disabling sequelae, including effort claudication and cold-induced vasomotor symptoms, were present in only 7 symptomatic cases due to incomplete removal of distal occlusive lesions. Anatomical results were rather disappointing, however, compared to clinical findings. Arterial patency of the proximal as well as distal upper extremity was achieved in only one-third (10/30) of cases with no distal pulses before surgery. Of note, only one of the four distal bypasses to the interosseous artery remained patent. All 30 cases with distal pulses before surgery remained so in the postoperative period.

REFERENCES

1. Sanders RJ, Craig H. Review of arterial thoracic outlet syndrome with a report of five new instances. *Surg Gynecol Obstet.* 1991;173:415–425.
2. Kieffer E, Jue-Denis P, Benhamou M, et al. Complications artérielles du syndrome de la traversée thoraco-brachiale: traitement chirurgical de 38 cas. *Chirurgie.* 1983;109:714–722.
3. Roos DB. Congenital anomalies associated with thoracic outlet syndrome. *Am J Surg.* 1976;132:771–778.
4. Wright IS. The neurovascular syndrome produced by hyperabduction of the arms. *Am Heart J.* 1945;2:1–19.
5. Short DW. The subclavian artery in 16 patients with complete cervical ribs. *J Cardiovasc Surg.* 1975;16:135–141.
6. Finkelstein JA, Johnston KW. Thrombosis of the axillary artery secondary to compression by the pectoralis minor muscle. *Ann Vasc Surg.* 1993;7:287–290.
7. Blank RH, Connar RG. Arterial complications associated with thoracic outlet syndrome. *Ann Thorac Surg.* 1974;17:315–324.
8. Swinton NW Jr, Hall RJ, Baugh JH, et al. Unilateral Raynaud's phenomenon caused by cervical-first rib anomalies. *Am J Med.* 1970;48:404–407.
9. Martin J, Gaspard DJ, Johnston PW, et al. Vascular manifestations of the thoracic outlet syndrome. A surgical urgency. *Arch Surg.* 1976;111:779–782.
10. Mercier C, Houel F, David G, et al. Les complications vasculaires des syndromes de la traversée thoraco-brachiale. *Chirurgie.* 1981;107:433–438.
11. Pietri J, Vierling JP, Kieny R, et al. Les complications artérielles au cours des anomalies congénitales du défilé costo-claviculaire. *J Chir.* 1968;95:329–352.
12. Baumgartner F, Nelson RJ, Robertson JM. The rudimentary first rib: a cause of thoracic outlet syndrome with arterial compromise. *Arch Surg.* 1989;124:1090–1092.
13. Dumeige F, André J, Vargas R, et al. Les complications vasculaires des anomalies de la première côte. *Chirurgie.* 1986;112:584–590.
14. Banis JC Jr, Rich N, Whelan TJ Jr. Ischemia of the upper extremity due to noncardiac emboli. *Am J Surg.* 1977;134:131–139.
15. Bouhoutsos J, Morris T, Martin P. Unilateral Raynaud's phenomenon in the hand and its significance. *Surgery.* 1977;82:547–551.
16. Cormier JM, Amrane M, Ward A, et al. Arterial complications of the thoracic outlet syndrome: fifty-five operative cases. *J Vasc Surg.* 1989;9:778–787.
17. Rob CG, Standeven A. Arterial occlusion complicating thoracic outlet compression syndrome. *Br Med J.* 1958;20:709–712.
18. Dorazio RA, Ezzet F. Arterial complications of the thoracic outlet syndrome. *Am J Surg.* 1979;138:246–250.
19. Fields WS, Lemak NA, Ben Menachem Y. Thoracic outlet syndrome: review and reference to stroke in a major league pitcher. *Am J Roentgenol.* 1986;7:809–814.
20. Judy KL, Heymann RL. Vascular complications of thoracic outlet syndrome. *Am J Surg.* 1972;123:523–531.
21. Simon H, Gryska PF, Carlson DH. The thoracic outlet syndrome as a cause of aneurysm formation, thrombosis, and embolization. *South Med J.* 1977;70:1282–1284.
22. Melliere D, Escourrou J, Becquemin JP, et al. Ischémies aigues des membres: complications tardives de cals hypertrophiques et de pseudarthroses. *J Chir.* 1981;118:641–645.
23. Wellington JL, Martin P. Post-stenotic subclavian aneurysm. *Angiology.* 1965;16:566–573.
24. Raphael MJ, Moazzez KH, Offen DN. Vascular manifestations of thoracic outlet compression: angiographic appearances. *Angiology.* 1974;25:237–248.
25. McCarthy WJ, Yao JST, Schafer MF, et al. Upper extremity arterial injury in athletes. *J Vasc Surg.* 1989;9:317–327.
26. Boughner DR, Roach MR. Effect of low frequency vibration on the arterial wall. *Circ Res.* 1971;29:136–144.
27. Dobrin PB. Post-stenotic dilatation. *Surg Gynecol Obstet.* 1991;172:503–508.
28. Ojha M, Johnston KW, Cobbold RSC. Evidence of a possible link between post-stenotic dilation and wall shear stress. *J Vasc Surg.* 1990;11:127–135.

29. Zarins CK, Zatina MA, Giddens DP, et al. Shear stress regulation of artery lumen diameter in experimental atherogenesis. *J Vasc Surg.* 1987;5:413–420.

30. Bertelsen S, Mathiesen FR, Ohlen-Schlaeger HH. Vascular complications of cervical rib. *Scand J Thorac Cardiovasc Surg.* 1968;2:133–139.

31. Gunning AJ, Pickering GW, Robb-Smith AHT, et al. Mural thrombosis of the subclavian artery and subsequent embolism in cervical rib. *Q J Med.* 1964;129:133–154.

32. Al Hassan HK, Sattar AM, Eklof B. Embolic brain infarction: a rare complication of thoracic outlet syndrome. A report of two cases. *J Cardiovasc Surg.* 1988;29:322–325.

33. De Villiers JC. A brachiocephalic vascular syndrome associated with cervical rib. *Br Med J.* 1966;2:140–143.

34. English R, Macauley M. Subclavian artery thrombosis with contralateral hemiplegia. *Br Med J.* 1977;2:1583.

35. Milazzo VJ, Hobson RW II. Axillosubclavian artery aneurysms. In: Yao JST, Pearce WH, eds. *Aneurysms: New Findings and Treatment.* Norwalk, Conn: Appleton & Lange; 1994;451–457.

36. Pairolero PC, Walls JT, Payne WS, et al. Subclavian axillary artery aneurysms. *Surgery.* 1981;90:757–763.

37. Vayssairat M, Fiessinger JN, Housset E. Les nécroses digitales du membre supérieur: 86 cas. *Nouv Presse Med.* 1977;6:931–934.

38. Porter JM, Rivers SP, Anderson CJ, et al. Evaluation and management of patients with Raynaud's syndrome. *Am J Surg.* 1981;142:183–189.

39. Vayssairat M, Fiessinger JN, Housset E. Phénomène de Raynaud: étude prospective de 100 cas. *Nouv Presse Med.* 1979;8:2177–2180.

40. Vayssairat M, Baudot N, Rouffy J. Phénomène de Raynaud et syndrome de la traversée thoraco-brachiale. In: Kieffer E, ed. *Les Syndromes de la Traversée Thoraco-brachiale.* Paris France: AERCV; 1989;165–168.

41. Sachatello CR, Ernst CB, Griffen WO Jr. The acutely ischemic upper extremity: selective management. *Surgery.* 1974;76:1002–1009.

42. Etheredge S, Wilbur R, Stoney RJ. Thoracic outlet syndrome. 1979;138:175–182.

43. Maiman MH, Bookstein JJ, Bernstein EF. Digital ischemia: angiographic differentiation of embolism from primary arterial disease. *Am J Roentgenol.* 1981;137:1183–1187.

44. Scher LA, Veith FJ, Haimovici H, et al. Staging of arterial complications of cervical rib: guidelines for surgical management. *Surgery.* 1984;95:644–649.

45. Van Dongen RJAM. Lesions of the subclavian artery: reconstructive procedures. In: Greep JM, Lemmens HAJ, Roos DB, et al, eds. *Pain in Shoulder and Arm.* The Hague, The Netherlands: Martinus Nijhoff; 1979;281–291.

46. De Weese JA, Green RM. Arterial complications of thoracic outlet syndrome: association with bony abnormalities and optimal method of treatment. In: Veith FJ, ed. *Current Critical Problems in Vascular Surgery.* St Louis, Mo: Quality Medical Publishing; 1993;5:379–383.

47. Salo JA, Varstela E, Ketonen P, et al. Management of vascular complications in thoracic outlet syndrome. *Acta Chir Scand.* 1988;154:349–352.

48. Traphagen DW, Marshall F. Subclavian artery thrombosis six years after rib resection. *Arch Surg.* 1961;83:700–701.

49. Harris JD, Jepson RP. Vascular complications of cervical ribs. *Aust N Z J Surg.* 1964;34:269–274.

50. Sullivan KL, Minken SL, White RI. Treatment of a case of thromboembolism resulting from thoracic outlet syndrome with intra-arterial urokinase infusion. *J Vasc Surg.* 1988;7:568–571.

V

The Diabetic Foot

18

The Role of Magnetic Resonance Imaging in the Management of Foot Abscess in the Diabetic Patient

Joseph R. Durham, MD

An accurate noninvasive means of diagnosing the presence, character, and precise location of an infection is an important component in helping to direct the timely treatment of the diabetic foot. Foot infection in the diabetic patient is a significant clinical problem with attendant high morbidity and mortality outcomes. In fact, diabetic foot infections occur in 15% of all diabetic patients,[1] account for approximately 20% of all diabetic hospital admissions in the United States,[2] and result in more in-hospital days than any other complication of diabetes.[3] Evaluation of the clinically infected diabetic foot can be quite challenging. An abscess or focus of necrotic tissue must be promptly drained and debrided to avoid life-threatening sepsis, ascending infection, and progressive local tissue destruction. Conversely, the empiric exploration of a foot that is found not to have an abscess or deep infection may result in irreparable harm to the diabetic foot.[4] Magnetic resonance imaging (MRI) has been a major advance in helping to direct the expedient care of the infected diabetic foot.

Effective noninvasive means of evaluating the diabetic foot for suspected infectious processes have been sought for years. Physical examination, plain radiographs, and three-phase radionuclide scanning (using technetium 99m or gallium 67) have been the principal diagnostic mainstays in evaluating musculoskeletal infections in the recent past.[5] Plain film radiographs are quite helpful in the identification of foreign bodies or soft tissue gas and can also demonstrate bony changes characteristic of advanced osteomyelitis; however, these simple studies suffer from a paucity of early findings in osteomyelitis and, except for tissue gas, do not yield any truly significant findings with soft tissue infections. Radionuclide scans are often helpful in the evaluation of osteomyelitis in the stable patient, but these scans are time consuming and not often relevant in the timely evaluation of the patient requiring possible prompt surgical intervention, as most require delayed imaging sessions at 24 hours. Moreover, the radionuclide scans are notorious for yielding false-positive and false-negative results in as many as 40% of those studied.[6] More recently, though, indium 111–labeled leukocyte scanning has resulted in improved sensitivity and specificity.[7,8] Scintigraphic techniques do not really document the presence of infection; rather, they merely detect any increase in capillary blood flow from inflammatory changes or any bone reaction or remodeling, whether the cause is traumatic or infectious. Unfortunately, such scans are particularly useless in the early postoperative period, since normal wound-healing processes yield positive findings with these techniques. Even the best results from radionuclide scanning provide poor spatial resolution with the attendant difficulty of localizing precisely any infectious focus.[9]

The use of computerized tomography (CT) has been a significant advance in assessing the location and extent of foot infections, especially in the diabetic population. Noninvasive, quick, and widely available, CT scanning provides excellent spatial resolution, making it invaluable in the localization of small sequestra, foreign bodies, and subtle foci of gas.[10] While CT scanning can usually localize an infectious process within the foot, it often fails to predict precisely the proximal extent of the infection; a gradual "zone of transition" between areas of definite infection and unequivocally normal tissue may extend over several centimeters, lending a certain degree of subjectivity to the interpretation of the most proximal margin of infected tissue.[6] The proximal extent of the infectious process may be of critical importance in predicting the likelihood of healing a foot amputation in the diabetic patient.[11] Furthermore, CT lacks discrimination in defining abnormal soft tissue densities within the diabetic foot; these findings may represent suppuration, reactive granulation tissue, edema, or fibrosis, underscoring the limited contrast discrimination of this radiological technique.[12] In spite of these significant limitations, CT scanning remains a worthwhile substitute for imaging of the diabetic foot when MRI is contraindicated or not available.

MRI provides a new means of "viewing" the depths of the diabetic foot noninvasively and offers several distinct advantages over those traditional diagnostic techniques outlined above. Most notable are the increased soft tissue contrast resolution, the multiplanar imaging capability, and the enhanced spatial resolution that are possible with MRI. The ability to image with equal resolution in multiple planes (including axial, coronal, sagittal, and any oblique planes) is a real improvement over CT scanning.[13] MRI has emerged as a valuable diagnostic tool and has significantly influenced the ability to manage diabetic foot infections in an efficient manner. The presence and extent of soft tissue inflammatory processes, as well as bony abnormalities, can be accurately identified. Precise localization of the extent of an infectious foot process not only can direct the need for surgical intervention, but also can assist in the planning of surgical incisions and the extent of any tissue debridement; moreover, reliable MRI results may obviate the need for *empiric* surgical exploration if a positive response to careful nonsurgical management can be anticipated.

MAGNETIC RESONANCE IMAGING TECHNIQUES

A description of quantum mechanics and the physical basis of MRI is beyond the scope of this chapter, but a brief review of MRI terminology is helpful in understanding the various spin-echo sequences needed for complete evaluation of the foot suspected of harboring an infectious process.[14] MRI employs no ionizing radiation. MR images are quite unique because they are derived from the actual chemical composition of tissues, rather than from the tissue density relationships that are assessed with standard radiological techniques. MRI is based on the interaction of radiowaves and hydrogen nuclei within tissues as a strong magnetic field is applied. The single proton of the hydrogen nucleus is the primary source of the MRI signal; in turn, water is the most common source of hydrogen nuclei contributing to the MR signal. The basic principle of MRI is dependent on the fact that a vector of any proton spin will become aligned, or "flipped," with the brief application of a defined magnetic field. The MRI signal is generated as these protons return to their original nonexcited random orientation. The data reconstructed into an MR image are actually voltage measurements of these MR signals. Data acquisition is the process of generating the MR signals and measuring them. The signals measured in MRI are called echoes because they reappear after a specific event, such as a 180° radio frequency (RF) pulse. The actual measurements start when the signal begins to grow into an echo. Typically, the echo forms halfway through the set of measurements. The time from the creation of an MR signal by an RF pulse to the peak of the echo is called the echo time (TE). Hundreds of MR signals are generated during the data acquisition. The time between consecutive MR signals for the same image is called the repetition time (TR). The size of an MR image refers to the number of pixels incorporated into the study, for example, an image matrix size of 256 × 128 (256 columns and 128 rows of pixels). The strength of the applied magnetic field is measured in tesla units (T).

Three basic types of contrast images are obtained on routine, or spin-echo, MR images: T1-weighted, T2-weighted, and proton density–weighted (relatively T2-weighted) images. The T1-weighted images are obtained via a TR of 500 to 800 milliseconds and a TE of 20 milliseconds. The T1-weighted images yield contrast that is most similar to that seen on the familiar CT scans; in this technique the dominant contrast comes from the fatty tissues. Fat appears as dark structure on CT images, and anatomic structures such as muscle, organs, and bone are visualized as gray to white on the black background. With T1-weighted MR images the tissue shades are opposite: fat produces a high signal intensity (white) and the anatomic structures appear in shades of gray to black.[13] T2-weighted images are obtained using a TR of 2,000 milliseconds and a TE of 80 milliseconds. Finally, the balanced proton density images (relatively T2-weighted images) are derived via a TR of 2,000 milliseconds and a TE of 20 milliseconds.

The image contrast and detail possible with MRI is derived from and reliant on the amount of free protons in the tissues, which, in turn, is proportional to the water content of the tissues.[15] Water results in decreased signal intensity on T1-weighted images and increased signal intensity on T2-weighted images. Thus, T2-weighted images are very sensitive for the presence of fluid; unfortunately, this does not always allow a definite anatomic distinction between soft tissue pathology and bone marrow processes, making the differentiation between superficial cellulitis or edema and osteomyelitis difficult in some cases.[15] To address this problem of decreased specificity, the standard spin-echo sequences of T1, T2, and proton density (relatively T2-weighted images) are often supplemented with short T1 inversion-recovery (STIR) images (TR, 1,500 milliseconds; TE, 30 milliseconds; inversion time, 100 milliseconds). The STIR technique suppresses the normal signals from the fat and results in an absence of signal in normal bone marrow; focally increased bone marrow signal on STIR sequences in conjunction with focally decreased marrow signal on T1-weighted images is diagnostic for osteomyelitis.[16] Moreover, signal intensity and tissue contrast are enhanced.[17]

MRI of the diabetic foot is readily accomplished using a 0.5- to 1.5-T head coil,[16] extremity coil, or loop gap resonator coil,[4,18] all of which are capable of yielding high-resolution images. The head coil has an 18- to 24-cm field of view, while the extremity and loop gap coils allow a smaller more focused field of view ranging from 12 to 24 cm.[19] A real advantage of MRI is that images may be obtained in multiple planes. This is typically achieved with two excitations using an image matrix size of 256 × 128. Five-millimeter–thick slices are obtained in axial, coronal, and sagittal planes; special oblique plane views may be obtained as required.

The evaluation of the diabetic foot for infectious complications requires *at least* both T1- and T2-weighted images. T2-weighted images reveal abscesses better than T1-weighted images alone due to the poor contrast between soft tissue and abscess foci on the T1-weighted studies. State-of-the-art investigative protocols typically employ four spin-echo sequences.[4,16,18] (1) T1-weighted images, (2) balanced proton density images (relatively T2-weighted images), (3) T2-weighted images, and (4) STIR images. More recent studies have investigated the utility of adding contrast enhancement to fat suppression techniques to improve the sensitivity and specificity of MRI in the evaluation of foot infections.[19] The most widely used MR contrast agent to date is the paramagnetic compound gadolinium (gadopentetate dimeglumine).[20,21] MR contrast agents alter the signal intensities of tissues by enhancing the relaxation of protons in the vicinity of the contrast media.[17]

Acquisition time for a complete meaningful MRI study of the diabetic foot varies from one institution to another. The actual physical location of the MR equipment in relation to the hospital, the availability of the MRI staff, the number of MR imagers, and the degree of interest of the radiology and surgical physicians all play a role in the time required to obtain the requested study. In the ideal setting in which multiple MR imagers are available and a prospective protocol is in effect, a complete study can be obtained within 60 to 90 minutes of the patient's initial clinical evaluation.[4,18]

MAGNETIC RESONANCE IMAGING DIAGNOSTIC CRITERIA

MRI can help differentiate among the various pathological conditions known to afflict the diabetic foot: edema, cellulitis, osteomyelitis, neuropathic joints, tenosynovitis, and abscesses. Previous studies have outlined the MRI findings characteristic of these diverse disorders and allow differential diagnosis in most instances. Soft tissue edema and cellulitis appear as diffuse ill-defined high-signal-intensity areas from within the soft tissue structure on T2-weighted (long TR, long TE) or short STIR images. Soft tissue edema cannot be differentiated from cellulitis by MRI techniques[21]; the clinical presentation is required to make this distinction. Distinguishing neuropathic joint disease from osteomyelitis can be challenging from both the clinical and radiological standpoints. This distinction is particularly important, though, due to the marked difference in therapy for these two disorders. Osteomyelitis appears as decreased signal intensity on T1-weighted (short TR, short TE) images and high signal intensity within the intramedullary space on long TR/TE sequences or STIR images, with or without evidence of cortical bone destruction.[21,22] Neuropathic joints are characterized by irregular destruction of the subchondral cortices of a joint accompanied by low signal intensity of the underlying trabecular bone on short TR/TE or relatively T1-weighted images with similar low signal intensity on T2-weighted images as well.[9] Tenosynovitis is recognized when high-signal-intensity fluid is found within tendon sheaths on T2-weighted images.[9]

Foot abscesses have unique properties on MRI. They are detected as well-defined soft tissue collections identified by high signal intensity on T2-weighted or STIR images, both of which indicate the presence of fluid. It is important to realize that the MRI appearance of fluid collections is the same whether or not the fluid is infected. Abscesses can usually be distinguished from soft tissue edema or cellulitis by the presence of a smooth discrete margin with a higher signal intensity than that of the surrounding edematous tissues.[18,21] Areas of cellulitis have ill-defined margins.[9] The differentiation between cellulitis and an abscess may be difficult to make in some patients due to decreased contrast between the abscess cavity and the surrounding abnormal signal in the adjacent soft tissues. Enhancement of the suspected abscess focus may be achieved with paramagnetic contrast agents such as gadolinium, which is sometimes useful in differentiating focal areas of cellulitis from an abscess (Fig. 18–1). Areas of cellulitis appear to be enhanced with the administration of gadolinium, while abscesses are defined by enhancement of the surrounding rim.[21,23] The abscess demonstrates a high-intensity enhancing rim around a central focus of low intensity on contrast-enhanced T1-weighted images. This rim enhancement is the result of central necrotic or devitalized tissue surrounded by a hyperemic zone.[19]

CLINICAL APPLICATIONS

Treatment of severe diabetic foot infections includes bedrest, intravenous antibiotics, and, if necessary, surgical debridement or drainage. Limitation of activity is important, for continued ambulation on an insensate infected diabetic foot can only lead to further tissue destruction and facilitation of the spread of infection along tissue planes and tendon sheaths. Antibiotic coverage must be broad spectrum until specific causative organisms are isolated and identified; at this point organism-specific antibiotic coverage may be selected. The presence of gangrenous nonviable tissue is usually readily apparent and the need for surgical debridement of these abnormal tissues is obvious and straightforward. The decision to use surgical therapy, either for debridement of

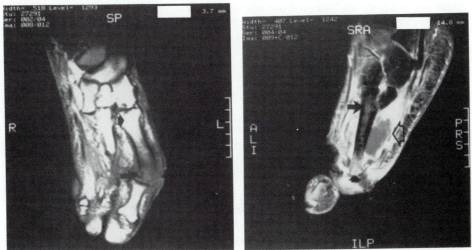

Figure 18–1. (A) A standard T1-weighted image of a patient suspected of having an acute diabetic foot infection. The normal bone marrow shows up as high signal intensity (short arrow). The bone marrow of the first metatarsal head has a low signal intensity (long arrow), suggestive of involvement by osteomyelitis. **(B)** A T1-weighted image of the same patient using the fat suppression (STIR) technique and intravenous gadolinium for contrast enhancement. The normal bone marrow returns a low-intensity signal (long arrow), while the focus of osteomyelitis has a high-intensity signal (short arrow). Note an area of low signal intensity surrounded by an area of high signal intensity representing an abscess within the soft tissue (open arrow). (*Reproduced by permission from Horowitz JD, Durham JR, Nease DB, et al. Prospective evaluation of magnetic resonance imaging in the management of acute diabetic foot infections. Ann Vasc Surg. 1993;7:44–50.*)

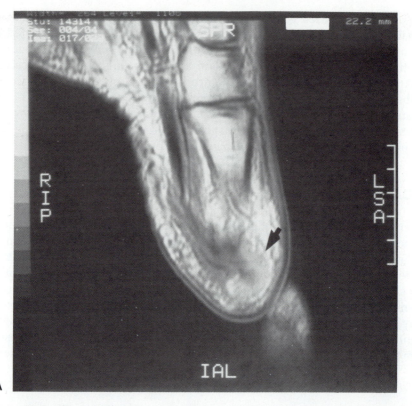

Figure 18–2. MRI study of a patient with a suspected deep-seated abscess of the left foot due to a mal perforans ulceration beneath the second metatarsal head. (**A**) On a proton density–weighted image, a zone of low signal intensity surrounded by a rim of high intensity is noted (arrow). (*Figure continues*)

devitalized tissue or for drainage of deep-seated infection, is made from the patient's presentation and the clinical findings.

The neuropathic diabetic foot can be quite challenging to evaluate, especially when an infection is suspected but is not obvious. Differentiation of a superficial cellulitis process from a deep infection is often difficult in the absence of an open or draining wound. In this setting surgical clinical judgment has directed the course of therapy. An aggressive surgical approach to the infected diabetic foot is usually rewarded with acceptable outcomes, provided that the arterial perfusion to the foot is normal. Timely drainage, debridement, and limited digital amputation in combination with aggressive revascularization have been shown to be successful in preserving functional diabetic feet.[24] However, a noninvasive means of assessing the deep structures of the foot is helpful not only in possibly avoiding an unnecessary surgical procedure when there is no abscess to drain, but also to assist in planning the optimal surgical approach when operative therapy is necessary.

There are three clinical situations in which MRI of the infected diabetic foot can have significant impact in directing patient management: preoperative evaluation of the foot with unsuspected abscess, preoperative evaluation of the foot with probable abscess, and postoperative evaluation of the foot following debridement and drainage. In the first setting the patient has an erythematous swollen foot with signs and symptoms of systemic toxicity. Unless there is an obvious draining open wound or

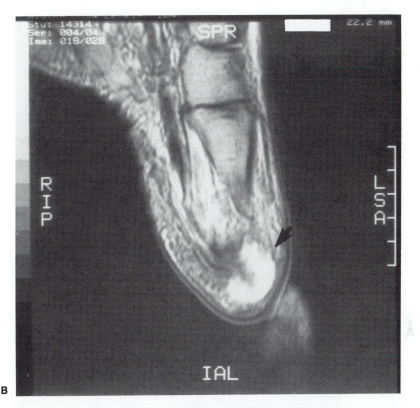

Figure 18–2. *(continued)*. (**B**) On the corresponding T2-weighted image the area of abnormality brightens significantly to a high-intensity signal, allowing diagnosis and localization of the abscess. *(Reprinted with permission from Durham JR, Lukens ML, Campanini DS, et al. Impact of magnetic resonance imaging on the management of diabetic foot infections.* Am J Surg. *1991;162:152.)*

a fullness of the plantar space, the distinction between an aggressive superficial cellulitis and a deep abscess can be quite difficult to make. Ready access to MRI can help to sort out this potential diagnostic dilemma. As long as the patient is hemodynamically stable, a prompt MRI study can be performed simultaneously with the aggressive resuscitation of the patient with appropriate intravenous fluids, electrolytes, and antibiotics. The diagnosis of cellulitis only with no evidence of a deeper abscess process allows confidence in pursuing a nonsurgical therapeutic course. Of course, if the patient's clinical course does not rapidly improve or if it deteriorates, a repeat MRI study may be performed or the patient may promptly be treated surgically as conditions mandate. Under no circumstance should an MRI study completely overrule the clinical judgment of the experienced surgeon in directing appropriate patient care. Occasionally, patients present with such severe systemic sepsis and hemodynamic compromise that even a short delay of 1 hour or so would be hazardous; in this instance emergent debridement and drainage of the infectious process must be undertaken as a lifesaving maneuver. The clinical appearance of the involved foot and the intraoperative findings must guide the location and extent of the surgical procedure.

The second preoperative situation that presents an opportunity to utilize MRI is in the planning of incisions and surgical approach. Having made the decision that operative intervention is necessary, the surgeon must decide how best to achieve

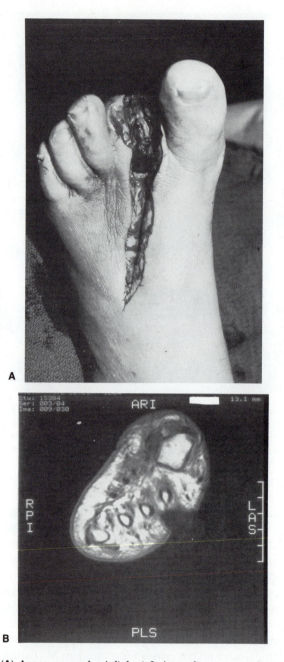

Figure 18–3. (A) Appearance of a left foot 2 days after a second ray amputation and aggressive debridement for treatment of a severe diabetic foot infection causing systemic sepsis and hypotension. The patient had persistent fever and leukocytosis in spite of an apparently adequate surgical debridement and drainage procedure with intensive intravenous antibiotic therapy. **(B)** An axial T1-weighted image with findings suggestive of edema. (*Figure continues*)

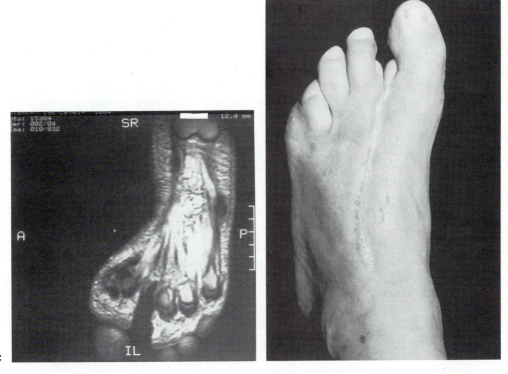

Figure 18–3. *(continued).* (**C**) A representative coronal T2-weighted image demonstrating findings compatible with soft tissue inflammation and edema, but without any evidence of discrete fluid collection or abscess. (**D**) Local wound care and intravenous antibiotics were continued and the patient gradually improved without the need for repeat surgical exploration. Appearance of the foot 4 months later, having healed completely.

drainage of all abscess collections. Not all abscesses are apparent on physical examination, and drainage of an obvious collection of pus may leave other unrecognized abscess pockets intact. While wide incision and debridement procedures minimize the risk of undrained pus collections, such an aggressive approach can damage the intrinsic architecture of the diabetic foot. Drainage of all pus is a surgical mandate, but this should be accomplished through strategically placed incisions in a manner that minimizes disruption of the normal tissue planes. Preoperative MRI studies can help accomplish this goal. The precise location and extent of significant abnormal fluid collections are readily apparent in the complete MRI study (Fig. 18–2). The most direct least injurious surgical approach can then be applied; moreover, normal portions of the foot may be left undisturbed with the confidence that no significant abscess cavities remain undetected. Some patients may present with a small superficial abscess that is amenable to drainage percutaneously or through a small well-placed incision. Complete drainage of all purulence through minimum tissue disruption allows faster convalescence and probably results in increased limb salvage rates.

A final application of MRI in the evaluation and treatment of diabetic foot infections is in the immediate postoperative period. Occasionally, patients have persistent fever and leukocytosis following what had been thought to be complete and thorough drainage of a foot abscess. Empiric re-exploration of the foot may be undertaken for possible additional pus drainage, but many of these reoperations result in negative findings. A novel approach in this setting is to obtain an MRI of the involved foot in search of an unrecognized or recurrent abscess. Identification of undrained pus allows pinpoint localization for minimally invasive drainage with good results.[4,18] Moreover, MRI documentation that there is no evidence of undrained pus or residual necrotic material allows continued nonoperative management with aggressive local wound care and culture-specific intravenous antibiotics (Fig. 18–3). Close observation in this setting is imperative, for recurrent infectious complications may develop *after* the MRI study is obtained. Failure to improve on the nonoperative regimen or worsening of the clinical picture should prompt repeat MRI evaluation or repeat surgical debridement and drainage.

The application of MR imaging to view noninvasively the depths of the diabetic foot has been shown to be quite accurate. In experienced hands the use of MRI to diagnose infectious foot problems has been quite impressive, with sensitivity rates of 94% to 100% and specificity rates of 77% to 100%,[16,25] and positive predictive values of 100% and negative predictive values of 96%.[18] MRI can detect unsuspected foci of infection or abscesses and can usually differentiate between a cellulitic process and an abscess. However, MRI can fail to detect or can misinterpret necrotic or infected muscle; it is by no means infallible. There appears to be a time window between the development of nonviable tissue and the onset of a detectable abscess focus. The clinical status of the patient and experienced surgical judgment must over-ride a negative MRI study when the patient deteriorates or fails to improve adequately on an appropriately aggressive nonoperative therapeutic course.

CONCLUSION

The use of MRI to evaluate the septic diabetic patient with an acute foot infection will not always influence the surgeon's decision as to whether operative treatment is required at the initial presentation; such decisions are usually reached on clinical grounds in the systemically septic patient. Conversely, in a reasonably stable patient MRI can probe the depths of the infected diabetic foot within 1 hour. Unsuspected or poorly localized abscess cavities can be pinpointed for optimal drainage through precisely planned skin incisions, resulting in minimal disruption of the normal intact tissue planes of the foot. Cellulitis can usually be differentiated from osteomyelitis or an abscess. Additionally, persistent postoperative fever and leukocytosis following debridement and drainage of a foot abscess can now be evaluated noninvasively with MRI, obviating the need for empiric surgical exploration. Avoidance of unnecessary surgical intervention allows maximum preservation of viable tissues and prevents further damage to the delicate architecture of the diabetic foot. Judicious use of MRI can result in accurate surgical drainage of abscess cavities and, at the same time, can avoid unnecessary surgical exploration of the tenuous diabetic foot. MRI allows the radiologist and the surgeon a degree of confidence in interpreting the findings in these complex cases that is not provided by other modalities. Further refinements in MRI technology will surely enhance the availability and value of this technique.

REFERENCES

1. Palumbo PJ, Melton LJ. Peripheral vascular disease and diabetes. In: Harris MI, Hamman RF, eds. *Diabetes in America* (NIH publication 85-1468). Bethesda, Md: National Institutes of Health; 1985;15:1–21.

2. Smith DM, Weinberger M, Katz BP. A controlled trial to increase office visits and reduce hospitalizations of diabetic patients. *J Gen Intern Med*. 1987;2:232–238.

3. Gibbons GW, Eiliopoulos GM. Infection of the diabetic foot. In: Kozak GP, Hoar CS, Rowbotham JL, et al, eds. *Management of Diabetic Foot Problems*. Philadelphia, Pa: WB Saunders Co; 1984;97–102.

4. Durham JR, Lukens ML, Campanini DS, et al. Impact of magnetic resonance imaging on the management of diabetic foot infections. *Am J Surg*. 1991;162:150–154.

5. Schults DW, Hunter GC, McIntyre KE, et al. Value of radiographs and bone scans in determining the need for therapy in diabetic patients with foot ulcers. *Am J Surg*. 1989;158:525–530.

6. Sartoris DJ, Devine S, Resnick D, et al. Plantar compartmental infection in the diabetic foot: the role of computed tomography. *Invest Radiol*. 1985;20:773–784.

7. Jacobson AF, Harley JD, Lipsky BA, et al. Diagnosis of osteomyelitis in the presence of soft-tissue infection and radiologic evidence of osseous abnormalities: value of leukocyte scintigraphy. *AJR*. 1991;157:807–812.

8. Newman LG, Waller J, Palestro CJ, et al. Leukocyte scanning with 111In is superior to magnetic resonance imaging in diagnosis of clinically unsuspected osteomyelitis in diabetic foot ulcers. *Diabetes Care*. 1992;15:1527–1530.

9. Beltran J, Campanini DS, Knight C, et al. The diabetic foot: magnetic resonance imaging evaluation. *Skeletal Radiol*. 1990;19:37–41.

10. Tang JSH, Gold RH, Bassett LW, et al. Musculoskeletal infection of the extremities: evaluation with MR imaging. *Radiology*. 1988;166:205–209.

11. Durham JR, McCoy DM, Sawchuk AP, et al. Open transmetatarsal amputation in the treatment of severe foot infections. *Am J Surg*. 1989;158:127–130.

12. Kerr R, Sartoris DJ, Fix CF, et al. Imaging of the diabetic foot. In: Frykberg RG, ed. *The High Risk Foot in Diabetes Mellitus*. New York, NY: Churchill Livingstone Inc; 1991;79–102.

13. Yucel EK, Kaufman JA. Magnetic resonance imaging and magnetic resonance angiography of aortic aneurysms. In: Yao JST, Pearce WH, eds. *Aneurysms: New Findings and Treatments*. Norwalk, Conn: Appleton & Lange; 1994;133–143.

14. Wood ML. Fourier imaging. In: *Magnetic Resonance Imaging*. Stark DD, Bradley WG, eds. St Louis, Mo: Mosby–Year Book Inc; 1990;21–35.

15. McEnery KW, Gilula LA, Hardy DC, et al. Imaging of the diabetic foot. In: Levin ME, O'Neal LW, Bowker JH, eds. *The Diabetic Foot*. 5th ed. St Louis, Mo: Mosby–Year Book Inc; 1993;341–364.

16. Yuh WTC, Corson JD, Baraniewski HM, et al. Osteomyelitis of the foot in diabetic patients: evaluation with plain film, 99m Tc-MDP bone scintigraphy, and MR imaging. *AJR*. 1989;152:795–800.

17. Physical basis of magnetic resonance imaging. In: Heiken JP, Brown JJ, eds. *Manual of Clinical Magnetic Resonance Imaging*. 2nd ed. New York, NY: Raven Press; 1991;1–69.

18. Horowitz JD, Durham JR, Nease DB, et al. Prospective evaluation of magnetic resonance imaging in the management of acute diabetic foot infections. *Ann Vasc Surg*. 1993;7:44–50.

19. Morrison WB, Schweitzer ME, Bock GW, et al. Diagnosis of osteomyelitis: utility of fat-suppressed contrast-enhanced MR imaging. *Radiology*. 1993;189:251–257.

20. Beltran J, Chandnani V, McGhee RA Jr, et al. Gadopentetate dimeglumine-enhanced MR imaging of the musculoskeletal system. *AJR*. 1991;156:457–466.

21. Spaeth HJ, Dardani M. Magnetic resonance imaging of the diabetic foot. *MRI Clin North Am*. 1994;2:123–130.

22. Erdman WA, Tamburro F, Jayson HT, et al. Osteomyelitis: characteristics and pitfalls of diagnosis with MR imaging. *Radiology*. 1991;180:533–539.

23. Dangman BC, Hoffer FA, Rand FF, et al. Osteomyelitis in children: gadolinium-enhanced MR imaging. *Radiology*. 1992;182:743–747.

24. Taylor LM Jr, Porter JM. The clinical course of diabetics who require emergent foot surgery because of infection or ischemia. *J Vasc Surg*. 1987;6:454–459.

25. Chandnani VP, Beltran J, Morris CS, et al. Acute experimental osteomyelitis and abscesses: detection with MR imaging versus CT. *Radiology*. 1990;174:233–236.

19

The Diabetic Neuropathic Foot Ulcer:

Pathogenesis, Management, and Prevention

Marvin E. Levin, MD

Diabetes is one of the oldest diseases known to mankind. The Ebers Papyrus of 1500 BC mentions its symptoms and suggests treatment. However, the history of gangrene of the foot goes back to Biblical time, when, in Chronicles II, the first case of gangrene of the feet, perhaps due to diabetes, is described: "In the 39th year of his reign, King Asa became affected with gangrene of his feet; he did not seek guidance from the Lord but resorted to physicians. He rested with his forefathers in the 41st year of his reign" (Chronicles XVI, 12–14).

Whether King Asa did indeed have diabetic gangrene is a moot point. Certainly, in Biblical times there was not much one could do for a foot lesion except pray. During the 1500s healing continued to depend on prayer alone. The famous surgeon Ambroise Paré said, "I dressed (the wound) and God healed him." Today the skills of physicians in multiple medical disciplines are significantly reducing amputation rates. With increasing awareness of diabetic foot problems and improved treatment, amputation rates will continue to decrease.

The diabetic foot is especially vulnerable to amputation because of the frequent complications of peripheral neuropathy (PN), infection, and peripheral arterial disease (PAD). A combination of this triad leads to the final cataclysmic events: gangrene and amputation.

The relationship among diabetic neuropathy, the insensitive foot, and foot ulceration was recognized by Pryce, a British surgeon, over a century ago. He stated that "It was abundantly evident that the actual cause of the perforating ulcer was peripheral nerve degeneration and that diabetes itself played an active part in the causation of the perforating ulcer".[1]

More than 56,000 major amputations due to diabetes were reported in 1987 in the United States.[2] Fifty percent of all nontraumatic amputations are performed on the diabetic. Fifteen percent of all diabetics will develop a foot ulcer during their lifetime.[3] Most of these are the result of PN and the insensate foot, which leads to painless trauma and ulceration.

Diabetic foot lesions are not very glamorous and do not generate as many publications as do other complications of diabetes. However, in the United States the annual incidence of lower extremity leg and foot ulcers is 200,000. Add to these 56,000 major amputations and we have over a quarter of a million lower extremity diabetic complications. This is greater than all other complications of diabetes combined: coronary artery disease, 101,000; stroke, 27,000; blindness, 6,900; and kidney failure, 5,900.[4]

Diabetic foot problems are a major cause of hospitalization and prolonged hospital stays. Twenty percent of all diabetic persons who enter the hospital do so because of foot problems.[5] In the series of Smith et al, foot problems were responsible for 23% of the in-hospital days over a 2-year period.[6] At the India Institute of Diabetes in Bombay, more than 10% of all admissions for diabetes are primarily for foot management. More than 70% required surgical intervention and in more than 40% of those interventions there was a toe or limb amputation.[7] In the United Kingdom more than 50% of bed occupancy of diabetics is due to foot problems.[8] It is obvious from these figures that throughout the world diabetic foot problems are a major cause of hospitalization, morbidity, and mortality.

PATHOGENESIS OF DIABETIC FOOT LESIONS

The signs and symptoms of either ischemia or neuropathy may predominate. However, neither is present to the total exclusion of the other. The clinical picture is therefore the result of complications stemming from a combination of both. PN is the leading cause of most diabetic foot lesions. A majority of patients who enter the hospital because of diabetic foot lesions do so because of ulceration secondary to painless trauma. The various pathways leading to ulceration—infection, gangrene, and amputations—are shown in Fig. 19–1.

The exact incidence of PN is difficult to assess. Most studies estimate the incidence of clinical neuropathy to be 10% to 20%. However, this percentage may increase to as much as 50% after 25 years of diabetes.

While most diabetic foot ulcers are due to PN and the insensate foot, it must be remembered that painful symptoms are common in patients with PN. The series of Veves et al has shown that painful symptoms are frequent in patients with PN, irrespective of the presence or absence of foot ulceration.[9] Diabetic patients may have an insensitive foot and still experience painful symptoms. Painful symptoms were present in 33% of the foot ulcer group.[9] Therefore, painful and painless PNs are not necessarily two separate clinical conditions and may coexist. It should also be kept in mind that when a patient with a diabetic foot ulcer which has been painless suddenly develops pain in the ulcer, it may be indicative of worsening infection.

The most important effect of PN on the diabetic foot is the loss of sensation, making the foot vulnerable even to trivial trauma. A break in the skin, even though it is inconspicuous and minuscule, can become a portal of entry for bacteria. Unsuccessfully treated infection leads to gangrene and amputation.

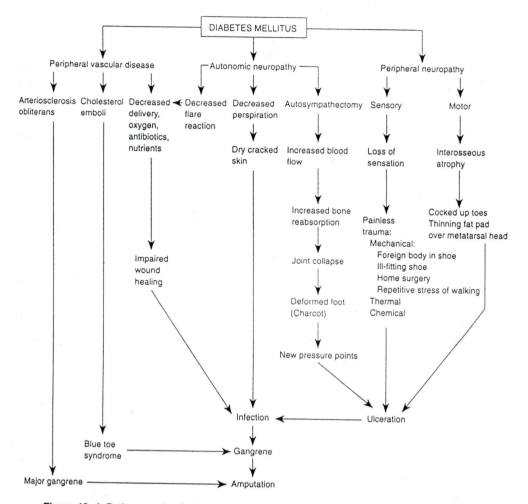

Figure 19–1. Pathogenesis of diabetic foot lesions. (*Adapted from Levin ME. Pathogenesis and management of diabetic foot lesions. In: Levin ME, O'Neal LW, Bowker JH, eds. The Diabetic Foot. 5th ed. St Louis, Mo: Mosby–Year Book Inc; 1993;17–60.*)

SPECIAL DIABETIC FOOT PROBLEMS

The Heel

The heel of the diabetic patient is particularly vulnerable to trauma. When the diabetic patient is required to have bed rest for any length of time, such as when hospitalized, particular attention must be paid to the heel. Because of loss of sensation, the patient tends to keep the heels in the same position. This results in pressure necrosis, causing the skin to break down. Infection and gangrene can follow. These patients should have their heels inspected at least once a day, preferably twice. If erythema is present, aggressive protective intervention must be instituted.

Prevention is critical. This is best achieved by turning the patient, using heel protectors, and using an air suspension mattress. The available heel protectors may not stay in place; therefore, frequent checks are required.

Foot Deformities

Foot deformities frequently lead to ulceration. Diabetics are particularly prone to develop cocked-up toes, which can result in pressure at the top of the tip of the toes. I refer to this as the "tip-top-toe syndrome." This deformity is frequently associated with a thinning or shifting of the fat pad under the first metatarsal head. These areas, the tops and tips of the toes, and the area under the first metatarsal head are therefore very vulnerable to ulceration and infection. The ideal treatment is prophylactic surgery to straighten these toes while the circulation is still good. When prophylactic surgery cannot be carried out, these patients should wear a shoe with a larger toe box or an in-depth shoe with a cushioned insole to protect the toes and the metatarsal head area. Bunions are common and frequently lead to ulceration and infection. Prophylactic surgery is the ideal treatment.

The Charcot foot is the classic diabetic foot deformity. The Charcot foot develops in four stages. In the first, or acute, stage the patient usually presents with a history of mild trauma and a hot red swollen foot with bounding pulses. This must be differentiated from cellulitis. Once infection has been ruled out and a diagnosis of Charcot foot has been established, the treatment is non–weight bearing. This is best accomplished with a contact cast. If the patient is allowed to ambulate, the second stage of the Charcot foot develops, with the breakdown of the bones of the foot, resulting in fractures. The x-ray at the time of the patient's initial visit may be perfectly normal. Calcification of the interosseous arteries is rarely found. The second stage develops in a 2- to 3-week interval. Repeat x-ray may show fractures, usually at the tarsometatarsal joint but not infrequently at the distal ends of the metatarsals. The third stage of the Charcot foot is characterized by foot deformity. The foot takes on a clubfoot appearance and a rocker-bottom configuration. Treatment at this stage requires the use of special molded shoes. If the patient continues to walk on unprotected feet, the fourth stage ensues, with development of a plantar ulceration in the area of the arch. The ulceration can become injected, leading to gangrene and amputation.[10]

Exercise for Diabetics with Foot Problems

Exercise is an important modality in the management of diabetes. However, in patients with PAD and PN, weight-bearing exercises, such as jogging, prolonged walking, the use of a treadmill, and step exercises, may need to be curtailed or avoided. The presence of an active foot ulcer is an absolute contraindication for weight-bearing exercise. Patients who have a previously healed ulcer must take special precautions when exercising. Scar tissue is not good tissue and is very vulnerable to the sheer forces of walking. Patients with PAD, PN, and an insensate foot can do a variety of non–weight-bearing exercises, such as swimming, bicycling, rowing, and chair and upper body exercises.

Diabetic persons, particularly those with PAD, PN, and previously healed ulcerations, should have specific detailed instructions in foot care and techniques for decreasing foot pressure before undertaking an exercise program.

Physical therapists and personnel in exercise centers should discuss with the referring physicians the type of exercise program suitable for the diabetic.

The Immunosuppressed Diabetic

The healing of foot ulcers in immunosuppressed renal transplant diabetics is markedly impaired. These patients also have a higher amputation rate.[11] In most kidney transplant series limb amputation is required for at least 15% of kidney recipients in the short term and one-third of the 10-year survivors.[12]

DIABETIC FOOT ULCERS

Ulcers occur in the diabetic foot because of repetitive stress on insensitive feet. When repetitive stress continues, the foot develops hot spots, callus build-up, pressure necrosis, and, ultimately, ulceration. Ulcerations occur most often at the site of the maximum pressure and excessive callus build-up, usually over the metatarsal heads, especially the first, and on the plantar surface of the hallux. Patients who develop ulcers have increased foot pressures.[13] Increased pressure can be the result of foot deformities. Decreased flexibility of the foot, probably due to glycosylation of tendons and ligaments, can also cause increased foot pressures. There are several techniques for decreasing plantar foot pressures in the diabetic. Removing a callus can reduce pressure at that site by at least 30%. Wearing cushioned shoes[14] and pressure-reducing hosiery[15] can also be beneficial. Patients should not go barefoot, not only because of possible trauma, but because pressures are significantly higher when walking barefoot than when wearing cushioned shoes. On a rare occasion it may be necessary to alleviate internal pressure, for example, by removing the sesmoid bones or metatarsal heads. When a patient presents with ulceration on the dorsum of the foot, it is due to trauma. When the presentation is on the side of the foot, it is most likely due to an ill-fitting shoe.

Persistent and untreated ulceration in the diabetic foot leads to lower limb amputation in 84% of all cases.[16]

Management of Diabetic Foot Ulcers

Table 19–1 lists the steps in the management of diabetic foot ulcers.[17] X-rays are necessary to rule out osteomyelitis, gas formation, the presence of foreign objects, and asymptomatic fractures. It is my feeling that any foot with ulceration or infection should be x-rayed.

Treatment of a diabetic foot ulcer requires establishment of the depth and degree of ulceration. What appears to be a superficial ulceration may be only the tip of the iceberg. There may be penetration deep into the tissues. Vigorous debridement of the ulcer must be done to establish the degree of penetration and to remove all necrotic tissue. Debridement should be carried out to healthy tissue. The ulcer following debridement will, in all probability, be larger than it was at presentation. Eschars should be completely removed. Whirlpool is not the method of choice for debridement. When the foot is insensitive, minor debridement can be carried out at the bedside. However, in many cases the patient must be taken to the operating room for adequate debridement under anesthesia. Taylor and Porter have demonstrated that aggressive foot debridement, and, when indicated, revascularization resulted in long-term salvage of 73% of threatened limbs even in high-risk patients.[18]

Biopsy should be considered when the ulcer appears at an atypical location (eg, not over the metatarsal heads or the plantar surface of the hallux), when it cannot be explained by trauma, and when it is unresponsive to aggressive therapy. On numerous occasions biopsies of atypical ulcers have revealed malignancies, both primary and metastatic.

Infection is a common and major complication of diabetic foot wounds. Infection leads to microthrombi formation, causing further ischemia, necrosis, and progressive

TABLE 19–1. MANAGEMENT OF DIABETIC FOOT ULCERS

I. Evaluation
   A. Clinical appearance
   B. Depth of penetration
   C. X-ray
      1. Foreign body
      2. Osteomyelitis
      3. Subcutaneous gas
   D. Location
   E. Biopsy
   F. Blood supply (noninvasive vascular studies)
II. Debridement, radical
III. Bacterial cultures (aerobic and anaerobic)
IV. Metabolic control
V. Antibiotics
   A. Oral
   B. Parenteral
VI. Do not soak feet
VII. Decrease edema
VIII. No weight bearing
   A. Bed rest
   B. Crutches
   C. Wheelchair
   D. Contact casting
IX. Improve circulation (vascular surgery)

Adapted from Levin ME. Pathogenesis and management of diabetic foot lesions. In: Levin ME, O'Neal LW, Bowker JH, eds. *The Diabetic Foot.* 5th ed. St Louis, Mo: Mosby–Year Book Inc; 1993;17–60.

gangrene. Massive infection is the most common factor leading to amputation. Lichter et al reviewed the laboratory results of a large series of patients with serious pedal infections.[19] In this series the sedimentation rates were significantly elevated (mean, 58.6 mm/h). Surprisingly, the mean white blood cell count was only 9,700. Therfore, one should not depend on these cell counts alone as a measure of the seriousness of the foot infection. As in other series, these investigators found the lesions to be polymicrobial, 72% having gram-positive cocci and 49%, gram negative. Nine percent had gram-negative anaerobes.[19] There is a high correlation among foot ulcers, infection, and other diabetic complications. Lichter et al found that 67% of these patients had retinopathy; 70%, nephropathy; 80%, PN; 91%, decreased pulses; 69%, hypertension; and 40%, atherosclerotic heart disease.[19]

The selection of an oral antibiotic or parenteral antibiotic for the treatment of a diabetic foot infection is based on medical judgment. It should be kept in mind that many diabetic foot infections contain gram-negative organisms. Therefore, the oral antibiotic chosen should be effective for gram-positive and gram-negative organisms. The criterion for hospitalization and treatment with parenteral antibiotics includes patients who are septic, febrile, and have leukocytosis and deep infection. The patient with what appears to be a minor infection on the plantar surface of the foot and evidence of infection on the dorsum of the foot, suggested by erythema and frequently edema, should be hospitalized. Even though the patient is not septic, there is a high probability that severe infection exists deep in the foot. Patients with infection and severe PAD should be hospitalized and evaluated for arterial bypass surgery. The worst scenario leading to amputation is ischemia and infection. Patients with PAD should be given parenteral antibiotics to achieve a higher concentration of antibiotics in the peripheral tissues than can be achieved by oral therapy alone. Furthermore, the antibiotic of choice frequently can only be given parenterally.

If an oral antibiotic is selected, it is my opinion that the diabetic patient should not merely be told to take the medication and return in 1 week. Infection in the diabetic can cause the patient's condition to deteriorate rapidly within 24 hours. It is therefore my recommendation that diabetics on oral therapy should be seen within a few days following institution of therapy. They must be carefully instructed to notify the physician at once should there be an increase in redness, drainage, pain, odor, or evidence of lymphangitis. While many of these patients have insensate feet, the development of pain is indicative of deep infection and requires immediate attention. The development of a bad odor also indicates worsening infection and frequently the presence of anaerobes.

It is very important that patients with infection monitor their blood sugar level closely. A rising blood sugar level strongly suggests worsening infection, even though other signs and symptoms are absent.

When infection is not responding to aggressive debridement and antibiotic therapy, the wound should be debrided again and recultured, as the flora may have changed. Chronic recurrent or resistant infection suggests that presence of osteomyelitis. Impending or developing gangrene also suggests possible progression of infection. Indications of worsening infection are noted in Table 19–2.

Osteomyelitis is a frequent complication of diabetic foot ulcers and infection. Osteomyelitis may be difficult to detect on a clinical basis. Newman and coworkers showed that in biopsy-proven osteomyelitis only one-third of the patients had clinically suspected osteomyelitis.[20] If bone is visible or the ulcer can be probed to bone, the probability of the presence of osteomyelitis is extremely strong. Scanning techniques for osteomyelitis are not always successful. The triple-phase scan with technetium lacks specificity.[21] Magnetic resonance imaging (MRI) is proving to be a helpful technique. However, Newman and coworkers[22] found the use of labeled-leukocyte indium 111 scanning techniques to be superior to MRI.[22] Bamberger, Daus, and Gerding established prognostic factors for preventing amputation in the face of osteomyelitis.[23] They found that in patients without necrosis, gangrene, or the presence of swelling, the use of antimicrobial therapy active against the isolated pathogens given intravenously for at least 4 weeks or combined intravenously and orally for 10 weeks predicted a good outcome without the need for ablative surgical procedures.[23]

TABLE 19–2. WORSENING INFECTION: INDICATIONS

Signs and symptoms
  Increased
    Drainage
    Erythema
    Pain
    Temperature
  Malodorous
  Lymphangitis
  Lymphadenopathy
  Gangrene
Laboratory measurements
  Increased
    Blood sugar
    White blood cell count
    Sedimentation rate

Lipsky et al have recently reviewed soft tissue and bone infection in the diabetic foot.[24]

Metabolic control is essential. It has been well demonstrated in a number of studies that leukocyte function is impaired in the presence of uncontrolled diabetes. Blood sugar levels should be kept below 200 mg/dL and as close to euglycemia as is reasonable.

Soaking the feet has no benefit, although it has been a traditional approach. Because of the insensitive foot, soaking may take place in water that is too hot, resulting in severe burns. Chemical soaks can result in chemical burns. Excessive soaking can lead to maceration and infection.[25]

Edema is frequently present. Elevation of the feet, no more than the thickness of one pillow, can be beneficial. Higher elevation may impede circulation.

Avoidance of weight bearing is essential. These patients have insensitive feet and because the ulcer is not painful, they continue to walk. The result is an increase in pressure necrosis, forcing bacteria deeper into the tissues and causing failure to heal. The use of crutches and wheelchairs is seldom successful in achieving total and consistent avoidance of weight bearing. Many patients with PN have ataxia, making the use of crutches potentially dangerous. The best method for avoidance of weight bearing in appropriately selected patients is the use of the contact cast. The contact cast allows the patient to be ambulatory but essentially avoids weight bearing by redistributing the weight and decreasing the pressure on the ulcerated area.[26,27]

When an ulcer does not heal despite good metabolic control, adequate debridement, parenteral antibiotic therapy, and avoidance of weight bearing, the impaired healing may be caused by vascular insufficiency. Mills et al found that all appropriately treated neuropathic ulcers and forefoot infections healed in patients with palpable pedal pulses. If foot pulses were absent and arteriography confirmed large-vessel occlusive disease, foot lesions and infections healed when concomitant revascularization was done.[28]

The worst scenario for impaired wound healing or the clearing of infection may be vascular insufficiency. Ankle or brachial indexes of less than 0.45 or transcutaneous oxygen pressure below 30 mm Hg and certainly those under 20 mm Hg are highly predictive that the infection will not resolve and that the ulcer will not heal. For example, Pecoraro and colleagues found a 39-fold increased risk of early wound failure if the average periwound transcutaneous oxygen pressure was under 22 mm Hg.[26] Vascular surgery should always be considered in these cases. The importance of peripheral arterial reconstruction was demonstrated by LoGerfo and associates. In 2,883 extreme distal arterial reconstructions, they found a statistically significant decrease in every category of amputation, a decrease that correlated precisely with increasing the rate of dorsal pedis artery bypass.[29]

Hyperbaric oxygen delivered by the hyperbaric chamber has been reported to be helpful in healing diabetic foot ulcers.[30] Hyperbaric oxygen delivered by hyperbaric boot is totally ineffective. It must be kept in mind that the hyperbaric oxygen is used in conjunction with all of the aggressive treatments outlined in Table 19–1. Experimental studies have suggested that a combination of topical growth factors and hyperbaric oxygen may be beneficial in improving wound healing.[31]

Topical Treatment of Foot Ulcers

The use of topical therapy goes back to ancient times, when an unbelievable number of substances were used to treat wounds, ranging from wine to human excreta (*Table-*

Talk, XCII "Of God's Works," Martin Luther, 1483–1546). Today the list of topical agents remains long and continues to grow. Currently, resins and enzyme therapy to aid in debridement are advocated by some. Although these are of some benefit, they represent adjunct therapy and should not be substituted for aggressive surgical debridement. It has been traditional to use povidone-iodine (Betadine), acetic acid, hydrogen peroxide, and sodium hypochlorite (Dakin's solution). Although these substances destroy surface bacteria, they are cytotoxic to granulation tissue and may delay wound healing.[32] It is therefore my belief that these substances should be either avoided or used only for a very brief period.

The benefits of topically applied antibacterial agents, silver sulfadiazine 1%, polymyxin B with bacitracin and neomycin, and gentamicin surlfate may be helpful.[32] Topical antibiotics alone may not be satisfactory, and the use of oral or parenteral antibiotics in conjunction with topical therapy is frequently necessary. Cleansing agents and types of dressings can make a difference in the rate of wound healing. Moist dressings seem to aid wound healing.[32]

Despite aggressive therapy and adequate circulation, some diabetic foot ulcers heal slowly or not at all. Current investigative studies with topically applied platelet-derived growth factors to these foot ulcers have shown these factors to be important adjunct therapy in wound healing.[33,34] Bentkover and Champion have shown the cost-effectiveness of wound care centers and the use of platelet releasate.[35] Platelet-derived wound-healing formula is an autologous solution extracted from the α-granules of the patient's platelets. This extract is applied to the ulcer daily by the patient in an outpatient setting. The platelet-derived wound-healing formula contains several growth factors. They are platelet-derived growth factor, angiogenesis factor,

TABLE 19–3. IMPEDIMENTS TO WOUND HEALING

1. Vascular
   a. Atherosclerosis
   b. Increased viscosity
2. Neurological
   a. Insensate foot
   b. Decreased flare reaction
3. Infection
   a. Inadequate debridement
   b. Poor blood supply
   c. Microthrombi
   d. Hyperglycemia
   e. Decreased polymorphonuclear neutrophil function
   f. Polymicrobial infection
   g. Changing bacteria
   h. Osteomyelitis
4. Immunosuppression
5. Mechanical
   a. Edema
   b. Weight bearing
6. Poor nutrition
   a. Low serum albumin level
7. Decreased growth factors
8. Poor patient compliance
9. Delayed treatment and referral

Adapted from Levin ME. Pathogenesis and management of diabetic foot lesions. In: Levin ME, O'Neal LW, Bowker JH, eds. *The Diabetic Foot.* 5th ed. St Louis, Mo: Mosby–Year Book, Inc; 1993;17–60.

epidermal factor, transforming growth factor β, and platelet factor 4. Recent work has been shown that interactions between growth factors and the extracellular matrix are of central importance in the process that causes wounds to close. Transforming growth factor β appears to be a central player in many of the steps of wound healing: inducing angiogenesis, acting as a chemoattractant for macrophages and fibroblasts, regulating self-proliferation, and stimulating extracellular matrix.[36] The impediments to wound healing are listed in Table 19–3.

Post-treatment Management of Healed Diabetic Foot Ulcers

Even when the diabetic foot ulcer has healed, the job is not complete. The underlying causes responsible for the ulcer, such as foot deformity, calluses, and increased pressure, are still present. In addition, scar tissue from previously healed ulcers is not strong tissue and is thus vulnerable to the shearing forces of walking. Special measures are therefore necessary to protect the vulnerable sites of previous ulceration. These include education of the patient in walking, for example, taking shorter steps and decreasing overall walking. Patients whose jobs require standing or walking, such as waiters, may need to change jobs. Therapeutic shoes play a very important role in preventing recurrence of these ulcers.

Special Shoes

The use of special therapeutic shoes is critical in preventing ulceration or recurrence. Patients who have cocked-up toes require a shoe with a bigger toe box. The patient with a markedly deformed foot, such as the Charcot foot, needs a specially molded shoe. An in-depth shoe with a plasticlike material, such as a plastazote insole, is frequently required to redistribute the weight away from the previously ulcerated site and thus prevent recurrence of ulcer. The importance of special shoes was clearly demonstrated in a study at King's College in London, which showed an 83% recur-

TABLE 19–4. TEAM MEMBERS INVOLVED IN THE CARE OF THE DIABETIC FOOT

1. Primary physician
2. Endocrinologist
3. Diabetologist
4. Podiatrist
5. Nurse educator
6. Physician's assistant
7. Enterostomal nurse
8. Infectious disease specialist
9. Neurologist
10. Vascular surgeon
11. Orthopedist
12. Physiatrist
13. Pedorthist
14. Orthotist
15. Physical therapist
16. Prosthetist
17. Occupational therapist
18. Social worker
19. Home care nurse

TABLE 19–5. PATIENT INSTRUCTIONS FOR CARE OF THE DIABETIC FOOT

1. Do not smoke.
2. Inspect the feet daily for blisters, cuts, and scratches. The use of a mirror can aid in seeing the bottom of the feet. Always check between the toes.
3. Wash feet daily; dry carefully, especially between the toes.
4. Avoid extremes of temperatures. Test water with hand, elbow, or thermometer before bathing.
5. If feet feel cold at night, wear socks. Do not apply hot water bottles or heating pads. Do not use an electric blanket. Do not soak feet in hot water.
6. Do not walk on hot surfaces such as sandy beaches or cement around swimming pools.
7. Do not walk barefoot.
8. Do not use chemical agents for removal of corns and calluses, corn plasters, or strong antiseptic solutions.
9. Do not use adhesive tape on the feet.
10. Inspect the insides of shoes daily for foreign objects, nail points, torn linings, and rough areas.
11. If your vision is impaired, have a family member inspect feet daily, trim nails, and buff calluses.
12. Do not soak feet.
13. For dry feet, use a very thin coat of lubricating oil or cream. Apply after bathing and drying the feet. Do not put oil or cream between the toes. Consult your physician for detailed instructions.
14. Wear properly fitting stockings. Do not wear mended stockings or stockings with seams. Change stockings daily.
15. Do not wear garters.
16. Shoes should be comfortable at the time of purchase. Do not depend on them to stretch out. Shoes should be made of leather. Purchase shoes late in the afternoon when feet are largest. Running or special walking shoes may be worn after checking with your physician. Purchase shoes from a shoe salesperson who understands diabetic foot problems.
17. Do not wear shoes without stockings.
18. Do not wear sandals with thongs between the toes.
19. In the winter take special precautions. Wear wool socks and protective footgear such as fleece-lined boots.
20. Cut nails straight across.
21. Do not cut corns and calluses: follow instructions from your physician or podiatrist.
22. See your physician regularly and be sure that your feet are examined at each visit.
23. Notify your physician or podiatrist at once should you develop a blister or sore on your foot.
24. Be sure to inform your podiatrist that you are diabetic.

Adapted from Levin ME. Pathogenesis and management of diabetic foot lesions. In: Levin ME, O'Neal LW, Bowker JH, eds. *The Diabetic Foot.* 5th ed. St Louis, Mo: Mosby–Year Book Inc; 1993;17–60.

rence of ulcers when patients returned to wearing regular shoes; with the use of special shoes, there was only a 17% recurrence of ulceration.[37]

TEAMWORK

The management of the diabetic foot requires the interaction of many medical disciplines (Table 19–4). A team approach is needed that will save the foot, not amputate it.

PATIENT EDUCATION

Of all the approaches to prevent ulceration and save the diabetic foot, the most important is patient education. Despite our current knowledge, physicians cannot totally prevent PAD and PN. However, the patient can be educated in proper foot care, and can learn how to prevent injury and detect lesions as early as possible.

At the time of the office visit and while the shoes and socks are off, the nurse or physician should review the do's and don'ts of foot care with the patient. This objective cannot be adequately accomplished simply by handing the patient a list of instructions. The instructions should be explained and questions should be encouraged and answered, so that the patient can attain a better understanding of the importance of foot care (Table 19–5). These instructions should be carried out at least once a year or even more often. The effectiveness of an educational program in reducing amputation has been noted by Malone and coworkers[38] and more recently by Litzelman.[39]

CONCLUSION

Diabetic foot ulcers are common. If treatment is delayed or improper treatment is given, these lesions can lead to infection, gangrene, and amputation. Physicians and clinics that avoid delay in the treatment of the diabetic foot ulcer, exercise aggressive therapy for these ulcers, provide revascularization when indicated, use therapeutic shoes, practice the team approach, and repeatedly educate patients in foot care have reduced their amputation rates by 50%.[37,40] This should be the goal of everyone who cares for patients with diabetes.

REFERENCES

1. Pryce TD. A case of perforating ulcers of both feet associated with diabetes and ataxic symptoms. *Lancet*. 1887;2:11–12.
2. Lower extremity amputations. In: *Diabetes Surveillance, 1980–1987*. Atlanta, Ga: Policy program research, Centers for Disease Control/Division of Diabetes Translation, US Department of Health and Human Services; 1990;23–25.
3. Palumbo PJ, Melton LJ III. Peripheral vascular disease and diabetes. In: *Diabetes in America: Diabetes Data Compiled in 1984*. (NIH publication 85-1468) Washington, DC: US Government Printing Office; 1985.
4. Bild D, Teutsch SM. The control of hypertension in persons with diabetes; a public health approach. *Public Health Rep*. 1987;102:522.
5. Block P. The diabetic foot ulcer: a complex problem with a simple treatment approach. *Mil Med*. 1981;146:644–646.
6. Smith DM, Weinberger M, Katz BP. A controlled trail to increase office visits and reduce hospitalizations of diabetic patients. *J Gen Intern Med*. 1987;2:232–238.
7. Sathe SR. Managing the diabetic foot in developing countries. *IDF Bull*. 1993;38(2):16–18.
8. Waugh NR. Amputations in diabetic patients: a review of rates, relative risks, and resource use. *Comm Med*. 1988;10:279–288.
9. Veves A, Manes C, Murray HJ, et al. Painful neuropathy and foot ulceration in diabetic patients. *Diabetes Care*. 1993;16:1187–1189.
10. Sanders LJ, Frykberg RG. Charcot foot. In: Levin ME, O'Neal LW, Bowker JH, eds. *The Diabetic Foot*. 5th ed. St Louis, Mo: Mosby–Year Book Inc; 1993;149–180.

11. Fletcher F, Ain M, Jacobs R. Healing of foot ulcers in immunosuppressed renal transplant patients. *Clin Orthop Relat Res.* 1993;296:37–42.

12. Friedman EA. Diabetic renal disease. In: Rifkin H, Porte D, eds. *Ellenberg and Rifkin's Diabetes Mellitus: Theory and Practice.* 4th ed. New York, NY: Elsevier; 1990;684–709.

13. Veves A, Murray HJ, Young MJ, et al. The risk of foot ulceration in diabetic patients with high foot pressure: a prospective study. *Diabetologia.* 1992;35:660–663.

14. Cavanagh PR, Ulbrecht JS. Biomechanics of the foot in diabetes mellitus. In: Levin ME, O'Neal LW, Bowker JH, eds. *The Diabetic Foot.* 5th ed. St Louis Mo: Mosby–Year Book Inc; 1993;199–232.

15. Murray HJ, Veves A, Young MJ, et al. Role of experimental socks in the care of the high-risk diabetic foot: a multicenter patient evaluation study. *Diabetes Care.* 1993;16:1190–1192.

16. Pecoraro RE, Reiber GE, Burgess EM. Pathways to diabetic limb amputation: basis for prevention. *Diabetes Care.* 1990;13:513.

17. Levin ME. Pathogenesis and management of diabetic foot lesions. In: Levin ME, O'Neal LW, Bowker JH, eds. *The Diabetic Foot.* 5th ed. St Louis, Mo: Mosby–Year Inc; 1993;17–60.

18. Taylor LM Jr, Porter JM. The clinical course of diabetics who require emergent foot surgery because of infection or ischemia. *J Vasc Surg.* 1987;6:454.

19. Lichter SB, Allweiss P, Harley J, et al. Clinical characteristics of diabetic patients with serious pedal infections. *Metabolism.* 1988;37:22–24.

20. Newman LG, Waller J, Palestro CJ, et al. Unsuspected osteomyelitis in diabetic foot ulcers. *JAMA.* 1991;266:1246–1251.

21. Littenberg B, Mushlin AI. The Diagnostic Technology Assessment Consortium. Technetium bone scanning in the diagnosis of osteomyelitis: a meta-analysis of test performance. *J Gen Intern Med.* 1992;7:158–163.

22. Newman LG, Waller J, Palestro CJ, et al. Leukocyte scanning with 111 In is superior to magnetic resonance imaging in diagnosis of clinically unsuspected osteomyelitis in diabetic foot ulcers. *Diabetes Care.* 1992;15:1527–1530.

23. Bamberger DM, Daus GP, Gerding DN. Osteomyelitis in the feet of diabetic patients: long-term results, prognostic factors, and the role of antimicrobial and surgical therapy. *Am J Med.* 1987;833:653–660.

24. Lipsky BA, Pecoraro RE, Wheat LJ. The diabetic foot: soft tissue and bone infection. *Infect Dis Clin North Am.* 1990;4:409–432.

25. Levin ME, Spratt IL. "To soak or not to soak." *Clin Diabetes.* 1986;4:44–45.

26. Pecoraro RE, Ahroni JH, Boyko EJ, et al. Chronology and determinants of tissue repair in diabetic lower extremity ulcers. *Diabetes.* 1991;40:1305–1313.

27. Sinacore DR, Mueller MJ. Total-contact casting in the treatment of neuropathic ulcers. In: Levin ME, O'Neal LW, Bowker JH, eds. *The Diabetic Foot.* 5th ed. St Louis, Mo: Mosby–Year Book Inc; 1993;283–304.

28. Mills JL, Beckett WC, Taylor SM. The diabetic foot: consequences of delayed treatment and referral. *South Med J.* 1991;84:970–974.

29. LoGerfo FW, Gibbons GW, Pomposelli FB Jr, et al. Trends in the care of the diabetic foot: expanded role of arterial reconstruction. *Arch Surg.* 1992;127:617–621.

30. Cianci P, Hunt TK. Adjunctive hyperbaric oxygen therapy in treatment of diabetic foot wounds. In: Levin ME, O'Neal LW, Bowker JH, eds. *The Diabetic Foot.* 5th ed. St Louis, Mo: Mosby–Year Book Inc; 1993;305–319.

31. Zhao L, Davidson JD, Wee SC, et al. Effect of hyperbaric oxygen and growth factors in rabbit ear ischemic ulcers. *Arch Surg.* In press.

32. Alvarez OM, Gilson G, Auletta MJ. Local aspects of diabetic foot ulcer care: assessment, dressings, and topical agents. In: Levin ME, O'Neal LW, Bowker JH, eds. *The Diabetic Foot.* 5th ed. St Louis, Mo: Mosby–Year Book Inc; 1993;259–281.

33. Knighton DR, Fiegel VD. Growth factors and repair of diabetic wounds. In: Levin ME, O'Neal LW, Bowker JH, eds. *The Diabetic Foot.* 5th ed. St Louis, Mo: Mosby–Year Book Inc; 1993;247–257.

34. Steed DL, Goslen JB, Holloway GA, et al. Randomized prospective double-blind trial in healing chronic diabetic foot ulcers: CT-102 activated platelet supernatant, topical versus placebo. *Diabetes Care.* 1992;15:1598–1604.

35. Bentkover JD, Champion AH. Economic evaluation of alternative methods of treatment for diabetic foot ulcer patients: cost effectiveness of platelet releasate and wound care clinics. *Wounds.* 1993;5(4):207–215.
36. Skerrett PJ. "Matrix algebra" heals life's wounds. *Science.* 1991;252:1064–1066.
37. Edmonds ME, Blundell MP, Morris ME, et al. Improved survival of the diabetic foot: the role of a specialized foot clinic. *Q J Med.* 1986;60:763–771.
38. Malone JM, Synder M, Anderson G, et al. Prevention of amputation by diabetic education. *Am J Surg.* 1989;158:520–524.
39. Litzelman DK, Slemenda CW, Langefeld CD, et al. Reduction of lower extremity clinical abnormalities in patients with non–insulin-dependent diabetes mellitus. *Ann Intern Med.* 1993;119:36–41.
40. Assal JP, Muhlhauser I, Pernant A, et al. Patient education as the basis for diabetes care in clinical practices. *Diabetologia.* 1985;28:602–613.

20

The Microbiology of Foot Infections in Diabetic Patients

Dale N. Gerding, MD

The 5% of patients with diabetes mellitus account for half of the 60,000 annual nontraumatic lower extremity amputations in the United States.[1] Sixty-eight percent of these patients have an active infection of the affected lower extremity at the time of amputation.[1] Lack of diabetes education and the presence of vibratory neuropathy in the extremities are the two greatest risk factors for ultimate amputation, emphasizing the potential for prevention by simple educational interventions.[1,2] When infection does occur, most can be successfully managed without limb loss even if the infection is deep in the soft tissues or involves the bones of the foot (osteomyelitis). Antimicrobial therapy alone or accompanied by local surgical incision and drainage are usually successful if the antimicrobial agent chosen is appropriate for the likely bacterial pathogens. The purpose of this discussion is to review the microbiology of foot infections in patients with diabetes in order to better direct antimicrobial selection.

SPECIMEN COLLECTION

The preferred means by which to obtain specimens for culture from foot ulcerations remains somewhat controversial. The choices range from simple cotton-tipped applicator swab of the ulcer to curettage of the ulcer base to needle aspiration into deep tissues via entry through intact antiseptically prepared skin adjacent to the ulcer.[3] Swab and curettage specimens yield somewhat higher numbers of species than needle aspirations, presumably because they contain organisms that colonize the surface as well as pathogens. Needle aspirations should lack contaminating bacteria and yield fewer species, but may miss pathogens if the needle is not inserted into the infected area of the deep tissues. Significantly more monomicrobial infections are diagnosed using needle aspiration or other surgical approaches using the aseptic technique.[4] Compared to cultures obtained by careful dissection of the amputated limb, there was no statistically significant difference in concordance of any of the specimens obtained by the three methods, thus leaving the choice to the clinician.[3] Swab specimens are not suitable for anaerobic culture unless a special anaerobic transport container is used. Needle aspirate and curettage specimens should also be placed in an anaerobic transport container to preserve anaerobic bacteria. In our studies we prefer to do both a swab culture and a deep needle aspiration if the ulcer appears to involve subcutaneous tissues, submitting the specimens in anaerobic transport containers for both aerobic and anaerobic culture in the laboratory.

MICROBIOLOGY OF UNCOMPLICATED INFECTIONS

The majority of foot infections are of the non–limb-threatening type and can be managed in the outpatient setting using oral antimicrobial therapy. The infections are classified as acute skin infection with ulceration, acute infection of a chronic ulcer, paronychia, superficial abscess, or cellulitis alone.[5] The microbiology of these infections is different from the more invasive limb-threatening infections. In previously untreated patients the uncomplicated infections are predominantly caused by aerobic gram-positive cocci, which are present in 94% of such lesions and are the sole pathogen in 43%. The most frequently isolated gram-positive organism is *Staphylococcus aureus*, followed by coagulase-negative staphylococci, *Streptococcus* sp, and enterococci. Among other aerobic bacteria, gram-negative bacilli are present in 23% of specimens, predominantly Enterobacteriaceae (*Klebsiella* sp, *Escherichia coli*, and *Proteus* sp) and occasionally *Pseudomonas*. Anaerobic bacteria are found in only 13% of specimens from these uncomplicated lesions, 87% are due solely to aerobic bacteria, and 46% are caused by a single organism.[5]

MICROBIOLOGY OF COMPLICATED INFECTIONS

Complicated foot infections are those that are deemed to be limb or life threatening. They usually include severe cellulitis, skin gangrene or necrosis, or involvement of the deep soft tissues, including necrotizing fasciitis, deep abscesses, and/or osteomyelitis. It is critically important in the management of these lesions that they be probed thoroughly to establish the extent of infection and that local incision and drainage be done if areas of abscess or necrosis are suspected. In contrast to the uncomplicated infections, these infections are polymicrobial in the majority of cases and contain a mean of 4.1 to 5.8 bacterial species per culture.[3,6,7] The mean number of aerobic species ranges from 2.9 to 3.5, and the mean number of anaerobic species ranges from 1.2 to 2.6.[3,6,7] The specific species isolated are shown in Table 20–1, as determined from four published series and my unpublished data.[3,4,6,7]

The majority of isolates (64%) are aerobic, and 64% of all isolates are gram positive, whether aerobic or anaerobic. An easy rule of thumb for remembering the microbiology of these infections is to assume that most infections will be mixed, polymicrobial, and consist of about two-thirds gram-positive and one-third gram-negative bacterial species, two-thirds of which will be aerobic and one-third of which will be anaerobic. Staphylococci are the most frequently isolated species among the aerobic gram-positives (18% of all isolates), followed closely by streptococci and enterococci. The anaerobic gram-positives are predominantly peptostreptococci, some of which were formerly called peptococci. Thus, in Table 20–1, the majority of organisms classified as peptococci when the studies were performed would today be called peptostreptococci, and this genus would constitute about 17% of all isolates. Clostridial species

TABLE 20–1. BACTERIOLOGY OF FOOT INFECTIONS IN PATIENTS WITH DIABETES MELLITUS AS OBTAINED BY ASPIRATION, BIOPSY, OR CURETTAGE[a]

Organism	No. of Isolates
Aerobic and facultative isolates	393
Gram-positive aerobes	249
Streptococcus sp	62
Staphylococcus aureus	59
Coagulase-negative staphylococci	54
Enterococcus sp	45
Gram-positive bacilli	29
Gram-negative aerobes	144
Proteus sp	39
Escherichia coli	19
Enterobacter sp	18
Klebsiella sp	16
Pseudomonas aeruginosa	13
Other gram-negative bacilli	37
Gram-negative cocci	2
Anaerobic isolates	222
Gram-positive anaerobes	143
Peptococcus sp	54
Peptostreptococcus sp	48
Clostridia sp	22
Other gram-positive anaerobes	19
Gram-negative anaerobes	79
Bacteroides fragilis group	39
Bacteroides melaninogenicus group	17
Other *Bacteroides* sp	13
Other gram-negative anaerobes	10

[a] Data were compiled from 614 isolates from 160 patients in references 3, 4, 6, and 7 plus the chapter author's unpublished data.

are a distant second to peptostreptococci among anaerobic gram-positive organisms and constitute 3% to 4% of all isolates.

For unclear reasons, the most frequently isolated gram-negative aerobic genus is *Proteus* sp, followed by *E coli*, *Enterobacter* sp, and *Klebsiella* sp. *Pseudomonas aeruginosa* is an infrequent primary pathogen, constituting only about 2% of all isolates. Among gram-negative anaerobic bacteria, *Bacteroides* sp are by far the most commonly isolated organisms and constitute about 11% of all isolates.

MICROBIOLOGY OF OSTEOMYELITIS

The organisms isolated from osteomyelitis of the foot in patients with diabetes are similar to those isolated from complicated foot infections in general. The isolates from two studies of a total of 71 patients are shown in Table 20–2.[8,9] The organisms are classified in the same manner as in Table 20–1. Most infections were polymicrobic, with an average of 2.8 bacterial species per patient. Proportionately fewer anaerobic species (18%) were isolated in osteomyelitis than in complicated foot infections in general; this may reflect an inadequate anaerobic technique in handling specimens or may be a significant clinical finding. Gram-positive aerobic species constituted 58% of all isolates, with staphylococci, enterococci, and streptococci predominating as in complicated foot infection in general. The similarity of species shown in Tables 20–1

TABLE 20–2. MICROBIOLOGY OF OSTEOMYELITIS OF THE FOOT IN 71 DIABETIC PATIENTS[a]

Organism	No. of Isolates
Aerobic and facultative isolates	160
Gram-positive aerobes	114
Staphylococcus aureus	30
Enterococcus sp/group D streptococci	29
Coagulase-negative staphylococci	21
Group B streptococci	14
Diphtheroids/*Corynebacterium* sp	10
Streptococcus sp	9
Bacillus sp	1
Gram-negative aerobes	46
Proteus sp	9
Enterobacter sp	8
Klebsiella sp	8
Pseudomonas aeruginosa	6
Morganella morganii	5
Serratia marcescens	3
Escherichia coli	3
Other gram-negative bacilli	4
Anaerobic isolates	35
Gram-positive anaerobes	26
Peptococcus sp	15
Clostridia sp	5
Peptostreptococcus sp	4
Other gram-positive bacilli	2
Gram-negative anaerobes	9
Bacteroides sp	5
Bacteroides fragilis group	4
Fungi	3
Yeast species	3

[a] Data were compiled from references 8 and 9.

and 20–2 may reflect the similar mechanism of deep soft tissue infection and osteomyelitis in these patients, namely, contiguous spread from cutaneous tissue to subcutaneous tissue to bone.

INTERPRETATION OF MICROBIOLOGICAL RESULTS

Because of the polymicrobial nature of the microbiology of cultures of foot infections, there are questions about how the results should be used and interpreted in the management of the patient. Specifically, a question often asked is, Is it necessary to treat every organism isolated from culture? This is a particularly important question if cultures contain highly resistant organisms such as *P aeruginosa*, enterococci, or methicillin-resistant staphylococci, which may require the addition of specific agents that will increase the complexity of the antimicrobial regimen or make oral therapy impossible. It is known that in a polymicrobial infection there is an interdependence of the micro-organisms such that certain organisms provide the environmental and metabolic conditions that allow others to survive. Thus, treatment of a portion of the bacterial species present may result in elimination of other species that may not be susceptible to the antimicrobial agent being used. In addition, the use of surgical incision and drainage may discourage the persistence of some bacterial species such as

TABLE 20–3. CLINICAL OUTCOME AND BACTERIOLOGICAL ELIMINATION OF MICRO-ORGANISMS ISOLATED IN MIXED CULTURE FROM FOOT INFECTIONS IN PATIENTS WITH DIABETES MELLITUS AND TREATED EMPIRICALLY WITH CEFTIZOXIME OR CEFOXITIN

Organisms	Ceftizoxime		Cefoxitin	
	Clinical[a]	Bacteriological[b]	Clinical[a]	Bacteriological[b]
Staphylococcus aureus	12/16	11/13	9/13	8/10
Enterococcus sp	8/9	4/7	4/9	2/9
Enterobacter cloacae	3/4	3/3	2/3	2/3
Pseudomonas aeruginosa	1/2	0/2	1/3	1/2

Adapted from Hughes CE, Johnson CE, Bamberger DM, et al. Treatment and long-term follow-up of foot infections in patients with diabetes or ischemia: a randomized, prospective, double-blind comparison of cefoxitin and ceftizoxime. *Clin Ther.* 1987;10(suppl A):36–49.
[a] Number clinically improved per number treated with the antimicrobial agent.
[b] Number of bacteriological eradications per number of bacteriologically evaluable cases.

anaerobes. There are some data available for the clinical and microbiological outcome of diabetic foot infections that have been managed with initial empiric therapy that was continued as long as the clinical response was good, without regard to the initial microbiological results; that is, no change in antimicrobial therapy was made solely on the basis of culture results, even if the cultures revealed organisms resistant to the treatment agent.[7] These data are summarized in Table 20–3 for a prospective blinded trial of ceftizoxime versus cefoxitin against four bacterial species of variable susceptibility to the study agents.

Both cephalosporins were active *in vitro* against *S aureus*, neither was active against enterococci or *P aeruginosa,* and ceftizoxime was active against *Enterobacter cloacae,* but cefoxitin was not.[7] Outcomes were generally good for infections from which *S aureus* was isolated, whether treated with ceftizoxime or cefoxitin (69% to 75% clinical response and 80% to 85% bacterial eradication; see Table 20–3). The response of infections that contained enterococci was clinically good for ceftizoxime (89%) but not for cefoxitin (44%), although neither agent showed high bacterial eradication rates (57% for ceftizoxime, 22% for cefoxitin). This may seem surprising, given that neither agent has any *in vitro* activity against enterococci, and illustrates the principle that it may not be necessary to have antimicrobial activity against all bacterial components of a mixed infection to achieve clinical success. The same observation holds for *P aeruginosa* and *E cloacae,* as shown in Table 20–3.

Culture results are of the greatest importance in patients who are clinically failing therapy and in those who have osteomyelitis. In the case of clinical failure, culture results are highly valuable in redirecting changes in antimicrobial selection to better match the bacterial susceptibility of the organisms present. In the case of osteomyelitis, the duration of therapy is long (4 weeks intravenous or 10 weeks intravenous and oral), and successful therapy has been correlated with the selection of antimicrobial agents that are active *in vitro* against the isolated organisms.[8] Thus, selection of an antimicrobial agent(s) for the treatment of osteomyelitis should include *in vitro* susceptibility of all the bacterial isolates to ensure the highest possible chance that the long period of required treatment will be successful.[8]

REFERENCES

1. Reiber GE, Pecoraro RE, Koepsell TD. Risk factors for amputation in patients with diabetes mellitus. *Ann Intern Med.* 1992;117:97–105.

2. Litzelman DK, Slemenda CW, Langefeld CD, et al. Reduction of lower extremity clinical abnormalities in patients with non–insulin-dependent diabetes mellitus. *Ann Intern Med.* 1993;119:36–41.
3. Sapico SL, Witte JL, Canawati HN, et al. The infected foot of the diabetic patient: quantitative microbiology and analysis of clinical features. *Rev Infect Dis.* 1984;6(suppl 1):S171–S176.
4. Wheat JL, Allen SD, Henry M, et al. Diabetic foot infections: bacteriologic analysis. *Arch Intern Med.* 1986;146:1935–1940.
5. Lipsky BA, Pecoraro RE, Larson SA, et al. Outpatient management of uncomplicated lower-extremity infections in diabetic patients. *Arch Intern Med.* 1990;150:790–797.
6. Louie TJ, Bartlett JG, Tally FP, et al. Aerobic and anaerobic bacteria in diabetic foot ulcers. *Ann Intern Med.* 1976;85:461–463.
7. Hughes CE, Johnson CE, Bamberger DM, et al. Treatment and long-term follow-up of foot infections in patients with diabetes or ischemia: a randomized, prospective, double-blind comparison of cefoxitin and ceftizoxime. *Clin Ther.* 1987;10(suppl A):36–49.
8. Bamberger DM, Daus GP, Gerding DN. Osteomyelitis in the feet of diabetic patients. *Am J Med.* 1987;83:653–660.
9. Wheat J. Diagnostic strategies in osteomyelitis. *Am J Med.* 1985;78(suppl):218–224.

21

Dorsalis Pedis Bypass in Diabetic Patients

Frank B. Pomposelli, Jr, MD, and
Frank W. LoGerfo, MD

Autogenous vein bypass grafts to the dorsalis pedis artery represent a technical advance that is highly suited to the management of atherosclerotic occlusive disease as it occurs in association with diabetes mellitus.[1] The pattern of occlusion commonly found in diabetes involves the tibial and peroneal arteries but spares arteries of the foot, especially the dorsalis pedis artery.[2] The propensity toward tibial peroneal involvement in diabetes mellitus was noted in prospective studies of amputation specimens[3] and more recently by arteriography.[4] One of the early impediments to extreme distal reconstruction in the diabetic probably resulted from the suggestion that there was an occlusive lesion in the microcirculation that prevented tissue perfusion.[5] All of the subsequent prospective studies have failed to confirm the existence of such a lesion. With this understanding of vascular disease in mind, therefore, it is logical to extend arterial reconstruction to the dorsalis pedis artery in patients with diabetes.

The precise role of any arterial reconstructive procedure in the management of the diabetic foot is complicated by the fact that polyneuropathy and infection often occur simultaneously with ischemia. Intrinsic muscle atrophy from motor neuropathy leads to foot deformities, creating pressure points under the metatarsal heads, the tips of the toes, etc. Sensory neuropathy diminishes awareness of pressure-related trauma or other injuries to the skin, establishing a portal of entry for bacteria. In addition, the neurogenic inflammatory response mediated by fine sensory C-fibers and neurokinins is blunted. Thus, the usual signs and symptoms of early infection are absent. Under these circumstances established deep-seated infections can occur before a diagnosis is made. These three pathogenic mechanisms—neuropathy, infection, and ischemia—account for the complex pathobiology and clinical presentation of the diabetic foot. Successful management of the ischemia and limb salvage require a clinical care plan that addresses all aspects of the underlying pathology. In general, this can be broken down into a few simple guidelines.

1. Promptly and thoroughly drain the infection and debride obviously necrotic tissue. This is the first order of business in the management of any diabetic foot problem.

2. Always evaluate for ischemia, even when infection and neuropathy are present. Often, because an ulcer is located beneath the metatarsal head, it is referred to as "neuropathic." Under these circumstances the single most important observation is the presence or absence of a clearly palpable dorsalis pedis or posterior tibial pulse at the ankle. If these pulses are not palpable, arteriography is recommended. Noninvasive tests may be of additional help, especially for baseline information; however, the presence or absence of a palpable pulse is a highly effective guide.

3. The arteriogram must be conducted so that the status of the foot arteries is determined even when the tibial and peroneal arteries are occluded. A common mistake is to terminate the arteriogram once the occluded tibial vessels are encountered, on the presumption that all of the distal vessels are also occluded. Intra-arterial digital subtraction arteriography is a simple and effective methodology,[6] although other techniques have their advocates.[7] Adequate hydration prior to the arteriogram will help diminish contrast-induced renal failure, particularly in patients with diabetes who have pre-existing renal insufficiency.

4. Arterial reconstruction should then be performed to restore maximum perfusion to the foot.

5. Secondary revision or closure of the open foot lesion can then be carried out, usually as a separate procedure. This might involve further debridement, toe amputations, occasional transmetatarsal amputation, local flaps, and, rarely, free flaps. With the fully vascularized foot, even in the presence of diabetes, all of these options become available.

Only within this broader context of understanding can the dorsalis pedis bypass be used effectively. The vascular surgeon undertaking vascular reconstruction to the dorsalis pedis artery must understand that this operation is only part of the overall surgical care necessary to obtain limb salvage. If the operation is approached as a technical exercise without proper attention to the role of infection and neuropathy, the results will be compromised.

PATIENT SELECTION

Once a patient has been evaluated by the aforementioned protocol and a patent dorsalis pedis artery is identified, consideration may be given to pedal bypass. It is, of course, important that the site of the anastomosis be free of necrosis or infection. Other than that, patients with necrosis of the forefoot, plantar aspect of the foot, or the heel are all suitable for reconstruction. The details on the arteriogram are important. Calcification may be seen on the plane films of the leg, including the dorsalis pedis artery in the foot; however, this observation should not be regarded as a contraindication to an attempt at arterial reconstruction, as the calcification itself is not an occlusive lesion. Distal lower extremity arteriography has been greatly enhanced by the widespread use of digital subtraction technology. This makes it possible for the angiographer to observe the distal vessels over an extended time course following contrast injection and capture the best images for hard copy. Although the resolution is compromised as compared with standard angiography, we have not found this drawback to be a significant problem in clinical decision making. Regardless of the method of arteriography, both anteroposterior and lateral foot views must be included with the infrageniculate portion of the arteriogram in order to obtain as complete a picture as possible of the locations of all stenosis and occlusions. The foot views should be obtained without excessive plantar flexion, as this can stop flow in the dorsalis pedis, and it may not be visualized. The pattern of occlusive disease on a given arteriogram may present several options for arterial reconstruction. Our goal is to restore palpable foot pulses whenever possible. When bypasses into the popliteal or tibial arteries will not achieve this goal, we preferentially extend the bypass to the foot—usually to the dorsalis pedis artery. Although this is our preferred approach, we will alter this plan based on factors such as conduit availability and extent of infection.

TECHNICAL CONSIDERATIONS

At this time autogenous vein is the only appropriate conduit for bypass to the dorsalis pedis artery. Beyond this, however, there is room for a great deal of flexibility on the part of the surgeon. Our experience has indicated that the outcome of dorsalis pedis bypass is not influenced by the use of *in situ*,[8] reversed, or translocated[9] nonreversed vein grafts. Each of these techniques has specific advantages that apply to different technical situations. One such consideration is the size discrepancy between the saphenous vein and the inflow and outflow arteries, which is most pronounced when constructing a pedal bypass from the common femoral artery. Using an *in situ* graft minimizes the size mismatch, eliminates the need to completely mobilize and harvest the vein, and avoids concerns about tunneling, twisting, etc. This is our preferred approach for dorsalis pedis bypass grafts originating from the common femoral artery. The drawback of the *in situ* technique is that it requires two parallel incisions in the foot, one to harvest the distal vein and one to expose the dorsalis pedis artery, which creates a bridge of skin and subcutaneous tissue at the ankle between the incisions. To minimize problems with skin necrosis, we mobilize the distal portion of the saphenous vein and bring it subcutaneously anterior to the tibia proximal to the skin bridge so that the conduit does not actually pass under the bridge. In addition, we use fine sutures instead of staples for skin closure of these incisions at the ankle and the foot. The skin staples tend to gather in too much skin and create unnecessary tension, which may lead to necrosis and dehiscence.

When the popliteal artery is used for inflow, it is our preference to harvest the more proximal vein with an incision beginning proximal to the ankle to avoid the parallel incisions on the foot. The vein is harvested to a point just above the knee, excised, and translocated. The valves in the vein graft can then be cut under direct vision with an angioscope in *ex vivo* fashion[10] and used nonreversed, or if the saphenous vein is actually larger at the ankle than it is at the knee, the vein graft can be used in the reversed configuration to provide optimum size matching. When harvesting lower leg vein, the graft can be placed back in the bed of the vein or additional tissue coverage is possible by tunneling the graft subfascially, which affords extra protection in the event of any problems with wound necrosis.

OUTFLOW CONSIDERATIONS

With a complete angiogram of the lower extremity circulation, it is usually possible to choose an outflow artery that will restore a palpable foot pulse. As a consequence of a compromised biology in the diabetic foot, as a general rule it is desirable to restore maximum perfusion to the foot. This can be accomplished with a bypass to an anterior or posterior tibial artery that is continuous with the foot or it can be accomplished with a bypass directly to one of the foot arteries, most often the dorsalis pedis. Bypass grafts to an isolated popliteal segment or to the peroneal artery will improve circulation to foot but will not restore maximum perfusion. In particular, some debate has centered around the choice between the peroneal artery and the dorsalis pedis for a vein graft.[11] Our preference is for the dorsalis pedis, since is it easily accessible, provides maximum perfusion to the foot, and provides equivalent, if not better, patency.[12] However, bypass to the dorsalis pedis is unnecessary when a more proximal bypass will restore foot pulses, and it should not be done when there is inadequate high-quality autogenous vein conduit to reach the foot. Calcification of the dorsalis pedis artery is common; however, we have rarely found it impossible to sew to these arteries. Occasionally, the artery is so calcified it cannot be occluded with elastic tapes, in which case we use intravascular occluders or simply let the artery bleed during the anastomosis.

INFLOW CONSIDERATIONS

As noted earlier, in patients with diabetes, the superficial femoral artery is frequently spared and the occlusion is confined to the tibial and peroneal vessel segments. Under these circumstances the superficial femoral or popliteal artery can be used for inflow. This results in a shorter vein graft and avoids the need for groin incisions, which can be problematic in these often obese patients. Several studies[13,14] have reported excellent long-term patency with lower extremity vein grafts originating from the popliteal artery, showing that concerns about progression of atherosclerotic disease in the superficial femoral artery as a cause of graft failure are unjustified. In general, we avoid using the popliteal artery as inflow if there is a diameter-reducing stenosis of greater than 30% proximal to the inflow site. There is a considerable margin for error in assessing popliteal inflow. An easily palpable pulse on physical examination, coupled with the angiogram, is a perfectly adequate assessment. Since the vein graft is going to a small artery with a relatively limited outflow bed, the increased flow demand on the popliteal artery is quite limited. Using these simple criteria, to the best of our knowledge, we have not had a postoperative graft thrombosis due to inadequate inflow.

RESULTS

From 1985 to 1992 we performed 384 consecutive bypasses to the dorsalis pedis in 367 patients. In 275 cases the dorsalis pedis artery was the only available outflow target and in 109 other pedal bypasses were done in preference to an isolated popliteal segment or a distal peroneal artery. Twenty-nine bypasses failed within 30 days. The perioperative mortality rate was 18%. In follow-up ranging from 1 to 83 months (mean, 20 months), primary and secondary patency rates at 5 years were 68% and 82%, respectively.[15] Separate analyses of *in situ* versus translocated vein grafts and grafts with inflow arising from the common femoral and more distal (usually popliteal) arteries demonstrated no difference in patency or limb salvage.[16] When the subset of patients presenting with acute infection and complicating ischemia were evaluated, graft patency and limb salvage rates were 92% and 98%, respectively, at 36 months. All patients had bypass delayed until active spreading infection was controlled, which took an average of 5 days. No patient lost a potentially salvageable limb during this time delay. Wound infection in this group was 12.5%.[17] Thus, bypass to the dorsalis pedis artery can be performed with a high rate of success and low mortality, certainly equivalent to that achieved with other lower extremity vein grafts.

CONCLUSION

Improvements in angiography and in the results of distal reconstruction have established extreme distal autogenous vein reconstruction to the foot vessels as a safe and effective treatment for limb-threatening ischemia. This has proven especially important for patients with diabetes mellitus, who are most likely to require these procedures due to the predilection of atherosclerotic lesions to involve the crural vessels with relative sparing of the foot vessels, especially the dorsalis pedis artery. Bypass grafts to the dorsalis pedis artery currently constitute approximately 25% of all lower extremity arterial reconstructions in our patients with diabetes. Our increased use of this procedure has correlated almost precisely with a decline in the incidence of all levels of amputations in our practice.[18] Success with this operation requires a familiarity with all techniques for autogenous vein reconstruction. Because nearly all of the patients undergoing dorsalis pedis bypass have diabetes, a thorough understanding of the pathobiology of diabetic foot problems is also essential to success. A carefully planned approach, including prompt control of infection, complete arteriography, and arterial reconstruction to maximize foot perfusion, affords a likelihood of successful limb salvage in diabetics that should equal or exceed that in nondiabetics.

REFERENCES

1. Pomposelli FB Jr, Jepsen SJ, Gibbons GW, et al. Efficacy of the dorsalis pedis bypass for limb salvage in diabetic patients: short term observations. *J Vasc Surg*. 1990;11:745–752.
2. Conrad MC. Large and small artery occlusion in diabetics and nondiabetics with severe vascular disease. *Circulation*. 1967;36:83–91.
3. Strandness DE Jr, Priest RE, Gibbons GE. Combined clinical pathological study of diabetic and nondiabetic peripheral arterial disease. *Diabetes*. 1964;13:366–372.
4. Menzoian JO, LaMorte WW, Paniszyn CC, et al. Symptomatology and anatomic patterns of peripheral vascular disease: differing impact of smoking and diabetes. *Ann Vasc Surg*. 1989;3:224–228.
5. Goldenberg SG, Alex M, Joshi RA, et al. Nonatheromatous peripheral vascular disease of the lower extremity in diabetes mellitus. *Diabetes*. 1959;8:261–273.
6. Blakeman BM, Littooy FM, Baker WH. Intra-arterial digital subtraction angiography as a method to study peripheral vascular disease. *J Vasc Surg*. 1986;4:168–173.
7. Veith FJ, Gupta SK, Samson RH, et al. Progress in limb salvage by reconstructive arterial surgery combined with new or improved adjunctive procedures. *Ann Surg*. 1981; 194:386–401.
8. Leather RP, Powers SR, Karmody AM. A reappraisal of the in situ saphenous vein arterial bypass: its use in limb salvage. *Surgery*. 1979;86:453–461.
9. Thompson RW, Mannick JA, Whittemore AD. Arterial reconstruction at diverse sites using nonreversed autogenous vein. *Ann Surg*. 1987;205:747–751.
10. Miller A, Stonebridge P, Tsoukas A, et al. Angioscopically directed valvulotomy: a new valvulotome and technique. *J Vasc Surg*. 1991;13:813–821.
11. Plecha EJ, Seabrook GR, Bandyk DF, et al. Determinants of successful peroneal artery bypass. *J Vasc Surg*. 1993;17:97–106.
12. Schneider JR, Walsh DB, McDaniel MD, et al. Pedal bypass versus tibial bypass with autogenous vein: a comparison of outcome and hemodynamic results. *J Vasc Surg*. 1993;17:1029–1040.

13. Veith FJ, Gupta SK, Samson RH, et al. Superficial femoral and popliteal arteries as inflow sites for distal bypasses. *Surgery.* 1981;90:980–990.
14. Sidawy AN, Menzoian JO, Cantelmo NL, et al. Effect of inflow and outflow sites on the results of tibioperoneal vein grafts. *Am J Surg.* 1986;152:211–224.
15. Pomposelli FB Jr, Marcaccio EJ, Gibbons GW, et al. Dorsalis pedis arterial bypass: durable limb salvage for foot ischemia in patients with diabetes mellitus. *J Vasc Surg.* In press.
16. Pomposelli FB Jr, Jepsen SJ, Gibbons GW, et al. A flexible approach to infrapopliteal vein grafts in patients with diabetes mellitus. *Arch Surg.* 1991;126:724–729.
17. Tannenbaum GA, Pomposelli FB Jr, Marcaccio EJ, et al. Safety of vein bypass grafting to the dorsal pedal artery in diabetic patients with foot infection. *J Vasc Surg.* 1992;15:982–988.
18. LoGerfo FW, Gibbons GW, Pomposelli FB Jr, et al. Trends in the care of the diabetic foot: expanded role of arterial reconstruction. *Arch Surg.* 1992;127:617–621.

22

Experience with Femoropopliteal
Bypass in Patients with Diabetic
End-Stage Renal Disease

*Anthony D. Whittemore, MD, Michael Belkin, MD, and
Magruder C. Donaldson, MD*

For the vast majority of patients with peripheral arterial insufficiency, infrainguinal reconstruction offers palliation of claudication and preservation of limbs threatened with critical ischemia and tissue necrosis. As illustrated in Table 22–1, autogenous infrainguinal reconstruction, including both primary and secondary procedures, provides a 70% primary and an 80% secondary patency rate after 5 years and a limb salvage rate of 90%.[1-3] These results from three large series in the recent literature are remarkably comparable in spite of the fact that some derive from the *in situ* technique, while others represent primarily reversed grafts although the proportion of claudicants varies greatly. Nevertheless the operative mortality remains low (2%), and the patient survival rate approximates 50% at 5 years. Our own 10-year experience demonstrates a 5-year patient survival rate of nearly 70% and a 10-year survival rate of 50%.[3] These series also include a large proportion of infrageniculate reconstructions, which achieve patency rates no different from those of femoropopliteal bypass. In particular, bypasses to the peroneal artery yield just as favorable an outlook as reconstructions to the tibial vessels. Evidence suggests that the diabetic population achieves similar results to people without diabetes with respect to distal bypass.

Although many patients with end-stage renal disease (ESRD) who require maintenance dialysis do very well for years, the overall survival rate among patients for whom dialysis is initiated at the ages of 55 to 64 years is 80%, 50% and 40%, at 1, 3, and 5 years, respectively.[4] For patients with diabetic nephropathy, however, survival statistics are dismal: only one in ten patients survive 5 years on dialysis initiated after the age of 65 years. The 5-year survival rate for younger diabetic patients who initiate dialysis at 55 to 64 years of age is only slightly better at 18%. The survival rate diminishes progressively to 4% after the age of 80 years. The survival statistics associated with diabetic ESRD are the lowest for any dialysis subpopulation thus far studied and may influence the management of associated peripheral vascular disease. From this collective experience, it is reasonable to infer that infrainguinal reconstruction for

TABLE 22–1. INFRAINGUINAL RECONSTRUCTION WITH AUTOGENOUS VEIN

| Author | Year | No. of Limbs | Operative Mortality (%) | 5-Year Cumulative | | Limb Salvage Rate (%) | Patient Survival Rate (%) |
| | | | | Graft Patency Rate (%) | | | |
				1°	2°		
Taylor et al[1]	1990	516	1	75	80	90	28
Bergamini et al[2]	1991	361	3	63	81	86	57
Donaldson et al[3]	1991	440	2	72	83	84	66
Weighted average		1,317	2	70	81	87	50

diabetic patients with ESRD provides satisfactory limb salvage, but overall survival is limited.

A number of reports in the literature each describe slightly different patient populations and therefore appropriately reflect varying results. During the past 15 years, our own experience with infrainguinal reconstruction for 56 patients with renal impairment (serum creatinine >2 mg) consisted of 70 reconstructions. The average age was 69 years, and associated risk factors included diabetes (53%) and coronary artery disease (70%). An additional 31 patients underwent primary amputation for extensive tissue necrosis or severe co-morbidity that rendered the patient nonambulatory, and a few declined surgical reconstruction. This latter group who underwent amputation was slightly younger than the average (65 years) but had a similar distribution of risk factors, including diabetes (48%) and coronary disease (62%). Their condition was generally more debilitated with severe co-morbidity as reflected in their high operative mortality (17%) and minimal subsequent 5-year survival rate (9%). In contrast, the overall operative mortality for the group that underwent reconstruction was 11%, and the 5-year survival rate was considerably higher at 40% for all patients with varying degrees of renal impairment (Table 22–2). No patient maintained on chronic hemodialysis, however, survived beyond 3 years.

Renal insufficiency was defined by the detection of a serum creatinine level in excess of 2 mg, which corresponds to a glomerular filtration rate of 20–40 mL/min as determined by iothalamate assays. Reconstruction was indicated for disabling claudication in 11 (16%) patients with minimal elevations. Most reconstructions were indicated for critical ischemia manifest as rest pain in 21 patients (30%) and tissue necrosis in the remaining 38 (54%). All reconstructions were carried out utilizing autogenous

TABLE 22–2. INFRAINGUINAL RECONSTRUCTION WITH AUTOGENOUS VEIN

| Indication | Number of Limbs | Operative Mortality (%) | Secondary Graft Patency Rate (%) | | Limb Salvage (%) | | Patient Survival Rate (%) | |
			2 y	5 y	2 y	5 y	2 y	5 y
Total	582	2.2	87	81	93	90	83	64
Critical ischemia	401	2.8	84	81	91	87	80	60
Diabetes	188	3.2	83	80	87	83	80	54
Renal insufficiency	70	11	83	77	87	80	60	40
Diabetes	27	9.0	87	65	84	63	47	21
ESRD	16	19	82	0	76	0	32	0

vein, most of which consisted of the greater superficial saphenous vein most often used in the *in situ* configuration. Most reconstructions were primary procedures, and nearly half (44%) were carried to the infrapopliteal level. The perioperative mortality proved significantly higher and the 5-year survival rate significantly lower for patients with renal impairment than for those with normal renal function. Overall graft patency and limb salvage rates, however, were in every way comparable with those for the general population, particularly if the patients with diabetes and those with ESRD were excluded.

Diabetic patients with renal impairment sustained a high operative mortality of 9% and a significantly reduced 5-year survival rate of 21% (Table 22–2). Short-term graft patency and limb salvage were again comparable to those for the general population, but the 5-year rates were significantly lower. Patients with ESRD, however, sustained the highest mortality, 19%, but still achieved acceptable short-term graft patency and limb salvage rates. Unfortunately, no patient with ESRD on hemodialysis survived long enough to establish longer-term graft patency and limb salvage rates. These discouraging results represent the most unfavorable end of the spectrum and again reflect our particular patient population.

Table 22–3 illustrates the operative mortality derived from recent reports of infrainguinal reconstruction in patients with ESRD, mortality figures that range from 4% to 19%. As anticipated, the 2-year patient survival proved equally dismal, ranging from 18% to 70%. Among survivors, however, limb salvage rates are reasonably consistent, ranging from 71% to 91%. These series are certainly not homogeneous, nor are they strictly comparable, particularly with regard to the age at initiation of hemodialysis, co-morbidity, and its relative acuity. For instance, one might expect a significant difference in morbidity and mortality among a young, stable outpatient dialysis population when compared with a tertiary hospital dialysis population who are older and whose initial admission more likely necessitated by acute co-morbidity. Age and the relative acuity of clinically significant co-morbidity are among the more important determinants of ultimate outcome following infrainguinal reconstruction. Other determinants include type of conduit, status of proximal inflow, and distal runoff. Sanchez et al[9] include five inflow procedures, and several include prosthetic as well as autogenous reconstructions. All series but ours include a number of patients with functioning transplants, and interestingly show no difference in outcome from those on hemodialysis. In general, then, while operative mortality and morbidity associated with infrainguinal reconstruction is higher in patients with ESRD than that observed in patients with normal renal function, the majority of patients with ESRD warrant an initial attempt at limb salvage bearing in mind the higher operative morbidity and reduced overall life expectancy.

As a logical extension of this conclusion, since only 21% of diabetic patients survived 5 years and no dialysis patient survived more than 3 years, some consideration of alternative methods of infrainguinal revascularization may be appropriate if such methods can provide a reasonable chance of limb salvage but at a diminished operative mortality. Although these methods may not provide the customary durability associated with conventional surgical reconstruction, shorter-term durability may represent a more realistic goal in these individuals with markedly limited survival. Since the diabetic dialysis patients with acute co-morbidity in our inpatient population demonstrate the most limited survival, such patients with advanced tissue necrosis and infection might be best served with a primary amputation rather than with a heroic effort at infrainguinal reconstruction, in which the time required for healing of these extensive lesions would consume a large amount of remaining life expectancy. This view is shared by others in reviewing similar experiences.[5,11]

TABLE 22–3. INFRAINGUINAL RECONSTRUCTION IN PATIENTS WITH END-STAGE RENAL DISEASE

Author	Year	No. of Patients	No. of Grafts	Rate of Diabetes (%)	30-day Mortality (%)	Graft Patency Rate (%) 1°	Graft Patency Rate (%) 2°	2-year Cumulative Limb Salvage Rate (%)	2-year Cumulative Patient Survival Rate (%)
Edwards et al[5]	1988	19	25	89	—	85	—	76	18
Chang et al[6]	1990	24	32	71	6	90	—	83	62
Harrington et al[7]	1990	39	52	56	8	68	—	91	47
Wasserman et al[8]	1991	37	42	54	4	71	81	78	70
Sanchez et al[9]	1992	47	69	70	14	—	56	70	46
Whittemore et al[10]	1992	11	16	75	19	22	82	76	32

Most patients with chronic renal insufficiency, however, including those with diabetes and those maintained on chronic hemodialysis warrant aggressive infrainguinal revascularization for critical ischemia, but with the understanding that operative morbidity is higher and overall survival rate lower than characteristic of patients with normal renal function.

REFERENCES

1. Taylor LM, Edwards JM, Porter JM. Present status of reversed vein bypass grafting: five-year results of a modern series. *J Vasc Surg.* 1990;11:193–206.
2. Bergamini TM, Towne JB, Bandyk DF, et al. Experience with in situ saphenous vein bypasses during 1981 to 1989: determinant factors of long-term patency. *J Vasc Surg.* 1991;13:137–149.
3. Donaldson MC, Mannick JA, Whittemore AD. Femoral-distal bypass with in situ greater saphenous vein. *Ann Surg.* 1991;213:457–465.
4. Byrne C, Vernon P, Cohen JJ. Effect of age and diagnosis on survival of older patients beginning chronic dialysis. *JAMA.* 1994;271:34–36.
5. Edwards JM, Taylor LM, Porter JM. Limb salvage in end-stage renal disease (ESRD). *Arch Surg.* 1988;123:1164–1168.
6. Chang BB, Paty PSK, Shah DM, et al. Results of infrainguinal bypass for limb salvage in patients with end-stage renal disease. *Surgery.* 1990;108:742–747.
7. Harrington EB, Harrington ME, Schanzer H, Haimov M. End-stage renal disease: is infrainguinal limb revascularization justified? *J Vasc Surg.* 1990;12:691–696.
8. Wassermann RJ, Saroyan RM, Rice JC, Kerstein MD. Infrainguinal revascularization for limb salvage in patients with end-stage renal disease. *South Med J.* 1991;84:190–192.
9. Sanchez LA, Goldsmith RN, Rivers SP, et al. Limb salvage surgery in end stage renal disease: is it worthwhile? *J Cardiovasc Surg.* 1992;33:344–348.
10. Whittemore AD, Donaldson MC, Mannick JA. Infrainguinal reconstruction for patients with chronic renal insufficiency. *J Vasc Surg.* 1993;17:32–41.
11. Dossa C, Shepard AD, Amos AM, et al. Results of lower extremity amputation in end stage renal disease. *J Vasc Surg.* [In press].

VI

The Blue
Toe Syndrome

23

Noninvasive Evaluation of Atherosclerotic Emboli

William H. Pearce, MD, and Stephen P. Wiet, MD

In recent years, our ability to identify the source of atheroemboli has improved with the development of new technology. Traditionally, patients with atheroembolism required complete arteriography (including the thoracic aorta) to identify the source. Unfortunately, arteriography in these patients may have induced further embolization of atherosclerotic debris with worsening of the distal ischemia. A minimally invasive method to identify the source of the atheroemboli avoids this complication and allows a more directed approach for the radiologist. For example, a transaxillary approach may be more appropriate than a transfemoral approach in a patient with ulcerated plaques of the infrarenal aorta. Finally, nonivasive techniques provide the opportunity to study in detail the natural history of aortic atherosclerosis and evaluated potential therapeutic interventions without high risk.

Atheroembolism represents the degeneration of an atherosclerotic plaque that produces either macroembolization of plaque material and clot or microembolization of cholesterol, fibrin, and platelet fragments. In either case, end artery occlusion occurs with ischemia and tissue necrosis. The important problem associated with atheroembolism is the propensity for recurrence; atheroembolism recurs in nearly 50% of patients at 1 year after the first embolism.[1,2] Recurrent atheroembolization results in a high incidence of tissue loss and amputation because of previous microvascular occlusion. The prevalence of atheroembolism is difficult to determine from the literature. Kealy in 1978 studied sections of the aorta and solid organs in 2,126 autopsies of patients older than 60 years of age.[3] Atheroembolism was found in nine men and seven women (0.79%) with a mean age of 76.7 years. Cholesterol crystals, which varied from 150μ to 1100μ in diameter, were found in the lumen of small arteries. The kidney was the most commonly involved solid organ (13/16), followed by the spleen (6/16), ileum (3/16), liver (2/16), brain (1/16), and colon (1/16). Peripheral vascular disease was found in 13% of patients with peripheral atheroembolism.[4]

The pathophysiology of atheroembolism is uncertain but is associated with uneven flow surfaces, such as coral reef aorta, the shaggy aorta syndrome, and ulcerative plaques. Basic research is being performed to define the natural history of plaque formation from fatty streaks to the complex plaques with central necrosis, plaque rupture, and thrombosis. Inflammation is an essential element of the atherosclerotic process. The exact antigenic stimulus is not known, but is thought to be cholesterol. An intense inflammatory response is found in the distal artery following embolization and is associated with the intraluminal cholesterol crystals.

The clinical syndrome of atheroembolism is variable. Peripheral cutaneous emboli (livido reticularis) and digital gangrene (blue toe syndrome) are the most commonly recognized manifestations of atheroembolization. However, isolated atheroemboli has been reported in the calf muscles without cutaneous manifestations.[5] More proximal atheroembolism may produce intestinal ischemia, pancreatitis, and renal failure.[6] Renal atheroembolism produces acute renal failure with eosinophilia and urine eosinophils. Wilson et al reported a 67% incidence of peripheral eosinophilia and a 90% incidence of eosinophiluria in patients with renal cholesterol emboli. Atheroemboli from the ascending aorta may produce ocular and cerebral symptoms in addition to lower extremity emboli. Amaurosis fugax, transient ischemic attacks, strokes, and Hollenhorst plaques are associated with atherosclerosis of the ascending aorta. In every instance, it is mandatory to identify the source of the atheroembolism as precisely as possible to direct subsequent therapy.

Any segment of the arterial tree may be the source of the atherosclerotic emboli. In general, however, the source of the debris is related to the degree and distribution of the atherosclerotic process. The majority of lower extremity atheroemboli arise from the aortoiliac segment with nonaneurysmal disease. A review of the literature and our own experience show that the aortoiliac segment is involved in nearly two thirds of patients (63%) and is related either to aneurysmal degeneration (13%) or ulcerative plaques (50%) (Table 23–1).[8–15] The femoropopliteal segment is the source in 34% and the thoracic aorta in 3%. Only recently has the thoracic aorta been recognized as an important source of both cerebral and peripheral emboli. In one autopsy series, the rate of atheroembolism following cardiac surgery increased significantly from 4.5% to 48% in the past 10 years.[16] Manipulation of the ascending thoracic aorta during coronary artery bypass surgery dislodges friable plaques with distal

TABLE 23–1. REVIEW OF THE LITERATURE ON ATHEROEMBOLISM[a]

Author	N	TA	AAA	Aortoiliac	Femoro-popliteal
Mehigan & Stoney[8]	12			5	7
Karmody et al[1]	31		6	2	23
Kealy[3]	16		7	9	
Kempczinski[2]	10	1		9	
Kwaan & Connolly[9]	15			15	
Perdue & Smith[10]	13			11	2
Brenowitz & Edwards[11]	4			4	
Schechter[12]	17		3	10	4
Crane[13]	3		1	2	
McFarland et al[14]	42			14	28
Jenkins & Newton[15]	15	1	2	6	6
Adamson et al[5]	2		2		
Northwestern (see Chapter 24)	82	6	12	45	19
TOTAL	**262**	**8** (3%)	**33** (13%)	**132** (50%)	**89** (34%)

[a] TA, thoracic aorta; AAA, abdominal aortic aneurysm.

embolization. Multiple atheroemboli occurred in 63% of patients, with the kidney and spleen the most commonly affected organs (10%).

COMPUTED TOMOGRAPHY

Computed tomography (CT) offers a new dimension to define arterial pathology and anatomy. Vascular CT examinations require specific protocols to maximize contrast enhancement by scanning during the intravascular phase of the constrast. Our current protocols for vascular CT scans include 5-mm section thickness (in special instances, 3-mm section thicknesses) with minimum interscan delay and dynamic table movement. The contrast agent is injected in an initial bolus of 50 mL followed by a maintenance infusion of 0.1 to 1.5 mL per second for a total volume of 100 to 150 mL. Unenhanced CT scans are performed to define arterial size, hemorrhage, and hematoma formation.

The CT scan provides a clear definition of the aorta beginning at the aortic root and extending to the aortic bifurcation. CT defines the characteristics of the arterial wall, including size and intraluminal morphology. Calcification of the arterial wall with laminated wall thrombus suggests ulceration with thrombus formation. In addition, CT provides images of adjacent anatomy and pathology. In patients with visceral atheroembolism, CT is able to define splenic and renal infarcts. Other abnormalities on CT scans that are consistent with atheroembolism are aortic aneurysms and aortic dissections.[17,18] CT images of aortic aneurysms include aortic enlargement, intraluminal thrombus, and calcification of the aortic wall (Fig. 23–1A,B). With large aneurysms, adjacent viscera may be displaced. Aortic dissections appear as a double-barreled lumen separated by an intimal flap. The sensitivity of CT is 94% when compared with magnetic resonance imaging (MRI) (98%) or transesophageal echocardiography (TEE) (97%) in the diagnosis of aortic dissection.[19] CT is also a sensitive method for detecting atherosclerotic occlusion. The arterial lumen is unopacified with calcium deposition seen within the arterial wall.

CT is an important primary diagnostic test for patients who present with suspected atheroembolization. A transfemoral angiogram may produce additional embolization with clinically significant adverse effects. In patients who present with aortic aneurysms and distal embolization, CT scans reveal mural thrombi that are irregular and star-shaped with fissures and multiple lumens.[20,21] A CT scan also provides important aortic morphology at the level of the renal arteries. Aortic thrombus that extends to the renal arteries may result in renal failure following aortic cross-clamping. To minimize renal emboli in these patients, it is important to clamp above the renal arteries and remove the thrombus. The clamp is then re-placed below the renal arteries.

Iliac and peripheral aneurysms are also readily imaged on standard and contrast-enhanced CT scans. Similar to aortic aneurysms, the CT findings of peripheral aneurysms are arterial dilatation, calcification, and intraluminal thrombus. CT scans of the popliteal fossa enable an accurate diagnosis of popliteal artery aneurysms, adventitial cysts, and entrapment.

MAGNETIC RESONANCE IMAGING

MRI is similar to CT in that both methods attempt to characterize the tissue contained within a small, defined area. The current advantage of MRI over CT is that MRI

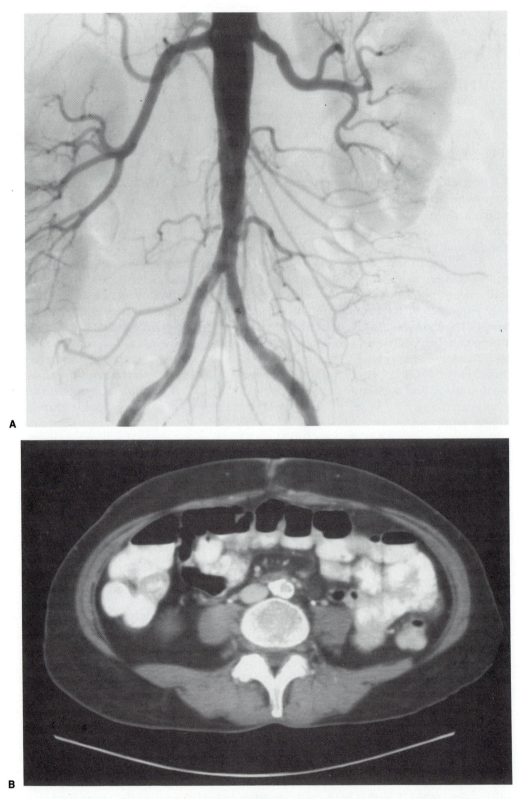

Figure 23–1. (A) Aortogram of a patient who presented with distal atheroembolism. Distal aortic narrowing. No ulcer scan. **(B)** CT scan of distal aorta demonstrating heavy aortic calcification (arrow). (*Figure continues*)

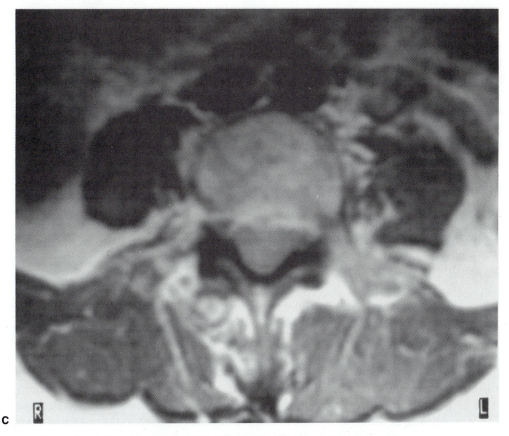

C

Figure 23–1. *(continued).* **(C)** MRI of same location. No calcification seen.

images can be reconstructed in multiple planes. However, three dimensional CT images are now possible with the development of ultrafast and spiral CT scanners. More important, MRI does not require contrast materials, which may contribute to renal failure. By pulsing the radio frequency, images of both the arterial and venous systems may be obtained. Magnetic resonance angiography is used for intracerebral/ extracerebral vascular disease and for assessment of peripheral arterial vascular occlusive disease. The value of MRI and MRA in atheroembolism is only now being explored. Combining MRI techniques and image analysis, Merickel et al[22] were able to reconstruct aortic segments in three dimensions. Wall volume was twice as thick as normal with no change in lumen size. This compensatory enlargement would not have been detected with conventional angiography on CT. Wesbey et al[23] using standard MRI techniques detected 92% of "nonocclusive" protrusional plaques. Purely calcified lesions were missed. Using a new proton MRI pulse, Wesbey et al were also able to detect fat and water within the aortic wall. Thus, MRI may be able to detect abnormal arterial lipid accumulation before complication occurs.

MRI is valuable in diagnosing conditions such as aortic aneurysms, aortic dissections, and coarctations.[20,23,24] Like CT, MRI has a very high sensitivity and specificity for the diagnosis of aortic dissections.[19] When both lumens are patent, flowing blood produces a double flow void. When there is differential flow, phase shift may be used to display differences in the flow between the two lumens. Aortic aneurysms appear as enlargements of the aorta on MRI and intraluminal clots may be visualized. The clear delineation of the intraluminal thrombus is not as good with MRI when compared with CT. Calcifications are not visualized with MRI (Fig. 23–1C). In patients with ulcerative plaques, coral reef formation, and other intimal irregularities, MRI appears to lack sensitivity because the resolution of MRI is approximately 1–2 mm. Therefore, only very large, irregular plaques can be reliantly demonstrated with this method. Recent reports suggest MRI may be an important tool to quantitate medial and intimal thickening.[22] However, the clear delineation of the luminal surface by MRI is inferior to that of CT, TEE, or angiography.

TRANSESOPHAGEAL ECHOCARDIOGRAPHY

TEE is an important technique for the diagnosis of intrathoracic aortic disease. Although TEE is not truly noninvasive, the technique appears to be safe and avoid any potential for producing further embolization. In several large series, the complication rate with TEE was low. This evaluation can be performed rapidly at any location within the hospital.[20,25,26]

With TEE, we have gained a greater appreciation of the thoracic aorta as a potential source of emboli, either to the cerebral circulation or to the peripheral arterial beds. TEE using either the monoplanar or biplanar technique provides high-quality, high-resolution images of the ascending aorta, aortic arch, and descending thoracic aorta. Amarenco et al[20] studied 500 consecutive patients with cerebrovascular disease and other neurologic problems. The prevalence of ulcerative plaques in the ascending aorta in patients with strokes with no known cause was 58% with an odds ratio of 5:7. The presence of ulcerative plaques was a risk factor independent of extracranial carotid artery disease. Cerebral infarctions in this group of patients were multiple, hemorrhagic, and frequently subcortical.

With the more generalized use of TEE, numerous abnormalities of the thoracic aorta have been identified that have produced distal emboli including the ligamentum arteriosum, ulcerative plaques, and protruding mobile atheromas.[27–29] Defining plaque mobility with TEE has played an important role in redefining our understanding of peripheral and cerebral emboli. Karalis et al[30] found mobile atherosclerotic debris in 6% of patients who underwent TEE for a variety of indications. In this subgroup of patients, 31% had a history of embolic events either to the cerebral circulation or peripheral circulation. In this study only 4% of age-matched controls who had no evidence of aortic disease had a history consistent with distal embolization. A pedunculated mobile atheroma carries the highest risk of distal embolization (73%) as compared with a smooth luminal plaque (12%) (Fig. 23–2). In one case-control study, 122 patients were referred for TEE for unexplained stroke, transient ischemic attack, or peripheral emboli.[31] Protruding atheromas were found in 10% of patients. The left brain was involved in 72%, right brain in 49%, and peripheral circulation in 10%. The presence of a protruding atheroma correlated highly with symptoms with an odds ratio of 3:2. The majority of these patients had asymptomatic disease, and the follow-up data, for this group are unknown. TEE is also superior to transthoracic echocardiography in identifying cardiac lesions that may produce central or peripheral emboli. A cardiac source of cerebral or peripheral emboli was found in 57% of TEE examinations compared with 15% of transthoracic echos. TEE was superior for identifying atrial septal aneurysms, patent foramen ovale, left atrial thrombus or tumor, and left atrial spontaneous echo contrast (low flow state).[32]

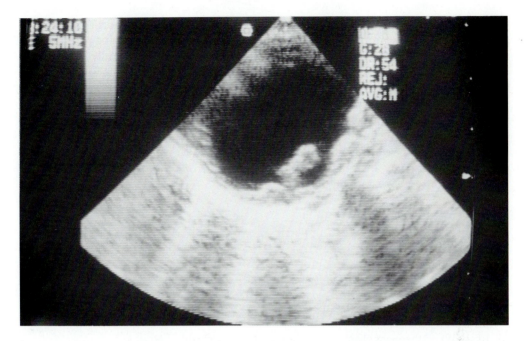

Figure 23–2. TEE demonstrating mobile protruding plaque.

CONCLUSION

Selecting the appropriate imaging modality for patients with evidence of cerebral or peripheral emboli depends on the patient's presenting symptoms. The entire arterial segment from the heart to the affected organ must be evaluated. In patients who present with bilateral cerebral symptoms, the initial test should be TEE. TEE gives a clear view of intracardiac structures and the ascending aorta and arch. The particular benefit is that no intraluminal manipulation need be performed. TEE provides a detailed view of the anatomy of the left atrium, the mitral value, and the aortic valve. With the advent of TEE the heart has been recognized as an occult source of emboli and a cause of stroke. TEE also may be important in determining the presence of atherosclerotic debri in the ascending aorta before coronary artery bypass surgery. In patients who present with a unilateral upper extremity atheroembolism, the source must be distal to the arch. In these patients, arteriography is mandatory. A duplex ultrasound scan may be used to identify subclavian arterial pathology, including aneurysms and intimal ulceration. However, arteriography is still needed to evaluate the degree of distal embolization. For patients who present with bilateral lower extremity atheroembolism, the source is probably distal to the left subclavian artery. In these patients, the selection of the imaging modality is variable. We have found that CT is particularly useful in the diagnosis of aortic aneurysm, aortic dissection, and laminated wall thrombus. If the use of contrast material is contraindicated, MRI is performed. Arteriography is performed only in anticipation of surgical intervention. If the CT scan does not demonstrate a source, TEE is performed to evaluate the descending thoracic aorta. We have found seven patients in whom TEE was more sensitive than CT in detecting mobile protruding atheromas. MRI is useful only in patients with aortic dissections or aortic aneurysms. To date MRI resolution has not been sufficient to allow the diagnosis of small mural thrombi. In patients who present with unilateral lower extremity atheroembolism, the source must be distal to the aortic bifurcation. Although a duplex scan may be used to define intraluminal morphology in the common femoral and superficial femoral arteries, arteriography is generally required.

In conclusion, the use of a particular imaging modality is tailored to the patient's symptoms and the anticipated surgical or medical intervention. Minimally invasive tests offer the potential to study the long-term consequences of asmyptomatic mobile protruding plaques. The development of new image analysis has made three-dimensional renderings of the luminal surface and wall characteristics possible using either MRI or duplex ultrasound. A three-dimensional image of the aortic wall and plaque provides new insights into the progression of atherosclerotic disease and plaque rupture with distal embolism.

REFERENCES

1. Karmody AM, Powers SR, Monaco VJ, Leather RP. "Blue toe" syndrome: an indication for limb salvage surgery. *Arch Surg.* 1976;111:1263–1268.
2. Kempczinski RI. Lower-extremity arterial emboli from ulcerating atherosclerotic plaques. *JAMA.* 1979;241:807–810.
3. Kealy WF. Atheroembolism. *J Clin Pathol.* 1978;31:984–989.
4. Thurlbeck W, Castleman B. Atheromatous emboli to the kidneys after aortic surgery. *N Engl J Med.* 1957;257:442–447.
5. Adamson AS, Pittman MR, Darke SG. Atheroembolism presenting as selective muscle embolisation. *J Cardiovasc Surg.* 1991;32:705–707.
6. Carvajal JA, Anderson WR, Weiss L, et al. Atheroembolism: an etiologic factor in renal insufficiency, gastrointestinal hemorrhages and peripheral vascular diseases. *Arch Intern Med.* 1967;119:593–599.
7. Wilson DM, Salazer TL, Farkough ME. Eosinophiluria in atheroembolic renal disease. *Am J Med.* 1991;91:186–189.
8. Mehigan JT, Stoney RJ: Lower extremity atheromatous embolization. *Am J Surg.* 1976;132:163.
9. Kwaan JHM, Connolly JE: Peripheral atheroembolism: an enigma. *Arch Surg.* 1977;112:987–990.
10. Perdue GD, Smith RB: Atheromatous microemboli. *Ann Surg.* 1969;169:954–959.
11. Brenowitz JB, Edwards WS: The management of atheromatous emboli to the lower extremities. *Surg Gynecol Obstet.* 1976;143:941–945.
12. Schechter DC: Atheromatous embolization to lower limbs. *NY State Med J.* 1979;79:1180–1186.
13. Crane C. Atherothrombotic embolism to lower extremities in arteriosclerosis. *Arch Surg.* 1967;94:96.
14. McFarland RJ, Taylor RS, Woodyer AB, Eastwood JB. The femoropopliteal segment as a source of peripheral atheroembolism. *J Cardiovasc Surg.* 1989;30:597–603.
15. Jenkins DM, Newton WD. Atheroembolism. *Am Surg.* 1991;57:588–590.
16. Blauth CI, Cosgrove DM, Webb BW, et al. Atheroembolism from the ascending aorta. *J Thorac Cardiovasc Surg.* 1992;103:1104–1112.
17. Papanlcolaou N, Wittenberg J, Ferrucci JT Jr, et al. Preoperative evaluation of abdominal aortic aneurysms by computed tomography. *AJR.* 1986;146:711–715.
18. Machida K, Tasaka A. CT patterns of mural thrombus in aortic aneurysms. *J Comput Assist Tomogr.* 1980;4:840–842.
19. Nienaber CA, Von Kodolitsch Y, Nicolas V, et al. The diagnosis of thoracic aortic dissection by noninvasive imaging procedures. *N Engl J Med.* 1993;328:1–9.
20. Amarenco P, Duyckaerts C, Tzourio C, et al. The prevalence of ulcerated plaques in the aortic arch in patients with stroke. *N Engl J Med.* 1992;326:221–225.

21. Baxter BT, McGee GS, Flinn WR, et al. Distal embolization as a presenting symptom of aortic aneurysms. *Am J Surg.* 1990;160:197–201.
22. Merickel MB, Berr S, Spetz K, et al. Noninvasive quantitative evaluation of atherosclerosis using MRI and image analysis. *Arteriosclerosis Thromb.* 1993;13:1180–1186.
23. Wesbey GE, Higgins CB, Hale JD, Valk PE. Magnetic resonance applications in atherosclerotic vascular disease. *Cardiovasc Intervent Radiol.* 1986;8:342–350.
24. Akins EW, Carmichael MJ, Hill JA, Mancuso AA. Preoperative evaluation of the thoracic aorta using MRI and angiography. *Ann Thorac Surg.* 1987;44:499–507.
25. Erbel R, Borner N, Steller D, et al. Detection of aortic dissection by transesophageal echocardiology. *Br Heart J.* 1987;58:45–51.
26. Barzilai B, Marshall WG, Saffitz JE, Kouchoukos N. Avoidance of embolic complications by ultrasonic characterization of the ascending aorta. *Circulation.* 1989;80:S275–S279.
27. Laperche T, Sarkis A, Monin JL, et al. The ligamentum arteriosum: an unreported origin of periperal emboli diagnosed by transesophageal echocardiography. *Am Heart J.* 1992;124:222–223.
28. Porembka DT, Johnson DJ, Fowl RJ, et al. Descending thoracic aortic thrombus as a cause of multiple system organ failure: diagnosis by transesophageal echocardiography. *Crit Care Med.* 1992;20:1184–1187.
29. Wiet SP, Pearce WH, McCarthy WJ, et al. Utility of transesophageal echocardiography in the diagnosis of disease of the thoracic aorta. *J Vasc Surg.* 1994;20:613–620.
30. Karalis DG, Chandrasekaran K, Victor MF, et al. Recognition and embolic potential of intraaortic atherosclerotic debris. *J Am Coll Cardiol.* 1991;17:73–78.
31. Tunick PA, Perez JL, Kronzon I. Protruding atheromas in the thoracic aorta and systemic embolization. *Ann Intern Med.* 1991;115:423–427.
32. Pearson AC, Labovitz AJ, Tatineni S, Gomez CR. Superiority of transesophageal echocardiography in detecting cardiac source of embolism in patients with cerebral ischemia of uncertain etiology. *J Am Coll Cardiol.* 1991;17:66–72.

24

Experience in the Management of Atherosclerotic Emboli

Richard R. Keen, MD, and James S. T. Yao, MD, PhD

Of all the manifestations of limb ischemia encountered by the vascular surgeon, diagnosis and treatment of extremity ischemia caused by atherosclerotic emboli is often a challenge. Atherosclerotic emboli can be difficult to manage for several reasons. Commonly, the diagnosis of atherosclerotic embolization is delayed, especially because many physicians are unaware of the protean presentations of atheroemboli. Blue toe syndrome and livedo reticularis, signs of microembolization, can be misdiagnosed as vasospasm, vasculitis, and dermatitis in the presence of palpable extremity pulses. By the time the limb-threatening nature of the ischemia due to atheroembolization is recognized, the small size of the fibrinoplatelet aggregates, thrombi, and cholesterol crystals may obliterate the vessels, making limb salvage procedures difficult. This chapter discusses experience in the diagnosis and management of atherosclerotic embolization.

HISTORY

Atheromatous embolization was recognized by pathologists long before its clinical significance was appreciated. The first documented case of atherosclerotic embolization was reported in a postmortem examination by Panum in 1862 in which an atheroembolus caused lethal coronary artery occlusion.[1] In 1896, Doch[2] reported the first case of atheroembolization recognized in the United States; this was also a case in which atheromatous debris occluded a coronary artery causing death. The hypothesis that visceral atheroemboli may originate from a severely diseased, atherosclerotic aorta was first made by Flory[3] in 1945. In examining a large number of autopsy specimens, Flory observed that bodies with the most extensive proximal aortic atherosclerosis had the greatest number of visceral and muscular atheroemboli. He tested this hypothesis by scraping atherosclerotic debris from diseased aortas, solubilizing it, and injecting it into rabbit ear veins, where pulmonary artery lesions developed that were identical to those found in human autopsy specimens. The first clinical case of macroscopic atheroembolization was reported by Venet and Friedfeld[4] in 1952. A calcified embolus to the femoral artery from a more proximal arterial source was

313

successfully treated by operative embolectomy. Atheroembolization occurring during operations on the aorta was first reported by Thurlbeck and Castleman[5] in 1957 in a patient with emboli to the renal parenchyma. Livedo reticularis and distal extremity gangrene due to atheroembolism were first recognized and reported by Hoye et al in 1959. The importance of livedo reticularis as a sign of atheroembolization was further emphasized by Kazmier et al[7] in 1966 in patients with abdominal aortic aneurysm.

The poor prognosis of atheroembolization that is not treated operatively was recognized both by Karmody et al[8] and Kempczinski.[9] In 1976, Karmody et al observed that infrainguinal atherosclerotic lesions that caused the blue toe syndrome had a recurrence rate of 80% within 6 weeks and a 60% incidence of tissue loss if the source lesion was not corrected with an operation.[8] In 1979, Kempczinski[9] reported that 75% of patients with atheroemboli of aortic origin treated with warfarin anticoagulation or antiplatelet agents, and no operative intervention, experienced recurrent atheroembolic events within 6 weeks.

PHYSICAL FINDINGS

Atherosclerotic arterial to arterial emboli can present as microscopic emboli (pulses intact), macroscopic emboli (pulse deficit), or as a combination of both macroscopic and microscopic emboli. Microscopic atheroembolization accounts for approximately one half of all cases. Combined micro- and macroemboli occur in about 20% of patients, and isolated macroscopic atheroemboli account for less than 40% of all cases.

The diagnosis of atheromatous microembolization is most often made when the characteristic physical findings—blue toes or livedo reticularis—are recognized in the setting of a history of the acute onset of digital pain and discoloration. Microemboli consist of fibrinoplatelet aggregates, cholesterol crystals, or thrombus and occlude 100μ to 200μ arterioles, triggering dermal and subcutaneous ischemia. Cholesterol emboli also initiate a specific vasculitic-type inflammatory reaction, marked by infiltration of the arteriolar wall with foreign-body giant cells, granulomatous inflammation, or necrotizing angiitis.[10] The digital pain characteristic of blue toe syndrome and the myalgias observed with microembolization to extremity muscles are distinct from the metatarsal pain seen with chronic lower extremity rest pain.

The blue toe syndrome refers specifically to emboli to lower extremity digital arterioles secondary to femoral or popliteal atherosclerotic lesions,[8] but blue toes and fingers also occur with microemboli of aortic or upper extremity arterial origin. The tenderness seen with digital atheroembolization is often much greater than that found in other causes of digital ischemia, probably because of the inflammatory component that can accompany atheroemboli. The skin discoloration that occurs after atheroembolic events is usually immediate, and the pain and tenderness usually present 24 to 48 hours later.

Livedo reticularis appear as a diffuse, petechial-type, violacious or erythematous reaction secondary to localized areas of ischemia. Sharp demarcations exist between the ischemic areas and the normally perfused skin. Livedo reticularis and blue digits can be confused with a vasculitis or dermatitis.[10,11] Livedo reticularis tends not to be as painful as the blue toe syndrome, although myalgias secondary to emboli to muscle tissue are more commonly seen with the embolic showers that characterize livedo reticularis.

A third presentation of microemboli is the relatively silent, progressive obliteration of distal extremity arterial circulation characteristic of emboli that originate from popliteal and subclavian artery aneurysms.[12] The ischemia seen with this third type of atheroembolization is usually severe and end-stage, often presenting as rest pain and seldom producing the findings of livedo reticularis or the blue toe syndrome, probably because of the different nature of the emboli debris. In contrast to the strong inflammatory reaction within the target arteriole seen with embolic cholesterol and fibrin plaques, the platelet aggregates and microscopic thrombi characteristic of popliteal and subclavian artery aneurysms do not trigger this same reaction. Instead, a gradual occlusion of the entire distal runoff of the extremity takes place, leading to eventual thrombosis of the larger axial arteries. Prior distal embolization is the most important prognostic factor in determining both long-term limb salvage in patients with popliteal artery aneurysms[13] and graft patency in patients undergoing upper extremity arterial reconstruction.[14] This form of atheroembolization is probably underappreciated and is not always recognized as a form of atherosclerotic embolization.

Macroscopic atheroemboli of noncardiac origin present with the classic findings of acute arterial occlusion. On clinical presentation and at the time of operative embolectomy, thrombolytic therapy, or pathologic examination, these emboli often cannot be differentiated from emboli of cardiac origin. Differentiating atherosclerotic emboli from cardiac emboli depends on examination of the potential embolic sources.

SOURCES OF ATHEROSCLEROTIC EMBOLI

From January 1983 to September 1994, we reviewed 137 patients with atherosclerotic emboli to the upper or lower extremities treated at Northwestern University Medical Center and found that the infrarenal aorta is the most common atheroembolic source (Fig. 24–1) (Table 24–1). Among 107 patients with lower extremity atheroemboli, aortoiliac occlusive disease was localized as the atheroembolic source in 56 patients (52%). Small aortic aneurysms were the source in 21 patients (20%), followed by lower extremity stenoses in 12 patients (11%). Shaggy thoracoabdominal aorta in 9 patients (8%), patent but degenerating bypass grafts in 7 patients (7%) (Fig. 24–2), and lower extremity arterial aneurysms in 2 patients (2%) were the remaining sources. Overall, atherosclerotic disease proximal to the inguinal ligament accounted for more than 80% of all lower extremity atheroemboli.

Limb-threatening upper extremity ischemia is relatively rare, but the proportion of cases of upper extremity ischemia that involve arterial atheroembolization is high. Atheroembolic events complicate nearly 70% of upper extremity aneurysms.[14] Although occlusive disease is the cause of most lower extremity atheroemboli, aneurysms are responsible for 50% of cases of upper extremity emboli (Table 24–2).

DIAGNOSTIC WORK-UP

The initial physical examination, specifically the pulse examination, guides the strategy for performing diagnostic tests. For patients with a new pulse deficit, aortoiliac arteriography with extremity runoff is the first imaging study performed. Aortography in these patients carries the risk of a procedure-related atheroembolic shower.[15,16] Aortography should be performed with great care, and a brachial approach should be considered. If aortography successfully localizes the source of the embolus, no further work-up needs to be performed, and operative repair of the embolic source

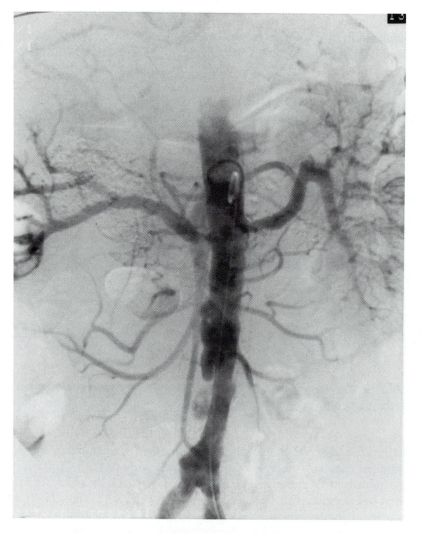

Figure 24–1. Aortogram of a 56-year-old man with acute embolic occlusion of the left popliteal artery reveals an ulcerated infrarenal aorta as the source of the embolus.

TABLE 24–1. SOURCES OF LOWER EXTREMITY ATHEROEMBOLI IN 107 PATIENTS SEEN AT NORTHWESTERN UNIVERSITY MEDICAL CENTER

Source of Emboli	No. of Patients	Percentage (%)
Thoracoabdominal aorta	9	8
Aortoiliac stenosis	56	52
Aortoiliac aneurysm	21	20
Lower extremity stenosis	12	11
Existing bypass graft	7	7
Lower extremity aneurysm	2	2

Derived from Keen RR, et al. *Surgical management of atheroembolization.* Paper presented at the Midwestern Vascular Surgical Society annual meeting, September 23–24, 1994, Cincinnati, Ohio.

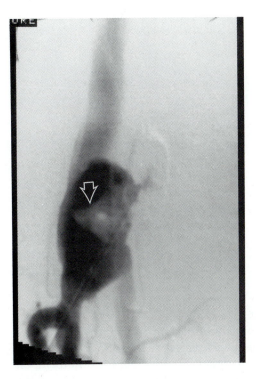

Figure 24–2. Aortogram of a 60-year-old man who sustained an embolus to his right common femoral artery to posterior tibial artery bypass graft, which originated from a previously placed aortofemoral bypass graft. Arteriogram reveals a thrombus-filled right femoral artery anastomotic pseudoaneurysm (arrow) as the source.

can be planned. The arteriogram also provides the anatomic details that may be needed in any lower extremity revascularization.

If aortography does not reveal the likely atheroembolic source in a patient with a new pulse deficit, contrast-enhanced computed tomography (CT) of the thoracic and abdominal aorta is the next text performed. If the CT scan suggests a suspicious lesion of the thoracic aorta, transesophageal echocardiography can confirm this. If the previously obtained arteriogram suggests a high-grade iliac or femoral artery stenosis, or if the CT scan suggests a femoral or popliteal artery aneurysm that could be the embolic source, an arterial duplex ultrasonic examination of the suspicious region should be completed. The increased velocity of blood flow through high-grade stenoses appears to be a common characteristic of embolic iliac and femoral atherosclerotic lesions. A duplex scan can also aid in the diagnosis of thrombus-lined femoral or popliteal artery aneurysms that may not be seen on arteriograms.

Our approach for patients who present with microembolization and intact axial pulses differs from that just described. For these patients, a contrast-enhanced CT scan of the thoracic and abdominal aorta is the initial diagnostic examination.[17] Microscopic emboli that cause livedo reticularis and blue digits appear to have a high chance of

TABLE 24–2. SOURCES OF UPPER EXTREMITY ATHEROEMBOLI IN 30 PATIENTS

Source of Emboli	No. of Patients	Percentage (%)
Arterial stenosis	6	20
Non-thoracic outlet aneurysm	8	27
Thoracic outlet stenosis/aneurysm	16	53

Derived from Keen RR, et al. *Surgical management of atheroembolization.* Paper presented at the Midwestern Vascular Surgical Society annual meeting, September 23–24, 1994, Cincinnati, Ohio.

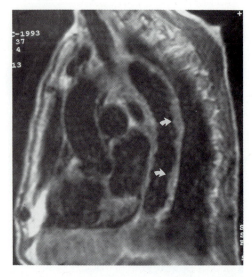

Figure 24–3. Magnetic resonance image demonstrates severe atherosclerosis of the descending thoracic aorta (arrows) in a 79-year-old man who presented with blue toes and renal insufficiency 6 months after aortobifemoral bypass. Transesophageal echocardiography revealed that this plaque was mobile.

originating from an atherosclerotic thoracic or abdominal aorta or from a small infrarenal aortic aneurysm. A properly timed infusion CT scan of the thoracic and abdominal aorta usually provides the necessary anatomic detail for localizing the atheroembolic source without the risk of intra-arterial catheter manipulations. If the examination localizes the embolic source as a severely atherosclerotic infrarenal aorta, a shaggy thoracic or thoracoabdominal aorta, or a small aortic aneurysm, aortography should not be performed unless specific indications exist. Microembolization to the renal parenchyma can lead to renal insufficiency that prohibits the use of intravenous contrast agents. In these patients, magnetic resonance imaging of the aorta may be useful in detailing atherosclerotic disease of the thoracic and abdominal aorta (Fig. 24–3).

Because most atherosclerotic emboli are microscopic and occur in patients with intact extremity pulses, contrast-enhanced CT of the thoracic aorta and abdominal aorta has become the initial, and often only, diagnostic test for a large number of our patients who present with atherosclerotic embolization. This diagnostic work-up proceeds simultaneously with the treatment of the ischemic complications of the embolic event. Similar to all cases of extremity ischemia secondary to acute arterial occlusion, the first treatment is anticoagulation with heparin. The primary role of heparin is the prevention of further embolic events, a prevention that can be life-saving if the source of the embolus is actually cardiac. In addition, heparin also serves to limit the thrombotic complications distal to the embolus.

Thrombolytic therapy will apparently have a role in management of emboli that originate as thrombi in popliteal and upper extremity aneurysms, although the indications are still evolving. Because the emboli from aneurysms usually consist of organized thrombi, these emboli should be amenable to treatment with thrombolytic agents, and several small series have confirmed the utility of thrombolysis in these cases.[18] Giddings[18] demonstrated the efficacy of thrombolytic therapy in patients with popliteal aneurysms who present with distal embolization. We have obtained similar results. Livedo reticularis and blue digits are less frequently improved with thrombolytic therapy. The new onset of microembolic complications has been reported with the initiation of thrombolytic therapy.[19]

OPERATIVE TREATMENT OF ATHEROEMBOLISM

The rationale for aggressive operative intervention in patients with extremity manifestations of atherembolization is the dismal outcome in patients who do not undergo an operation. Short-term recurrence rates for extremity atheroembolization exceeding 75%[8,9] and tissue loss rates exceeding 60%[8] have been discussed, and the long-term survival in these patients, not surprisingly, is poor. For patients not undergoing an operation, Hollier et al[20] observed only one survivor among nine patients (11%) at 5 years' follow-up.

Although most patients with atheroembolization can be operated on with low morbidity and mortality, enthusiasm for pursuing operative intervention is tempered somewhat by the high mortality and morbidity that accompany surgical therapy in these patients. Among 96 patients operated on for extremity atheroemboli at Northwestern University Medical Center, 6 patients died (6% perioperative mortality). Perioperative renal failure secondary to renal atheroemboli appears to be the critical event that determines postoperative complications. Dialysis-dependent renal failure developed in 8% (5/65) of our patients who underwent aortic operations. Bauman et al[21] observed similar mortality and renal failure rates of 5% and 8%, respectively, in 62 patients.

In our series, the patients at highest risk for perioperative complications were those operated on for infrarenal aortic atheroembolic disease who had thrombus or irregular plaque extending above the level of the renal arteries on CT scans. All six deaths occurred in this group of patients. Although some of these patients presented with evidence of preoperative renal atheroembolization, intraoperative renal atheroembolization due to plaque or thrombus disruption at the time of suprarenal clamp placement could also be implicated. Green et al[22] postulated a similar mechanism to explain the demonstrated advantage of supraceliac as opposed to suprarenal clamping in patients with difficult infrarenal aneurysms. The single most important risk factor in their series was the presence of atherosclerotic debris in the nonaneurysmal juxtarenal segment where the proximal clamp was placed.[22] In addition to supraceliac clamp placement above the level of the atherosclerotic disease, selective, temporary renal artery clamping immediately before proximal aortic clamp placement can also reduce intraoperative renal atheroembolization.[23]

Additional operative techniques have been shown to decrease the incidence of extremity atheroembolization at the time of operation.[17] Distal clamping before proximal clamping decreases the risk that any plaque or thrombus that disrupts at the time of proximal clamp placement will embolize to the extremity arteries. In aortoiliac occlusive disease, the most common source of atheroemboli, the posterior common iliac artery plaque usually extends to the iliac bifurcation. Separate clamping of the external iliac and hypogastric arteries, rather than the distal common iliac artery, is associated with an incidence of intraoperative embolism of less than 1%.[24] Systemic heparin administered prior to the time of arterial clamp placement, irrigation with heparin-saline solution prior to completing the final anastomosis, and flushing of inflow and backbleeding of the outflow also serve to limit the incidence of intraoperative embolization of plaque or thrombus.

Even with attention to these judicious operative techniques, intraoperative embolization can occur, because sometimes it is not possible to place a clamp proximal to the atheroembolic segment (Fig. 24–4). The decreased renal function that accompanies renal atheroembolization is often reversible.[25] However, the acute loss of renal function

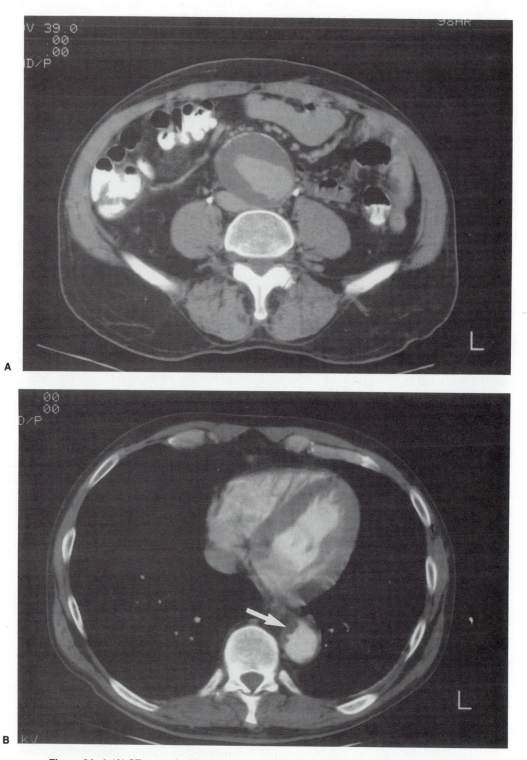

Figure 24–4. (A) CT scan of a 59-year-old man with a 5-cm thrombus-lined infrarenal aortic aneurysm who sustained intraoperative atheroemboli characterized by postoperative extremity, buttock, and flank livedo reticularis. **(B)** Thrombus is noted to extend proximally from the aneurysm all the way to the midthoracic aorta (arrow).

at the time of an aortic operation makes postoperative fluid management challenging. The treatment for patients who sustain intraoperative embolization at the time of operative repair consists of dextran in the early postoperative period followed by heparin, once the risk of postoperative retroperitoneal bleeding is decreased.

Because most atheroemboli originate in the infrarenal aorta and iliac arteries, definite operative treatment can be offered to these patients with the expectation of excellent clinical results. Atherosclerotic occlusive disease of the infrarenal aortoiliac segment that presents with atheroembolization is best managed by aortoiliac or aorto-femoral bypass. More focal disease can be managed successfully with endarterectomy and patch angioplasty. In our series, 55 patients with lower extremity atheroemboli were treated with aortic tube or bifurcation grafts, and 21 patients were treated with endarterectomy and patch angioplasty. Femoropopliteal bypass was performed in a smaller number of patients. Most upper extremity atheroembolic lesions require arterial bypass for treatment, but 20% of these lesions were treated with endartectomy and patch angioplasty in the Northwestern series.[14]

Atheroembolization has a predilection for patients with multiple organ failure. The reasons for this association between severe illness and atheroemboli are not clear, but Flory[3] discovered 50 years ago that the frequency of atheroembolization correlated closely with the severity of diffuse aortic atherosclerosis found at autopsy. In our series of 137 patients with extremity atheroemboli, operations were performed on 112 (82%) patients. Twenty-five patients (18%) were thought to be either at too high a risk for operative treatment or else refused operation. Arterial exclusion and extra-anatomic reconstruction is a reasonable option for patients with thoracic or abdominal aortic disease who are at too high a risk for direct aortic reconstruction.[26–28] Hollier et al[20] observed that external iliac artery exclusion and axillofemorofemoral bypass decreased the incidence of visceral atheroembolization, in addition to treating lower extremity atheroemboli. A possible explanation for this finding is the 18% decrease in mean aortic flow velocity, resulting in decreased aortic shear, following extra-anatomic reconstruction.[20]

Percutaneous transluminal angioplasty (PTLA) has become a primary interventional method for treating non-atheroembolic iliac occlusive disease, but its role in atheroembolic disease is not clear. PTLA has been used to treat atheroembolic lesions of the iliac and femoral arteries,[29] but no prospective studies have been performed comparing PTLA with standard operative therapy in atheroembolic disease. Because of the inherent instability of plaques that present with emboli, any endovascular intervention would appear to be fraught with risks of further embolic events occurring at the time of catheter manipulation. For this reason, we treat aortoiliac atheroembolization with PTLA only when the patient refuses operative therapy. Operations on the iliac arteries can be performed with minimal risk because they can usually be performed through oblique lower quadrant retroperitoneal incisions.

Atheroembolic disease of the thoracic aorta can be a particularly difficult problem to treat. For patients with disease localized to a short segment of the thoracic aorta, segmental repair with an interposition tube graft if the patient is at low risk is appropriate.[30] Diffuse disease characterized as the "shaggy aorta" is a more perplexing problem. Long-term anticoagulation with warfarin does not appear to be efficacious and often aggravates the underlying pathologic condition, leading to recurrent episodes.[31,32] For patients with atheroembolization from a thoracic source that is not treatable with an operation, we initiate dextran infusion followed by aspirin.

An operation is very effective in terminating the progression of the extremity ischemia. After operative treatment, only 10% of our patients required subsequent transmetatarsal or leg amputation, and another 10% eventually required digital amputation. These amputations are usually the sequelae of the atheroembolization that occurred prior to the definitive operation. Lumbar sympathectomy has been used in the treatment of the extremity ischemia that can occur with atheroemboli,[20,33] but its effectiveness has not been documented. Recurrent embolic episodes during postoperative follow-up occur in less than 2% of patients.[21] Embolic episodes in an arterial distribution different from the original atheroembolic source do occur, confirming the often systemic nature of this condition.

Atheroembolization to the renal parenchyma can occur at the time of attempted renal artery angioplasty.[16] Renal atheroembolization is often characterized by severe postprocedure hypertension.[34] The cause of the hypertension is excessive renin secretion due to emboli obstructing the preglomerular renal arterioles. The decreased renal perfusion pressure activates the renin-angiotensin axis, causing hypertension, while the decreased perfusion pressure leads to decreased renal excretory function. The hypertension that accompanies renal atheroembolization should be treated with agents other than angiotensin-converting enzyme inhibitors, because perfusion pressure in the efferent arterioles needs to be maintained to optimize renal parenchymal perfusion. Angiotensin-converting enzyme inhibitors can dilate the efferent arterioles and further decrease perfusion pressure, aggravating the renal insufficiency. Eosinophilia is seen in 80% of patients with renal atheroemboli and can aid in the diagnosis of this event.[35] Eosinophilia is otherwise uncommon in acute renal insufficiency. Atheroemboli can be seen at renal biopsy.

CONCLUSION

The mechanisms that cause some atherosclerotic plaques to embolize and others to remain stable are not known. The primary risk factors observed in patients who sustain atheroembolic events are similar to those seen in all patients with atherosclerosis. The processes responsible for disruption of the fibrous plaque that covers most atherosclerotic plaques are probably the key events that lead to atheroembolization.

REFERENCES

1. Panum PL. Experimentelle beitrage zur lehre von der embolie. *Virchows Arch Pathol Anat.* 1862;25:308–310.
2. Doch G. Some notes on coronary arteries. *M S Reporter.* 1896;75:1–7.
3. Flory CM. Arterial occlusions produced by emboli from eroded aortic atheromatous plaques. *Am J Pathol.* 1945;21:549–565.
4. Venet L, Friedfeld L. Avulsion and embolization of a calcific arterial plaque: femoral embolectomy. *Surgery.* 1952;32:119–122.
5. Thurlbeck WM, Castleman B. Atheromatous emboli to the kidneys after aortic surgery. *N Engl J Med.* 1957;257:442–447.
6. Hoye SJ, Teitelbaum S, Gore I, Warren R. Atheromatous embolization a factor in peripheral gangrene. *N Engl J Med.* 1959;261:128–131.
7. Kazmier FJ, Sheps SG, Bernatz PE, Sayre GP. Livedo reticularis and digital infarcts: a syndrome due to cholesterol emboli arising from atheromatous abdominal aortic aneurysm. *Vasc Dis.* 1966;3:12–24.
8. Karmody AM, Powers SR, Monaco VJ, et al. "Blue-toe" syndrome: an indication for limb salvage surgery. *Arch Surg.* 1976;3:1263–1268.

9. Kempczinski RF. Lower-extremity arterial emboli from ulcerating atherosclerotic plaques. *JAMA*. 1979;241:807–810.

10. Richards AM, Eliot RS, Kanjuh VI, et al. Cholesterol embolism: a multiple disease masquerading as polyartreitis nodosa. *Am J Cardiol*. 1965;5:696–707.

11. Cappiello RA, Espinoza LR, Adelman H, et al. Cholesterol embolism: a pseudovasculitic syndrome. *Semin Arthritis Rheum*. 1989;18:240–246.

12. Kempczinski RF. Atheroembolism. In: Kempszinski RF, ed. *The Ischemic Leg*. Chicago: Year Book; 1985:81–93.

13. Lilly MP, Flinn WR, McCarthy WJ, et al. The effect of distal arterial anatomy on the success of popliteal aneurysm repair. *J Vasc Surg*. 1988;7:653–660.

14. Mesh CL, Yao JST. Upper extremity bypass: five-year follow-up. In: Yao JST, Pearce WH, eds. *Long-Term Results in Vascular Surgery*. Norwalk Conn: Appleton & Lange; 1993:353–365.

15. Baxter BT, McGee GS, Flinn WR, et al. Distal embolization as a presenting symptom of aortic aneurysms. *Am J Surg*. 1990;160:197–201.

16. Gaines PA, Kennedy A, Moorhead P, et al. Cholesterol embolisation: a lethal complication of vascular catheterisation. *Lancet*. 1988;1:168–170.

17. Keen RR, Yao JST. Aneurysms and embolization: detection and management. In: Yao JST, Pearce WH, eds. *Aneurysms: New Findings and Treatments*. Norwalk, Conn: Appleton & Lange; 1994:305–313.

18. Giddings AEB. Influence of thrombolytic therapy in the management of popliteal aneurysms. In: Yao JST, Pearce WH. eds. *Aneurysms: New Findings and Treatments*. Norwalk, Conn: Appleton & Lange; 1994:493–508.

19. Bhardwaj M, Goldweit R, Erlebacher J, et al. Tissue plasminogen activator and cholesterol crystal embolization. *Ann Intern Med*. 1989;11:687–688.

20. Hollier LH, Kazmier FJ, Ochsner J, et al. "Shaggy" aorta syndrome with atheromatous embolization to visceral vessels. *Ann Vasc Surg*. 1991;5:439–444.

21. Baumann DS, McGraw D, Rubin BG, Allen BT. An institutional experience with arterial atheroembolism. *Ann Vasc Surg*. 1994;8:258–265.

22. Green RM, Ricotta JJ, Ouriel K, DeWeese JA. Results of supraceliac aortic clamping in the difficult elective resection of infrarenal abdominal aortic aneurysm. *J Vasc Surg*. 1989;9:125–134.

23. Starr DS, Lawrie GM, Morris GC Jr. Prevention of distal embolism during arterial reconstruction. *Am J Surg*. 1979;138:764–769.

24. Imparato AM. Abdominal aortic surgery: prevention of lower limb ischemia. *Surgery*. 1983;93:112–116.

25. McGowan JA, Greenberg A. Cholesterol atheroembolic renal disease. *Am J Nephrol*. 1986;6:135–139.

26. Kaufman JL, Saifi J, Chang BB, et al. The role of extraanatomic exclusion bypass in the treatment of disseminated atheroembolism syndrome. *Ann Vasc Surg*. 1990;4:260–263.

27. Friedman SG, Krishnasastry KV. Eternal iliac ligation and axillary-bifemoral bypass for blue toe syndrome. *Surgery*. 1994;115:27–30.

28. Kazmier FJ. Shaggy aorta syndrome and disseminated atheromatous embolization. In: Bergan JJ, Yao JST, eds. *Aortic Surgery*. Philadelphia: WB. Saunders; 1989:189–194.

29. Jenkins DM, Newton WD. Atheroembolism. *Am Surg*. 1991;57:588–591.

30. Rubin BG, Allen BT, Anderson CB, et al. An embolizing lesion in a minimally diseased aorta. *Surgery*. 1992;112:607–610.

31. Bruns FJ, Segel DP, Adler S. Case report: control of cholesterol embolization by discontinuation of anticoagulant therapy. *Am J Med Sci*. 1978;275:105–108.

32. Hyman BT, Landas SK, Ashman RF, et al. Warfarin-related purple toes syndrome and cholesterol microembolization. *Am J Med*. 1987;82:1233–1237.

33. Mehigan JT, Stoney RJ. Lower extremity atheromatous embolization. *Am J Surg*. 1976;132:163–167.

34. Dahlberg PJ, Frecentese DF, Cogbill TH. Cholesterol embolism: experience with 22 histologically proven cases. *Surgery*. 1989;105:737–746.

35. Kasinath BSM, Corwin HL, Bidani AK, et al. Eosinophilia in the diagnosis of atheroembolic renal disease. *Am J Nephrol*. 1987;7:173–177.

25

Treatment of Blue Toe Syndrome with Intra-Arterial Injections of Prostaglandin E$_1$

Juan C. Parodi, MD

The blue toe syndrome is caused by the embolization of atherosclerotic debris and cholesterol, usually arising from the abdominal aorta. This microembolization is often multiple and recurrent. Components of the embolic material include fibrin, platelets, blood cells, and cholesterol crystals. Atheroembolism is frequently misdiagnosed because many microemboli remain clinically silent. Massive or recurrent microembolization, however, may produce profound ischemia. Atheromatous embolization is one of the most challenging diagnostic and therapeutic problems for vascular surgeons. Atheroembolism probably creates a vicious circle that perpetuates the ischemic process. Activation of leukocytes and complement initiate tissue damage. Platelet aggregation and release of 5-hydroxy-tryptamine and thromboxane promote intravascular coagulation, which further aggravate the initial insult.[1]

Management of microembolization includes removing the source of the emboli; if the condition is severe, treatment of the microcirculation should be considered. Medical management includes the use of heparin, dextran, papaverine, urokinase, vasodilators, high doses of corticosteroids,[2,3] and lumbar sympathectomy, among others. Unfortunately, results are not uniformly good. Often atheroembolism produces tissue loss or even death.

Keen and Yao[3] reported on a series of 15 patients with spontaneous distal embolization as an initial presenting symptom of abdominal aortic aneurysm (AAA). Twenty percent required major amputation and 33% minor amputation. Progressive renal failure occurred 33% with a mortality of 13%. In 1985, because of the failure of standard treatment of atheromatous embolization, at Instituo Cardiovascular de Buenos Aires, Argentina, we initiated a study of intra-arterial prostaglandin E$_1$ (PGE$_1$) therapy in patients with severe microembolization. This report is based on our experience treating 16 patients affected by severe atheroembolism with intra-arterial PGE$_1$.

Prostaglandins were discovered in 1930 by Kurzrock and Lieb.[4] von Euler in 1934, coined the term *prostaglandin* because he mistook the substance for a secretory product of the prostate. PGE$_1$ has several biologic activities that make it a suitable drug for maintaining patency of the microcirculation. Prostanoids have been used extensively in Europe since 1973 to treat peripheral arterial disease.[5-7] Prostanoids used in clinical studies include prostacyclin (PGI_2), PGE_1, and the chemically stable prostacyclin analogue, iloprost. PGI_2 is chemically unstable and needs to be given at high pH, which has the potential to cause vascular damage. PGE_1 is used intra-arterially because one passage through the lungs inactivates it. Once the decision to treat the patient is made, a 3-F size multiperforated catheter is advanced percutaneously via common femoral artery into the popliteal artery in an antegrade manner. Mild analgesia is used. Heparin is administered (500 U per hour intravenously) during the intra-arterial injection. Alprostadil (Prostin Pediatric; Upjohn, Kalamazoo, Mich), 250 μg diluted in 200 mL of normal saline solution, is administered with an automatic injector every 2 to 4 hours depending on the vasodilator effect of PGE_1. In one patient with renal involvement, the catheter was placed in the suprarenal aorta. The injection is repeated, according to the response, either on the same day or on subsequent days. In the present series, the total dose varied from 1,000 to 8,000 μg of PGE_1, and treatment lasted 1 to 5 days. One patient received a second series of injections 1 week after the first series.

MATERIAL AND METHODS

Since 1985, 16 patients admitted to our clinic with the diagnosis of blue toe syndrome were treated with intra-arterial injections of PGE_1. Criteria for inclusion in the trial included all the following features: (a) persistent pain resistant to medication; (b) severe ischemia with risk of tissue loss; (c) presence of distal pulses or positive Doppler signal. Patients with asymptomatic or mild microembolization were not included in this series.

In this analysis we are considering only those patients suffering from occlusion of small arteries (muscular and dermal). Distal pulses or Doppler signals were present in all patients. Macroemboli that necessitated surgical removal of occluding material were excluded. Visceral arteries were affected in some patients, aggravating the condition greatly. Spinal cord ischemia was seen in massive microembolization from the abdominal aorta. Other potential clinical findings, not seen by us but described in the medical literature[2] are adrenal infarction and penile gangrene.

Fifteen patients were men and one was a woman. The average age was 68 years (range, 58–76 years). The clinical presentation included livedo reticularis, blue toes, blue finger (thoracic outlet syndrome), skin necrosis, leg pain, weight loss, abdominal pain, hematuria, anuria, spinal cord injury, and uncontrollable hypertension (Table 25–1). The most common source of atheroemboli was the abdominal aorta (Table

TABLE 25–1. CLINICAL PRESENTATION

Signs and Symptoms	No. of Patients (%)
Severe limb pain	16 (100)
Livedo reticularis	16 (100)
Elevation of creatine phosphokinase	16 (100)
Abdominal pain	4 (25)
Uncontrollable hypertension	4 (25)
Renal failure requiring dialysis	4 (25)
Weight loss	2 (12)
Paraparesis	1 (6)

TABLE 25–2. CAUSES OF ATHEROEMBOLYSM

Causes	No. of Patients
Related to AAA	
Spontaneous	6
Following resection	1
Endoluminal graft	3
Iatrogenic	3
Thoracic outlet syndrome	1
Popliteal	1
Iliac stenosis	1
TOTAL	16

25–2) followed by the subclavian artery, popliteal artery, and iliac artery. Treatment of the source of the atheroemboli was by arterial replacement, endoluminal graft, or stent (Table 25–3).

Endoluminal treatment was performed using the technique described by the author.[8] The aneurysm or the atheromatous aorta is excluded by placing a Dacron graft over the inner surface of the diseased artery. The Dacron graft is fixed in place by two Palmaz balloon expandable stents attached to the ends of the graft. One patient underwent aortic stent graft placement because of a "shaggy aorta."

CLINICAL EXPERIENCE

Sixteen patients were treated with intra-arterial injection of PGE_1. They were grouped according to the source of emboli. Sources of microemboli were defined with aortography and computed tomography. Histologic studies of skin and muscle were performed on two patients. Catheter entrance was percutaneous through the brachial artery to prevent further embolization when lower extremities were affected (15 patients) or the femoral retrograde approach was needed to study upper extremities (1 patient).

We used the criteria for diagnosis of AAA as a source of emboli, as reported by Keen and Yao.[3] They described CT findings in patients who sustained spontaneous microembolization from an AAA as (a) irregular luminal surface, (b) multiple lumens, (c) heterogeneity of the thrombus, (d) calcification within the thrombus, (e) fissures extending from the lumen into the thrombus, and (f) noncontiguous areas of intraluminal thrombus. In seven of the 15 patients reported, an aortogram failed to depict the presence of an AAA.

TABLE 25–3. TREATMENT OF THE SOURCE OF EMBOLISM[a]

Procedure	No. of Patients
AAA resection	3
AAA endoluminal treatment	3
Aortobifemoral bypass	2
Resection of cervical rib	1
Resection of popliteal aneurysm	1
Iliac stenting	1

[a] AAA, abdominal aortic aneurysm.

RESULTS

In the two cases of massive microembolization caused by endoluminal treatment of aneurysms, the intra-arterial injection of PGE_1 gave only temporary and partial improvement of perfusion. Both patients died of multiorgan failure. One patient developed parapareses from spinal cord emboli. One patient affected with an AAA and recurrent renal and lower limb microembolization was successfully treated with a stented graft after distal ischemia was relieved with PGE_1. He was anuric and on dialysis. Immediately after the aneurysm was excluded, the patient started to make urine. Unfortunately, he suffered a massive pulmonary embolism and died.

The improvement in renal function immediately after aneurysm exclusion in two patients indicated that continuous microembolization is an important factor in renal failure, and perhaps interruption of this continuous shower of microemboli will improve renal function.

The other 13 patients had relief of the distal ischemia and had only minor tissue loss. Long-term follow-up information was available for seven of the 13 survivors, and all of them had favorable outcomes. Persistent causalgia-like pain 6 months after treatment was a complaint of one patient, who had clinically significant distal embolization. The 30-day mortality was 18%.

DISCUSSION

Atheroembolism is a rare condition that is becoming more common as the number of endovascular procedures increases. In addition, the aging of the population increases the incidence of shaggy aortas and aortic aneurysms, other causes of atheroembolism. The widespread use of anticoagulants and thrombolytic agents may unmask the presence of such conditions that initiates the shower of atheroembolism. Anticoagulants may precipitate atheroembolism by preventing the formation of a protective thrombus. Streptokinase and urokinase may dissolve overlying thrombus.[2]

Sources of arterioarterial embolization can be divided into either spontaneous or iatrogenic. Spontaneous microembolization occurs as a results of several conditions, including proximal aneurysms (thoracic, abdominal, iliac, femoral, or popliteal), complicated atheromatous plaques, and intimal ulcers. Aneurysms of the upper extremities embolize more frequently than aneurysms of the lower extremities.[9]

Dahlberg et al[2] in 1989 reported on 22 histologically proven cases of atheroembolism not caused by aneurysms. Eight patients had peripheral embolism and 14 had visceral atheroembolism with or without peripheral embolism. Precipitating factors in this series were angiographic procedures and anticoagulation. Iatrogenic causes include endovascular instrumentation, either diagnostic or therapeutic, and surgical procedures applied to treat occlusive disease or aneurysmal disease.

Until now, the treatment of atheroembolism has been limited to controlling the source of embolization. In most instances, removing the source of the emboli was sufficient, and the consequences of embolization subsided leaving little residual. However, atheroembolism may produce tissue or limb loss and on occasion the death of the patient. We have tried corticosteroids in high doses, heparin, local urokinase, papaverine, sodium nitroprusside, nitroglycerin, and sympathectomy, all with poor results. The encouraging results with PGE_1 in Buerger's disease induced us to try the drug for severe atheroembolism.

TABLE 25–4. EFFECTS OF PROSTAGLANDIN E₁ (ALPROSTADIL)

Vasodilatation

Inhibition of white cell function
   Macrophage activation
   Neutrophil chemotaxis and release of oxygen radicals
   Leukotrienes and lysosomal enzymes

Inhibition of coagulation
   Platelet adhesion and aggregation
   Activation of factor X
   Promotion of fibrinolysis

Modification of the erythrocyte deformability and aggregation

Cytoprotection[a]

Inhibition of the proliferative and mitotic activity of vascular smooth muscle cells

[a] Cytoprotection is an ill-defined pharmacologic property of PGE_1. The drug preserves myocardial function in isolated heart preparations and in intact animals after ischemia-reperfusion injury. A membrane-stabilizing action is also suggested in animal experiments.

PGE_1 (Table 25–4) is a potent vasodilator that activates fibrinolysis and inhibits leukocyte migration and activation. Therefore, leukocyte release of leukotrienes, oxygen free radicals, and proteolytic enzymes is also inhibited. In addition, PGE_1 provokes platelet disaggregation and inhibits platelet release of thromboxane and 5-hydroxytryptamine. PGE_1 increases the deformability of the red blood cells and has an antiproliferative action of vascular smooth muscle cells. Finally PGE_1 is protective of the endothelium by unknown mechanics.[10–12]

PGE_1 is transported in the bloodstream bound to albumin (81% to 99%). Seventy to ninety percent of the drug administered intra-arterially is metabolized in the lung during the first passage, and metabolites are eliminated by the kidneys. Carlson et al[13] found that vasodilatation was persistent in time in spite of the short action of the PGE_1. Dormandy[14] suggested that intermittent treatment with prostaglandin augments endogenous prostanoid activity. This observation could be another explanation for the persistence of the changes induced by the drug. Absence of side effects other than pain and swelling makes this treatment attractive. The clinical effect takes place in a few minutes. Pain relief and capillary filling are evident almost immediately after the injection of PGE_1 (Table 25–5). Iloprost, a stable PGI_2, can be used intravenously. It has the advantage of avoiding arterial puncture. Gruss[15] reported on his experience with intravenous PGE_1 in patients with postoperative trash foot; there was only one treatment failure among eight patients.

The relationship between stented graft and microembolization deserves special comment. Atheroembolization is the most dreaded complication of the use of stented grafts for endoluminal treatment of AAA.[8] However, endoluminal exclusion of AAA is an emerging tool to treat microembolization from aneurysms. At first glance, it

TABLE 25–5. SIDE EFFECTS OF PGE₁

Effect	Rate (%)
Local pain in the treated limb	100
Swelling of the limb	10
Hematoma, false aneurysm, infection at the site of arterial puncture[a]	
Headaches, anorexia, diarrhea[a]	

[a] Reported by others[6] in longer periods of treatment.

seems unreasonable to use a therapy for a condition that can be caused by the proposed technique. The explanation for this dispute is that aneurysms that embolize spontaneously are usually small.[3,8] Small aneurysms have straight iliac arteries, and aortic aneurysms are usually non-tortuous. Conversely, aneurysms that embolize during endoluminal treatment are very large, tortuous, and have iliac arteries that were elongated.

CONCLUSION

Intra-arterial injection of PGE$_1$ appears to be an effective treatment of severe microembolization when all other treatments have failed. No conclusions can be reached in regard to the effect of PGE$_1$ on visceral microembolization because of the small number of patients. Dramatic response in severe distal ischemia caused by atheroembolism motivated the report of these initial results because other treatments are usually ineffective. The side effects and complications of the proposed method are minimal (see Table 25–2). Surgical or endoluminal treatment of the primary source of atheromatous embolization should be performed to prevent recurrence. Prevention of embolization is recommended by judicious use of endoluminal diagnostic and therapeutic methods when needed.

REFERENCES

1. Ernst E, Hammersschmidt DE, Bagge U, et al. Leukocytes and risk of ischemic diseases. *JAMA*. 1987;257:2318–2324.
2. Dahlberg PJ, Frecentese DF, Cogbill TH. Cholesterol embolism: experience with 22 histologically proven cases. *Surgery*. 1989;105:737–747.
3. Keen RR, Yao JST. Aneurysms and embolization: detection and management. In: Yao JST, Pearce WH, eds. *Aneurysms: New Findings and Treatment*. Norwalk, Conn: Appleton & Lange; 1994:305–314.
4. Kurzrock L, Lieb CC. Biochemical studies of human semen. *Proc Soc Exp Biol Med*. 1930;28:268.
5. Carlson LA, Erikson I. Femoral artery infusion of prostraglandin E$_1$ in severe peripheral vascular disease. *Lancet*. 1973;1:155.
6. Altstaedt H, Berzewski B, et al. Treatment of patients with peripheral arterial occlusive disease fontaine stage IV with intravenous iloprost and PGE$_1$: a randomized open controlled study. *Prostaglandins Leukotriene Essential Fatty Acids*. 1993;49:573–578.
7. Gruss JD, Vargas MD. Use of prostaglandins in arterial occlusive diseases. *Int Angiol*. 1984;3:7–16.
8. Parodi JC, Barone HD. Transfemoral placement of aortic graft in aortic aneurysm: clinical experience in patients. In: Yao JST, Pearce WH, eds. *Aneurysms: New Findings and Treatment*. Norwalk, Conn: Appleton & Lange; 1994:341–352.
9. Pearce WH, Tropea BI, Baxter BT, Yao JST. Arterial complications in the thoracic outlet. *Semin Vasc Surg*. 1990;3:236–241.
10. Sinzinger H, Rogatti W. Prostaglandin E$_1$ in der therapieder peripheren arteriellen durch blutungsstorung. *Wien Klin Wochenschr*. 1991;103:558–565.
11. Krais T, Muller B. Iloprost in peripheral vascular disease. *Cardiovas Drug Rev*. 1991;9:158–171.
12. Hirai M, Nakayama R. Haemodinamic effects of intra-arterial and intravenous administration of prostaglandin E$_1$ in patients with peripheral vascular disease. *Br J Surg*. 1986;73: 20–23.

13. Carlson LA, Ericsson M, Ericsson U. Prostaglandin E_1 in peripheral arteriographies. *Acta Radiol Diagn.* 1972;14:583.

14. Dormandy JA. *European consensus document on critical limb ischemia.* European Working Group on Critical Limb Ischemia. Berlin, Germany: Springer-Verlag; 1989.

15. Gruss JD. Experience with PGE_1 in patients with postoperative trash foot. *Vasa[Suppl].* 28:57–60.

VII

Correction of Inflow Lesions for Lower Extremity Ischemia

26

Current Techniques in the Assessment of Aortoiliac Inflow

D. Eugene Strandness, Jr, MD

In terms of incidence, it would appear that aortoiliac atherosclerosis is second to that found in the superficial femoral artery. From a clinical standpoint involvement at this level is an important cause of severe intermittent claudication. However, when aortoiliac disease is found in combination with disease in the superficial femoropopliteal segment and below the knee, critical ischemia is frequently present. The implications, depending on the level of involvement, are entirely different, and the evaluation process must be varied to conform to the questions that need resolution.

The traditional approach, which is still of great value, is the history followed by a carefully performed physical examination. The physical examination revolves around the detection of bruits with or without associated pulse deficits. Before considering some of the more direct approaches to resolving the status of the aortoiliac inflow to the legs, it is necessary to review some of the important factors relating to exercise that are relevant to this discussion.

From a hemodynamic standpoint, atherosclerosis results in a gradual buildup of material within the lumen that in its most severe form leads to total occlusion. A most important question relates to the point where the developing stenosis is sufficient to lead to the development of symptoms with exercise. Exercise increases the need for flow to an amount determined by the workload and the amount of ischemia that develops.[1] For most applications, the degree of narrowing necessary to produce a pressure and flow reduction is referred to as the *critical* stenosis.[2] This is determined under resting flow conditions. However, it is well known that lesions can exist that do not produce a pressure drop at rest but do so with the flow increase needed by exercise.[3] From a clinical standpoint, these patients have "disappearing" pulses.

Patients with the less than critical stenosis who had intermittent claudication have the following findings:

1. They give a history typical of intermittent claudication.
2. Pulses are palpable at the level of the foot and are thought to be normal.
3. A bruit often is detected over the iliac artery on the symptomatic side.
4. With exercise to the point of leg pain, the pulses at the level of the foot disappear.

5. If a bruit was present, it would be accentuated by the increase in flow required of the exercise. If a bruit was not detected under resting flow conditions, it would most certainly be present immediately after exercise.[4]

Given this scenario, the diagnosis would be quite clear. Furthermore, it would be very likely that the lesion would be a stenotic one and not a total occlusion. In this setting, given the success with transluminal angioplasty, the patient would be scheduled for the procedure at the time the arteriogram was to be performed. However, this is not the most common problem seen; furthermore, there are situations in which the determination of the hemodynamic significance of a lesion can be difficult and very important.

ISOLATED AORTOILIAC DISEASE

The involvement of the aortoiliac system can lead to the most severe intermittent claudication that we observe.[1] This is because the entire limb, hips, and buttock can be deprived of normal arterial input. This means that during the course of exercise, the entire limb is ischemic, as contrasted to just the calf muscles in cases of superficial femoral artery occlusion. During exercise, the parts of the limb farthest away from the heart are the most ischemic and are the last to be repaid the oxygen debt that occurs with exercise. In general, the ankle–brachial index will be less than 0.9 but greater than 0.5, which is common with single segment disease.

The findings are usually straightforward at physical examination with a reduction in the amplitude of the femoral pulse with or without an associated bruit. Because one is never certain on the basis of the physical examination alone whether the disease is confined to the aortoiliac segment, it is necessary to carry out some further testing. Although the extent of disease also can be determined at the time of arteriography, there is evidence that a duplex ultrasonic (US) scan can be performed. The duplex US scan should help the clinician:

1. Assess the location of the arterial lesion.
2. Determine if the lesions are stenotic lesions or total occlusions.
3. Plan the therapy on the basis of the findings.[5]

If the lesion is confined to the aortoiliac segment, the only determination remaining is whether the therapy to be provided be endovascular or direct arterial surgery. There would seem to be little disagreement at the present time about the treatment of stenotic lesions in this area. The results with balloon angioplasty are sufficiently good to warrant this as the preferred form of therapy. Both the short-and long-term results are sufficiently good balloon angioplasty should be performed rather than surgery. The problem becomes more complex in cases of total occlusion, particularly if the segment is long and associated with marked calcification.

MULTILEVEL DISEASE

The problem from a diagnostic standpoint is multilevel disease in which the decision is to intervene at the aortoiliac level either as a primary procedure or in combination with a procedure distal to the inguinal ligament. It must be remembered that this pertains only to instances in which the lesions in the aortoiliac area are stenoses in which the determination of hemodynamic significance is the most important question that needs to be answered.

Hemodynamic significance can be determined in many ways, but it is important to remember that if one uses arteriography alone, considerable errors can occur. Sumner and Strandness[6] in a study that examined outcome after reconstruction noted that in patients with both proximal and distal disease, correction of the aortoiliac disease alone did not result in improvement in 19% of patients. This rate is obviously unacceptable and does not represent a failure of the reconstruction but reflects the hemodynamic significance of the lesions in the aortoiliac region that were mistakenly bypassed. Many methods have been proposed to minimize this problem, including segmental limb pressures, pulse volume recordings, duplex US scanning, and finally intraarterial pressure recordings done at the time of arteriography or in the operating room.[7]

To be useful the diagnostic methods employed must be able to document the presence and levels of involvement by atherosclerosis. Segmental pressures in theory should provide some information, but they have serious limitations, some of which are as follows[8]:

1. A low pressure from any level of the limb does not tell the examiner anything about the nature of the lesion itself (stenosis vs occlusion).
2. The pressures are artifactually high, particularly at the upper thigh level. This is due to the mismatch between the circumference of the thigh and that of the cuff.
3. A pressure drop from the upper thigh to above the knee that exceeds 20 mm Hg is suggestive of disease in the superficial femoral artery but can be misleading both as to the presence of a lesion and its length and nature (stenosis vs occlusion). This can be very important from a therapeutic standpoint.

Role of Duplex Ultrasonic Scanning

With the availability of duplex US scanning, we can directly examine the suspected areas of involvement at any level of the circulation. The criteria originally described by Jager et al[9] are still usable in practice although some investigators have slightly modified the criteria that can be used. Before reviewing the application of this method, it is important to emphasize that duplex US scanning for peripheral arterial disease should only be done when the patient is considered a candidate for some form of intervention. It is in this setting that it can be most profitably used so assess areas of involvement and assess hemodynamic status.

The hemodynamics of the arterial system must be understood if one is to properly use duplex US scanning. This is because imaging per se is not sufficient either to detect areas of involvement or to assess their hemodynamic significance. The principles most important to remember are as follows[10]:

1. The lower extremity arterial bed under resting conditions is a high-resistance circuit where reverse flow should normally be seen to the level of the pedal arteries at the ankle. Thus the absence of reverse flow at any level of the lower limb is abnormal, signifying the presence of arterial disease proximal to the recording site.
2. The normal velocity patterns seen are triphasic (forward-reverse-forward) flow.[11]
3. There is a gradual decrease in the peak systolic velocity as one proceeds down the limb.[12]

4. Although it is possible to record absolute velocities along the course of any peripheral artery, the range of normal values is so wide that this measurement has little value particularly in the detection of minimal disease.

5. All studies in both normal and abnormal situations *must* be done with a constant angle of incidence of the sound beam with the long axis of the artery. We have shown that the preferable angle for such studies is 60°. While it is true that most modern instruments can provide what is referred to as angle-corrected velocity, this is best termed *angle-adjusted velocity*.[13]

The scanning procedure normally includes the entire arterial system from the level of the abdominal aorta to the arteries below the knee. Because most important impediment to ultrasound is the presence of air in the bowel, these studies are usually scheduled in the early morning after the patient has fasted all night. In performing the scan, the technologist uses findings to be of assistance in the scanning process. The most important of these is the type of waveforms being recorded and the changes that take place when the sample volume is moved from segment to segment. The change in the peak systolic frequency (velocity) from one segment of artery to the next is the most important finding. The criteria at which my colleagues and I have arrived at through our validation studies are as follows[9,14]:

1. A triphasic waveform is very likely to be found distal to normal arteries or those with minimal disease (<50%).

2. At sites of narrowing there is an increase in peak systolic velocity that reflects the degree of narrowing as follows:
   a. Minimal wall disease—no change in peak systolic velocity but minor increase in the amount of spectral broadening (1% to 19%).
   b. 20% to 49% stenosis—an increase in the peak systolic velocity of 30% to 100% from the previous segment. The reverse flow component may be preserved but there is spectral broadening.
   c. 50% to 99% stenosis—a greater than 100% increase in the peak systolic velocity, loss of the reverse flow component, and marked spectral broadening.
   d. Total occlusion—loss of signal from visualized arterial segment.

Color Doppler US, which is the most recent addition to the technology of duplex US scanning can be used both as a pathfinder for the arteries of interest and also can be used profitably in a qualitative sense to document the location and degree of stenosis.[15,16] However, with most current systems, one must not use the color alone to document the velocity changes because the Color Doppler tends to underestimate the changes that are occurring. One must use both the color and the fast Fourier transform method of spectrum analysis to be certain of the presence of stenosis and to estimate its severity. The criteria that have been tested with the color system are as follows:

1. The triphasic flow response. Because the reverse flow component noted in normal arteries can be seen in color by the sudden transition to blue in late systole, if found it is suggestive that the arteries proximal to that point are hemodynamically normal.

2. Because turbulence induces random flow, the color changes are dramatic, representing the admixture of colors associated with multiple flow vectors with different directions relative to the sound beam. It is probably valid to

assume that such changes are associated with greater than 50% diameter-reducing stenosis.

3. Another feature of color Doppler US is that turbulence induces arterial wall vibration, which is responsible for the detected bruit. Because this vibration can be transmitted to the soft tissues, it can also be seen in the color display. When the vibration is detected in conjunction with turbulence, it can be assumed that a pressure and flow reducing stenosis may be present.

4. Occlusions are recognized by absence of flow and by the appearance of collateral arteries which by virtue of their change in direction away from the transducer produce a sudden color change to an apparently higher velocity (Doppler angle is 0°).

The experience with color Doppler US suggests that it may save time in the examination and that it is also very useful below the knee, which is often a quite difficult area to examine with conventional black-and-white duplex US systems.

Implications of Duplex US Findings on Decision Making

The manner in which both the noninvasive and invasive diagnostic studies are used depend entirely on the clinical presentation and the questions that need to be answered. It has been known for a considerable period of time that the interpretation of angiographic images in the aortoiliac area can be difficult. Even with multiple views of this segment, the correlation between what is seen and what is present hemodynamically can be very difficult. Thiele and I[17] reported on the comparison between arteriographic recordings and intra-arterial pressure recordings in 73 aortoiliac segments. In 39 of the segments, significant pressure drops were recorded at the time of arteriography. Two vascular surgeons reviewed the arteriograms without prior knowledge of the pressure-gradient results. The results of this study were as follows:

1. Reader 1 identified 34 aortoiliac segments as being hemodynamically significant. In 24 cases they were.
2. Reader 2 identified 37 arteries as significant. In 27 cases, this was verified by the pressure recordings.
3. For those 34 aortoiliac segments that did not have a significant pressure gradient, reader 1 correctly identified 27 and reader 2, 24.

This study confirmed our clinical impressions that visual classification of arteriographically visualized stenoses is not a simple matter. Furthermore, if one depends entirely on such estimates, serious clinical errors can be made. What can one do to improve the accuracy of the screening process and ensure proper direction for the patient?

The use of segmental pressures and simple continuous-wave Doppler US at the level of the common femoral artery can be of some help, but the information is not specific enough to make the necessary distinctions in many cases. What is needed is to identify the features that will point the physician in the correct direction. It is here where duplex US scanning can have an important impact. I use this information as follows:

1. If the velocities recorded from the aorta and the iliac arteries are normal, one can rule out this area as a cause of hemodynamic abnormalities.
2. If an occlusion is detected, one can be very certain it exists and plan therapy on the basis of the status of the disease in the opposite iliac artery segment and that below the knee.

3. If a less than 50% stenosis is found, the femoropopliteal segment is patient, and the patient describes intermittent claudication, one should measure the pressure gradient across the suspected area before and after the injection of a vasodilating agent such as papaverine.

4. If greater than 50% diameter-reducing stenosis is detected but the femoropopliteal segment is normal, one can proceed with a transluminal angioplasty, measuring pressure gradients before and after the procedure.

A patient with multilevel disease is more difficult to evaluate because an accurate delineation of sites of increased resistance to flow is necessary. However, in this setting, it is also important to base the studies and their interpretation on the clinical presentation. The most reasonable classification is as follows:

1. Intermittent claudication alone. With multilevel disease, the claudication is usually very severe. It is also true that if complete relief of the problem is desired, all levels of disease that are hemodynamically significant must be treated. However, if there is significant disease in the aortoiliac area, correction of this problem alone may result in considerable improvement. The availability of transluminal angioplasty for the iliac arteries has created a new opportunity for patients in this category. For example, if there is a tight aortoiliac stenosis and a superficial femoral occlusion, it may be possible to treat the proximal lesion by angioplasty and the femoral lesion by bypass grafting. This simplifies treatment considerably for patients while offering complete relief of their symptoms.

2. Critical ischemia. For a patient with ischemic rest pain alone, improvement in inflow to the level of the profunda femoris artery may be all that is required. However, with ulceration and gangrene, maximal blood flow may be needed to ensure healing and avoid an amputation. Again as in No. 1, correction of the proximal lesion by angioplasty followed by a bypass is the most direct and successful approach to this problem.

Given the foregoing classification, my current approach is as follows. If the patient is a candidate for intervention on the basis of the clinical presentation, I proceed with a duplex US scan. If this does not show aortoiliac disease, attention can be directed to the arteries distal to the groin. If the proximal arterial segments are diseased but still patent, I recommend balloon angioplasty as the first procedure. If only the proximal segment of the arterial system is involved, no further therapy is needed at that time. If there is additional disease distal to the inguinal ligament, it would have to be treated with the final decision depending on the clinical status of the patient.

How does this approach work and does it have an impact on the decision-making process and outcome? To test this hypothesis, I enlisted the cooperation of six well-known vascular surgeons to review data provided to study this question.[18] The data from both arteriography and duplex US scanning along with the clinical history and ankle/brachial index was provided to each surgeon. The duplex US and arteriographic results were transferred to an anatomic diagram and submitted in a random manner in two batches. The surgeons were allowed to choose from a treatment plan that offered eight different options, which were as follows:

1. Angioplasty
2. No intervention
3. Endarterectomy
4. Aortobifemoral bypass

5. Femorofemoral bypass
6. Femoropopliteal bypass
7. Combined aortofemoral and femoropopliteal bypass
8. Other

The interobserver agreement between different surgeons was quite good ($\kappa = 0.70$). However, when the interobserver κ statistic was considered, it was not as high ($\kappa = 0.56$). It is of interest that there was considerable disagreement in 43% of the cases in which the data available from the duplex US scan and arteriogram were essentially identical. We concluded that a considerable part of the decision-making process was based more on experience and preference and not on the data per se. Legemate et al[19] also addressed the potential for arteriography to be replaced by duplex US scanning. In their studies of the aortoiliac segment, the sensitivity was 92% and the specificity was 98%. For the detection of occlusions in the aortoiliac system, both the sensitivity and specificity were 100%.

Another potential advantage of duplex US scanning is its ability to facilitate selection of patients who, on the basis of the location of their disease and its severity, might be candidates for angioplasty. My colleagues and I[5] studied this prospectively on 110 arteriograms that had been preceded by the performance of duplex US scanning. From this group, 50 patients (45%) were scheduled for angioplasty on the basis of the results of the scan. The procedure was successfully performed on 47 (94%) of the patients. This approach was helpful not only to the radiologist but also to the patients, who were informed before the event as to what to expect and what the outcome might be. I believe this is a very good approach.

REFERENCES

1. Sumner DS, Strandness DE Jr. The relationship between calf blood flow and ankle pressure in patients with intermittent claudication. *Surgery.* 1969;65:763–771.
2. May AG, VandeBerg L, Deweese JA, Rob CG. Critical arterial stenosis. *Surgery.* 1963; 54:250–259.
3. Carter SA. Response of ankle systolic pressure to leg exercise in mild or questionable arterial disease. *N Engl J Med.* 1972;287:578–582.
4. Carter SA. Arterial asuccultation in peripheral vascular disease. *JAMA.* 1981;246:1682–1686.
5. Edwards JM, Coldwell DM, Goldman ML, Strandness DE Jr. The role of duplex scanning in the selection of patients for transluminal angioplasty. *J Vasc Surg.* 1991;13:69–74.
6. Sumner DS, Strandness DE Jr. Aortoiliac reconstruction in patients with combined iliac and superficial femoral arterial occlusion. *Surgery.* 1978;84:348–355.
7. Thiele BL, Bandyk DF, Zierler RE. A systematic approach to the assessment of aortoiliac disease. *Arch Surg.* 1983;18:477–485.
8. Strandness DE Jr, Bell JW. Peripheral vascular disease: diagnosis and objective evaluation using a mercury strain gauge. *Ann Surg.* 1965;161[Suppl]:1–35.
9. Jager KA, Phillips DJ, Martin R, et al. Noninvasive mapping of lower limb arterial lesions. *Ultrasound Med Biol.* 1985;11:515–521.
10. Strandness DE Jr, Sumner DS. *Hemodynamics for Surgeons.* New York: Grune & Stratton, 1975.
11. Strandness DE Jr. *Duplex Scanning in Vascular Disorders.* 2nd ed. New York: Raven Press, 1993.
12. Strandness DE Jr. Hemodynamics of the normal arterial and venous system. In: Strandness DE Jr, ed. *Duplex Scanning in Vascular Disorders.* New York: Raven Press; 1993;45–79.
13. Phillips DJ, Beach KW, Primozich JP, Strandness DE Jr. Should results of ultrasound Doppler studies be reported in units of frequency or velocity? *Ultrasound Med Biol.* 1989;15:205–212.

14. Kohler TR, Nance SC, Cramer MM, et al. Duplex scanning for diagnosis of aortoiliac and femoropopliteal disease: a prospective study. *Circulation.* 1987;76:1074–1080.

15. Hatsukami TS, Primozich JP, Zierler RE, Strandness DE Jr. Color Doppler characteristics in normal lower extremity arteries. *Ultrasound Med Biol.* 1992;16:167–171.

16. Hatsukami TS, Primozich JP, Zierler RE, et al. Color Doppler imaging of lower extremity arterial disease: a prospective validation study. *J Vasc Surg.* 1992;16:527–533.

17. Thiele BL, Strandness DE Jr. Accuracy of angiographic quantification of peripheral atherosclerosis. *Prog Cardiovasc Dis.* 1983;26:223–236.

18. Kohler TR, Andros G, Porter JM, et al. Can duplex scanning replace arteriography for lower extremity arterial disease? *Ann Vasc Surg.* 1990;4:280–287.

19. Legemate DA, Teeuwen C, Hoeneveld H, et al. The potential for duplex scanning to replace aortoiliac and femoropopliteal angiography. *Eur J Vasc Surg.* 1989;3:49–54.

27

Use of the Palmaz Stent in Stenting of the Iliac Arteries

Julio C. Palmaz, MD

The use of percutaneous transluminal balloon angioplasty is now a standard interventional procedure in the treatment of segmental iliac artery stenosis. Several reports on long-term results have established the validity of this procedure.[1,2] The recent development of an expandable stent has provided a further adjunctive technique in maintaining the patency of the balloon angioplasty, especially in patients with recurrent stenosis or diffuse narrowing of the external iliac artery. The efficacy of the stent to overcome the limitations of conventional percutaneous balloon angioplasty has been emphasized by several investigators.[3–5] To evaluate the use of an expandable stent (Palmaz stent) in the treatment of iliac artery disease, a multicenter trial was initiated in August 1987, to evaluate the safety and efficacy of this technique. Nearly 7 years have elapsed since the beginning of this trial. This report summarizes the results of this multicenter trial, which have been reported previously.[6]

DESIGN OF THE STUDY

Seventeen centers participated in this multicenter trial (Table 27–1). The criteria for patient selection, the procedural guidelines, and the method of follow-up evaluation were established under a protocol approved by the U.S. Food and Drug Administration and the institutional review boards and ethics committees of the institutions involved.

The device under evaluation is a balloon-expandable stent manufactured by Johnson and Johnson Interventional Systems (Warren, NJ). The device is currently approved for the clinical treatment of iliac artery disease in the United States and most other countries. The protocol, patient selection, indications, contraindications, and procedure guidelines for the use of the device have been previously described in detail.[7–9] The criteria for evaluation of the clinical results followed the guidelines proposed by Rutherford et al.[10]

TABLE 27–1. CENTERS THAT PARTICIPATED IN THE MULTICENTER TRIAL

Alexandria Hospital, Alexandria, Virginia
Arizona Heart Institute, Phoenix, Arizona
Hospital of the University of Pennsylvania, Philadelphia, Pennsylvania
Incor, Sao Paulo, Brazil
Indiana University Hospitals, Indianapolis, Indiana
Miami Vascular Institute, Miami, Florida
Scripps Clinic, San Diego, California
Shadyside Hospital, Pittsburgh, Pennsylvania
St. Vincent's Hospital, Indianapolis, Indiana
Thomas Jefferson University Hospital, Philadelphia, Pennsylvania
Terrebone Hospital, Houma, Louisiana
University of Freiburg Hospital, Freiburg, Germany
University of Minnesota Hospital, Minneapolis, Minnesota
University of Mainz, Mainz, Germany
University of Texas Health Science Center, San Antonio, Texas
Washington Hospital, Washington, DC
Western Pennsylvania Hospital, Pittsburgh, Pennsylvania

PATIENT POPULATION

A total of 486 patients entered the trial with a total of 587 procedures available for analysis. The mean age of these patients was 62.9 ± 10 years, with patients in their 60s being the largest group. Seventy-five percent of the patients were men, and 25% were women. A history of smoking was found in 94.4% of the patients, 22.9% had diabetes mellitus, 50.4% had coronary disease, and 18.2% had cerebrovascular disease. Hypertension was found in 52% of the patients.

The lower extremity ischemia was ranked in stages (Table 27–2).

LESION CHARACTERISTICS DEFINED BY ARTERIOGRAM

The average length of the iliac artery lesion treated was 3.2 ± 3.1 cm, and 62.6% of the patients had a lesion equal to or shorter than 3 cm. Longer lesions were present in fewer patients, 1.6% (eight patients) having lesions equal to or longer than 15 cm. The mean stenotic lesion was 82 ± 16%, and 13.5% of the lesions amounted to complete occlusion. Most of the lesions (40.8%) were in the 80% to 90% category. Most

TABLE 27–2. CLINICAL STAGES OF ISCHEMIA

Stage	Symptoms
0	Asymptomatic
1	Mild claudication (≥500 yards)
2	Moderate claudication (50–500 yards)
3	Severe claudication (<50 yards)
4	Rest pain
5	Nonhealing ulcer
6	Major tissue loss, foot not viable

of the patients with a less severe degree of stenosis were those with inflow and outflow disease in whom iliac revascularization was part of a combined treatment involving iliac stenting and lower extremity bypass surgery. Twenty-seven such patients accounted for 5.5% of the trial population. The mean luminal pressure gradient across the stenosis to be treated was 39.1 ± 24 mm Hg.

STENT PLACEMENT AND FOLLOW-UP EVALUATION

Stents were placed in the iliac artery in 405 patients, and 81 patients had bilateral placements. Of these, 59 had both iliac arteries treated with stents at the same sitting, and the other 22 patients had iliac stenting on two separate occasions. The common iliac artery was the site for stent placement in 66.5%, and the external iliac artery in 19% of the patients. Both common and external iliac arteries were treated in 13.1% of the patients, and 1.4% received stents in the distal aortic lumen.

The patients were followed up by clinical examination, hemodynamic measurement, and angiography as described previously.[7-9] The average clinical and hemodynamic follow-up period was greater than 1 year (13.3 ± 11 months); the largest group of patients was followed-up for 6 months. Sixty-nine (16.3%) of the patients had more than 24 months of follow-up study.

Two hundred and one patients had an arteriographic follow-up study an average of 8.7 ± 5.7 months after stent placement (range, 1 to 35 months). Stenosis was defined as a 50% or greater narrowing of the stented vessel. The clinical outcome of the procedure was evaluated by the Kaplan-Meier product-limit method (BMPD statistical software, Los Angeles, Calif). Validity of an observation was set at a standard error <0.1. Statistical evaluation between categories was assessed by the Wilcoxon test, and the significance level was set at $P \leq .05$.

RESULTS

Stent Placement

Most patients (52.4%) received one stent because the most frequent lesion length was shorter than 3.0 cm. The number of stents placed in the entire series is shown in Table 27–3. An average of 1.9 ± 1.3 stents were used per patient (range, one to eight stents).

TABLE 27–3. NUMBER OF STENTS PLACED IN PATIENTS IN THE CURRENT SERIES

No. of Stents	Percentage of Patient Population[a]
1	52.4
2	28.7
3	9.2
4	4.6
5	2.7
6	1.0
7	0.8

[a] Percentages do not total 100 because of rounding.

Hemodynamic Measurement

After stenting, the mean pressure gradient across the treated area was reduced to 1.3 ± 2.9 mm Hg. The mean ankle–brachial index increased from 0.62 ± 0.2 before stenting to 0.8 ± 0.2 soon after, and it was 0.8 ± 0.2 at the latest follow-up examination.

Clinical Outcome

Similar ranking was used before treatment and at the time of discharge for patients with stent placement alone or in combination with bypass surgery on the lower extremity. Three hundred fifty-seven (74.7%) patients had no symptoms, 5% had stage 1, 13.4% stage 2, 2.9% stage 3, 1.9% stage 4, and 2.1% stage 5 lower extremity ischemia. The longest time of follow-up averaged 13.3 ± 11 months (range, 1 to 39 months). At the latest follow-up evaluation of the clinical status of the lower extremity, 67.1% of patients had no symptoms, 7.1% had stage 1, 15% stage 2, 5% stage 3, 2.3% stage 4, 2.3% stage 5, and 1.2% stage 6 lower extremity ischemia.

The evaluation of clinical success by the product-limit method, as defined by the retention of at least one-stage improvement in the ischemic ranking system, indicated a success rate of 99.2% immediately after treatment, 90.9% at 12 months, 84.1% at 24 months, and 68.6% at 43 months (Fig. 27–1). Comparison of survival curves between patients with and without diabetes mellitus indicated a statistically significant difference in retention of improvement at 3 years (Wilcoxon test $P < .00001$) (Fig. 27–2).

The overall limb loss rate was 1.9%. Five below-knee amputations were performed 15 days and 1, 2, 3, and 4 months, respectively. Four additional above-knee amputations were performed 1, 6, 15, and 16 months, respectively. No stent thrombosis was present in any of the amputees.

The 30-day mortality was 1.9% (nine patients). Twenty-seven patients (6.2%) died more than 30 days after treatment. One year after treatment, the overall mortality was 6.1%. Cardiovascular causes were responsible for 63% of deaths. Neoplasm was the reason in 19.4%, infection in 8.3%, and miscellaneous causes in an additional 8.3% of the patients.

Analysis of Arteriographic Findings

Patients with poor runoff vessels had poorer results than those with good runoff (Wilcoxon test $P = .0013$). Patients with recanalized complete iliac artery occlusion did better than those with stenosis; 87.7% of the patients with stented occlusion were classified at 40 months as having successful results compared with 66.6% of those

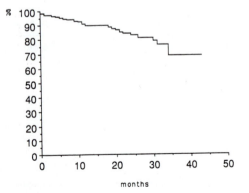

Figure 27–1. Product limit statistics on overall success of the treatment. (*Reprinted, with permission, from Palmaz JC, Laborde JC, Rivera FJ, et al. Stenting of the iliac arteries with the Palmaz stent: experience from a multicenter trial. Cardiovasc Intervent Radiol. 1992;15:291–297, copyright Springer-Verlag New York Inc., 1992.*)

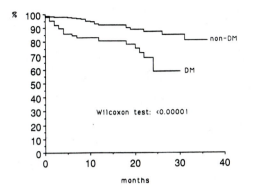

Figure 27–2. Product limit statistics of clinical success in patients with and without diabetes mellitus. DM, diabetes mellitus. (*Reprinted, with permission, from Palmaz JC, Laborde JC, Rivera FJ, et al. Stenting of the iliac arteries with the Palmaz stent: experience from a multicenter trial. Cardiovasc Intervent Radiol. 1992;15:291–297, copyright Springer-Verlag New York Inc., 1992.)*

with stenosis. The statistical comparison did not, however, achieve significance (Wilcoxon test $P = .13$).

Among 201 patients who underwent arteriographic follow-up study, the angiographic patency rate was 91.9%. Including the complete occlusions, the mean loss of luminal diameter was 15 ± 16%. Restenosis occurred in 15 common iliac and one external iliac artery stents. In two patients, restenosis occurred in both common and external iliac stents. Restenosis was diagnosed 1 month or sooner after stent placement in seven patients (1.4%) and 1 month in eight patients (1.8%). Arteriography depicted progression of atherosclerotic disease at a site distant to the stent in 4.5% of the patients during the first year, in 5.5% of the patients during the second year, and in 5.8% during the third year of treatment.

Complications

The overall complication rate in this series was 9.9% (Table 27–4). Eight percent of the complications were procedure-related and largely localized to the entry site. The remaining 1.9% were related to the stent itself. Acute thrombosis soon after stent placement occurred in five instances. Two pseudoaneurysms adjacent to the stented site developed in two patients who had laser recanalization of complete chronic occlusions followed by stent placement. One was treated conservatively and the other was treated by distal ligation of the iliac artery and femorofemoral bypass. Four stent thromboses were recanalized with thrombolytic therapy and balloon angioplasty. One patient underwent aortofemoral bypass. The incidence of complications was similar at all clinical trial sites.

CONCLUSION

Current commercially available stents are the Cook Z stent (Bloomington, Ind), the Schneider Wallstent (Minneapolis, Minn), the Medi-tech Strecker stent (Watertown, Mass), and the Johnson and Johnson Palmaz stent (Warren, NJ). Each stent has its own technical advantage. In a study by Hausegger et al,[11,12] three stents (Palmaz, Wallstent, and Strecker) were found to be effective in the treatment of complicated iliac disease. The Palmaz stent is currently the only one approved in the United States as an iliac artery stent. Most reports on the use of iliac artery stents are not standardized. Richter et al[13] demonstrated that stenting may improve the results of iliac angioplasty, but longer follow-up is needed to confirm this observation. To address the safety and efficacy of this device, this multicenter trial was organized to

TABLE 27–4. COMPLICATIONS OF STENT PLACEMENT FOR ILIAC ARTERY DISEASE IN 486 PATIENTS (587 PROCEDURES)

Procedure-Related		Stent-Related	
Complication	*n*	*Complication*	*n*
Groin hematoma	8	Acute thrombosis	5
Distal embolization	6	Pseudoaneurysm	2
Groin pseudoaneurysm	4	Dislodgment	4
Iliac artery pseudoaneurysm	1		
Aortic extravasation	1		
Groin arteriovenous fistula	1		
Retroperitoneal hematoma	2		
Surgical arteriotomy bleed	1		
Puncture site thrombosis	2		
Puncture site laceration	4		
Angioplasty site rupture	4		
Subintimal dissection	5		
Contrast-material–induced renal failure	4		
Death (contrast reaction)	2		

Reprinted with permission, from Palmaz, JC, Laborde JC, Rivera FJ, et al. Stenting of the iliac arteries with the Palmaz stent: experience from a multicenter trial. *Cardiovasc Intervent Radiol.* 1992; 15:291–297, copyright Springer-Verlag New York Inc., 1992.

record the acute occlusion rate, patency, and complications. The clinical experience in iliac stenting reported in the literature is summarized in Table 27–5.[13-19]

The present study yielded valuable information about the natural history of iliac artery disease and how it can be affected by intraluminal stent placement. As expected,

TABLE 27–5. CLINICAL EXPERIENCE IN ILIAC ARTERY STENTING*

Stent	No. of Patients	Acute Occlusion (%)	Patency (%)	Complication Rate (%)
Palmaz				
US multicenter[13]	401	1	94.1	11
European multicenter[14]	159	1.3	93.1	3.1
Henry et al[15]	56	0	97	3.5
Average	616[a]	1	94.1	8.5
Wallstent				
Vorwerk & Guenter[16]	68	3	93.3	12
Guenter et al.[17]	91	2.2	83.5	20
Zollikofer et al[18]	26	0	96	7.8
Average	185[a]	2.2	88.6	9.2
Gianturco Z				
Kichikawa et al[19]	10[a]	0	100	0

* Stents and authors are listed by number of cases reported.
[a] Values representing total number of patients.
Adapted, with permission, from Palmaz JC, Laborde JC, Rivera FJ, et al. Stenting of the iliac arteries with the Palmaz stent: Experience from a multicenter trial. *Cardiovasc Intervent Radiol.* 1992;15:291–297, copyright Springer-Verlag New York Inc., 1992.

most patients are male smokers in their 60s. Both hypertension and coronary artery disease were common, and about one fifth have cerebrovascular disease or diabetes mellitus. The most common lesion treated was a short (≤ 3 cm), high-grade ($82 \pm 16\%$) common iliac artery stenosis causing a large pressure gradient (39 ± 24 mm Hg). Survival statistics of clinical success showed a steady decline in the cumulative success rate, only 67% of the patients retaining benefit 43 months after treatment. Progression of atherosclerotic disease proximal or distal to the treated site appeared to be a factor, and the incidence is about 5% per year. This observation is supported by the fact that all amputations were performed on patients with patent stents at the time of amputation. As expected, diabetes mellitus and poor runoff had an important effect on the long-term outcome.

The higher treatment success rate among patients with recanalized occlusions as opposed to those with stenoses is of interest. Probably a larger group of patients is needed for more accurate statistical analysis. It is also of interest that all clinical failures among recanalized occlusions occurred within 8 months of stenting, with no failure thereafter. This suggests that re-endothelialization may take this long to be complete after stenting.

The complication rate (9.9%) of stent placement in this series was comparable to that of iliac balloon angioplasty.[2,20-22] Most of the complications at the entry site were due to the use of a large delivery system. It is expected that these complications will be reduced when a smaller diameter of balloon-expandable stent is available. Pseudoaneurysm can be prevented if laser or atherectomy is not used.

In conclusion, this multicenter trial supports the use of balloon-expandable stenting of the iliac artery as a safe and effective procedure for the treatment of atherosclerotic iliac artery disease. Whether iliac balloon angioplasty with a stent fares better than balloon angioplasty without a stent, however, remains unanswered. A comparative trial is probably needed to address this question.

Acknowledgment
This chapter is a summary of the final results of a multicenter trial, previously reported in greater detail in Palmaz JC, Laborde JC, Rivera FJ, et al. Stenting of the iliac arteries with the Palmaz stent: experience from a multicenter trial. Cardiovasc Intervent Radiol. *1992;15:291–297, copyright Springer-Verlag New York Inc, 1992.*

REFERENCES

1. Kalman PG, Sniderman KW, Johnston KW. Technique and six-year follow-up of percutaneous transluminal angioplasty to treat iliac artery occlusive disease. In: Yao JST, Pearce WH, eds. *Long-term Results in Vascular Surgery.* Norwalk, Conn: Appleton & Lange; 1993; 201–212.
2. Gallino A, Mahler F, Probst P, Nachbur B. Percutaneous transluminal angioplasty of the arteries of the lower limbs: a 5-year follow-up. *Circulation.* 1984;70:619–623.
3. Bonn J, Gardiner GA, Shapiro MJ, et al: Palmaz vascular stent: initial clinical experience. *Radiology.* 1990;174:741–745.
4. Palmaz JC, Garcia OJ, Schatz RA, et al. Placement of balloon-expandable intraluminal stents in iliac arteries: first 171 procedures. *Radiology.* 1990;174:969–975.
5. Long AI, Page PE, Raynaud AC, et al. Percutaneous iliac artery stent: angiographic long-term follow-up. *Radiology.* 1991;180:771–778.
6. Palmaz JC, Laborde JC, Rivera FJ, et al. Stenting of the iliac arteries with the Palmaz stent: experience from a multicenter trial. *Cardiovasc Intervent Radiol.* 1992;15:291–297.
7. Palmaz JC, Richter GM, Noeldge G, et al. Intraluminal stents in atherosclerotic artery stenosis: preliminary report of a multicenter study. *Radiology.* 1988;168:727–731.

8. Rees CR, Palmaz JC, Garcia OJ, et al: Angioplasty and stenting of completely occluded iliac arteries. *Radiology.* 1989;172:953–959.

9. Palmaz JC, Encarnacion C, Garcia OJ, et al. Aortic bifurcation stenosis: treatment with intravascular stent. *JVIR.* 1991;2:319–323.

10. Rutherford RB, Flanigan PD, Gupta SK, et al. Suggested standards for reports dealing with lower extremity ischemia. *J Vasc Surg.* 1986;4:80–94.

11. Hausegger KA, Cragg AH, Lammer J, et al. Iliac artery stent placement: clinical experience with a Nitinol stent. *Radiology.* 1994;190:199–202.

12. Hausegger KA, Lammer J, Hagen, B, et al: Iliac artery stenting: clinical experience with the Palmaz stent, Wallstent and Strecker stent. *Acta Radiol.* 1992;33:292–296.

13. Palmaz JC: Update on clinical experience with peripheral vascular stents. Presented at International Congress IV of the Arizona Heart Institute, February 13, 1991, Phoenix, Arizona.

14. Richter GM, Noeldge G, Roeren T, et al: First long-term results of a randomized multicenter trial: iliac balloon-expandable stent placement versus regular percutaneous transluminal angioplasty. (Abstract.) *Radiology.* 1990;177(P):152.

15. Henry M, Beron R, Amicabile C, et al. Palmaz-Schatz stents in the treatment of peripheral vascular diseases. (Abstract.) *J Am Coll Cardiol.* 1991;17:302A.

16. Vorwerk D, Guenther RW. Mechanical revascularization of occluded iliac arteries with use of self-expandable endoprotheses. *Radiology.* 1990;175:411–415.

17. Guenther RW, Vorwerk, D, Antonucci F, et al. Iliac artery stenosis or obstruction after unsuccessful balloon angioplasty: treatment with a self-expandable stent. *AJR.* 1991; 156:389–393.

18. Zollikofer CL, Antonucci F, Pfyffer M, et al. Arterial stent placement with use of the Wallstent: mid-term results of clinical experience. *Radiology.* 1991;179:449–456.

19. Kichikawa K, Uchida H, Yoshioka T, et al. Iliac artery stenosis and occlusion: preliminary results of treatment with Gianturco expandable metallic stents. *Radiology.* 1990;177:799–802.

20. Borozan PG, Schuler JJ, Spigos DG, Flanigan DP: Long-term hemodynamic evaluation of lower extremity percutaneous transluminal angioplasty. *J Vasc Surg.* 1985;2:785–793.

21. Johnston KW, Rae M, Hogg-Johnston SA, et al. Five-year results of a prospective study of percutaneous transluminal angioplasty. *Ann Surg.* 1987;206:403–413.

22. Waltman AC, Greenfield AJ, Novelline RA, et al. Transluminal angioplasty of the iliac and femoropopliteal arteries. *Arch Surg.* 1982;117:1218–1221.

28

Acute Aortic Occlusion

Alexander D. Shepard, MD, and Calvin B. Ernst, MD

Acute aortic occlusion (AAO) is an uncommon but well-recognized vascular catastrophe. The sudden interruption of lower extremity blood flow coupled with an acute increase in cardiac afterload, usually in a patient with pre existing compromised myocardial function, predictably results in a high morbidity and mortality. Recent reports have documented a mortality of 30% to 60% for AAO, making this entity just as lethal as a ruptured abdominal aortic aneurysm.[1-6] Prompt recognition and aggressive surgical management are necessary for a successful outcome.

ETIOLOGY

AAO most commonly involves the infrarenal abdominal aorta. Suprarenal AAO has been reported, but is rare, few patients surviving to diagnosis.[6] The infrarenal abdominal aorta is most frequently involved because of its smaller caliber and its greater predilection for atherosclerotic disease.

Acute occlusion of the infrarenal aorta is usually caused by either a large embolus lodging at the aortic bifurcation or thrombosis of a diseased aortoiliac segment. In a review of AAO in 46 adult patients treated at the Henry Ford Hospital over the last 40 years, embolism was the cause in 30 (65%) patients, and thrombosis was the cause in 16 (35%).[5]

Embolic Occlusion

Most emboli originate from the heart. The most common conditions producing cardiac thrombus were atrial fibrillation, congestive heart failure, mitral valve disease, and myocardial infarction (Table 28–1). Unusual causes included aortic mural thrombi or atheroemboli and tumor emboli.[7,8]

Thrombotic Occlusion

Severe aortoiliac occlusive disease is the most common cause of thrombotic AAO; it accounted for 12 of 16 (75%) cases in our study. Other causes included hypercoagulability (2 cases), abdominal aortic aneurysm (1 case), and aortic dissection (1 case). Patients with occluded aortic aneurysms usually have concomitant clinically significant iliac

TABLE 28–1. EMBOLIC ACUTE AORTIC OCCLUSION: ASSOCIATED CARDIAC ABNORMALITIES, HENRY FORD HOSPITAL*

Abnormality (n = 30)	No. of Patients	Percentage
Atrial fibrillation	21	70
Congestive heart failure	13	43
Valvular disease	12	40
Rheumatic heart disease	7	23
History of MI	9	30
History of multiple MIs	4	13
Recent MI (<2 weeks)	4	13
Postop mitral commissurotomy	4	13
Left ventricular aneurysm	2	7

* MI, myocardial infarction.
Modified with permission from Dossa CD, Shepard AD, Reddy DJ, et al. Acute aortic occlusion: a 40 year experience. *Arch Surg.* 1994;129:603–608.

occlusive disease.[9] A transient state of hypoperfusion related to congestive heart failure or dehydration may be the precipitating event in patients with occlusive disease.[6] Blunt abdominal trauma leading to an aortic intimal tear is a rarely reported cause of acute aortic thrombosis.[10]

PATHOPHYSIOLOGY

The hemodynamic and metabolic consequences associated with AAO are similar to those attendant with infrarenal aortic cross-clamping. A rapid rise in peripheral vascular resistance produces an acute increase in cardiac afterload with an increase in left ventricular stroke work and myocardial oxygen consumption, which is poorly tolerated in an unprepared patient with marginal cardiac reserve. Cardiac decompensation with ventricular dilatation, arrhythmias, and even cardiac arrest can result. Distal ischemia leads to anaerobic metabolism in the lower extremities, which can only be tolerated for 2 to 3 hours before serious metabolic consequences begin to occur (e.g., lactic acidosis, hyperkalemia). These profound metabolic and hemodynamic derangements are in large part responsible for the high mortality associated with AAO.

INCIDENCE

The frequency with which AAO has been diagnosed appears to have changed over the last 40 years. During the first three decades of our study 9 to 10 patients with AAO were seen each decade, embolism exceeding thrombosis as the most common cause of AAO (Fig. 28–1). Over the last 10 years, however, we have treated 17 patients with AAO, 11 of which were thrombotic in etiology. The reasons for these changes are unclear. The decrease in the incidence of embolic occlusions may be a result of the decreasing incidence of rheumatic heart disease as well as wider recognition of the importance of chronic anticoagulation in patients with atrial fibrillation and valvular heart disease. The increased frequency of thrombotic AAO may simply be the result of the growing population of older patients with atherosclerotic disease. This change in the pattern of AAO has not been previously noted.

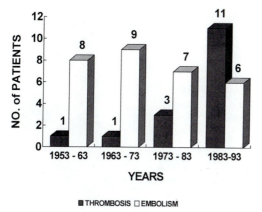

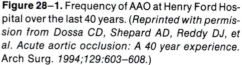

Figure 28–1. Frequency of AAO at Henry Ford Hospital over the last 40 years. (*Reprinted with permission from Dossa CD, Shepard AD, Reddy DJ, et al. Acute aortic occlusion: A 40 year experience.* Arch Surg. *1994;129:603–608.*)

CLINICAL PRESENTATION

The average age of patients presenting with AAO in our study was 59 years (range, 39 to 77 years) similar to that in other recent reports.[3,11] Women (59%) outnumbered men (41%) by a small margin. Co-morbidities included cardiac disease (74%), hypertension (48%), history of tobacco use (33%), diabetes mellitus (26%), and cerebrovascular disease (24%).

Patients typically presented with signs and symptoms of acute arterial occlusion involving both lower extremities. All patients complained of the acute onset of lower extremity pain and/or paresthesias and more than 80% had lower extremity weakness or paralysis. Femoral and distal pulses were absent. The lower extremities were cold with mottling to the level of the calves or higher in the majority. In 30% of patients, cyanosis extended to the umbilicus.

Despite these findings, AAO is occasionally misdiagnosed. Since most patients present with acute neurologic complaints, including pain, paresthesias, weakness, and paralysis, treating physicians may overlook the obvious signs and symptoms of AAO and focus on possible neurologic causes. Five patients in our study were first referred to a neurologist or neurosurgeon before the correct diagnosis was made. Others have reported a similar pattern of confusion and referral.[2,6]

DIAGNOSIS

The diagnosis of AAO is usually made on clinical grounds. Whereas some authors have advocated diagnostic aortography,[1,3,12] others have not found it useful and believe that it only delays definitive therapy.[2,11,13] In our study, 24 of 46 patients (52%) underwent translumbar or transaxillary aortography. In 20, the occlusion was confined to the infrarenal aorta with sparing of the renal arteries (Fig. 28–2). Two patients with embolic occlusion had simultaneous emboli to the superior mesenteric and left renal arteries. One patient with aortic thrombosis had thrombus extending to the level of the left renal artery, and one patient had an aortic dissection. Both patients with visceral emboli had abdominal pain in addition to lower extremity symptoms and were the only two patients to complain of abdominal pain. None of these concomitant visceral/renal occlusions were treated at the time of aortic operation, however, because of hemodynamic instability secondary to recent myocardial infarctions in two patients and poor general medical condition in the third. Aortography thus proved useful for

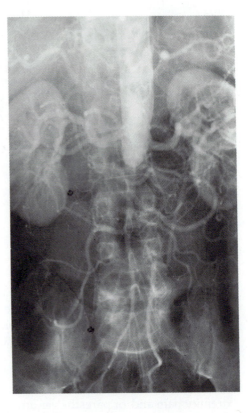

Figure 28–2. Typical aortogram of AAO involving the infrarenal abdominal aorta with sparing of the renal arteries.

definitive therapy only in the patient with aortic dissection. Patients with AAO for whom we currently consider preoperative aortography are those who present with acute renal failure and/or abdominal pain, findings that suggest the possibility of concomitant renal and/or visceral involvement, and the occasional patient with pre-existing aortoiliac disease. Aortography should be performed expeditiously and only in well-hydrated patients because of the renal insult brought about by contrast media.

Distinguishing between embolic and thrombotic AAO is not always easy. Women are more likely than men to have embolic AAO.[5,11,14] In our study, 70% of embolic occlusions occurred in women (Table 28–2). Although reasons for this difference are unclear, it may be that the smaller-caliber female infrarenal aorta traps emboli that would travel farther in the larger-diameter male aorta. Patients with emboli also have a higher incidence of serious heart disease compared with those with thrombotic AAO and not infrequently give a history of prior arterial emboli.[5,11] In our experience, patients with thrombotic AAO were more frequently tobacco abusers and diabetics, but they did not have a significantly higher incidence of intermittent claudication compared to those with embolic occlusions.

Typically, patients with embolic AAO present for medical evaluation earlier than patients with thrombotic AAO.[3,5] The median duration of ischemia in our study, defined as the interval between onset of symptoms and revascularization, was 7 hours for the embolic group and 17 hours for the thrombotic group. The most likely reason for this difference is a lesser degree of collateral circulation development in patients with embolic AAO, leading to the earlier manifestation of ischemic symptoms. There was no difference between the two groups in our study in the incidence of severe ischemia at the time of presentation, defined as the presence of lower extremity paralysis and/or anesthesia. Forty-one percent of the embolic group had severe isch-

TABLE 28–2. ACUTE AORTIC OCCLUSION: EMBOLISM VS THROMBOSIS, HENRY FORD HOSPITAL

	Embolism (n = 30)	Thrombosis (n = 16)	P Value
Risk Factors			
Female sex	21 (70)[a]	6 (38)	.058
Heart disease	30 (100)	4 (25)	.001
Prior arterial embolism	4 (13)	0	.201
Cigarette smoking	4 (13)	11 (69)	.001
Diabetes	5 (17)	7 (44)	.077
Claudication	9 (30)	9 (56)	.116
Hypertension	12 (40)	10 (63)	.217
Duration of Ischemia (median)	7 h	17 h	.15
Severe Ischemia[b]	11/27 (41)	8/15 (53)	NS

[a] Values in parentheses are percentages.
[b] Severe ischemia = lower extremity paralysis and/or anesthesia on presentation; information not available on all patients.
Modified with permission from Dossa CD, Shepard AD, Reddy DJ, et al. Acute aortic occlusion: a 40 year experience. *Arch Surg.* 1994;129:603–608.

emia compared with 53% of the thrombotic group. Both patients with spinal cord ischemia, however, had thrombotic AAO. Despite these differences, clinical differentiation between embolic and thrombotic occlusion is not always possible preoperatively and is not necessary prior to initiation of treatment.

TREATMENT

Once the diagnosis of AAO has been made, 10,000 units of heparin solution is given intravenously. Anticoagulation prevents propagation of thrombus and maintains patency of critical collateral pathways. Central venous access should be obtained prior to heparin therapy to facilitate safe conversion to a pulmonary artery catheter. Heparin solution should be withheld temporarily in the rare patient in whom preoperative aortography is desired. Patients with AAO require aggressive monitoring with a pulmonary artery catheter, radial artery catheter, and urinary bladder drainage to assess hemodynamics and guide resuscitation. Particular attention should be paid to the patient's cardiac status, and measures must be taken to control concomitant heart failure, myocardial ischemia, and arrhythmias. A brisk urine output, >100 mL/h, should be maintained in patients with severe lower extremity ischemia to reduce the risk of renal dysfunction from possible myoglobinuria. Intravenous sodium bicarbonate to alkalinize the urine and mannitol are helpful adjuncts when myoglobinuria is suspected. Patients should be promptly prepared for operation without prolonged resuscitative efforts.

Nonoperative treatment with continued high-dose heparin sodium anticoagulation is occasionally appropriate for patients at high risk with minimal limb ischemia. Intra-arterial catheter-directed thrombolysis is another potential therapeutic modality, although its role in the treatment of AAO has not yet been clearly defined. Two factors militating against routine thrombolysis are the advanced degrees of ischemia in most patients and the amount of the clot burden. However, in patients with less advanced ischemia, particularly those with prohibitive operative risks, intra-arterial thrombolysis may have a role. We have used thrombolysis successfully in one patient with an acute aortobifemoral graft occlusion. Rarely, patients present with advanced, irreversible limb ischemica manifest by rigidity of major muscle groups. In this situation, primary, bilateral above-knee amputation is the only appropriate treatment.

Operative Therapy

The abdomen, both lower extremities, and usually the right chest and axilla are prepared and draped to permit possible aortic reconstruction, extra-anatomic bypass, and distal limb exploration and fasciotomy as necessary. If the distal limb musculature is firm or doughy, fasciotomy should be considered before revasculariztion. Bilateral femoral artery explorations should be performed on all patients with an initial attempt at retrograde balloon catheter thromboembolectomy (Fig. 28–3). Local anesthesia can be used for patients at high risk. Brisk, pulsatile arterial inflow must be achieved, otherwise early reocclusion is likely. Reduced inflow is secondary to either retained thrombus or severe aortoiliac occlusive disease and mandates further therapy. Blood loss with this procedure can be considerable, and the use of an autotransfusion device is helpful.

Retrograde catheter thromboembolectomy is successful in restoring flow for most patients with embolic AAO. Distal limb thromboembolectomy should also be performed to remove distal clot. If catheter thromboembolectomy is unsuccessful, further intervention depends on the patient's condition. Transaortic thromboembolectomy or aortic reconstruction can be performed on patients at good risk and axillobifemoral bypass can be reserved for patients at high risk. With embolic occlusion, transabdominal embolectomy can usually be performed through a limited extraperitoneal approach

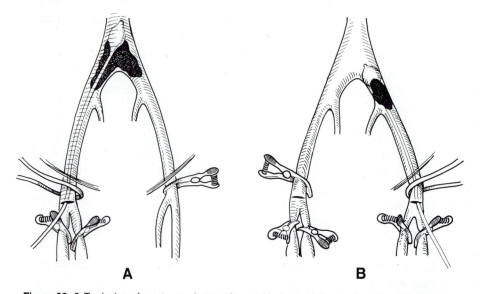

A   **B**

Figure 28–3. Technique for retrograde transfemoral balloon catheter aortic thrombectomy/embolectomy. When thrombosis is the most likely cause of the occlusion, longitudinal arteriotomies are preferred because of the high probability that arterial reconstruction will be required. (**A**) A large (6-F) catheter is passed retrograde into the aorta and withdrawn. (**B**) The same procedure is performed through the contralateral femoral artery. (*Reprinted with permission from Shepard AD, Ernst CB. Arterial embolectomy and arteriovenous fistula repair. In: Nora PF, ed. Operative Surgery. Philadelphia, Pa: W.B. Saunders, 1990.*)

under epidural anesthesia. If there is any doubt as to etiology, midline exposure is preferred. Extracted clot should be examined both grossly and histologically to confirm its composition and source.

In thrombotic AAO, retrograde catheter thrombectomy is rarely successful. The one patient with a successful outcome in our thrombotic group had an underlying hypercoagulable state. Most patients with thrombotic AAO require some form of arterial reconstruction. Aortofemoral bypass is favored over axillobifemoral bypass for stable patients at good risk. In the performance of aortic reconstruction, care must be taken in manipulating and clamping the aorta immediately below the renal arteries because of the frequent propagation of clot to this level and the risk of dislodging debris into the renal arteries. Under these circumstances, we have found temporary supraceliac aortic clamping sometimes to be a safer alternative. After transection of the infrarenal aorta and thrombectomy of the proximal stump, the clamp can be moved to an infrarenal location.

Regardless of the revascularization method used to treat AAO, reperfusion of the legs represents the most critical part of the procedure and should be carefully controlled. The metabolic derangements attendant with reperfusion of severely ischemic limbs can result in myocardial depression, arrhythmias, and cardiac arrest. Careful communication with the anesthesia team is necessary for proper timing of administration of sodium bicarbonate and mannitol. Once flow has been restored, the distal lower extremities are assessed for perfusion and possible compartment compression syndrome. With embolic AAO completion arteriography is helpful in identifying residual distal thromboemboli, which might preclude a good result. Fasciotomies should be performed as necessary.

Postoperative Management

Postoperatively, attention is focused on the patient's cardiac function, the lower extremities, and the possible sequelae of the reperfusion syndrome. Patients with moderately severe to severe ischemia should be observed for development of myoglobinuria and appropriate measures should be instituted if it is found. Acute renal failure in this setting carries a very high mortality.[3] Macro- and microembolism of lower extremity venous thrombi can result in pulmonary insufficiency and adult respiratory distress syndrome. Heparin anticoagulation should be maintained in all patients with embolic occlusion and converted to lifelong warfarin therapy to prevent early and late recurrent emboli.[5,11,15] A short course of heparin therapy may be beneficial in patients with thrombotic occlusion who have impaired distal perfusion following arterial reconstruction. In patients with embolic AAO, embologenic conditions should be sought and, when possible, corrected. Mitral valve repair was used to correct a cardiac source of emboli in almost 40% of survivors of embolic occlusion.

RESULTS

The mortality for AAO remains high despite advances in anesthetic management, operative technique, and postoperative care (Table 28–3). Over the first three decades of our study, the mortality was a fairly constant 40%, and only over the last 10 years did it drop to 24%. The mortality for embolic AAO was slightly higher than for thrombotic occlusion in our study (37% vs 31%), $P = NS$. In the compilation of the results of several recent series, however, the mortality for thrombotic AAO appeared to be higher than that for embolic AAO (43% vs 34%) (Table 28–3). Deaths in our

TABLE 28–3. ACUTE AORTIC OCCLUSION: RECENT PUBLISHED SERIES[a]

Author	Year	No. of Patients	Sex Ratio (M:F)	No. of Cases of Embolism	No. of Cases of Thrombosis	Mortality (%)	Limb Salvage Rate in Survivors (%)	Rate of Recurrent Emboli (%)
Busuttil[11]	1983	26	1:15	26	0	23 E+	98	27
Littooy[3]	1985	18	14:4	10	8[b]	40 E / 63 T▲	94	ND
Babu[6]	1987	34	17:17	0	34	50 T	94	—
Webb[1]	1988	10	9:1	ND	ND	50	90	ND
Meagher[2]	1991	8	5:3	1	7	63	ND	—
Tapper[4]	1992	26	13:13	13	13	30 E / 23 T	98	8
Dossa[5]	1994	46	19:27	30	16	37 E / 31 T / 34 E / 43 T	96	43

[a] ND, no data; E, embolic; T, thrombotic.
[b] Two of eight patients had an aortic graft occlusion.

study were most commonly due to cardiac events, as expected, given the high incidence of cardiac disease in these patients and the sustained increase in cardiac afterload associated with sudden occlusion of the infrarenal aorta. Recurrent emboli were also an important cause of early deaths. Three of five patients (17%) with embolic AAO who had early (<30 days) recurrent emboli died, two following with superior mesenteric artery emboli, and one following a carotid embolus.

The morbidity associated with AAO is also substantial and was not significantly different between patients with embolism and patients with thrombosis in our study (Table 28–4). Cardiac complications and reperfusion sequelae are the most common reported complications. Limb morbidity was surprisingly low in several reports, limb salvage rates exceeding 95% in survivors (Table 28–3). Excluding the one patient in our study who underwent primary, bilateral amputations, only four limbs were lost in three patients. Fasciotomies were performed on six patients, three of whom had persistent problems with ischemic neuropathy.

Studies detailing the long-term outcomes of survivors of AAO are limited. Considering the high incidence of cardiac disease among these patients, however, late survival appears reasonable. Busuttil et al[11] noted a 5-year survival rate of 55.6% among patients with embolic AAO, which is similar to the 70% rate in our analysis. Patients with thrombotic AAO had a 75% 5-year survival rate in our study. In contrast, Tapper et al[4] reported only a 50% 1-year survival rate and a 20% 10-year survival rate in their experience with 26 AAO patients.

Recurrent arterial embolism appears to be an important problem in patients with embolic AAO and underscores the importance of continued long-term anticoagulation. Busuttil et al[11] reported a 27% incidence of re-embolization, although none of these episodes apparently occurred during the initial AAO hospitalization. In our study, 43% of patients with embolic occlusions experienced recurrent emboli, including 37% (7/19) of survivors. Three of these late recurrent emboli resulted in a second episode of AAO. All late recurrent emboli in our study occurred despite sodium warfarin

TABLE 28–4. ACUTE AORTIC OCCLUSION: MORTALITY AND MORBIDITY, HENRY FORD HOSPITAL*

	Embolism (*n* = 30)	Thrombosis (*n* = 16)
Mortality	11 (37)	5 (31)
Cardiac	4 (13)	4 (25)
Recurrent arterial emboli	3 (10)	-----
Renal failure	2 (7)	0
Other[a]	2 (7)	1 (6)
Morbidity		
Cardiac	6 (20)	7 (43)
Reperfusion sequelae[b]	11 (37)	7 (44)
Renal failure[c]	1 (3)	1 (6)
Limb complications	7 (23)	5 (31)
Paraplegia	0	2 (12)

* Values in parentheses are percentages.
[a] Other = nonocclusive mesenteric ischemia, nonembolic stroke, sepsis.
[b] Reperfusion sequelae = myoglobinuria, adult respiratory distress syndrome.
[c] Renal failure = requirement for dialysis.
Modified with permission from Dossa CD, Shepard AD, Reddy DJ, et al. Acute aortic occlusion: a 40 year experience. *Arch Surg.* 1994;129:603–608.

administration, although no patient had a therapeutic prothrombin time at the time of readmission. In all, five of 12 recurrent emboli (both early and late) resulted in death.

FACTORS AFFECTING OUTCOME

To determine the impact of the severity of ischemia and its duration on outcome, we analyzed these relationships in our 46 patients. The severity of ischemia was defined by the neurologic status of the lower extremities when the patient was initially examined by a vascular surgeon. Patients with no sensory or motor deficits had no hospital mortality (Table 28–5). Conversely, patients who presented with any neurologic deficit other than mild sensory changes had high mortalities, regardless of whether deficits were moderate or severe. Limb morbidity, including compartment syndrome, ischemic neuropathy, and/or amputation, developed only in patients who presented with lower extremity paralysis. Paradoxically, the duration of ischemia prior to revascularization had an inverse relationship with mortality. Patients with symptoms lasting 6 hours or less before revascularization had a mortality of 57%, whereas among those with symptoms that lasted longer than 6 hours mortality was 29% (Table 28–6). There were, however, a greater number of patients with severe ischemia in the short ischemic duration group. This analysis confirmed that survival and functional results in patients with AAO were determined by the severity of ischemia rather than its duration. This observation, made by others,[11] contradicts prior studies of peripheral arterial embolism, which emphasized duration rather than severity of ischemia.[16–18]

The introduction of the balloon thromboembolectomy catheter in 1964 had no significant impact on the mortality of embolic AAO in our study despite the advantages of transfemoral embolectomy over transabdominal aortic embolectomy. Six of 16 (38%) patients who underwent catheter embolectomy died, compared with four of nine (44%) who underwent transabdominal embolectomy. However, operative stress for the transabdominal group may have been reduced by exposing the aorta through a

TABLE 28–5. EFFECT OF INITIAL LOWER EXTREMITY NEUROLOGIC DEFICIT ON MORTALITY, HENRY FORD HOSPITAL

	No. of Patients	No. of Deaths	Mortality (%)
Sensory Deficit			
None	4	0	0
Moderate[a]	19	7	37
Severe[b]	13	5	38
Unknown	10	4	40
Motor Deficit			
None	7	0	0
Paresis	17	8	47
Paralysis	18	6	33
Unknown	4	2	50

[a] Moderate = diminished sensation to light touch.
[b] Severe = anesthetic.
Modified with permission from Dossa CD, Shepard AD, Reddy DJ, et al. Acute aortic occlusion: a 40 year experience. *Arch Surg.* 1994;129:603–608.

TABLE 28–6. EFFECT OF DURATION OF ISCHEMIA ON MORTALITY, HENRY FORD HOSPITAL

Symptom Interval	No. of Patients	Etiology		Severe Ischemia	No. of Deaths	Mortality (%)
		Embolism	Thrombosis			
≤6 h	14	11	3	7/11 (63%)[a]	8	57
						$P = .10$
>6 h	28	16	12	11/27 (41%)[b]	8	29

[a] Information not available on three patients.
[b] Information not available on one patient.
Modified with permission from Dossa CD, Shepard AD, Reddy DJ, et al. Acute aortic occlusion: a 40 year experience. *Arch Surg.* 1994;129:603–608.

small extraperitoneal flank incision and by selective use of spinal or epidural anesthesia.

CONCLUSION

AAO is a vascular surgical emergency with a high morbidity and mortality, even when diagnosed promptly and treated appropriately. The early mortality of AAO results from both the advanced cardiac disease present in most patients and the physiologic insult associated with sudden aortic occlusion. Nevertheless, reasonable long-term outcomes justify a continued aggressive approach to diagnosis and treatment.

REFERENCES

1. Webb KH, Jacocks MA. Acute aortic occlusion. *Am J Surg.* 1988;155:405–407.
2. Meagher AP, Lord RSA, Graham AR, Hill DA. Acute aortic occlusion presenting with lower limb paralysis. *J Cardiovasc Surg.* 1991;32:643–647.
3. Littooy FN, Baker WH. Acute aortic occlusion: a multifaceted catastrophe. *J Vasc Surg.* 1986;4:211–216.
4. Tapper SS, Jenkins JM, Edwards WH, et al. Juxtarenal aortic occlusion. *Ann Surg.* 1992;5:443–450.
5. Dossa CD, Shepard AD, Reddy DJ, et al. Acute aortic occlusion: a 40 year experience. *Arch Surg.* 1994;129:603–608.
6. Babu SC, Shah PM, Sharma P, et al. Adequacy of central hemodynamics versus restoration of circulation in the survival of patients with acute aortic thrombosis. *Am J Surg.* 1987; 154:206–210.
7. Harris RW, Andros G, Dulowa LB, Oblath RW. Malignant melanoma embolus as a cause of acute aortic occlusion: report of a case. *J Vasc Surg.* 1986;3:550–553.
8. Newman HA, Cordell AR, Prichard RW. Intracardiac myxomas: literature review and report of six cases, one successfully treated. *Am Surg.* 1966;32:219–230.
9. Johnson JM, Gaspar MR, Movius HJ, Rosental JJ. Sudden complete thrombosis of aortic and iliac aneurysms. *Arch Surg.* 1974;108:792–794.
10. Lassonde J, Laurendeau F. Blunt injury of the abdominal aorta. *Ann Surg.* 1981;194:745–748.
11. Busuttil RW, Keehn G, Miliken J, et al. Aortic saddle embolus: a twenty-year experience. *Ann Surg.* 1983;197:698–706.
12. Matolo NM, Cheung L, Albo D Jr., Lazarus HM. Acute occlusion of the infrarenal aorta. *Am J Surg.* 1973;126:788–793.
13. Drager SB, Riles TS, Imparato AM. Management of acute aortic occlusion. *Ann Surg.* 1979;138:293–295.
14. Porter JM, Acinapura AJ, Silver D. Aortic saddle embolectomy. *Arch Surg.* 1966;93:360–364.
15. Elliott JP, Hageman JH, Szilagyi DE, et al. Arterial embolization: problem of source multiplicity, recurrence and delayed treatment. *Surgery.* 1980;88:833–845.
16. Haimovici H. Peripheral arterial embolism: a study of 330 unselected cases of embolism of the extremities. *Angiology.* 1950;1:20–45.
17. Albright HL, Leonard FC. Embolectomy from the abdominal aorta. *N Engl J Med.* 1950;242:271–277.
18. Levy JF, Butcher HR Jr. Arterial emboli: an analysis of 125 patients. *Surgery.* 1970;68:968–973.

29

Preliminary Experience with Endovascular Stented Grafts for Limb-Threatening Aortoiliac Occlusive Disease

Michael L. Marin, MD, and Frank J. Veith, MD

Aortobifemoral bypass represents the best current treatment of extensive aortoiliac occlusive disease.[1-6] Such reconstructions have been effective and durable in the treatment of lower extremity ischemia. Unfortunately, aortoiliofemoral bypass grafting is not perfect. Between 10% and 20% of all aortofemoral bypass grafts may be expected to develop at least one graft limb thrombosis over a 10-year period. Such failures frequently necessitate reoperation, which is often associated with an increased morbidity over primary procedures.[2,4] Patients who undergo reoperative aortoiliac surgery who also have serious co-morbid medical illnesses, including renal, pulmonary, and cardiac insufficiencies, are at increased risk for a perioperative complication.

Alternative interventional procedures to open aortic reconstruction include the use of percutaneous transluminal angioplasty and intravascular stenting.[7-13] These procedures, which may be performed without major anesthesia, have been shown to be effective for treating short, segmental, occlusive disease of the iliac arteries. However, balloon angioplasty has not proven durable for the treatment of multiple and long segment arterial occlusive diseases in the aortoiliac segment.[7,14]

An alternative method to treat long segment aortoiliac disease without standard, open aortofemoral grafting employs endovascular stented grafts to bridge the vascular pathology. Stented grafts represent a combination of intravascular stent, angioplasty, and prosthetic graft technologies to produce a new device that may be inserted in a minimally invasive manner. These devices can be inserted under general, regional, or local anesthesia; require less operative dissection; minimize local tissue trauma; and are associated with reduced blood loss and a more rapid post procedure recovery. This chapter reviews the development of endovascular stented grafts and their potential for the treatment of aortoiliac occlusive disease.

Intravascular stented grafts were first conceived of in 1969 by Dotter, the originator of percutaneous angioplasty.[15] At the time of that seminal report, Dotter also suggested that stents could be used for the treatment of a variety of arterial lesions, including aneurysms and arteriovenous fistulas. Subsequent feasibility studies, which showed the potential utility of stented graft devices, were carried out by a number of workers in experimental animals using a variety of stent and graft materials.[16–18] Recent clinical applications of endovascular stented grafts have included the treatment of abdominal aortic and peripheral artery aneurysms[19,20] and penetrating arterial injuries.[21]

The first clinical application of endovascular stented grafts for the treatment of arterial occlusive disease was by Volodos et al, who used a self-expanding, spring-type stent device covered with a Dacron graft material to treat an aortoiliac obstruction.[22] This device was effectively used to treat a long segment of occluded artery by dilating and relining the vessel. Following this report, several other devices have been used to treat a variety of occlusive arterial lesions within the aortoiliac and femoropopliteal arteries.[23,24] While the applications of endovascular stented grafts may extend to markedly different arterial lesions, the same general principles and techniques of graft insertion apply to all. These include remote arterial access site, less trauma to the surrounding artery, minimal anesthetic requirements, and repair of the arterial pathology from within the vessel lumen.

TECHNIQUE

Stented graft procedures for the treatment of arterial occlusive disease employ three basic techniques for endoluminal reconstruction (Fig. 29–1). These include guide wire passage through the diseased arterial segment, its balloon dilation, and finally, insertion and deployment-fixation of the graft.

Arterial Access

The arterial pathology to be treated with a stented graft is approached from a remote site. Direct access is obtained by one of two methods. If the access vessel is patent, it may be approached through a percutaneous puncture technique. However, many patients with extensive limb-threatening aortoiliac occlusive disease have occluded access arteries. The presence of an occluded vessel at the site of arterial access does not preclude the ability to perform an endovascular stented graft procedure. When occluded vessels are present, they can be approached by open, surgical exposure of

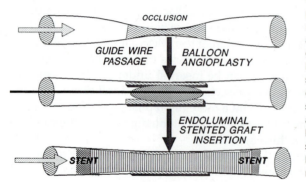

Figure 29–1. Summary of the steps involved in transluminal stented graft repair for arterial occlusive disease. A stenotic or narrowed segment within the arteries is first crossed with an angiographic wire. The entire stenosis is then balloon dilated. Next, the endovascular stented graft composed of a prosthetic conduit coupled with two intra-arterial stents is inserted within a guiding sheath and placed into the arterial system. After balloon expansion of the individual stents, the new endovascular graft relines the diffusely dilated, diseased arterial segment.

the access artery (Fig. 29–2A). Once the occluded vessel is identified, recanalization guide wires (often with hydrophilic coatings) are inserted directly into the central axis of the occluded vessel and guided under fluoroscopic control cephalad through the patent artery by means of directional catheters (Fig. 29-2B).

Arterial Dilation

Once the recanalization wires have established a connection between the remote access site and the patent segment of the proximal artery, diffuse arterial dilation is performed with angioplasty balloons inserted over the guide wire (Fig. 29–2C). Such dilation allows the formation of a widened tract through the atheromatous arterial wall. This will facilitate the insertion of the sheath containing the new endovascular graft within this tract.

Stented Graft Insertion

When a new luminal tract has been created within the wall of the occluded or diseased artery, a carrier system composed of a guiding catheter or sheath containing an endovascular stented graft is inserted over the previously placed wire and advanced under fluoroscopic control to the patent proximal arterial segment. After angiographic confirmation of the position of the stented graft, the graft is fixed into position by a stent attachment device (Fig. 29–2D). The attachment device provides a watertight seal between the proximal end of the graft and the patent portion of the proximal artery. The distal end of the endovascular graft is then ready for suture anastomosis or stenting to the patent portion of an outflow artery. When performed with sutures, this procedure may be accomplished by a standard end-to-side or end-to-end open arterial anastomosis. Alternatively, the endovascular stented graft may be sutured to the patent portion of the outflow artery by means of an endoluminal anastomotic technique (Fig. 29–2E).

All procedures must be followed by a completion arteriogram to inspect for technical adequacy of the procedure and patency of the outflow arteries without embolization.

CASE REPORTS

A summary of the endovascular stented graft reconstructions in two patients with limb-threatening ischemia is presented in Figure 29–3. The following are the highlights from these cases:

Patient 1

Patient 1 was transferred from another hospital for treatment of gangrene of the right foot. He had a complicated course following colon surgery. An attempted closure of a sigmoid colostomy for a perforated diverticular abscess had resulted in a colonic anastomotic dehiscence and necrotizing faciitis of the abdominal wall. Multiple, small intestinal–cutaneous fistulas had developed along with a colocutaneous fistula. Marked skin loss and cellulitis of the skin covering the flanks and groins were present. Severe aortoiliac and femoropopliteal occlusive disease in association with a left foot infection had necessitated a left above-knee amputation before transfer to our institution. Iliac and femoropopliteal occlusive disease was responsible for right limb-threatening ischemia and foot gangrene (Fig. 29–4A,B). The intestinal fistulas and

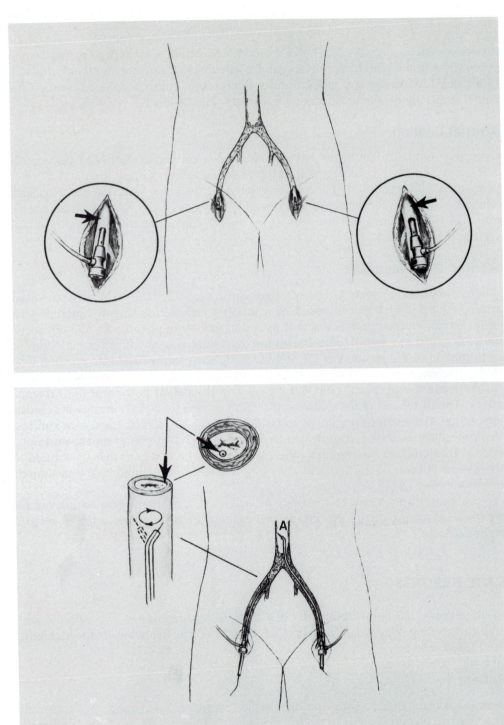

Figure 29–2. Steps required to perform an endovascular stented graft repair for aortoiliac occlusive disease. (**A**) Bilateral femoral cutdowns are performed and introducer catheters are inserted into the exposed, patent common femoral arteries (arrow). It is through these introducer catheters that all subsequent interventions on the occluded segment of the vascular system are accomplished. (**B**) By way of the previously placed introducer catheters, directional catheters then guide hydrophilic wires through the arterial stenoses into the patent artery above (A = aorta). *Inset,* the ideal plane of dissection is in the intra-intimal segment (arrow). Recanalization in the deep portions of the media may make re-entry into the patent abdominal aorta difficult. (*Figure continues*)

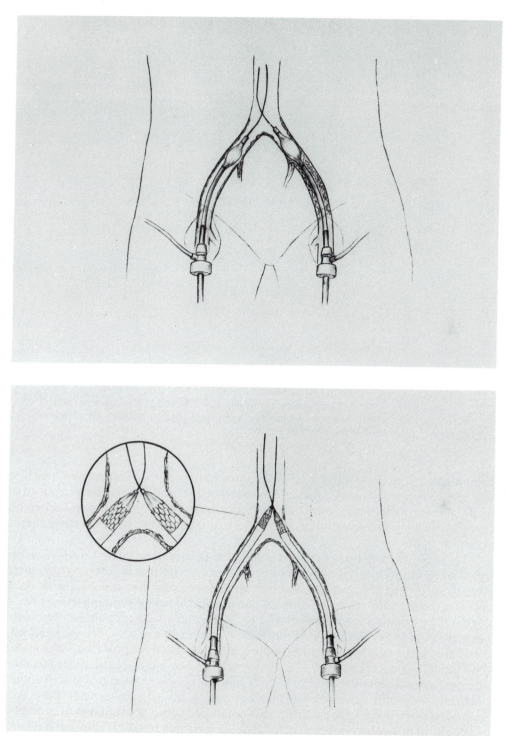

C

D

Figure 29–2. (*continued*). (**C**) After recanalization, balloon dilation is performed over the wire along the entire length of the occluded or diseased arterial segment. (**D**) After balloon dilation, endovascular stented grafts are simultaneously inserted through both newly dilated iliac systems. Their final proximal position is confirmed with fluoroscopy. (*Figure continues*)

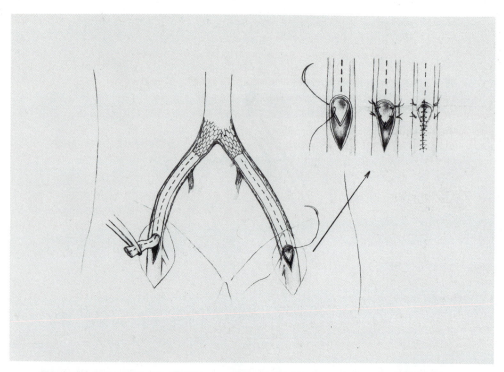

E

Figure 29–2. (*continued*). (**E**) The proximal stents of both endovascular iliac grafts are dilated, creating a watertight seal between the graft, the stent, and the aortic wall. *Inset,* the distal end of each graft is then endoluminally anastomosed to the common femoral artery. An endoluminal anastomosis consists of a series of 6–0 tacking silk or polypropylene U sutures placed within the prosthetic graft.

abdominal wall necrosis precluded an anterior transperitoneal surgical approach to the aorta for arterial reconstruction. Cellulitis of the skin of the flanks and groin made alternative retroperitoneal, femorofemoral, and axillofemoral approaches for revascularization hazardous. These limitations prompted the use of a transfemoral approach to the aorta.

Through an arteriotomy in the proximal superficial femoral artery (SFA) below the inflamed right groin, a 0.035-inch hydrophilic guide wire was inserted retrograde to cross the occluded SFA and diseased common femoral and iliac arteries to access the abdominal aorta. After over-the-wire balloon dilation of the new endovascular tract, a 30-mm long Palmaz stent was deployed to fix a 6-mm × 30-cm polytetrafluoroethylene (PTFE) graft at the aortoiliac junction. A second 20-mm long Palmaz stent was inserted to secure the lower portion of the graft in the distal external iliac artery above the inguinal ligament (Fig. 29–4C). A third 6-mm × 32-cm stented graft device was then inserted prograde into the predilated SFA, and the graft was fixed to the above-knee popliteal artery with a 20-mm long Palmaz stent (Fig. 29–4D). The cephalic portion of the graft was sewn to the proximal SFA with a standard suture anastomosis. Restoration of a popliteal pulse and resolution of the right leg ischemia resulted. The graft has been patient for 12 months.

Patient 2

Patient 2 had three previous left lower extremity revascularizations for limb-threatening ischemia. The last revascularization was 4 years before the present admis-

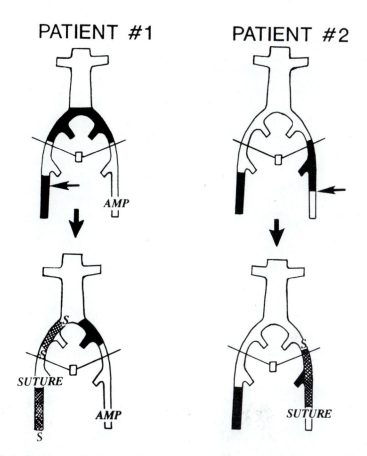

Figure 29–3. Summary of endovascular stent graft reconstruction in two patients. *Top,* before the procedures (arrows = sites of arterial access). *Bottom,* after procedure. (AMP = amputated; S = stent; thatched area = grafted region.)

sion and was associated with a deep left groin and retroperitoneal infection that resolved but was followed 3 years later by graft occlusion. Laboratory analysis for a hypercoagulable state was negative. The current admission was for an acute anterior wall myocardial infarction. At the time of admission to the coronary care unit, severe left foot ischemia with gangrene and infection was present in conjunction with absent femoral and pedal pulses in both lower extremities. Arteriograms demonstrated an occlusion of the distal left external iliac artery with reconstitution of the distal SFA (Fig. 29–5A).

Because of the risks concomitant with a complex peripheral revascularization within 10 days of an acute myocardial infarction and the extreme urgency associated with the pedal sepsis and gangrene, a stented graft was inserted through a mid-SFA arteriotomy under local anesthesia. After balloon dilatation of an endovascular tract created between the external iliac and SFAs, a 6-mm PTFE graft was inserted and fixed to the external iliac artery with a 30-mm long Palmaz stent. Preservation of terminal external iliac artery collateral branches was achieved by placing that portion of the stent not covered by prosthetic graft across the ostia of these collaterals (Fig. 29–5B). This allowed continued circulation to the branches through the uncovered interstices of the stent. The distal portion of the graft was anastomosed to the distal SFA by means of standard vascular surgical techniques. Restoration of pedal pulses

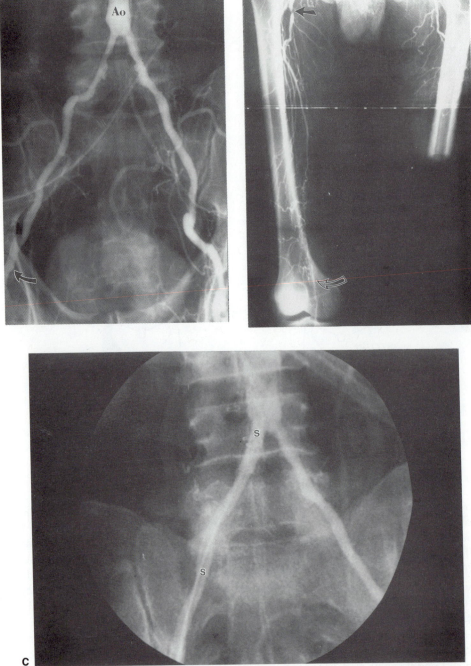

Figure 29–4. Preoperative femoral arteriograms of Patient 1 performed through a left transfemoral arterial puncture. (**A**) Diffuse aortoiliac disease that displayed a segmentally increasing pressure gradient of 80 mm Hg between the aorta (Ao) and the right common femoral artery (arrow). (**B**) Tight stenosis of the deep femoral artery (arrow) and an occlusion of the superficial femoral artery with reconstitution of the above-knee popliteal artery (open arrow). (**C**) After endoluminal insertion of a right aortoiliac stented graft, normal flow was restored to the right femoral artery. No pressure gradient between the aorta and the common femoral artery could be detected after graft insertion (s = location of endovascular stents). (*Figure continues*)

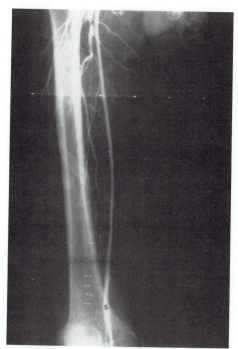

Figure 29–4. (*continued*). (**D**) Completion angiogram after insertion of a superficial femoral to popliteal artery stented graft. The balloon expandable stent attaches the graft to the above-knee popliteal artery (s = location of stent).

D

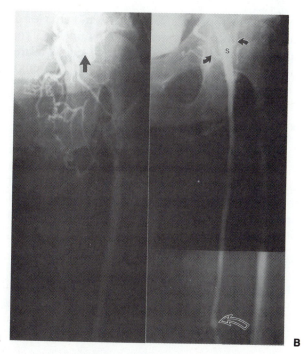

A

B

Figure 29–5. (**A**) A femoral arteriogram of Patient 2 demonstrating occlusion of the left external iliac artery at its junction with the common femoral artery (arrow). (**B**) After insertion of a stented graft through the left superficial femoral artery, circulation to the left foot is re-established. There is preservation of terminal external iliac collateral vessels (arrows). (s = location of stent; open arrow = site of distal sewn anastomosis.)

was associated with complete resolution of the gangrene, and the graft has been patent for 11 months.

CONCLUSION

Preliminary studies have shown that endovascular stented grafts are effective for the treatment of a variety of arterial lesions, including aneurysms, occlusions, and penetrating traumatic injuries.[19-24] Although the pathology of these three arterial lesions varies dramatically, the principles behind the techniques for endovascular stented graft repair of these lesions are very similar. Endovascular stented graft procedures allow remote access to the vascular system, intravascular insertion of a stent and graft combination, and repair of the arterial pathology from within the arterial lumen. Using this technique, treatment of aortoiliac occlusions requires a long segment angioplasty of the arterial segment. After diffuse arterial dilation, an endovascular stented graft may be inserted to reline the diffusely dilated arterial segment.

There are several theoretic advantages to using endovascular stented grafts. Because the procedures are performed from a remote arterial access site using minimal operative dissection, less anesthesia is required. In addition, there is no need for extensive incisions or periarterial dissection in the area of arterial occlusion, which may result in substantial trauma to surrounding tissues. The occlusion is repaired in an "anatomical" manner so that axillary arteries or the contralateral femoral artery will not be jeopardized, as might be the case with extra anatomic bypasses. Dissections in scarred or infected groins may be avoided. In the case of aortoiliac reconstruction, the avoidance of a transabdominal or retroperitoneal incision eliminates the potential for prolonged intestinal dysfunction, pulmonary complications, and large fluid shifts, which may be responsible for cardiac and pulmonary failure. Preservation of sexual function in younger patients can also be anticipated with the avoidance of aortic dissection.

There are many unknowns with this new approach. The long-term behavior of the dilated portion of the native arteries extrinsic to the graft remains unclear. The potential for arterial recoil, disease progression, and a hyperplastic response in the atheromatous plaque extrinsic to the endovascular graft are of concern. Although these problems have not been encountered during our preliminary clinical applications of this technique, their potential remains.

Endovascular stented grafts appear to be an important advance in the management of complex aortoiliac occlusive disease and may have particular merit in the treatment of patients with serious co-morbid medical illnesses or those with failed previous aortoiliac reconstructions. In these situations, stented grafts represent a way to re-establish arterial continuity without extensive operative procedures and associated morbidities. Long-term follow-up and careful comparisons with standard operative and endovascular techniques will be needed before widespread application of this procedure can be advocated.

Acknowledgments
Supported by grants from the U.S. Public Health Service (HL 02990-01), the James Hilton Manning and Emma Austin Manning Foundation, The Anna S. Brown Trust, and the New York Institute for Vascular Studies.

REFERENCES

1. Brewster DC, Darling RC. Optimal methods of aortoiliac reconstruction. *Surgery.* 1978;84:739–748.
2. Szilagyi DE, Elliott JP Jr, Smith RF, et al. A thirty-year survey of the reconstructive surgical treatment of aortoiliac occlusive disease. *J Vasc Surg.* 1986;3:421–436.
3. Brothers TE, Greenfield LJ. Long-term results of aortoiliac reconstruction. *J Vasc Intervent Radiol.* 1990;1:49–55.
4. Nevelsteen A, Wouters L, Suy R. Long-term patency of the aortofemoral Dacron graft: a graft limb related study over a 25-year period. *J Cardiovasc Surg.* 1991;32:174–180.
5. Poulias GE, Doundoulakis N, Prombonas E, et al. Aorto-femoral bypass and determinants of early success and late favourable outcome: experience with 1000 consecutive cases. *J Cardiovasc Surg.* 1992;33:664–678.
6. Rutherford RB. Aortobifemoral bypass, the gold standard: technical considerations. *Semin Vasc Surg.* 1994;7:11–16.
7. Johnston KW, Rae M, Hogg-Johnston SA, et al. 5-year results of a prospective study of percutaneous transluminal angioplasty. *Ann Surg.* 1987;206:403–413.
8. Martin EC. Percutaneous therapy in the management of aortoiliac disease. *Semin Vasc Surg.* 1994;7:17–22.
9. Tegtmeyer CJ, Hartwell GD, Selby JB, et al. Results and complications of angioplasty in aortoiliac disease. *Circulation.* 1991;83[Suppl 1]:I53–I60.
10. Liermann D, Strecker EP, Peters J. The Strecker stent: indications and results in iliac and femoropopliteal arteries. *Cardiovasc Intervent Radiol.* 1992;15:298–305.
11. Palmaz JC, Laborde JC, Rivera FJ, et al. Stenting of the iliac arteries with the Palmaz stent: experience from a multicenter trial. *Cardiovasc Intervent Radiol.* 1992;15:291–297.
12. Hausegger KA, Cragg AH, Lammer J, et al. Iliac artery stent placement: clinical experience with a nitinol stent. *Radiology.* 1994;190:199–202.
13. Vorwerk D, Gunther RW. Stent placement in iliac arterial lesions: three years of clinical experience with the Wallstent. *Cardiovasc Intervent Radiol.* 1992;15:285–290.
14. Johnston KW. Iliac arteries: reanalysis of results of balloon angioplasty. *Radiology.* 1993;186:207–212.
15. Dotter CT, Transluminally-placed coilspring endarterial tube grafts: long-term patency in canine popliteal artery. *Invest Radiol.* 1969;4:329–332.
16. Balko A, Piasecki GJ, Shah DM, et al. Transfemoral placement of intraluminal polyurethane prosthesis for abdominal aortic aneurysm. *J Surg Res.* 1986;40:305–309.
17. Mirich D, Wright KC, Wallace S, et al. Percutaneously placed endovascular grafts for aortic aneurysms: feasbility study. *Radiology.* 1989;170:1033–1037.
18. Laborde JC, Parodi JC, Clem MF, et al. Intraluminal bypass of abdominal aortic aneurysm: feasibility study. *Radiology.* 1992;184:185–190.
19. Parodi JC, Palmaz JC, Barone HD. Transfemoral intraluminal graft implantation for abdominal aortic aneurysms. *Ann Vasc Surg.* 1991;5:491–499.
20. Marin ML, Veith FJ, Panetta TF, et al. Transfemoral endoluminal stented graft repair of a popliteal artery aneurysm. *J Vasc Surg.* 1994;19:754–757.
21. Marin ML, Veith FJ, Panetta TF, et al. Transluminally placed endovascular stented graft repair for arterial trauma. *J Vasc Surg.* 1994;20:466–473.
22. Volodos NL, Shekhanin VE, Karpovich IP, et al. Self-fixing synthetic prosthesis for endo-prosthetics of the vessels. *Vestn Khir.* 1986;137:123–125.
23. Marin ML, Veith FJ, Panetta TF, et al. Transfemoral stented graft treatment of occlusive arterial disease for limb salvage: a preliminary report. (Abstract.) *Circulation.* 1993;88:I11.
24. Cragg AH, Dake MD. Percutaneous femoropopliteal graft placement. *J Vasc Intervent Radiol.* 1993;4:455–463.

VIII

Infrainguinal Revascularization for Lower Limb Ischemia

30

Magnetic Resonance
Angiography in the Evaluation of
Ischemic Extremities

William M. Abbott, MD, and John A. Kaufman, MD

BACKGROUND

A comprehensive diagnosis is extremely important in the overall modern management of peripheral arterial occlusive disease and ischemic symptoms in the lower extremities. A high degree of accuracy in diagnosis is paramount and serves as the cornerstone of an effective and durable treatment plan. Great changes have occurred over the past 20 years in the general approach to the care of patients with arterial occlusive disease, and clearly the evolution of diagnostic modalities, specifically the objective studies, has been an extremely important part of this.

Two basic principals are involved in the diagnosis of arterial occlusive disease: assessment of the physiology and assessment of the anatomy of the circulation. Arterial occlusive disease is a hemodynamic disorder that causes functional and physiologic abnormalities in the circulatory system. Arterial occlusive disease is also caused by anatomic derangements in the major and minor arterial pathways. There is considerable difference in the general approach to each of these diagnostic entities, that is, physiology and anatomy.

Traditionally, physiology has been evaluated hemodynamically in the noninvasive vascular laboratory. Noninvasive technologies to assess pressure and blood flow and related abnormalities and parameters have been an active field of development for the past 20 years. A large number of approaches have been advocated for the measurement of hemodynamic abnormalities, but there are now reasonably standardized protocols that are used in most vascular laboratories in the United States. The field has also further matured by the development of formalized training in the vascular laboratory for both technologists and physicians and the registration of vascular technologists through a certifying examination and the Registered Vascular Technologist designation. Finally, accreditation of the vascular laboratories themselves has recently been implemented through an Intersocietal Commission for the Accreditation of Vascular Laboratories. Until the present time, the physiologic testing methods have been primarily the responsibility of vascular surgeons because the development of the tests was mandated in the early 1970s by a subcommittee of the American Heart Association, which was composed largely of vascular surgeons.

In contrast, the demonstration of the anatomy has been primarily in the hands of radiologists since the 1970s. Contrast-enhanced arteriography has been available since the late 1920s,[1] but again, in the early 1970s documentation of the anatomy through arteriography, as we now know it, became more formalized. This was also due to technologic advances through the development of rapid-sequence multiple exposure filming, improved resolution of imaging modalities, and improved contrast agents, catheters, and ultimately digital subtraction technology. In the 1960s most arteriography was performed by the vascular surgeon caring for the patient as part of the overall evaluation. These were single-exposure images at one or two levels and often were obtained in the operating room. This practice had disappeared, however, by the early 1970s with the technologic advancements detailed earlier and the development of the subspecialty of vascular radiology. As in vascular surgery, radiologic training programs developing subspecialization in this area were created and accredited. With this turn of events came a marked improvement in the quality of anatomic documentation through conventional contrast-enhanced arteriography.

Technology, however, has not been stagnant. Although, the contrast-enhanced arteriogram remains the mainstay and standard of reference in the 1990s for the anatomic diagnosis of all forms of arterial disease, the field is changing rapidly. Two factors have driven these changes. One is the cost. Contrast-enhanced arteriography is time-consuming and hence is expensive. X-ray film is expensive, as are the contrast agents. Staffing time adds greatly to this cost. The procedures are extremely labor-intensive and actually rival the cost of some interventional procedures, both radiologic and surgical. Related to cost are complications. Because these procedures, albeit not in a major way, are still invasive there is a decided and unavoidable complication rate. Complications, of course, have a great impact on cost, and considerable morbidity is involved. In a study of 1,000 arteriographic procedures performed at the Massachusetts General Hospital (MGH), the overall complication rate was 7.5%.[2]

Major and minor arterial complications included damage to the vessel directly at the arterial puncture site and at remote locations. They included hemorrhage, thrombosis, false aneurysm, an occasional arteriovenous fistula and arterial rupture. Another major complication was contrast-material's induced renal insufficiency, which occurred in 3% of patients. Although not common, this renal insufficiency can be a serious problem in a small fraction of patients, especially those in whom underlying renal insufficiency is a problem. This problem may occur in as many as 15% of patients referred for an arteriogram for occlusive disease.[3] It is also a particular problem in the diabetic population, which is a substantial fraction (30% to 40%) of the total number of patients with arterial occlusive disease necessitating intervention.

Two new modalities in the diagnosis of arterial occlusive disease diagnostic have developed somewhat simultaneously: duplex ultrasonic (US) scanning and magnetic resonance imaging (MRI) or magnetic resonance angiography (MRA). There is a continuing active effort to use US imaging in combination with Doppler flow velocity measurements, so-called duplex or triplex US scanning (with color added), for the diagnosis of arterial occlusive disease. Although this is extremely important work and there are centers that perform it well, this modality has not yet had widespread utilization in the United States.[4] At the MGH, we have had only preliminary experience with duplex US scanning for innate occlusive disease, because the other modality (MRA) has proven to be so much better. In addition, we have found US to be technically difficult in heavy patients, and above the inguinal ligament the problems with resolution and intestinal gas prevent adequate imaging in a frustratingly high percentage of patients.

The most exciting development is the adaptation of the principals of MRI to techniques that result in the ability to perform angiography. This field has advanced rapidly in the last several years. Excellent-quality imaging using the magnetic resonance technology has become available at most medical centers. The advantages of MRI are that it is totally noninvasive and that one can reconstruct images of vessels in more than one plane as a static continuous column of blood. Because the principal MRI keys on the physical changes due to flowing blood, in theory at least, it has the advantage of being able to give better-quality imaging in extremely low flow situations as compared to radiographic contrast material. Contrast material becomes vastly diluted after injection from a proximal site and must travel through extensive collateral pathways to reach the peripheral bed.

A number of studies in the literature illustrate the potential quality and utility of MRA. Some advocates of the modality even maintain that MRA may eventually replace contrast-enhanced arteriography in a high percentage, if not all, patients. That fact remains to be seen. Of course, it must be stated that magnetic resonance cannot be achieved in all patients, certainly at least not at present. As noted herein, some patients are not candidates for study with the existing technology for various reasons, but even that may change with further development.

THEORETIC ADVANTAGES OF MAGNETIC RESONANCE ANGIOGRAPHY

The ideal vascular imaging technique would be rapid, accurate, painless, risk free, applicable to all patients, easy to interpret, and inexpensive. Most of the currently available imaging techniques fulfill only a few of these criteria, with the more invasive, riskier modalities generally having the highest accuracy.[5] MRA is certainly not the ideal imaging technique, because it is not rapid, is not applicable to all patients (i.e., those with pacemakers), and is not inexpensive. It does, however, have several characteristics that suggest it will have an important role in vascular imaging in the future.

The risks of MRA are virtually nonexistent, provided patients are properly screened before the examination. Specific contraindications to MRI include pacemakers, metallic intracranial aneurysm clips, and metallic intra-aural or intraocular objects.[6] Patients with most prosthetic cardiac valves can be imaged safely because the deflection of the valve within the magnetic field is minor in comparison with forces of normal cardiac activity.[6] In general, most patients are suitable candidates for MRI. Furthermore, the examination is painless, requiring only that the patient remain still during image acquisition. However, claustrophobia does prevent satisfactory completion of the examination in as many as 10% of patients.

The most compelling feature of MRA is that imaging is based on flow rather than opacification with contrast material.[5] This accounts for the noninvasive, painless nature of the examination, because there is no need to catheterize a vessel or inject contrast material. Two-dimensional time-of-flight (2-D TOF) MRA, the most commonly used technique in peripheral MRA, images blood as it flows into a slice of tissue that has been prepared by suppressing the signal from the stationary background tissues. The blood entering the slice appears bright, whereas the background tissues are dark. Blood that travels in a direction perpendicular to the imaging plane produces the brightest signal, because it spends the least amount of time within the section. Blood that travels in the plane of the section looses signal, because it remains within the section for the longest time and experiences the same suppression as the background tissues. To image only arterial blood, a saturation pulse can be applied to the venous blood just before it enters the section, so that it appears as dark as the background.

The intensity of the signal from the blood depends on the character and velocity of the flow. Slow-moving, non-pulsatile blood produces the most intense signal (Fig. 30–1). These are the precise flow characteristics of blood distal to severe occlusive disease. The typical pulsatile flow present in normal vessels is subject to some loss of signal because of the changes in velocity that occur during image acquisition. This is the explanation for the seemingly paradoxic situation in which normal vessels may not image as well as diseased vessels. This phenomenon is usually self-evident from the images and is not confused with atherosclerotic disease (Fig. 30–2). Stagnant or turbulent flow, such as within aneurysms, images poorly, in part because the sluggish blood becomes subject to the same signal suppression as the background tissues.

BACKGROUND STUDIES

The intense signal generated by non-pulsatile flow, independent of the need for contrast material, suggested to many investigators that MRA should be able to demonstrate flow in the presence of severe occlusive disease. Although the first successful MRA image of the lower extremities was obtained in 1985 by Wedeen et al[7] at the MGH, 5 years elapsed before the clinical feasibility of MRA of the peripheral vasculature was demonstrated by means of a variety of techniques by Steinberg et al.[8] In 1991, Mulligan et al[9] compared 2-D TOF MRA with color Doppler and found that US had a superior correlation with conventional contrast-enhanced angiography. These results, although disappointing, did not dampen interest in 2-D TOF angiography. It seemed to us that the long scanning times used in that study and other technologic problems due to less than state-of-the-art equipment did not result in a fair assessment. That opinion has subsequently proven to be true.

That point is illustrated in the study by Owen et al[10] in 1992, who reported that 2-D TOF MRA actually depicted 22% more vessels than conventional contrast-enhanced angiography in 25 lower legs (Fig. 30–3). This study was somewhat limited by the small number of patients, the fact that the conventional angiographic techniques employed adjunctive measures to improve visualization of the distal vessels in only 8 patients, and that digital subtraction angiography was utilized in only three patients.[10] Nevertheless, this was an important contribution because it emphasized the potential role of MRA in imaging the distal runoff vessels. The iliofemoral arterial segments were evaluated by Yucel et al[11] at the MGH in 1993 and were reported in a prospective comparison of 2-D TOF MRA and conventional contrast-enhanced angiography. In this study, we identified arterial occlusions and stenoses of greater than 50% diameter with a 92% sensitivity and an 88% specificity. This study was also limited, however, in that it was small in size and the infrapopliteal vessels were totally excluded from analysis. Nevertheless, the ability of 2-D TOF MRA to image the lower extremity vessels in the presence of occlusive disease was confirmed.

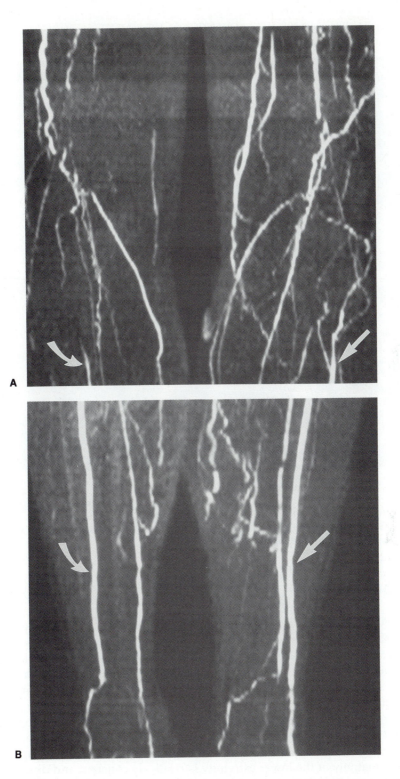

Figure 30–1. (A) Maximum intensity projection (MIP) of a 2-D TOF MRA of the popliteal region of a patient with bilateral occlusions of the superficial femoral and popliteal arteries. Many collateral vessels are seen, with proximal reconstitution of the right peroneal artery (curved arrow) and the left anterior tibial artery (straight arrow). **(B)** MIP of the 2-D TOF MRA of the calves of the same patient as in **A.** Note the intense signal in the reconstituted right peroneal artery (curved arrow) and the left anterior tibial artery (straight arrow). The right posterior tibial and left peroneal arteries are diffusely diseased.

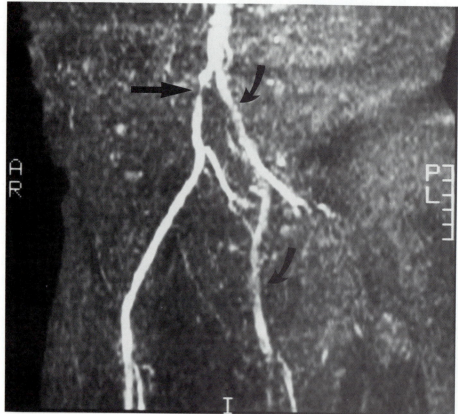

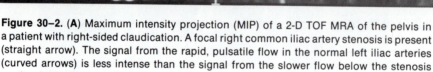

Figure 30–2. (A) Maximum intensity projection (MIP) of a 2-D TOF MRA of the pelvis in a patient with right-sided claudication. A focal right common iliac artery stenosis is present (straight arrow). The signal from the rapid, pulsatile flow in the normal left iliac arteries (curved arrows) is less intense than the signal from the slower flow below the stenosis on the right. (*Figure continues*)

TECHNIQUE

A proper MRA study of the lower extremities has many of the prerequisites of a conventional contrast-enhanced angiogram. First, an accurate history is essential to ensure that the study is performed and interpreted correctly. For example, the study has to be modified to image a femorofemoral transpubic graft, which would be difficult to see on standard axial sections because of saturation of in-plane flow. Second, coverage of the area of interest with adequate overlap requires the same planning as a cut-film runoff. Because of a limited field of view, MRA is performed one position at a time. If appropriate overlap is not obtained, focal lesions can be easily missed. Last, the interpreting physician must have expertise in vascular imaging. Although the arterial anatomy of the lower extremity is relatively constant and disease patterns are somewhat predictable, failure to recognize an important variant such as a persistent sciatic artery would be detrimental.

MRA of the lower extremities can be performed without specialized software or hardware by modifying the same 2-D TOF sequences that are used in carotid imaging.[12] The section thickness is increased to 2.0 to 2.9 mm in the extremities, which improves the signal-to-noise ratio (although there is some sacrifice in resolution). Images are

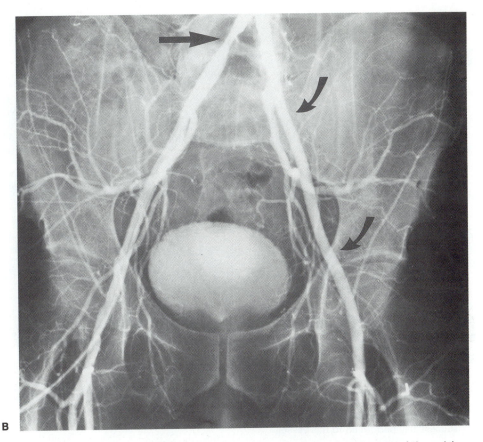

B

Figure 30–2. (*continued*). (**B**) Conventional contrast-enhanced angiogram of the pelvis from the same patient as in **A.** The gradient across the right common iliac artery stenosis (straight arrow) was 30 mm Hg at rest. Note that the left iliac arteries are normal (curved arrows).

acquired in a sequential and consecutive manner, starting distally. To mask the venous flow, a saturation pulse tracks at a fixed distance (usually 15 to 20 mm) inferior to each section. The pelvis and thighs can be imaged satisfactorily in the bore of the magnet (the body coil). For the lower legs and feet, higher-resolution images are obtained if either the extremity or the head coil is used. A typical examination would require five stations to cover the arterial anatomy from the renal arteries to the toes. With 7 minutes required for each angiographic sequence (100 to 110 sections), plus an additional 5 minutes for set-up and scouting, the average five-station study can be completed in less than 1 1/2 hours. The parameters of a typical 2-D TOF sequence would also include first-order flow compensation, a field of view of 16 to 32 cm, 29 msec (repetition time) and 6.7 msec echo time, and a flip angle of 45° to 60°.[10,11]

Image display is an important aspect of MRA, because more than 500 individual axial sections (raw data) can be generated during a single study. The interpretation of this volume of data would be inordinately difficult without the aid of fast, sophisticated postprocessing software. The most widely available technique is maximum intensity projection (MIP) display.[13] This algorithm projects only the brightest pixels from each axial section onto a coronal image, leaving the dark background. The MIP images appear remarkably similar to reversed digital subtraction angiograms, with bright

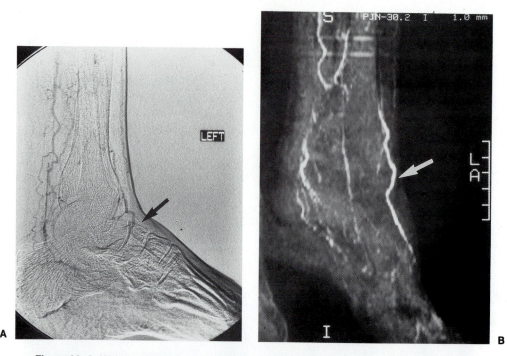

Figure 30–3. (A) Lateral digital subtraction angiogram of the left foot in a patient referred for severe rest pain, tissue loss, and unreconstructible anatomy. Only a short segment of the anterior tibial artery (arrow) was visualized in the distal lower leg, with occlusion at the ankle joint. **(B)** Lateral maximum intensity projection (MIP) of a 2-D TOF MRA of the same foot as in **A** demonstrates a patent dorsalis pedis artery (arrow). A distal bypass was successfully performed to this vessel.

blood displayed on an almost black, featureless background. However, because the algorithm does not correct for motion and other artifacts, the raw data can never be dispensed entirely.[14,15] For example, loss of signal from a metal artifact that is obvious on the axial sections could easily be mistaken for a stenosis from the coronal MIP images (Fig. 30–4).

MASSACHUSETTS GENERAL HOSPITAL RETROSPECTIVE STUDY

Because of the limitation of the aforementioned studies, the Division of Vascular Surgery and Radiology at the MGH decided to review their experience to date. Cambria et al[16] reported a retrospective evaluation of MRA in the diagnosis and management of lower extremity occlusive disease between March 1990 and April 1992. The studies of 24 patients with both MRA and conventional contrast-enhanced arteriography were compared. In these 24 patients, 180 possible arterial segments were available for comparison for imaging study agreement. In actual fact, because of various problems, including incomplete studies and prior amputation, this number was actually 175. The four segments compared were iliac arteries, common femoral arteries, superficial femoral/popliteal arteries, and infrapopliteal arteries. The two studies in each segment were correlated and results were tabulated into one of the following four categories consisting of: (1) agreement for insignificant (<50%) stenosis; (2) agreement for significant (>50%) stenosis; (3) disagreement with MRA overestimating stenosis or false positive; and (4) disagreement with MRA underestimating the degree of stenosis or false-negative. Sensitivity, specificity, and positive-negative predictive values for MRA were thereby generated. In addition, the κ statistic, which is a measure of agreement beyond chance, was calculated from the data in each table, that is, for each segment.

The results of that study are depicted in Tables 30–1 and 30–2. It can be seen in Table 30–1 that overall, MRA had a sensitivity of 100%, a specificity of 97%, a positive predictive value of 95%, and a negative predictive value of 100%. The overall agreement was 98%, which resulted in a κ statistic of .96. This value shows a statistically significant agreement at the $P < .001$. The accuracy and the agreement were equally good among all five of the arterial segments, further shown in Table 30–2. Image findings were confirmed intraoperatively; for several patients in fact, magnetic resonance was used as the sole modality for diagnosis. It is important to emphasize that the agreement was equally good at the more proximal as opposed to the more distal locations. That is, it was highly informative for arterial segments below the inguinal ligament. The conclusion of this study was that MRA seems to be an accurate modality in demonstrating relevant arterial anatomy in patients with peripheral arterial occlusive disease. Furthermore, in selected patients, it may eliminate the need for contrast-enhanced arteriography in the planning and execution of lower extremity arterial revascularization.

MASSACHUSETTS GENERAL HOSPITAL PROSPECTIVE STUDY

The study just detailed also had some limitations because of its size and its retrospective nature. However, because of the tantalizingly positive results, the same authors have designed and are now performing a prospective blinded comparison of MRA and contrast-enhanced arteriography in patients with occlusive disease at the MGH. Patients presenting with symptomatic arterial occlusive disease undergo both studies, performed by a single vascular radiologist. At the present time 75 patients have been enrolled, and it is planned that 150 patients will be entered before the study is completed. MRA images and contrast-enhanced arteriograms of each patient are then reviewed independently by different vascular radiologists. The treating vascular surgeon develops an operative plan based on both imaging studies as well as lower extremity noninvasive studies and the history and physical examination. For the study protocol a nontreating vascular surgeon reviews only the MRA image plus the supporting data from lower extremity noninvasive studies and the pertinent history and physical examination for each patient. He or she then determines an operative plan. This process is repeated with only the contrast-enhanced arteriogram plus supporting data interpreted by a different nontreating vascular surgeon. The data analysis will then include not only a comparison of the accuracy of diagnostic information itself but also the surgical planning that emanated from each of the two modalities. The purpose of this study is to conclusively prove whether MRA can replace contrast-enhanced arteriography for some patients, and if it can, which patients. At this intermediate juncture, it is clear to us, who are also investigators in this study, that the power and usefulness of this technology is great and that the goals of the study will be achieved. The results seem similar to those from studies at the MGH of similar design to evaluate the utility of MRA as compared with contrast-enhanced aortography in the diagnosis of aneurysmal disease. In a preliminary study of 23 patients,[17] the accuracy of MRA for identifying the proximal site of aortic occlusion and significant renal, celiac, and superior mesenteric artery stenosis was high; the specificities and

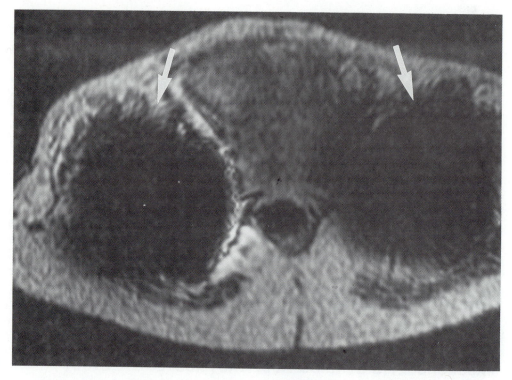

A

Figure 30–4. (A) Single axial section from a 2-D TOF MRA of the thighs in a patient with bilateral hip prostheses. Large signal voids due to metal artifact obliterate the vascular signal (arrows). (*Figure continues*)

sensitivities both were greater than 89%. In the prospective study the results are even better (Petersen, MJ, unpublished observations).

FUTURE CONSIDERATIONS

Several technical improvements are necessary to improve the quality and increase the accessibility of MRA. The pelvis remains a problematic area because of signal loss in aneurysms and tortuous vessels. Although a number of strategies have been proposed to overcome this limitation, a uniformly applicable technique has yet to be devised.[18,19] The length of time required for performing a complete study needs to be reduced, both for patient comfort and to help decrease the demands on a limited resource. Technical modifications such as cardiac gating, variable flip angles, larger image matrices, and specialized vascular coils should increase image quality.

One of the most important tasks in the future will be to determine the precise role of MRA in the management of peripheral vascular disease. After the validity of the technique is established, the outcomes of patients who are operated on solely on the basis of MRA will have to be compared with those of patients who undergo conventional contrast-enhanced angiography. Because of the slowly progressive nature of occlusive vascular disease, this will require the participation of multiple institutions over several years in order to be able to detect any significant differences in outcomes. Such a study will require a far greater degree of standardization of imaging techniques than currently exists.

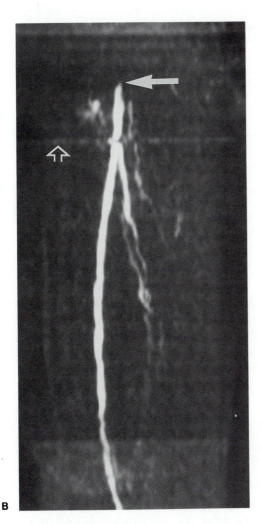

B

Figure 30–4. (*continued*). (**B**) Maximum intensity projection (MIP) of a 2-D TOF MRA of the left thigh in a patient with a hip prosthesis. There is absence of signal in the proximal superficial femoral artery (closed arrow). The etiology of the signal loss is not evident from this image. Note also the misregistration of a single section (open arrow) because the leg moved during image acquisition.

The cost-effectiveness of MRA will need to be proven before it can achieve wide clinical acceptance in the present economic environment. Given the limitations of MRI as we understand it today, it can be anticipated that some percentage of patients will continue to proceed to conventional contrast-enhanced angiography following MRA in order to clarify an anatomic issue, obtain an intra-arterial pressure measurement, or undergo a percutaneous intervention. If this percentage is large, then MRA, despite its many advantages, may not be a cost efficient study to perform on many

TABLE 30–1. RESULTS OF MAGNETIC RESONANCE ANGIOGRAPHY (MRA) IN RELATION TO ARTERIOGRAPHY: ALL SEGMENTS COMBINED*

Contrast-Enhanced Arteriography	MRA	
	Normal	*Diseased*
Normal	107	3
Diseased	0	65

*MRA sensitivity = 100%
MRA specificity = 97%
Agreement = 98%
κ = .96; $P < .001$

TABLE 30–2. COMPARISON OF MAGNETIC RESONANCE ANGIOGRAPHY AND CONTRAST-ENHANCED ANGIOGRAPHY BY ARTERIAL SEGMENT

Segment	Agreement (%)
Iliac arteries	94
Common femoral arteries	97
Superficial femoral/popliteal arteries	100
Infrapopliteal arteries	100

patients. As with analysis of outcomes, this extremely complex issue cannot be resolved until the technique is standardized and can be performed with consistent results.

CONCLUSION

Although MRA is exciting in concept, its exact utilization and application remains to be demonstrated. The preliminary data are encouraging, but definitive data, albeit forthcoming, are not yet available. Presuming a positive result in ongoing studies, however, the technology will need to be standardized and an outcomes type study performed to evaluate the proper place of MRA in vascular surgery.

REFERENCES

1. Pearse HF, Warren S. The roentgenographic visualization of the arteries of the extremities in peripheral vascular disease. *Ann Surg.* 1931;94:1094–1102.
2. O'Moore PV, Denham JS, Steinberg FL, et al. The complications of angiography: a prospective study. Abstract. *Radiology.* 1988;169:P317.
3. Gupta SK. Discussion of Cambria RP, et al. *J Vasc Surg.* 1993;17:1050–1057.
4. Moneta GL, Yeager RA, Antonovic R, et al. Accuracy of lower extremity arterial duplex mapping. *J Vasc Surg.* 1992;15:275–284.
5. Mistretta CA. Relative characteristics of MR angiography and competing vascular imaging modalities. *J Magn Reson Imaging.* 1993;3:685–698.
6. Shellock FG, Kanal E. Screening patients before MR procedures. In: *Magnetic Resonance: Bioeffects, Safety, and Patient Management.* New York: Raven Press; 1994:91–100.
7. Wedeen VJ, Meuli RA, Edelman RR, et al. Projectile imaging of pulsatile flow with magnetic resonance. *Science.* 1985;230:946–948.
8. Steinberg FL, Yucel EK, Dumoulin CL, Souza SP. Peripheral vascular and abdominal applications of MR flow imaging techniques. *Magn Reson Med.* 1990;14:315–320.
9. Mulligan SA, Matusda T, Lanzer P, et al. Peripheral arterial occlusive disease: prospective comparison of MR angiography and color duplex US with conventional angiography. *Radiology.* 1991;178:695–700.
10. Owen RS, Carpenter JP, Baum RA, et al. Magnetic resonance imaging of angiographically occult run off vessels in peripheral vascular disease. *N Engl J Med.* 1992;326:1577–1581.
11. Yucel EK, Kaufman JA, Geller SC, Waltman AC. Atherosclerotic occlusive disease of the lower extremity: prospective evaluation with two-dimensional time of flight MR angiography. *Radiology.* 1993;187:637–641.
12. Keller PJ, Saloner D. Time-of-flight flow imaging. In: Potchen EJ, Haacke EM, Siebert JE, Gottschalk A, eds. *Magnetic Resonance Imaging.* St. Louis, Mo: Mosby: 1993.
13. Kaufman JA, Yucel EK, Waltman AC, et al. MR angiography in the preoperative evaluation of abdominal aortic aneurysms: a preliminary study. *J Vasc Intervent Radiol.* 1994;5:489–496.

14. Anderson CM, Saloner D, Tsuruda JS, et al. Artifacts in maximum-intensity-projection display of MR angiograms. *AJR.* 1990;154;623–629.
15. McCarty M, Gedroyc WMW. Surgical clip artefact mimicking arterial stenosis: a problem with magnetic resonance angiography. *Clin Radiol.* 1993;48:232–235.
16. Cambria RP, Yucel EK, Brewster DC, et al. The potential for lower extremity revascularization without contrast arteriography: experience with magnetic resonance angiography. *J Vasc Surg.* 1993;17:1050–1057.
17. Edelman RR. MR angiography: present and future. *AJR.* 1993;161:1–11.
18. Prince MR, Yucel EK, Kaufman JA, et al. Dynamic Gd-DTPA enhanced 3DFT abdominal MR angiography. *J Magn Reson Imaging.* 1993;3:877–881.
19. Mulligan SA, Doyle M, Matsuda T, et al. Aortoiliac disease: two-dimensional inflow MR angiography with lipid suppression. *J Magn Reson Imaging.* 1993;3:829–834.

31

Not All *In Situ* Bypasses Are Created Equal

Robert P. Leather, MD, Benjamin B. Chang, MD,
R. Clement Darling III, MD, and Dhiraj M. Shah, MD

There is a widely held misconception that all *in situ* bypass techniques produce comparable results. Since the resurrection of *in situ* bypass by the introduction of "valve incision" as the least traumatic method of rendering bicuspid venous valves incompetent, many surgeons have introduced their own variations of technique. In Europe, *in situ* bypass has been largely performed by means of retrograde sequential valve disruption with the instruments of Hall–Gruss and Cartier–Chevalier (Langeron). These instruments have two serious disadvantages. First, the mechanism that produces valvular incompetence, namely, blunt tearing or avulsion of the valve leaflets. Second, these instruments are usually introduced and withdrawn through the distal divided end of the vein, which is invariably the portion of the vein smallest in diameter and most likely to be further narrowed by spasm when manipulated. These factors increase the likelihood of circumferential endothelial injury. Although the use of such instruments in this way is seductive in its simplicity, analysis shows that femoropopliteal bypasses using either veins less than 4 mm in outer diameter (OD) or longer, low-flow bypasses carried to the crural arteries for limb salvage, carries a 15% to 20% 30-day failure rate.

A technique that combines the safe use of both types of instruments will be reviewed. The review encompasses more than 1900 *in situ* bypasses with a primary 30-day failure rate of 4.6% (secondary rate <4%) in veins 2.5 mm OD or larger.

HISTORY AND EVOLUTION OF TECHNIQUES

An *in situ* bypass was first performed in 1959 at St. Mary's Hospital in London by Charles Rob at the suggestion of visiting vascular fellow from Oslo, Norway, Karl Victor Hall. They believed the operation of femoropopliteal bypass might be facilitated if the saphenous vein were left *in situ* and the valves disrupted, rendering them incompetent. The instrument used was the blunt end of an internal varicose vein stripper. Although arterial flow was achieved at the distal end of the vein, the patency of this bypass was short-lived. We have termed this technique *valve fracture*. Although quickly abandoned by Rob and Hall, it was extensively tried in North America and continued to be championed by Connolly and Stemmer.[1] Despite their enthusiastic reports in 1965 and 1970, the study that had the greatest impact on this procedure was performed by Barner et al in 1969.[2] They compared their results with *in situ* bypass using the Rob fracture technique with those achieved with excised reversed vein grafts. They found a very high incidence of early failure and late stenosis in the *in situ* bypasses and concluded that this procedure was inferior to standard reversed vein bypass. Their study, primarily because it reflected the experience at large with this technique, profoundly influenced the thinking of those interested in infrainguinal bypass and was largely responsible for bringing the concept of *in situ* bypass into disrepute and forestalling its further evaluation in North America. Thus, after the initial wave of enthusiasm in the 1960s, *in situ* bypass by the valve fracture technique was almost universally abandoned because of poor and unpredictable results without a conscious effort to investigate the reasons for failure.

At the same time, Hall on his return to Oslo independently developed another method of performing an *in situ* bypass by excising the valve leaflets by means of a transverse venotomy in each valve sinus. This technique, which we have termed *valve excision* was first reported in a preliminary manner in 1962.[3] This was followed by a larger series in 1964 that documented the excellent results with this technical approach.[4] Hall continued to use this method until 1968, amassing a series of 252 bypasses.[5] It seems incredible that these reports were completely ignored, perhaps because the procedure was perceived to be too complex, tedious, time-consuming, and technically demanding at a time when most femoropopliteal bypasses were relatively short (to the above-knee segment). By 1970, only Hall and Cartier persisted with the *in situ* bypass, at this time both using similar instruments for serial transluminal retrograde valve disruption, that is, the Hall valve stripper[6] and the Cartier–Chevalier valve stripper as reported by Langeron.[7] In 1972 Gruss et al adopted the Hall stripper, reporting their results in 1982 and 1987.[8]

Thus, in the decade between its abandonment (Barner et al 1969)[2] and its resurrection (Leather et al 1979),[9] there were only five surgical groups with any interest and experience in this technique. This is not only surprising but virtually unbelievable considering the appeal of the very basic nature of the concept of using the greater saphenous vein *in situ*. One would have expected that innate intellectual curiosity would have involved many times this small number.

With the advent of wider successful application of reversed saphenous vein bypass grafts to the tibial arteries, I returned in 1972 to the use of the saphenous vein *in situ* using a valve excision technique of Hall. In the course of struggling with this method and in spite of using 3.5-power operating loupes, I found that visualizing the valve leaflets through the transverse venotomies proved to be difficult and taxing, because the leaflets are gossamer thin and transparent. Because these leaflets are more readily identified with a fine nerve hook as suggested by Hall, it was inevitable that a leaflet would be picked up with the scissors blade used to excise it and cut down the middle. The leaflet would be bisected and the valve rendered incompetent. Thus, serendipitously, the technique of valve incision was discovered, and its effectiveness rapidly became apparent.

Valve incision was originally achieved by use of a scissors introduced through the open proximal end of the vein and, in more remote valve locations, by transverse venotomy at the valve site. Subsequently, appropriate side branches proximal to the valve site were used in combination with a specially designed narrow-shanked scissors to allow consistent and safe valve incision.

The modification and adaptation of the valvulotome described by Mills and Ochsner[10] for valvulotomy in reversed coronary artery bypass vein grafts eased the problem of gaining instrument access to valve sites by allowing valve incision from below, thereby minimizing the potential for endothelial injury. However, in spite of this and the use of two operative teams, an inordinate amount of time was spent in the preparation of the thigh segment of the saphenous vein when left *in situ*, that is, from the level of the medial accessory branch in the proximal incision to immediately below the knee, the portion of the vein largest in diameter and usually not well tapered.

In Europe, *in situ* bypass has been largely performed by means of retrograde serial valve disruption with the instruments of Hall and Cariter, both of which are of similar principle. These instruments have two serious disadvantages. The first is the mechanism that produced valvular incompetence, namely, blunt tearing or avulsion of the valve leaflets. Second and more important is that these instruments must be introduced and withdrawn through the distal divided end of the vein, which is invariably the portion of the vein not only smallest in diameter but also most likely to be further narrowed by spasm when manipulated. These factors increase the likelihood of circumferential endothelial injury or denudation. The effects of this type of injury may be concealed in part by high flow rates as evidenced by reasonable patency rates in bypasses using veins 4 mm OD or larger performed for claudication and/or limb salvage to the popliteal arterty with good runoff. However, when femoropopliteal bypasses using veins 4 mm OD or smaller,[11] or longer low-flow bypasses to the crural arteries for limb salvage are analyzed, there is a 15% to 20% 30-day failure rate, and the overall results are the same or worse than those historically obtained with reversed vein bypass grafts.[12–15]

In an effort to combine the ease of use of such instruments, thus expediting the procedure by minimizing the need for surgical exposure of the entire vein in the thigh and maintaining the proven increased operability, vein use, and patency of the method of valve incision, a precision injection molded polystyrene intraluminal valve cutter was developed.[15] This instrument achieves safe, consistent serial valve incision without mandatory exposure of each valve site.

Making the instrument detachable allows its introduction *and* retrieval through the large proximal end of the saphenous vein. In addition, the cutter should be used only in the thigh portion of the vein, where it can float freely in the larger vein, thereby minimizing the potential for endothelial injury. To provide both the functionally closed valve cusps for the blades to engage and a fluid medium for flotation of the valve cutter, a pressure gradient produced by flow of blood ideally at systemic pressure can be provided by construction of the proximal anastomosis, if there is a branch in the saphenous bulb large enough to allow easy introduction and retrieval of the cutter. Equally safe, effective, and far more expedient is a pressurized fluid column produced by a pneumatic transfusion cuff set at a safe pressure of 200 to 300 mm Hg over a compliant plastic bag containing either freshly drawn autogenous heparinized blood or dextran solution delivered to a catheter attached directly to the cutter. Thus, in preparation of the saphenous vein as an *in situ* bypass conduit, all three types of instruments may be used—the scissors or antegrade valvulotome introduced through the open proximal end of the vein to cut the valves down to the medial accessory branch; the valve cutter incising valves in the medial and distal thigh portion of the saphenous vein; and the retrograde valvulotome to cut the remaining valve from the knee to the point of distal transection of the vein.

The evolution of instruments and constraints of their use to achieve valve incision was guided by an overriding concern about minimizing the risk for endothelial injury while producing an incompetent valve. Our data show that particularly with the addition of the intraluminal valve cutter, there was no penalty in performance despite the greater potential for circumferential endothelial abrasion, the most devastating form of injury.[16] The high incidence of venous anomalies[17] (up to 30% of double systems) and smaller veins distally (>50%, <3.5 mm OD) makes the use of a cylindrical transluminal retrograde valve disrupter such as the Hall, Cartier, or LeMaitre strippers hazardous.

For the same reasons, the use of preoperative venous anatomic assessment either by venography or duplex ultrasonic (US) scanning is not only advisable but also mandatory, particularly if a valve cutter is to be used safely. A duplex US venous map provides the relevant information for the careful planning and execution of this procedure.[18] Without this map, attempts to define such anatomic variations surgically may result in excessive dissection, increasing the risk not only for injury to the vein but also for wound complications. Experience with more than 2,000 duplex US mappings has proven its safety, reliability, and utility in the performance of *in situ* bypass as well as in vein harvesting.

As more surgeons became involved in performing the *in situ* bypass, many introduced their own ideas and variations of technique. Many of these changes were made in an attempt at simplifying the procedure but unfortunately at the expense of either patency or utilization of smaller veins (<3.5 mm OD). Common to virtually all is the use of the Mills valvulotome or an obturator-style cutter-disrupter. The Mills valvulotome is the safest instrument for valve incision, largely because of the limited contact area of this instrument with the endothelium. This is borne out by the excellent results, that is, less than a 5% 30-day failure rate, whether used with the vein exposed or with angioscopic guidance. To a great extent how this instrument is used is the surgeon's preference or bias. Use of the angioscope requires accommodation and training with a new or foreign instrumentation, which requires not only a large initial investment ($60,000 to $75,000) but an ongoing disposable-replacement expense ($400 to $500 per procedure). Although application of this approach produces comparable results, our experience with the method that has evolved in Albany and has essentially not been changed in more than a decade, is simpler, safe, and reliable with all anatomic venous variations.

Several other instruments are available for performing *in situ* bypasses. These instruments (Hall, Cartier, LeMaitre, Bush) all utilize a cylindrical disrupter-cutter introduced through the distal divided end of the greater saphenous vein. Injury to the endothelial monolayer is produced primarily by the passage of these instruments retrograde along the wall of the distal, smaller end of the saphenous vein without the aid of distending intraluminal pressure. In addition, the frequency of missed valves is higher because of the increased likelihood of a valve leaflet's being placed against the sinus wall.[19] Thus, results with these instruments are satisfactory only in a high-flow situation (i.e., femoropopliteal) with larger veins (≥4 mm OD). When applied to smaller veins going to more distal tibial or pedal arteries, the importance of this degree of injury increases. In these distal bypasses, with their inherently lower flow volumes and velocities, these instruments exhibit an unacceptably high 30-day failure rate. Therefore, although the use of these other techniques is simplistic and seductive, their inherent limitations make their application questionable, especially with smaller veins and more distal outflow tracts.

Technically, the crucial issue in using the greater saphenous vein *in situ*, and the primary reason for its excision and reversal for femoral to distal arterial bypass, is to remove the valvular obstruction to arterial flow. All other considerations aside, leaving the saphenous vein *in situ* appears to be the most reliable method of achieving endothelial preservation, provided the valves can be rendered incompetent without injury to this very friable endothelial cell monolayer. The objective is to accomplish this maneuver with a minimum of operative manipulation of the vein and especially of the endothelial surface with particular avoidance of circumferential longitudinal shear. The simplest, most expedient, and least traumatic method of rendering the bicuspid venous valve incompetent is to cut the leaflets in the major axes, thus bisecting them. This is the essence of the valve incision technique.

A clear concept of venous valve function is important to an understanding of the problems encountered with valve lysis. The normal closing mechanism in a symmetric venous valve is initiated by tension along the leading edge of the valve leaflet caused by expansion of the valve sinus from the raised intraluminal pressures. This brings the edge of the leaflet toward the center of the lumen so that flow forces it into the closed competent position. In any segment of vein where a valve is mechanically opened from below by passage of any instrument, that is, a valvulotome, or a lumen-filling cylinder catheter, in the proximal direction, the potential exists for a valve leaflet to be pushed against the wall and to remain temporarily adherent to it in the open position. This is most likely to occur in asymmetric valves. In such valves, the normal closing mechanism may not be operative, so the valve may remain open for an indefinite period. The subsequent closure, either spontaneous or induced, of the artifically opened valve leaflet by manipulation, for example, palpation of the pulse in the area, results in partial or even complete obstruction of arterial flow. Therefore, before the distal anastomosis is performed, deliberate attempts should be made to precipitate closure of any incompletely lysed valves by the following maneuver. With the distal vein open and free flow observed, or high flow via a fistula distally, a sponge is rolled along the *in situ* conduit from top to bottom. When the cutter is used, the most frequent location of a missed valve is the junctional segment immediately distal to the point of the lowest cutter travel and the level of exposure of the vein. This segment should be checked routinely with the valvulotome, since, in the absence of flow, an undiminished pulse can be transmitted through even an intact valve in a static hydraulic column.

The simple expedient of assessing flow from the distal divided end of the saphenous vein before construction of the distal anastomosis is reliable in detecting any proximal hemodynamically significant lesions. If there is steady, undiminished pulsatile flow, it is unlikely that such a lesion is present proximally.

Most branches of the saphenous vein drain the superficial subcutaneous tissue, and their orifices are generally guarded by a competent valve, thus preventing flow away from the arterialized saphenous vein. Only valveless branches immediately become arteriovenous (AV) fistulas. However, these branches are usually small and generally undergo spontaneous thrombosis postoperatively. This thrombosis is signaled by the development of a superficial phlebitis, the extent of which is determined by the size of this iatrogenic AV malformation. Although occasionally a large area of induration results, it is sterile and self-limiting and invariably resolves within a few days. Even if such superficial veins remain patent, the loss of distal arterial flow is generally small and does not threaten the continued patency of a bypass. As a rule, only branches with sufficient flow to visualize the deep venous system with radiopaque dye on the completion angiogram need be ligated.

The effects of AV fistulas on *in situ* saphenous vein bypass hemodynamics and patency has been of great concern to some, even to the point of regarding these as a frequent cause of *in situ* bypass occlusion. From the onset more than 15 years ago, it has been our practice to ligate only fistulas that conduct enough dye at completion angiography to visualize the deep venous system. Most of the residual subcutaneous iatrogenic AV malformations produced undergo spontaneous thrombosis. We have studied more than 600 such bypasses longitudinally using duplex US scanning to assess overall hemodynamic function. The results indicate a steady reduction in fistula flow with no overall effect on distal perfusion. There is a small group of patients in whom high fistula flow is poorly tolerated, usually those with limited inflow capacity due to proximal stenosis or a small vein (<3 mm OD). In most patients, however, the flow capacity of the *in situ* conduit far exceeds the volume demanded by a fistula and adequate, undiminished distal perfusion.

The allegation that fistulas are a potential cause of occlusive bypass failure has not been our experience. The probable cause of failure in this setting is endothelial injury to the distal vein, the portion of the *in situ* conduit proximal to the fistula remaining patent because of flow to the fistula. For these reasons, we regard fistulas as at most an annoyance to the patient and the surgeon, but not as a crucial determinant of thrombosis of the bypass.

SURGICAL TECHNIQUE

After preparation and sterile draping of the entire extremity, warm (37°C) papaverine solution (60 mg/500 mL Plasmalyte or normal saline solution) is injected percutaneously into the subcutaneous tissue adjacent to the saphenous vein along its course below the knee.[20] The proximal saphenous vein, which lies immediately deep to the superficial fascia, is then exposed, and papaverine solution is infiltrated into the surrounding tissue to minimize spasm.

Although the common femoral artery has been considered the proper site for proximal anastomosis of all distal bypasses, there is evidence that use of the superficial femoral artery in the limb salvage patient population is equally satisfactory. Furthermore, technical circumstances such as a previous surgical scar or exposure of the common femoral artery or its encasement with circumferential calcification make either the deep femoral (profunda femoris) or the superficial femoral artery a valid alternative inflow source. In spite of its less accessible anatomic location, the deep femoral artery is usually less invested with thick or calcified plaque than either the common or superficial femoral artery and, therefore, frequently provides the most satisfactory site for proximal anastomosis.

The deep femoral artery is best approached from the medial aspect (with the surgeon on the opposite side of the table) by incision of the subcutaneous tissue immediately lateral to the saphenous vein down to the underlying investing myofascia (Fig. 31-1). Dissection laterally in this fusion plane to the superficial femoral artery is bloodless. The fascia is incised over the superficial femoral artery and, if it is occluded, a segment of 3 to 5 cm can be excised, thus facilitating exposure of the deep femoral artery. If it is patent, a plane is developed between the femoral vein and the superficial femoral artery. The lateral circumflex femoral vein is divided and the proximal deep femoral artery lies immediately deep to it.

Once the most satisfactory site of proximal anastomosis has been determined, the length of the proximal saphenous vein required to reach it is known. If the common femoral artery is to be used as the inflow source, a complete dissection of the saphenous bulb and secure ligation of its branches are carried out. If additional length is required

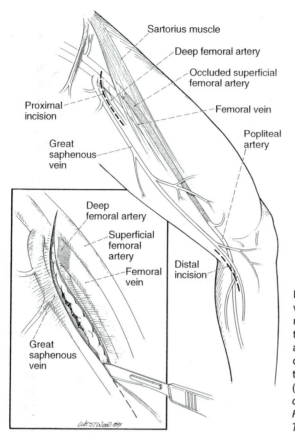

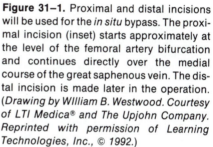

Figure 31–1. Proximal and distal incisions will be used for the *in situ* bypass. The proximal incision (inset) starts approximately at the level of the femoral artery bifurcation and continues directly over the medial course of the great saphenous vein. The distal incision is made later in the operation. (*Drawing by WIlliam B. Westwood. Courtesy of LTI Medica® and The Upjohn Company. Reprinted with permission of Learning Technologies, Inc.,* © *1992.*)

to facilitate anastomosis to the common femoral artery, a portion of the anterior aspect of the common femoral vein is removed in continuity with the saphenous bulb.

The value leaflets at the saphenofemoral junction are excised, removing only the transparent portion, leaving the usually prominent insertion ridge intact. The second valve invariably present 3 to 5 cm distal to this can be incised easily with a retrograde valvulotome through a side branch distal to the valve before the vein is divided. As an alternative it can be either a scissors or an antegrade valvulotome through the open end of the vein, as is the valve immediately distal to the medial accessory branch (Fig. 31–2). These valves are identified by gently distending the vein through its open end with dextran or heparinized blood and are cut with scissors while the valve is held in the functionally closed position by fluid trapped between the open end of the saphenous vein and the valve with the thumb and index finger around the shank of the scissors. The plane of closure of the valve cusps is invariably parallel to the skin. This dictates the orientation of all instruments with relation to the valve cusps.

If a valve cutter cannot be used, the location of the next valve site is determined by advancing a 6-F catheter, the infusion running under 200 mm Hg pressure, until it impacts in the valve sinus. This location is marked on the skin, and the proximal anastomosis is carried out. The saphenous vein is thus arterialized. If the cutter is to be used, a 3-to-5-cm incision is made 5 mm posterior to the position of the main saphenous vein below the knee marked preoperatively on the skin. A predetermined branch seen on the venogram or duplex US map is identified and used to gain access to the lumen of the saphenous vein. A No. 3 Fogarty catheter is introduced into

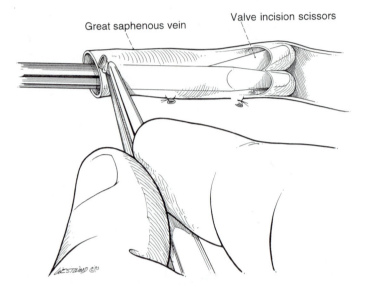

Figure 31–2. Valve incision scissors are inserted into the great saphenous vein, and the nearer valve leaflets are incised perpendicular to their plane of closure. The valves along the remaining bypass segment of the vein will be divided with the valve cutter or the retrograde valvulotome. (*Drawing by William B. Westwood. Courtesy of LTI Medica® and The Upjohn Company. Reprinted with permission of Learning Technologies, Inc.,* © *1992.*)

the saphenous vein through this side branch and passed proximally with the leg straightened to exit through the open end of the vein. The catheter is then divided at an acute angle at the 20- or 30-cm mark, whichever is closest to the open end of the vein. The valve cutter (2 or 3 mm) is screwed onto the catheter and a 6-F or 8-F catheter is then secured to the cutter with a loop of fine suture.

The leading cylinder of the cutter is drawn into the vein, providing a partial obturator obstruction to venous flow while allowing visualization of the cutting blade and minimal resistance in torque, thus allowing precise orientation of the cutting edges at 90 degrees to the plane of closure of the valves, that is, to the plane of the overlying skin surface. The catheter-cutter assembly is then drawn slowly distally while the dextran solution or blood is introduced through the catheter at 200 to 300 mm Hg pressure with a pressure seal provided by a 1-mm Silastic (polymeric silicone) vessel loop secured by a small hemostat around the most proximal end of the saphenous vein (Fig. 31–3). This pressurized fluid column snaps each successive valve to the closed position so that the cusps are efficiently engaged by the blades of the cutter. A slight but definite resistance is felt as the cutter encounters each valve and cuts the leaflets. Greater resistance than this should be managed by turning the cutter through 45 degrees and making another attempt at advancement. If this does not produce the desired result, the cutter should be withdrawn, dismounted, and the area of impaction exposed directly.

The cutter is advanced through a predetermined safe distance, generally to the knee-joint level, and is then withdrawn to the femoral exposure. The cutter is dismounted and the catheter removed from the saphenous vein. Proximal anastomosis of the saphenous vein to the selected inflow artery is performed (Fig. 31–4). The pulsatile impulse thus provided makes the location of the next competent valve readily apparent.

The remaining valves are incised with a retrograde valvulotome introduced through a side branch or the distal end of the vein. In passing the valvulotome

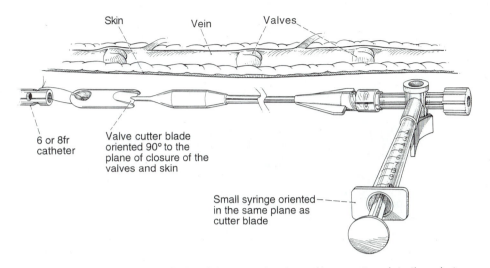

Figure 31–3. The leading cylinder of the cutter has been drawn partway into the vein to limit blood loss, and a 6- or 8-Fr catheter is attached with a suture loop to the opposite end. (*Drawing by William B. Westwood. Courtesy of LTI Medica® and The Upjohn Company. Reprinted with permission of Learning Technologies, Inc.,* © *1992.*)

intraluminally to and from a valve site, it is important that any pressure on the vein wall resulting from its curving path be exerted on the shaft of the instrument rather than on the projecting blade tip. This lessens the likelihood that the blade will become lodged in the side branch and lacerate the vein wall. This instrument is designed in such a way that it engages a leaflet, centers itself, and cuts the leaflet in its longitudinal axis. It is then readvanced, carefully rotated through 180 degrees, and withdrawn, thus engaging the remaining leaflet (Fig. 31–5). However, before the cutting force is applied to the tip of the valvulotome, the tip should be maneuvered toward the center of the vein lumen by depression of the vein itself. This maneuver allows division of the remaining leaflet without the risk of entering a side branch, which is invariably present, close to all valve sinuses.

Unobstructed pulsatile arterial flow is thus brought to the desired level. Before transection and mobilization of the distal vein, exposure of the anticipated outflow anastomotic site is carried out. This is desirable not only to minimize the warm ischemia time of the endothelium but also to assess the appropriate length required, always allowing an additional 1 to 2 cm so that the manipulated and thus traumatized terminal points can be excised and discarded.

After completion of the distal anastomosis, flow in the bypass as well as the outflow vessel is confirmed and a quantitative appraisal is made by the use of a sterile Doppler US probe. A completion angiogram is then performed with radiopaque reference markers (19-gauge needles in their plastic containers attached to the skin by sterile adhesive strips, a radiologic strip marker, or skin clips) to correlate roentgenographic position of the fistulas with the surface anatomy.

RESULTS

Of 2,695 consecutive distal bypasses, the ipsilateral greater saphenous vein was absent in 440 (16%). Of 2,109 attempted *in situ* bypasses, 1,853 (88%) were completed *in situ in toto* and an additional 162 (6%) were completed with short segments of reversed

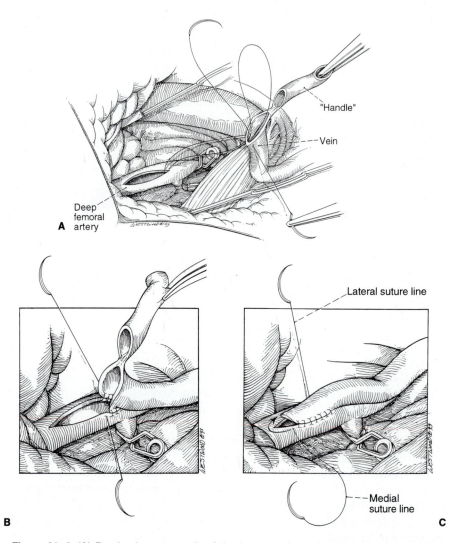

Figure 31–4. (A) Proximal anastomosis of the bypass vein to the deep femoral artery is carried out by the "open parachute" technique, which allows for accurate and atraumatic placement of each individual suture in the heel portion of the anastomosis. A single, double-needle suture of 7-0 polypropylene is used. **(B)** After placement of as many sutures as the length of suture material allows, the vein is drawn down to the artery. The handle will be excised. **(C)** Arterialization of the saphenous vein is completed by continuing the medial suture line clockwise around the arteriotomy to meet the lateral suture line at the midpoint of the arteriotomy. (*Drawing by William B. Westwood. Courtesy of LTI Medica® and The Upjohn Company. Reprinted with permission of Learning Technologies, Inc.,* © *1992.*)

vein graft (partial *in situ* bypass). In 85 (3%) limbs, the vein was inadequate by virtue of size and/or disease. Life Table analysis of secondary patency of bypasses for limb salvage to the popliteal level is shown in Table 31–1 and to the infrapopliteal level in Table 31–2.

Early detection of stenoses and correction of defects with *in situ* conduits before occlusion occurs can be achieved by a comprehensive surveillance program. Our patients are seen and examined every 3 to 4 months up to the second year and

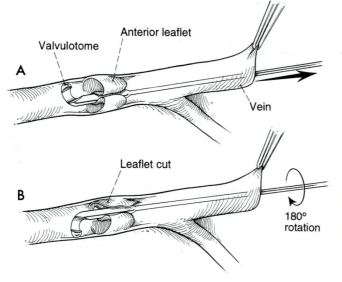

A

Valvulotome

Anterior leaflet

Vein

B

Leaflet cut

180°
rotation

Figure 31–5. Before any intraluminal instrumentation is carried out, the mobilized segment of vein is dilated with dextran solution at a controlled pressure of 200 mm Hg. (**A**) A retrograde valvulotome is introduced through the distal end of the vein, and as it is withdrawn, it cuts one valve leaflet. (**B**) The valvulotome is re-advanced, rotated 180 degrees, and again withdrawn, cutting the second leaflet. (*Drawing by William B. Westwood. Courtesy of LTI Medica® and The Upjohn Company. Reprinted with permission of Learning Technologies, Inc.,* © *1992.*)

every 6 months thereafter. Each examination includes pulse volume recordings and segmental pressures and audible Doppler assessment along the course of the bypass. Direct visualization of the conduit and estimates of volume flow by duplex US scanning, both at rest and after reactive hyperemia induced by 3 minutes of tourniquet occlusion, have been used and evaluated.

Among 1,853 *in situ* conduits constructed, 110 stenotic lesions developed in 88 patients. Seventy-five percent of these occurred within the first 12 months (82/110). Thirty-seven occurred in the distal mobilized segment, 34 in the proximal mobilized segment, and 39 in the midportion of the bypass conduit. Stenotic lesions tend to occur with increased frequency in smaller veins. Forty-five (10%) occurred in 470 veins 3.0 mm OD or less as compared with 45 (3%) in 1,338 veins 3.5 mm OD or larger. All of these stenoses were treated operatively by vein patch angioplasty, and all but five remained patent beyond 30 days. There were 94 residual AV fistulas that

TABLE 31–1. POPLITEAL *IN SITU* BYPASSES FOR SALVAGE: SECONDARY PATENCY

Interval (months)	No. of Bypasses at Risk	No. of Occlusions	Interval Patency (%)	Cumulative Patency (%)
0–1	484	20	0.956	0.956
2–12	408	17	0.951	0.909
13–24	263	8	0.966	0.878
25–35	202	2	0.988	0.868
37–48	138	7	0.944	0.819
49–60	105	1	0.989	0.810
61–72	72	2	0.967	0.784
73–84	49	1	0.978	0.766
85–96	39	0	1.000	0.766
97–108	27	2	0.918	0.704
109–120	20	0	1.000	0.704

TABLE 31–2. TIBIAL *IN SITU* BYPASSES FOR SALVAGE: SECONDARY PATENCY

Interval (months)	No. of Bypasses at Risk	No. of Occlusions	Interval Patency (%)	Cumulative Patency (%)
0–1	1212	47	0.958	0.958
2–12	970	45	0.943	0.903
13–24	567	16	0.967	0.873
25–36	377	11	0.966	0.843
37–48	250	8	0.962	0.811
49–60	168	3	0.979	0.794
61–72	116	1	0.990	0.787
73–84	84	2	0.971	0.763
85–96	50	1	0.976	0.745
97–108	31	0	1.000	0.745
109–120	18	2	0.871	0.649

required ligation under local anesthesia 3 days to 54 months after the initial procedure (5%). There were 85 occlusions within 30 days (immediate patency rate, 96%) and 69 deaths in the same period (operative mortality, 3.7%).

CONCLUSION

In situ bypasses require careful preparation. Merely retaining the saphenous vein *in situ* does not substitute for sustained care, patience, and attention to detail as well as consistent, meticulous surgical technique aided by optical magnification. Before attempting to adopt this technique, a surgeon should see it performed by an experienced operating team. In addition, familiarity with the use and feel of all instruments should be gained *ex vivo* on discarded valve-bearing vein segments from aortocoronary bypass procedures, vein-stripping operations, or autopsy specimens before one uses them on ischemic limbs.

REFERENCES

1. Connolly JE, Stemmer GA: The non-reversed saphenous vein bypass for femoral popliteal bypass for occlusive disease. *Surgery.* 1970;68:602–609.
2. Barner HB, Judd DR, Kaiser GC, et al: Late failure of arteriologic "in situ" saphenous vein. *Arch Surg.* 1969;99:781.
3. Hall KV: The great saphenous vein used in-situ as an arterial shunt after extirpation of the vein valves: a preliminary report. *Surgery.* 1962;51:492–495.
4. Hall KV: The great saphenous vein used "in situ" as an arterial shunt after vein valve extirpation. *Acta Chir Scand.* 1964;128:245–257.
5. Hall KV, Rostad H: In situ vein bypass in the treatment of femoro-popliteal atherosclerotic disease: a ten year study. *Am J Surg.* 1978;136:158.
6. Skagseth E, Hall KV: "In-situ" vein bypass. *Scand J Thorac Cardiovasc Surg.* 1973;7:53–58.
7. Langeron P, Puppinck P, Cordonnier D: La technique de la greffe veineuse in situ dans la chirurgie arterielle restauratrice des membres inferieurs. *J Chir.* 1978;115:171.
8. Gruss JD, Bartels D, Vargas H, et al. Arterial reconstruction for distal disease of the lower extremities by the in-situ vein graft technique. *J Cardiovasc Surg.* 1982;23:231–234.

9. Leather RP, Powers SR, Karmody AM: A reappraisal of the "in-situ" saphenous vein arterial bypass. *Surgery.* 1979;86:453–460.
10. Mills N, Oschner JL: Valvulotomy of valves in saphenous vein grafts before coronary artery surgery. *J Thorac Cardiovasc Surg.* 1976;71:878–879.
11. Moody AP, Edwards PR, Harris PL: In situ versus reversed femoropopliteal vein grafts: long-term follow-up of a prospective, randomized trial. *Br J Surg.* 1992;79:750–752.
12. Fietze-Fischer B, Gruss JD, Bartels D, et al: Prostaglandin E_1 as an adjuvant therapy in the event of femoropopliteal and crural great saphenous vein in situ bypass surgery. *Vasa.*[Suppl]1987;17:23–25.
13. Denton MJ, Hill D, Fairgrieve J: In situ femoropopliteal and distal vein bypass for limb salvage: experience of 50 cases. *Br J Surg.* 1983;70:358–361.
14. Harris PL, How TV, Jones DR: Prospective randomized clinical trial to compare in situ and reversed saphenous vein grafts for femoropopliteal bypass. *Br J Surg.* 1987;74:252–255.
15. Leather RP, Corson JD, Karmody AM: Instrumental evolution of the valve incision method of "in-situ" saphenous vein bypass. *J Vasc Surg.* 1984;1:113–123.
16. Sayers RC, Watt PAC, Muller S, et al.: Structural and functional smooth muscle injury after surgical preparation of reversed and non-reversed (*in situ*) saphenous vein bypass grafts. *Br J Surg.* 1991;78:1256–1258.
17. Shah DM, Chang BB, Leopold PW, et al. The anatomy of the greater saphenous venous system. *J Vasc Surg.* 1986;3:273–283.
18. Darling RC III, Kupinski AM. Pre-operative evaluation of veins. *Semin Vasc Surg.* 1993;3:6.
19. Parent FN II, Gandhi R, Wheeler JR, et al. Angioscopic evaluation of valvular disruption during in situ saphenous vein bypass. *Ann Vasc Surg.* 1994;8:24–30.
20. LoGerfo FW, Quist WC, Crawshaw HW. An improved technique for endothelial morphology in vein grafts. *Surgery.* 1981;90:1015.

32

Ischemic Limb Salvage by Revascularization and Free Tissue Transfer

Jack L. Cronenwett, MD, and Lawrence B. Colen, MD

Improved techniques for lower extremity bypass surgery usually result in successful limb salvage despite initially severe ischemia.[1] Venous bypass grafts to the distal tibial and pedal arteries have particularly benefited diabetic patients, who have a predominance of infrapopliteal occlusive disease.[2] Despite these advances, however, some patients present with such extensive tissue loss that primary wound healing cannot be anticipated even after a successful arterial reconstruction. These large ulcers usually expose tendon and bone and are often accompanied by chronic infection. They are particularly prone to develop in diabetic patients with severe peripheral neuropathy, often on the weight-bearing plantar surface.[3] Even though an arterial bypass might be technically feasible, these patients have traditionally required below-knee amputation.

In the absence of peripheral ischemia, plastic surgeons have successfully used free tissue transfer with microvascular techniques to obtain soft-tissue coverage of large defects in the leg and foot.[4] A high rate of success for free tissue transfer has been reported to close large wounds caused by trauma or extirpative surgery, and after debridement of bone or soft tissue infection. Furthermore, vascularized flaps have been shown to increase local antibiotic delivery, oxygen tension, neutrophil function, and generally to help eradicate chronic infection, even in ischemic regions.[5]

The availability of distal leg arterial reconstruction and microvascular free tissue transfer provides an opportunity to obtain limb salvage in patients with extensive, ischemic tissue loss who would normally require amputation.[6] A number of centers have reported dramatic limb salvage by combining both revascularization and free tissue transfer in selected patients. This chapter reviews the indications, techniques, and results of this approach.

PATIENT SELECTION

Even in a tertiary referral center, the need for free tissue transfer is infrequent, being required after less than 5% of our infrainguinal arterial revascularizations. This occurs for several reasons. First, most patients have ischemic tissue loss or gangrene of the toes or forefoot, which is readily treated by toe or transmetatarsal amputation. Second, patients with heel and hindfoot ulcers usually present early, when tissue loss is minimal, such that primarily healing can occur after revascularization, possibly aided by split-thickness skin grafts (STSG). Finally, some patients present with such extensive gangrene and infection, or without a suitable distal target artery, that primary, major amputation is mandatory. There does exist, however, a small group of patients who present with extensive tissue loss of the mid-hindfoot or lower leg who are candidates for revascularization plus free tissue transfer. In general, the best candidates for this approach are those who would predictably not achieve ambulation after a primary amputation. This includes patients with a previous contralateral amputation or diabetic patients with a high likelihood of subsequent contralateral amputation.

Optimal Cases for Revascularization Plus Free Tissue Transfer

Diabetic, Neurotrophic Ulcers

More than 75% of our patients who require this combined technique are diabetic and present with large, chronically infected neurotrophic ulcers. Most of these ulcers are located on the weight-bearing surface of an insensate foot, where debridement and STSG are usually not successful. Local rotation flaps may be jeoparidzed by marginal blood flow, even after revascularization. Most of these local flaps are based on antegrade blood flow through the posterior tibial artery and its medial and lateral plantar branches. If a distal bypass is performed to the dorsal pedal artery, such options are unavailable. For some of these patients, free tissue transfer can provide a more effective alternative than amputation, even though the transferred free flap is insensate. Because the remainer of the diabetic foot is also insensate, the usual diabetic foot precautions also help protect the free flap. Although recurrent ulcers have been reported in diabetic patients with heel free flaps, this occurs only after several years of walking on the flaps, and can be repaired with a second free flap.[7,8]

Post-Traumatic, Infected Ulcers

Nondiabetic patients who are candidates for free tissue transfer after leg revascularization are usually those with chronic, underlying infection and large soft-tissue defects that have resulted from trauma, surgery, or burns, on a severely ischemic limb. Multiple previous attempts at closure have often been undertaken for these patients but have been unsuccessful because of the combination of exposed bone or tendon and chronic associated infection. In these cases it is necessary to perform aggressive debridement of the infected soft tissue and bone, often resulting in a larger soft-tissue defect with exposed bone, which frustrates attempts at STSG coverage alone. Application of a free flap, however, allows adequate debridement and supplies well-vascularized tissue coverage to an area of chronic infection. This approach has been shown to eradicate local infection and promote healing.[5] Some of these patients may not have "traditional" indications for distal arterial reconstruction; that is, rest pain and distal ischemic tissue loss may not be present. If these patients have subclinical arterial disease, however, with inadequate arterial inflow at the popliteal-tibial level, revascularization is required to support free flap coverage of these proximal soft-tissue defects.

Open, Midfoot Amputations

Free tissue transfer may be useful to obtain closure of open transmetatarsal or transtarsal amputations after distal reconstruction for advanced forefoot ischemia. In these cases, extensive bone exposure at the amputation site may preclude STSG coverage, making free tissue transfer a possible alternative to more proximal, major amputation. This is especially useful in patients with contralateral amputations.

Isolated, Nutrient Flaps

It has also been proposed that free tissue transfer may provide a nutrient flap to the distal extremity if based on an isolated bypass when no target artery is present in the distal leg. At least five successful operations have now been reported in which distal bypass grafts have been performed with free flaps as the only outflow.[9,10] Our experience indicates that viability of the adjacent foot is essential since a nutrient free flap may remain viable but will not provide collateral circulation to adjacent tissue for some time after transfer. To illustrate this, two cases have now been reported in which a below-knee amputation was required despite a viable pedal free flap because the adjacent foot remained severely ischemic.[7,11] Thus, while outflow through a distal leg free flap appears sufficient to maintain patency of a vein bypass anastomosed only to the free flap, ultimate success appears to require an otherwise viable foot adjacent to the soft-tissue defect being covered. In such cases, after free flaps have been in place for several years, there does appear to be neovascularization of the tissue adjacent to the free flap, as demonstrated in one late arteriogram from our series (Fig. 32–1).

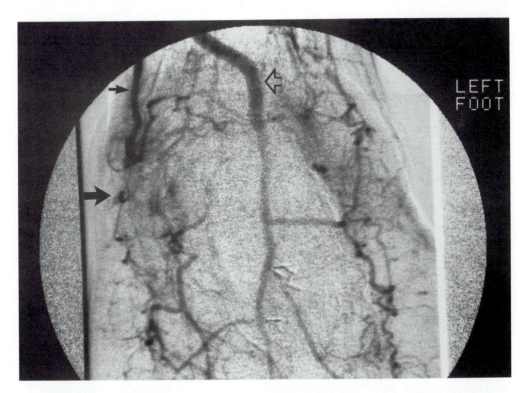

Figure 32–1. Arteriogram of the hindfoot of patient who underwent a scapular free flap transfer to cover a heel defect 2 years previously. The large open arrow shows the dorsal pedal artery. The small closed arrow shows the free flap artery, which was anastomosed more proximally to the distal vein graft. The large black arrow shows neovascularization at the edge of the scapular flap communicating with the adjacent foot.

Poor Cases for Revascularization Plus Free Tissue Transfer

High-Risk Patients

Patients who require distal arterial reconstruction for extensive tissue loss frequently have associated coronary artery disease and must be regarded as at high risk. Often these patients are diabetic and unable to walk, which may mask the normal warning symptom of angina. Free tissue transfer and distal arterial reconstruction, whether performed sequentially or as part of the same operation can be associated with substantial morbidity and mortality due to systemic complications of atherosclerosis. Thus, the most important contraindication to undertaking this combined approach is severe associated coronary disease, in the presence of which primary amputation would be a lower-risk alternative. Patients who undergo distal arterial reconstruction often undergo preoperative cardiac evaluation and special perioperative monitoring and management to minimize cardiac complications. Such precautions need to be equally rigorous during the subsequent free flap transfer, if this is performed separately.

Noncompliant Patients

Diabetic patients with large ulcers on the weight-bearing heel are good candidates for free tissue transfer only if they are well motivated to practice careful foot care postoperatively. Even nondiabetic patients who undergo free tissue transfer must observe similar precautions, including elevation of their leg to avoid edema and special protection to avoid trauma. Thus, a relative contraindication for this combined procedure is a non-motivated patient or one who cannot understand the importance of these special precautions.

Non-Ambulatory Patients

Because the purpose of free tissue transfer is to preserve limb length and ambulation, this procedure is not appropriate for non-ambulatory patients, for whom primary amputation is less complicated and more cost-effective.

Small, Forefoot Ulcers

Free tissue transfer is not necessary for patients with small ulcers, especially ulcers on the toes or forefoot, where primary healing may occur or where the lesions may be well managed by local amputation, with or without rotation or advancement flaps to obtain bone coverage.[3] The goal of any reconstructive procedure performed on the foot should be the maintenance of bipedal ambulation. When this goal can be achieved by successful forefoot or midfoot amputation, these simpler procedures should be selected.

TECHNICAL CONSIDERATIONS

When a patient presents with extensive lower extremity tissue loss, the initial assessment must include an evaluation of the arterial circulation. Doppler waveform examination and segmental arterial pressure measurements provide optimal screening to determine if ischemia is present. Transcutaneous oxygen tension or toe pressure measurement may be helpful for a diabetic patient with calcified, noncompressible tibial arteries. This initial evaluation may disclose borderline ischemia in a patient without obvious ischemic symptoms but with chronic tissue loss associated with osteomyelitis or previous trauma. Alternatively, severe leg ischemia may be apparent, with associated rest pain and marked skin trophic changes. Before free tissue transfer, however, arteriography of the lower extremity is required to delineate the optimal site for free flap arterial anastomosis. In addition, we have routinely used duplex ultrasound (US) to help localize a relatively disease-free area of the recipient leg artery to minimize the technical difficulty of the microvascular anastomosis. Duplex US assessment of potential recipient veins for free flap transfer has been useful as well.

The minimal arterial inflow necessary to support a free flap has not been established. Given the magnitude of this procedure and the risk to the patient, however, it is not appropriate to base a free flap on less than optimal inflow. Thus, it has been our practice to recommend arterial reconstruction before free tissue transfer whenever the ankle–brachial index is less than 0.7, the transcutaneous oxygen tension less than 30 mm Hg, or whenever biphasic Doppler waveforms were not present at the level of planned free flap arterial anastomosis. An occasional indication for distal arterial reconstruction before free flap transfer is a severely calcified tibial artery, which although patent, might jeopardize a successful flap anastomosis. In these patients, construction of a vein graft from a more normal proximal artery is appropriate, either to the free flap alone or to a distal target artery. Most patients who undergo free tissue transfer plus arterial reconstruction require a tibial-level venous bypass, although some patients may be effectively treated with more proximal bypass or balloon angioplasty, with the free flap then based on a patent popliteal or tibial artery.

A variety of flaps can be used for free tissue transfer. We have most frequently used the serratus anterior muscle flap because of the long pedicle length based on the thoracodorsal artery. Free muscle transfer (and STSG) is optimal for patients with osteomyelitis because this technique has proven effective in the definitive treatment of bone infection. Ulcers without osteomyelitis can be covered with fascial or muscle flaps or fasciocutaneous flaps, the specific choice dictated by the length of the vascular pedicle required and the size and location of the defect. We have used flaps harvested from above the waist whenever possible to reduce the likelihood of atherosclerotic involvement of the flap pedicle artery. Latissimus dorsi and rectus abdominis flaps are particularly useful for covering large soft-tissue defects, whereas serratus anterior and scapular flaps are useful for locations that require a long pedicle. If the recipient artery is severely calcified, a Carrel-type patch for the thoracodorsal artery can be made from its connection with the subscapular or circumflex scapular artery to facilitate a wide anastomosis. When it is desirable to avoid general anesthesia, we have also used ulnar fasciocutaneous flaps, which can be harvested under axillary block and implanted using epidural anesthesia.

Free flap transfer may be delayed after arterial reconstruction or performed during the same operative procedure. The optimal timing for individual patients depends on several factors. If both procedures are performed during the same operation, this may increase complications due to prolonged general anesthesia but avoids the need for two separate anesthetics. In either case, expert anesthesia is required to minimize complications in these high-risk patients. If the durability of an arterial reconstruction is questionable, delaying the free tissue transfer is recommended. This might apply to patients with a marginal quality vein graft, a poor distal target artery, or other suboptimal circumstances for arterial reconstruction. Delaying the free tissue transfer then allows postoperative assessment of the adequacy of the arterial reconstruction, including duplex US surveillance, to ensure that no graft defects are present that would also threaten the viability of the free flap. For patients with severe localized infection, extensive debridement is often required at the time of the arterial reconstruction, and the adequacy of this debridement may need to be reassessed postoperatively. This can best be accomplished before free tissue transfer. For these reasons, we have usually delayed free tissue transfer for several days, up to 1 to 2 weeks, after arterial reconstruction.[6] For some patients, however, simultaneous procedures may be optimal.[11,12] This is especially true if the soft-tissue defect encompasses the area where a vein graft will be placed, in order to allow immediate coverage of the arterial graft. Also, simultaneous performance of the arterial reconstruction and free flap hastens rehabilitation, decreases length of stay, and reduces cost. This approach is optimal for patients at good risk with optimal arterial reconstruction and limited infection.

Arterial revascularization combined with free tissue transfer requires a carefully coodinated effort by vascular and plastic surgeons. The arterial reconstruction must be performed with consideration for the planned anastomotic site of the free flap artery. Whenever possible, the free flap is best anastomosed directly to the distal vein graft. Thus, the distal graft anastomosis must be sufficiently near the soft-tissue defect to accommodate the length of the free flap pedicle. A two-team approach is recommended for free tissue transfer to simultaneously dissect the flap, debride the wound, and expose the recipient artery and vein if this is not being done during the same operation as the arterial bypass. Microvascular anastomoses are performed using an operating microscope with the use of interrupted 9–0 polypropylene suture. Arterial anastomoses are constructed end-to-side, whereas venous anastomoses are usually constructed end-to-end to a deep vein adjacent to the recipient artery. Low-molecular-weight dextran is used perioperatively and aspirin is used postoperatively in an attempt to improve graft pedicle patency. Postoperatively, patients are kept at bedrest with the extremity elevated for 2 weeks and then are gradually allowed to increase extremity dependency, progressing to ambulation during the third and fourth postoperative weeks. Compressive elastic wrapping and heat-molded shoe inserts are used to protect the operative site from unnecessary trauma.

RESULTS OF TREATMENT AT DARTMOUTH-HITCHCOCK MEDICAL CENTER

We have reviewed our experience with 21 consecutive patients who underwent arterial reconstruction plus free tissue transfer for ischemia plus extensive tissue loss during a recent 6-year period. All these patients had chronic ischemic ulcers that would traditionally have been impossible to heal despite revascularization, because of their large size (>5 cm diameter), exposure of tendon or bone, underlying osteomyelitis, or location on the weight-bearing surface. Of these 21 patients, 13 were men and 8 were women, with a mean age of 62 years (range, 33 to 79 years). Most of these patients were diabetic (76%), more than half of whom required insulin therapy. Most patients had associated ischemic heart disease, and many had complications of advanced diabetes, such as renal failure. A total of 22 separate ulcers was treated in these 21 patients (one patient had bilateral heel ulcers). These soft-tissue defects had been present from 3 to 15 months, except for those of one patient with tibial osteomyelitis, which had been present for more than 50 years. Nearly all the patients (95%) had undergone previous, unsuccessful attempts at wound closure with local flaps or STSG. Although all ulcers were associated with severe ischemia, the primary underlying cause was considered to be diabetic neuropathy in 10 patients, direct trauma in five, chronic osteomyelitis in two, non-healing surgical incisions in two, and three other miscellaneous causes, such as burns. The heel and hindfoot was the most common location involved (14 ulcers), followed by the lower leg (five ulcers) and ankle (three ulcers). The mean size of these ulcers was 5 by 8 cm. The smallest ulcer was 2 by 3 cm on the weight-bearing heel, and the largest ulcer was 6 by 25 cm on the pretibial region at the site of chronic osteomyelitis.

Preoperative evaluation disclosed severe arterial insufficiency in all patients. In the patients with compressible tibial arteries, the mean ankle–brachial index was 0.34. All other patients had poor monophasic or aphasic Doppler ankle waveforms and skin changes consistent with advanced arterial disease. Previous contralateral below-knee amputation had been required in 24% of patients who were ambulatory with a prosthetic limb.

Bypass grafts to the tibial or peroneal arteries were usually required to achieve adequate revascularization in these predominantly diabetic patients. Femorotibial or femoroperoneal bypass was performed on nine limbs, popliteal-pedal bypass was performed on six limbs, and femoropopliteal bypass on six limbs. One patient underwent balloon angioplasty of a focal tibial artery stenosis. All bypass grafts except one femoropopliteal graft were autogenous vein grafts. Several patients had required previous inflow procedures.

A total of 26 free flaps were placed in these patients. The serratus anterior muscle flap was most frequently used (10 flaps), followed by the scapular fasciocutaneous flap (six flaps), and the latissimus dorsi muscle (four flaps). Three rectus abdominis muscle flaps were used, and temporalis fascia, gracilis muscle, and ulnar forearm flaps each were used once. In 82% of patients, the free flap was done as a separate procedure, at a median interval of 11 days after the arterial reconstruction. In 42% of patients the free flap artery was anastomosed directly to the distal vein graft; 58% of the anastomoses were anastomosed directly to tibial arteries.

After a mean follow-up period of 32 months, the primary patency rate of the infragenicular bypass procedures in these patients was 81%. Four secondary procedures were required to establish 95% assisted-primary patency. No grafts occluded. One graft partially occluded in a patient in whom the distal saphenous vein was anastomosed both to a serratus anterior muscle flap on the heel and to the distal peroneal artery. The branch of this graft to the peroneal artery occluded (based on duplex US scanning) and the foot became ischemic. This ultimately led to below-knee amputation, despite a patent bypass to the viable free flap. None of the free flaps in our experience were lost to arterial graft failure. Frequent outpatient surveillance with duplex US scanning was performed to detect graft stenoses, so that these could be repaired before graft occlusion. Duplex US surveillance of the free flap artery and anastomosis was also possible, but none of these required late correction.

During the same 32-month average follow-up period, 85% of free flaps healed successfully after initial placement. This included 62% that healed primarily and 23% that healed after minor wound revisions. In 12% of cases, the initial free flap failed because of venous thrombosis. In each case these were successfully replaced with a second free flap, which healed primarily. Finally, one free flap (4%) remained viable but did not achieve healing, because of ongoing foot ischemia in the patient described earlier who required a below-knee amputation.

Of the 21 patients treated in this series, one postoperative death occurred from myocardial infarction within 30 days of free flap placement. Three additional patients experienced uncomplicated myocardial infarction, testifying to the high cardiac risk of this population. Among the 20 surviving patients, 95% of their ulcers healed, and one early below-knee amputation was required, as discussed earlier. Only one late amputation was required, more than 1 year after free flap placement, because of poor limb function despite a functioning free flap. Overall in these 21 patients, there was a 5% operative mortality, a 9% incidence of major amputation, and an 86% long-term limb salvage rate after a mean follow-up period of 32 months. The overall Life Table survival rate was only 50% after 4 years, however, nearly all patients dying of complications of advanced atherosclerosis or diabetes. This long-term survival rate compares with an average survival rate of 3 years in comparable patients after major amputation.[13,14] Noteworthy, however, is that these free flap recipients were ambulatory with functional flaps until the time of death.

Of the 20 surviving patients with 21 treated ulcers in this series, 35% were subsequently able to walk without assistance, and an additional 50% were able to walk by using a crutch or cane. Patients with ulcers on the weight-bearing surface of the foot or those with previous contralateral amputation were less likely to achieve completely independent ambulation, and more often required a crutch. Three patients (15%) remained non-ambulatory, one because of the early below-knee amputation, and two because of severe cardiac disease that prevented ambulation. Thus, 81% of these patients treated with revascularization plus free tissue transfer successfully achieved long-term ambulation.

ILLUSTRATIVE CASE REPORTS

Patient 1

A 52-year-old insulin-dependent diabetic man on dialysis presented with a large ulcer on the heel of his insensate foot. He had poor monophasic distal waveforms and an ankle–brachial index of 0.3. He underwent a femoropopliteal *in situ* saphenous vein graft with debridement of the right heel. After one additional debridement, he underwent a scapular free flap transfer to cover the right heel, which by now had a 5 by 6 cm defect exposing the calcaneous (Fig. 32–2A). The circumflex scapular artery was anastomosed to the medial calcaneal artery, and the scapular vein to the posterior-tibial vein. The posterior tibial artery was patent from the vein graft to the medial calcaneal artery, which provided a convenient recipient artery immediately adjacent to the ulcer. Postoperatively the patient was able to walk on this flap (Fig. 32–2B). Severe foot ischemia of the opposite leg developed, and the patient required a contra-lateral below-knee amputation 6 months later. He was then able to walk with assistance until his death 5 years later due to congestive heart failure and complications of renal failure. This case illustrates the most frequent use of free tissue transfer in our experience, namely, coverage of a diabetic neurotrophic ulcer on the heel after lower extremity revascularization.

Patient 2

A 71-year-old man with chronic lower extremity occlusive disease presented 2 weeks after first experiencing leg pain due to an embolus to the common femoral and deep femoral arteries. He underwent embolectomy of these arteries with restoration of blood flow; the superficial femoral and popliteal arteries were chronically occluded. Calf fasciotomy was performed, but because of the duration of ischemia, the anterior compartment muscles were nonviable. After subsequent debridement of this muscle, attempted closure with a STSG was unsuccessful. A 7 by 12 cm chronically infected defect in the tissue of the lower leg tissue resulted (Fig. 32–3A). Vascular laboratory studies revealed ischemia of the lower extremity, which led to arteriography and revascularization with a femoral–proximal peroneal bypass with *in situ* saphenous vein. After further debridement of the anterior compartment, this patient underwent

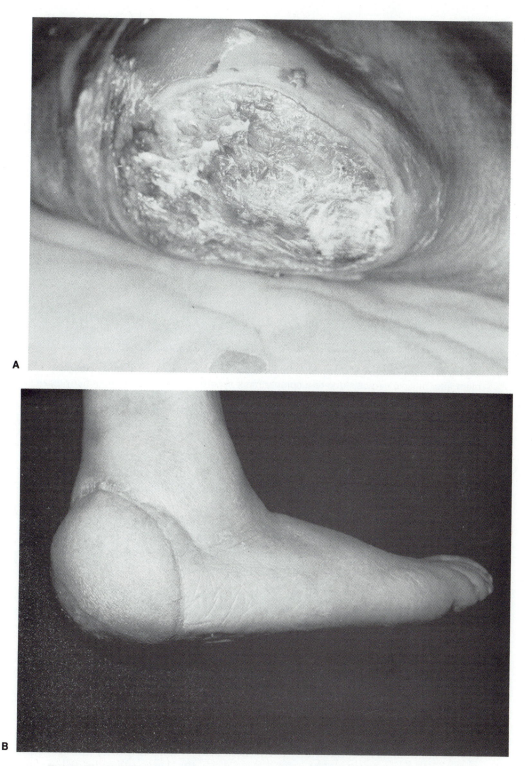

Figure 32–2. (A) This large heel ulcer developed in a diabetic patient with an insensate foot. After debridement, the calcaneous was extensively exposed. (**B**) After femoropopliteal bypass, a scapular free flap was transferred to cover this defect, which resulted in healing and ambulation for this patient who subsequently required a contralateral below-knee amputation.

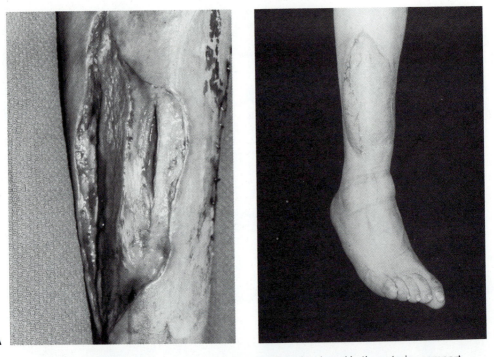

Figure 32–3. (A) This large, chronically infected defect developed in the anterior compart-ment after muscle necrosis due to a compartment syndrome. Because of the underlying ischemia, a distal bypass was required in this nondiabetic patient. **(B)** After revasculariza-tion, a scapular free flap was used to close this anterior compartment defect, resulting in complete healing.

transfer of a scapular free flap to cover this defect with the circumflex scapular artery anastomosed to the anterior tibial artery. The wound healed primarily and remained healed for 3 years before the patient died of a myocardial infarction (Fig. 32–3B). This case illustrates the use of free tissue transfer in a nondiabetic patient who had a large proximal soft-tissue defect due to leg ischemic complications. In this case, the collateral circulation between the peroneal and anterior tibial arteries was excellent, which allowed the vein graft to be placed in a separate muscle compartment before the free flap was placed.

Patient 3

A 62-year-old insulin-dependent diabetic woman presented with an ulcer on the lateral aspect of her right foot. This was debrided three times in her local hospital, yielding a 4 by 6 cm non-healing soft-tissue defect (Fig. 32–4A). After arteriography she underwent femoral–to–distal posterior tibial bypass with an *in situ* saphenous vein, with additional debridement of necrotic tissue on the right foot. She subsequently underwent transfer of a serratus anterior muscle flap with STSG to cover this defect. The thoracodorsal vessels were anastomosed directly to the saphenous vein graft and to the posterior tibial vena comitantes. The patient achieved healing after minor wound problems were treated with an Unna boot (Fig. 32–4B). Unfortunately, the patient died of a stroke 8 months later but was able to walk without assistance in the interim after free flap transfer. This case illustrates the use of free tissue transfer to cover midfoot defects, the usefulness of the long pedicle of the serratus anterior flap, and

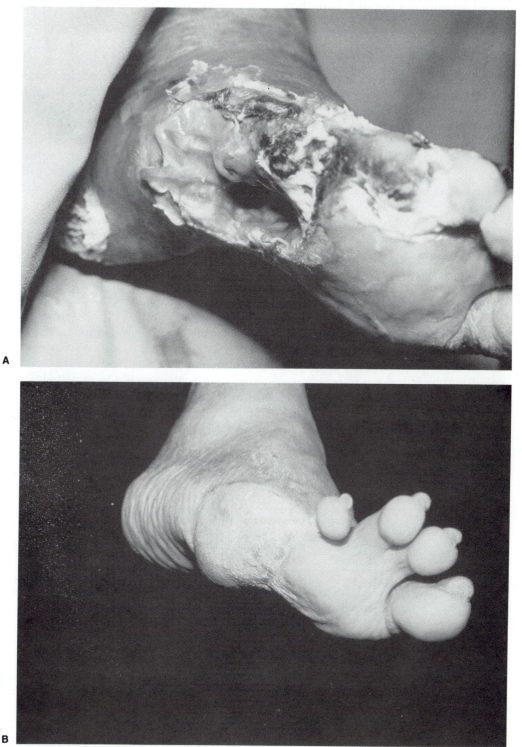

Figure 32–4. (A) Large, non-healing midfoot defect in an insulin-dependent diabetic after several debridements of a small neurotrophic ulcer. This chronically infected ulcer now exposed considerable bone and tendon, and its location prevented a transmetatarsal amputation. **(B)** After femoral–to–ankle level posterior tibial vein graft, a serratus anterior muscle flap with split-thickness skin graft was used to cover this defect, resulting in complete wound healing and eradication of local infection.

the opportunity to base such flaps directly on the vein used for distal arterial reconstruction.

Other Results and Comments

A number of other centers have also reported excellent results after revascularization and free tissue transfer for treating extensive ischemic tissue loss in the lower extremities (Table 32–1). In a total of 69 limbs with large ulcers treated by this combined approach, an 80% limb salvage rate has been obtained for at least 6 months. This was accomplished with an average operative mortality of only 2%. In at least half the patients in all series, a distal, tibial-level vascular reconstruction was required, emphasizing the frequency of diabetic disease in these patients. The preference for performing simultaneous operations varied, from 0 to 88%, with an average of 36% in these reported patients.

The outcome of revascularization plus free tissue transfer in patients with extensive tissue loss compares favorably with the rehabilitation achieved after primary below-knee amputation. Although a matched, comparable group of patients is not available, approximately 67% of patients achieve ambulation after unilatral below-knee amputation,[14,17] whereas only 30% achieve ambulation after bilateral below-knee amputation.[14] Among diabetic patients there is a high expected incidence of subsequent contralateral amputation, reported to be as high as 50% during 2-year follow-up.[18] Among our patients, 33% required a contralateral amputation after free tissue transfer. Because 25% had already undergone a contralateral amputation, nearly 50% of these patients had one major amputation. Thus, achieving more than 80% ambulation by free tissue transfer is substantially better than would be expected had bilateral below-knee amputations been performed in half of this group.

We have not subjected our results with revascularization plus free tissue transfer to a cost-effectiveness analysis. Undoubtedly, the cost of extensive lower extremity

TABLE 32–1. RESULTS OF REVASCULARIZATION PLUS FREE TISSUE TRANSFER FOR EXTENSIVE ISCHEMIC TISSUE LOSS OF LOWER EXTREMITIES

Center	n	Percentage Undergoing Tibial Bypass[a]	Percentage Undergoing Simultaneous Operation[b]	>6 Month Limb Salvage Rate (%)	30-day Mortality (%)
University of Louisville[15]	4	100	0	100	0
University of California[12]	7	100	71	71	14
Temple University[7]	8	50	0	88	0
Allentown–Lehigh Valley[16]	8	100	88	75	0
University of Rochester[11]	20	60	50	90	0
Dartmouth-Hitchcock	22	73	14	91	5
Weighted Average	[69]	74	36	87	2

[a]Versus popliteal or more proximal level bypass.
[b]Revascularization and free tissue transfer during same operation.

tissue loss is high, whether treated by primary amputation and prosthesis or by revascularization plus free tissue transfer. In the former situation, lower rehabilitation potential and higher costs of chronic care may compensate for the greater direct cost of surgical treatment and prolonged hospitalization after free tissue transfer.

CONCLUSION

Distal revascularization combined with free tissue transfer is applicable to only a few patients who present with lower extremity tissue loss. Thus, careful patient selection is critical to achieve successful results. There are a number of advantages to free tissue transfer. Adequate debridement of chronically infected tissue is possible; adequate bulk is restored to weight-bearing surfaces; local infection is better controlled; and neovascularization from the free flap may improve local tissue perfusion. Because of the high potential for perioperative morbidity and mortality, however, patients must be carefully screened, monitored, and managed perioperatively. Furthermore, the short life expectancy of this patient group requires careful selection to ensure optimal benefit after these complicated procedures. Given these caveats, however, revascularization plus free tissue transfer has achieved long-term ambulation in more than 80% of patients in our experience who would previously have been candidates only for major amputation. Close collaboration between plastic and vascular surgeons has made these results possible, and reproducible in a number of tertiary centers. This technique represents an important advance to improve limb salvage and ambulation for selected patients with leg ischemia combined with extensive tissue loss.

REFERENCES

1. Magnant JG, Cronenwett JL, Walsh DB, et al. Surgical treatment of infrainguinal arterial occlusive disease in women. *J Vasc Surg.* 1993;17:67–78.
2. Schneider JR, Walsh DB, McDaniel MD, et al. Pedal bypass versus tibial bypass with autogenous vein: a comparison of outcome and hemodynamic results. *J Vasc Surg.* 1993;17:1029–1040.
3. Morain WD, Dellon AL, MacKinnon SE, Colen LB. Current concepts in plastic surgery for the diabetic. *Adv Plast Reconstr Surg.* 1987;4:1–36.
4. Swartz WM, Mears DC. The role of free-tissue transfers in lower extremity reconstruction. *Plast Reconstr Surg.* 1985;76:364–373.
5. Eshima I, Mathes SJ, Paty P. Comparison of the intracellular bacterial killing activity of leukocytes in musculocutaneous and random pattern flaps. *Plast Reconstr Surg.* 1990;86:541–547.
6. Colen LB. Limb salvage in the patient with severe peripheral vascular disease: the role of microsurgical free-tissue transfer. *Plast Reconstr Surg.* 1987;79:389–395.
7. Cronenwett JL, McDaniel MD, Zwolak RM, et al. Limb salvage despite extensive tissue loss: free tissue transfer combined with distal revascularization. *Arch Surg.* 1989;124:609–615.
8. Greenwald LL, Comerota AJ, Mitra A, et al. Free vascularized tissue transfer for limb salvage in peripheral vascular disease. *Ann Vasc Surg.* 1990;4:244–254.
9. Mimoun M, Hilligot P, Baux S. The nutrient flap: a new concept of the role of the flap and application to the salvage of arteriosclerotic lower limbs. *Plast Reconstr Surg.* 1989;84:458–467.
10. Shestak KC, Hendricks DL, Webster MW. Indirect revascularization of the lower extremity by means of microvascular free-muscle flap: a preliminary report. *J Vasc Surg.* 1990; 12:581–585.

11. Serletti JM, Hurwitz SR, Jones JA, et al. Extension of limb salvage by combined vascular reconstruction and adjunctive free-tissue transfer. *J Vasc Surg.* 1993;18:972–980.

12. Caresi KF, Anthony JP, Hoffman WY, et al. Limb salvage and wound coverage in patients with large ischemic ulcers: a multidisciplinary approach with revascularization and free tissue transfer. *J Vasc Surg.* 1993;18:648–655.

13. Bodily DC, Burgess EM. Contralateral limb and patient survival after leg amputation. *Am J Surg.* 1983;146:280–282.

14. Couch NP, David JK, Tilney NL, Crane C. Natural history of the leg amputee. *Am J Surg.* 1977;133:469–473.

15. Briggs SE, Banis JC Jr, Kaebnick H, et al. Distal revascularization and microvascular free tissue transfer: an alternative to amputation in ischemic lesions of the lower extremity. *J Vasc Surg.* 1985;2:806–811.

16. Chowdary RP, Celani VJ, Goodreau JJ, et al. Free-tissue transfers for limb salvage utilizing in situ saphenous vein bypass conduit as the inflow. *Plast Reconst Surg.* 1991;87:529–535.

17. Hobson RW II, Lynch TG, Jamil Z, et al. Results of revascularization and amputation in severe lower extremity ischemia: a five-year experience. *J Vasc Surg.* 1985;2:174–185.

18. Kucan JO, Robson MC. Diabetic foot infections: fate of the contralateral foot. *Plast Reconstr Surg.* 1986;77:439–441.

33

Techniques to Extend Prosthetic Graft Patency:

The Use of a Venous Collar

John H.N. Wolfe, MS, FRCS, and
Mark R. Tyrrell, PhD, FRCS

In western societies critical limb ischemia is estimated to affect 500 to 1,000 people per million population each year. The prognosis for these patients is poor—approximately 18% of patients are dead after 1 year and 33% after 3 years.[1] Although these mortalities may improve slightly in the future, these figures portray an elderly group of patients who frequently have widespread end-stage arterial disease and are therefore unlikely to live for prolonged periods. The aim of the vascular surgeon is, therefore, to maintain the patient's independence and dignity by avoiding amputation, because this often leads to immobility and confinement within the patient's home.

Relief from critical ischemia can be achieved by aortoiliac or femoropopliteal intervention in approximately 70% of patients, but in the remainder a crural graft is required if amputation is to be avoided. There is little doubt that autologous vein is currently the best conduit available. Before resorting to a prosthetic graft the surgeon should therefore seek adequate lengths of vein in either the long or short saphenous system and in either cephalic or basilic systems in the arms. In some surgeons' practices this will completely preclude the need for a prosthetic femorocrural graft. However, with our increasingly interventional approach to arterial disease, many patients have undergone previous coronary artery bypass grafting or femoral-distal reconstruction with the result that veins have been utilized as grafts or thrombosed as a result of infusion lines. As a result of this most of us are occasionally faced with patients in whom adequate lengths of autologous vein are unavailable if a full-length graft to the ankle is required. When expanded polytetrafluoroethylene (ePTFE) became available, there was a natural tendency to turn to "the graft on the shelf" rather than rely on the more demanding vein-harvesting techniques but there is now conclusive evidence that ePTFE is inferior to vein—so much so that many surgeons believe that these operations should not be attempted in the absence of vein.[2]

The reasons for the discrepancy between vein and prosthetic graft patency at the crural level are complex and controversial, but they must include the increased thrombogenicity of the prosthetic material. In addition, anastomosing the rigid, large-diameter ePTFE to a small-diameter tibial vessel is demanding of the surgeon and the materials. These factors will cause early failure, but the attrition rate for ePTFE grafts remains high throughout the first 2 years. This is partly attributable to the formation of stenotic myointimal hyperplasia. It has been suggested that this process is greater in ePTFE than vein grafts.[3] Two techniques that interpose a segment of vein at the distal anastomosis have been accredited with surprisingly good patency rates in the infrapopliteal segment.[4,5] These results encouraged us to study the vein collar and develop modifications that may further improve the results.

EXPERIMENTAL EVIDENCE

The Elastic Properties of Vein

We examined the venous elastic properties of 16 specimens of normal vein and nine specimens containing a short interposed segment of re-orientated vein.[6] In the latter case a short central segment of vein specimen was excised and opened along its length to produce a rectangular sheet, which was rotated through 90 degrees. The re-oriented vein sheet was then replaced in the middle of the specimen by continuous suturing with 7–0 polypropylene sutures.

To assess the elastic properties of the wall we measured strain as a function of distending pressure. This was achieved using apparatus comprising two pressure reservoirs that instantly deliver a preset pressure at the switch of a three-way tap, which distends the segment of vein at the end of the delivery tube. The dimensional changes of the vein were then measured against a scale by means of a camera placed at a fixed distance.

Each specimen was inflated to a baseline pressure of 10 mm Hg for 5 minutes and then photographed. The pressure was then increased to 150 mm Hg for an additional 5 minutes before a second photograph was taken. The pressure was relieved, and after a rest period the process was repeated. The relative strains produced in the longitudinal and circumferential dimensions (normal specimens) and the normally orientated and re-oriented circumferences (surgically manipulated specimens) were compared by means of the Wilcoxon matched-pairs test for nonparametric data. The longitudinal strain was, on average, 7.2 times the circumferential strain produced by the increase in distending pressure ($P < .002$). The re-orientated segments distended more than normal vein. These results show that vein is anisotropic, so that when the vein is re-oriented as a collar around the distal anastomosis the compliant characteristics of the vein are maximized.

Flow Through End-to-Side Anastomosis

To explore the possibility that the Miller collar and Taylor patch increase total graft flow by an elastic reservoir mechanism we perfused 10 anastomoses of each of the three types (direct ePTFE to artery, Miller collar, Taylor patch). These were constructed using ePTFE and cadaver internal mammary artery and perfused with time-expired human blood. A double-headed pinch roller pump was able to stimulate pulsatile flow triggered by a simulated electrocardiogram, a pressure measuring device, and a Sarns water circulator to ensure a constant (37°C) perfusate temperature.

Each anastomosis was constructed using 40-cm lengths of 6-mm externally supported thin-wall ePTFE and cadaver internal mammary artery. A long saphenous vein was used for the collars and patches. After construction, each anastomosis was embedded in Silastic (polymeric silicone) foam (using a purpose-made mold) with 2 to 3 mm of artery protruding from either end. Once set, the Silastic foam and contained anastomosis were removed from the mold and the ePTFE was attached to the perfusion circuit. All specimens were perfused under conditions of pulsatile (pressure 120/ 80 mm Hg, pulse rate 100 min^{-1}) and then constant (pressure 100 mm Hg) flow (Fig. 33–1).

Flow was estimated by timed collections over 30 seconds on three occasions, the mean value being taken as representative. After flow testing the circumference of the internal mammary artery was gauged by cutting 2-mm "doughnuts" of artery open. The diameter was then calculated for samples from both the heel and the toe of the anastomoses.

There was no significant difference in total anastomotic flow for any technique when comparing pulsatile and constant flow. Furthermore, neither the Miller collar nor the Taylor patch delivered significantly greater flow than direct ePTFE-arterial anastomoses under either pulsatile or constant flow. This was the result that we expected but was at variance with a previous report suggesting that flow might be increased by the interposed vein collar.[7]

We then correlated proximal and distal flow with the vessel diameter and the heel and toe of the anastomosis. There was good correlation between flow and diameter using both the Miller collar and Taylor patch techniques, but with direct ePTFE-arterial anastomosis there was *no* correlation between flow and vessel wall diameter.

As a result of this last finding we proceeded to the third experiment, which was to perform casts of these anastomoses to try to identify the reason for the problem with the direct arterial-ePTFE anastomosis.

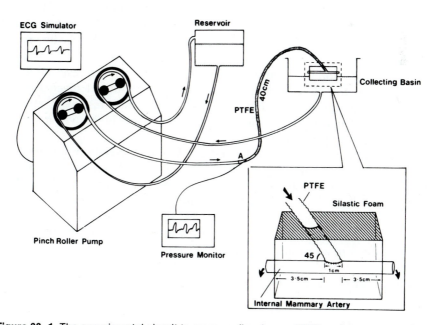

Figure 33–1. The experimental circuit to measure flow in an ePTFE graft anastamosed to internal mammary artery and embedded in Silastic foam. (*Reproduced with permission from Tyrrell MR, Chester JF, Vipond MN, et al. Experimental evidence to support the use of interposition vein collar/patches in distal PTFE anastomoses. Eur J Vasc Surg. 1990;4:95–101.*)

Casts of Anastomoses

We made casts of the anastomoses to assess the arterial distortion that they produce. This was achieved by inflating 10 additional anastomoses of each type with a silicone-based polymer at 100 mm Hg pressure. Each cast was then examined intact and by inspection of serial transverse sections. To assess the cross-sections in the immediate vicinity of the anastomotic heel and toe for distortion, we divided their maximal and minimal diameters—the more closely the resulting figure approached 1, the more nearly round was the specimen. There was distortion in 30% of the direct ePTFE-artery anastomoses and significantly greater oval distortion in these direct anastomoses as compared with the Miller collar and Taylor patch ($P = .01$).

CONCLUSIONS FROM EXPERIMENTAL EVIDENCE

Our conclusions from these experiments are that if a vein is wrapped around the anastomosis, the compliant characteristics will be maximized but this *does not* act as an elastic reservoir that discharges blood during diastole. We have also shown that there is some inevitable distortion of the anastomosis when the rigid ePTFE is anastomosed directly to the artery but that this problem is overcome by the interposition of the vein collar.

Several authors have indicated that there is benefit to be gained from matching the elastic properties of grafts with the recipient artery. One possible reason why an end-to-side anastomosis of a totally rigid material to an anisotropic tube (eg, artery) may be deleterious is that the immobilization of one-half of its wall may cause the graft to indent the anastomosis, since the compliant artery can distend with each pulse. This would result in distortion of the recipient vessel during systole and injure the vessel wall by repeated localized flexion. The interposition of a vein segment between the ePTFE and artery may ameliorate these problems. Our data suggest that the re-orientated vein segment takes maximum advantage of the elastic properties of the venous wall.

Another suggestion was that the venous collar or patch increases total graft flow and thus reduces the likelihood of thrombosis. The proposed mechanism for this hypothesis is that the venous chamber acts as an elastic reservoir, storing small volumes of blood in peak systole for passage during diastole. However, our findings *do not* support this hypothesis.[1]

We were somewhat surprised to find the lack of correlation between flow and vessel size in the case of the direct ePTFE-arterial anastomosis. This finding implies that the direct anastomotic technique incurs an additional, unpredictable element of resistance. For that reason we conducted the final experiment to visualize any technical flaws that were not apparent externally. The revelation that the ePTFE tends to protrude into the lumen at the critically narrow apex of the anastomosis presents an explanation. Even in a technically perfect anastomosis, there is some oval distortion of the recipient artery. A perfect circle has a greater cross-sectional area for any given circumference, and therefore oval distortion constitutes a stenosis.

CLINICAL STUDIES

A distal prosthetic bypass graft has inevitable problems. A long, relatively large-diameter tube with an artificial and alien flow surface is anastomosed to a small vessel with a high resistance and low runoff capacity. The volume of blood carried by this distal graft, and therefore its velocity, tends to be low, and there is a thrombotic "threshold" at which occlusion is likely to occur.[8] The thrombotic velocity threshold of ePTFE is much higher than that of vein, and this makes the conduits much more likely to thrombose. A second factor is the exposure of blood to the artificial flow surface. The amount of this exposure is increased by a high circumference–to–cross-sectional area ratio; it is therefore greater in tubes of small diameter. In normal laminar flow the blood elements are protected from contact with the flow surface by an acellular marginal zone, but this breaks down under conditions of high velocity, at which point the flow becomes turbulent. This is determined by the Reynold's number. The critical Reynold's number is that number above which turbulence is likely to occur. There are thus two conflicting problems. To avoid turbulence throughout the cardiac cycle it is necessary to ensure that the average blood velocity is below the critical Reynold's number, but the velocity must be maintained above the thrombotic threshold to avoid occlusion. For the time being little can be done about these conflicting factors. Therefore we have to concentrate on the third factor—the configuration and properties of the distal anastomosis itself.

The problems examined in the experimental study address the causes of early failure. We believe that these experiments have shown that the collar has advantages over the direct anastomosis. There is, however, also the problem of later failure, and unless the collar affects the development of anastomotic intimal hyperplasia, it is unlikely that the intermediate patency rates will be improved. Suggs et al[9] suggest in their *in vivo* studies in a dog model that intimal hyperplasia is reduced by the interposition of a venous collar. Our own clinical evaluation of patients does not support this hypothesis, but the disposition of myointimal hyperplasia does change. There is little doubt that the maximal amount of intimal hyperplasia occurs between ePTFE and the vein collar and spares the artery. The stenotic process therefore occurs in an area where the luminal reduction is less critical. One might therefore expect a collar to have greater benefit in crural vessels than in more proximal grafts, where the outflow artery has a greater diameter. Of the various reasons why a collar might improve patency rates, this is probably the most important.

CLINICAL STUDIES

It is difficult to compare results between units. In our hands full-length ePTFE grafts (70 cm) to the lower third of the calf were very unsuccessful. In fact, the results were sufficiently poor in a small number of patients for it not to be considered worthwhile continuing this practice. We were then introduced to the venous collar. Figure 33–2 shows the results, which demonstrate that one can expect approximately half the grafts to be running at 3 years (but these are secondary patency rates).[4] Graft failure invariably led to amputation in this group of patients, so limb salvage and graft patency have identical Life Table curves. We have not, therefore, considered it possible to perform a randomized trial between venous collars and direct ePTFE anastomoses for femorocrural grafts. We have, however, been involved in a study by the Joint Vascular Research Group of Britain randomizing above-knee and below-knee of ePTFE grafts between collar and direct anastomoses. These results require further follow up, which should be complete toward the end of 1994. In Sweden investigators embark on a randomized study of collar versus direct anastomosis for femorocrural grafts.

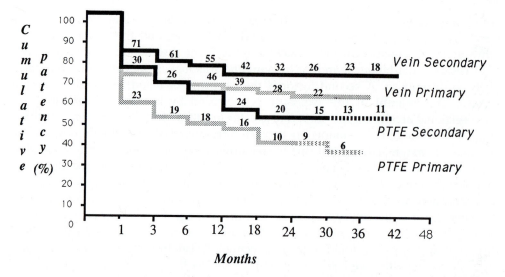

Figure 33–2. Life Table analysis of 89 femorocrural autologous vein grafts and 41 PTFE grafts shows primary and secondary patency curves. (*Reproduced with permission from Cheshire NJW, Wolfe JHN, Noone MA, et al. The economics of femorocrural reconstruction for critical leg ischaemia with and without autologous vein. J Vasc Surg. 1992;15:167–170.*)

The comparison between ePTFE grafts with a collar and vein grafts is important. Our results are shown in Figure 33–2. In this way a more direct comparison can be made between the efficacy of the two techniques, although we must accept that many patients who undergo a crural graft with ePTFE and a collar have already had a previous procedure with autologous vein. Our figures suggest that there is a difference in patency rate and limb salvage rate of 20% to 25% between the two techniques. If one assumes that this can be extrapolated to other surgeons' practice, then they are in a position to guess the approximate patency rates they might achieve.

In conclusion, therefore, 20% to 30% of these patients will be dead within 3 years and of those who survive approximately one-half will have a functioning graft and a viable limb. Our comparative figures for direct anastomosis with ePTFE to crural vessel in the lower third of the calf have a negligible patency rate and our vein grafts are approximately 20% to 25% better than ePTFE grafts with a collar.

TECHNIQUE

The proximal anastomosis is performed using a parachute technique and 6–0 polypropylene suture. The graft is tunneled directly to the lower third of the calf *without* a counterincision by means of a specially constructed long Meadox tunneler.

We then find a segment of either arm or leg vein and slit this along its length to form a rectangle. The depth of the "boot" should only be approximately 3 to 4 mm, and any redundant width should be removed. We then perform the anastomosis using a modified technique that allows more hemodynamic flow at the toe of the boot.

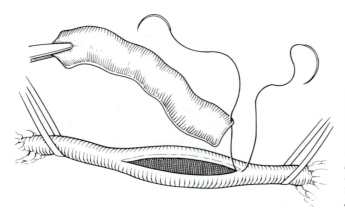

Figure 33–3. The segment of vein is slit along its longitudinal axis and anastamosed to the apex of the arteriotomy. *(With permission from Wolfe JHN, Tyrrell MR. New prosthetic venous collar anastamotic technique combining with the best of other procedures. Br J Surg. 1991;78:1016–1017.)*

An arteriotomy is performed in the crural vessel that should be at least 2 cm in length. We believe that this long incision is an important aspect of the success of this procedure. There should be an excess of vein so that a mosquito forceps can be applied to one end of the vein to anchor and control this segment while the anastomosis is being performed. Magnification loupes are essential. The distal edge of the vein is anastomosed to the apex of the arteriotomy with a 7–0 polypropylene suture (Fig. 33–3). The distal edge of the vein is then anastomosed to one side of the arteriotomy using the shorter end of the double-ended suture (Fig. 33–4). The far edge of the venous sheet is then draped around the arteriotomy and sewn down with the longer end of the doubled-ended suture (Fig. 33–5). Great care must be taken to ensure that there is no nipping at the heel of the suture line, because proximal flow is as important as distal flow in these very distal grafts. By positioning the mosquito forceps correctly, it is possible to align the anastomosis without difficulty so that the assistant can concentrate on the anastomosis itself.

The venous sheet is then anastomosed along the anterior edge until eventually the sutures meet the first corner of the graft (Fig. 33–6). Redundant vein is resected using Pott's scissors. At this stage it is essential that the two suture ends are tied in order to secure the suture line between vein and artery. The shorter end is cut and the longer suture used to sew the vein boot to itself. The boot is then completed by cutting back the heel to allow the ePTFE graft to be anastomosed to the collar at a 30-degree angle to the artery (Fig. 33–7). Once the boot has been completed, the anastomosis between ePTFE and vein is quite simple (Fig. 33–8).

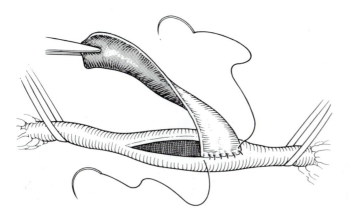

Figure 33–4. The distal edge of vein sewn along the proximal edge of the arteriotomy. *(With permission from Wolfe JHN, Tyrrell MR. New prosthetic venous collar anastamotic technique combining with the best of other procedures. Br J Surg. 1991; 78:1016–1017.)*

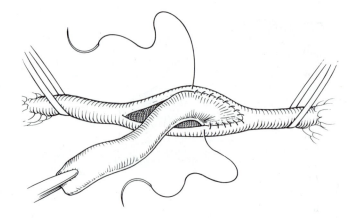

Figure 33–5. The longer end of suture is then used to anastamose along the distal edge of the arteriotomy. (*With permission from Wolfe JHN, Tyrrell MR. New prosthetic venous collar anastamotic technique combining with the best of other procedures.* Br J Surg. *1991; 78:1016–1017.*)

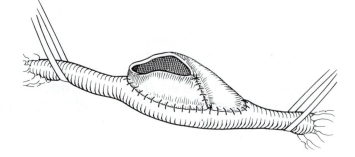

Figure 33–6. The suturing continues around the heel and the vein segment cut as marked. (*With permission from Wolfe JHN, Tyrrell MR. New prosthetic venous collar anastamotic technique combining with the best of other procedures.* Br J Surg. *1991;78:1016–1017.*)

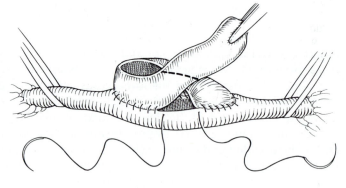

Figure 33–7. The vein segment is then sewn to itself to complete the boot. The heel of the boot is then cut away to allow a good fit for the PTFE graft. (*With permission from Wolfe JHN. Polytetrafluoroethylene (PTFE) femorodistal bypass. In: Jamieson CW, Yao JST, eds.,* Vascular Surgery, *5th edition. London: Chapman & Hall Medica, 1994, p. 339.*)

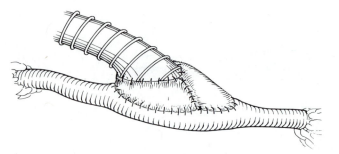

Figure 33–8. The completed amastamoses. (*With permission from Wolfe JHN, Tyrrell MR. New prosthetic venous collar anastamotic technique combining with the best of other procedures.* Br J Surg. *1991;78:1016–1017.*)

REFERENCES

1. Michaels JA. Choice of material for above-knee femoro-popliteal bypass graft. *Br J Surg.* 1989;76:7–14.
2. Bell PRF. Are distal vascular procedures worthwhile? *Br J Surg.* 1985;72:335.
3. DeWeese JA. Anastomotic intimal hyperplasia. In: Sawyer PN, Kaplutt NJ, eds. *Vascular Grafts.* New York, NY: Appleton-Century-Crofts; 1978:147–152.
4. Cheshire NJ, Wolfe JHN, Noone M, et al. The economics of femoro-crural reconstruction for critical leg ischemia with and without autologous vein. *J Vasc Surg.* 1992;15:167–175.
5. Taylor RS, McFarland RJ, Cox MI. An investigation into the causes of failure of PTFE grafts. *Eur J Vasc Surg.* 1987;1:335–343.
6. Tyrrell MR, Chester JF, Vipond MN, et al. Experimental evidence to support the use of interposition vein collars/patches in distal PTFE anastomoses. *Eur J Vasc Surg.* 1990;4:95–101.
7. Beard JD, Beneviste GL, Miller JH, et al. Haemodynamics of the vein interposition cuff. *Br J Surg.* 1986;73:823–824.
8. Sauvage LR, Walker MW, Berger KE, et al. Current arterial prostheses: experimental evaluation by implantation in the carotid and circumflex coronary arteries of the dog. *Arch Surg.* 1979;114:687–691.
9. Suggs WD, Henriquez MF, De Palma RG. Vein cuff interposition prevents juxta-anastomotic neointimal hyperplasia. *Ann Surg.* 1988;207:717–722.

34

Advances in the Treatment of the Severely Ischemic Limb:

The Use of Anastomotic Vein Patches

A. Loh, FRCS, and R. S. Taylor, MS, FRCS, FRCS (Edin)

Autogenous vein has been the preferred graft for arterial reconstruction since the use of the reversed saphenous vein was first described by Kunlin[1] in 1949. However, sufficient vein may not be available, particularly for infrapopliteal bypass, and the alternative means employing a prosthetic graft. One of the best currently available is the polytetrafluorethylene (PTFE) graft, but unfortunately the results reported have remained poor in comparison with vein and more so for anastomoses to tibial and peroneal vessels. In 1982 McFarland and Taylor[2] described the insertion of a vein patch into the distal PTFE-arterial anastomosis as a method of improving patency rates. Subsequently in a large prospective but uncontrolled series published in 1992, Taylor et al[3] achieved a 1-year patency of 81% for distal PTFE grafts, in contrast to most published results which ranged from 21% to 58%.

This chapter highlights the problems of revascularization using PTFE alone and describes the results obtained using anastomotic vein patches. New experimental data as to why these modifications should improve results are reported.

HISTORICAL BACKGROUND: USE OF PTFE FOR LOWER LIMB BYPASS GRAFTING

Results of Using PTFE Alone

Although autogenous vein is the first choice of graft for peripheral arterial reconstruction, it has been estimated that nearly 30% of patients undergoing primary infrainguinal revascularization and approximately 50% having secondary procedures,[4] do not have a vein of sufficient length or caliber, particularly if the distal anastomosis is beyond the popliteal trifurcation. Patients may have undergone earlier operative procedures requiring the use of vein, for example coronary bypass grafting; the veins

TABLE 34–1. CUMULATIVE PRIMARY PATENCY RATES FOR PTFE GRAFTS TO CRURAL ARTERIES FOR LIMB SALVAGE ONLY WITHOUT VEIN INTERPOSITION[a]

Author	Year	n	Percentage cumulative patency (y)				
			1	2	3	4	5
Cranley & Haffner[5]	1982	13	35(2)	35(1)	35(1)	35(1)	ND
Christenson et al[6]	1985	54	54(27)	52(25)	49(24)	49(22)	49(15)
Hobson et al[7]	1985	41	21(6)	12(3)	12(3)	12(2)	12(1)
Veith et al[8]	1986	98	46(39)	34(22)	30(16)	12(3)	ND
Rafferty et al[9]	1987	76	31(16)	21(10)	19(9)	17(6)	14(3)
Flinn et al[10]	1988	75	58(37)	45(20)	37(7)	37(5)	ND
Whittemore et al[11]	1989	21	25(4)	12(1)	12(1)	12(1)	12(1)
Johnson & Squires[12]	1991	37	37(36)	26(11)	21(8)	7(6)	0
Londrey et al[13]	1991	33	38(17)	26(7)	7(4)	7(1)	0

[a]The values in parentheses are numbers of patent grafts at risk at the start of each period.
ND, no data.

may be varicosed or previously stripped; or in the case of arm veins, may have been damaged by intravenous infusions.

In the absence of suitable vein, the alternative is the use of a prosthetic graft. Nowadays the most frequently employed prosthesis is the PTFE graft first introduced to Great Britain in 1976. Unfortunately, the results reported for PTFE are poor in comparison with vein; this is particularly so for anastomoses to the infrapopliteal vessels. Reported cumulative patency rates for direct anastomosis of PTFE alone to these vessels are summarized in Table 34–1. All patients in these series had grafts placed for limb salvage. Results from recent reports[14] with PTFE alone have a patency rate of 43% at 1 year (range, 21% to 60%) and 30% at 3 years (range, 14% to 38%). Comparable figures using vein were 75% (range, 47% to 100%) and 62% (range, 47% to 71%), respectively.

Causes of Failure

The disappointing results are due to several factors. In an analysis of 159 consecutive PTFE grafts, Taylor et al[15] highlighted four main causes of failure: extension of disease, anastomotic hyperplasia, kinking, and technical faults.

Extension of disease in the arteries proximal or distal to the anastomoses, either as stenoses or occlusions, was difficult to quantify until the era of graft thrombolysis. Table 34–2 summarizes the available information regarding progression of disease as a cause of failure in PTFE grafts. In Taylor's series[15] progression of disease accounted

TABLE 34–2. PROGRESSION OF DISEASE AS A CAUSE OF PTFE GRAFT FAILURE

Author	Year	Progression of distal disease (% of failed grafts)	Progression of inflow disease (% of failed grafts)
Veith et al[16]	1980	42	ND
O'Donnell et al[17]	1984	64	17
Sterpetti et al[18]	1985	48	8
Ascer et al[19]	1987	24	7
Taylor et al[15]	1987	22	8
Quinones-Baldrich et al[20]	1991	42	23

ND, no data.

for 30% of failures. Most of these were due to distal disease, although just under one-third were related to inflow problems.

The problem of graft kinking has yet to be adequately documented. Several workers describe it as an occasional but important cause of graft failure. In Taylor's series[15] it was thought to account for 13% of cases. Figure 34–1 shows kinking of an unsupported PTFE graft that was only detected at arteriography with the knee flexed.

Early graft failures (within 1 month of operation) are due to either technical errors or the presence of inadequate runoff vessels. It has been shown that the former can largely be avoided by a completion arteriogram. In our series of 159 grafts my associates and I detected nine with arteriographic defects that almost certainly would have led to failure if not immediately corrected; most of these were filling defects at the distal anastomosis.[15] The surgical difficulties of anastomosing a relatively stiff prosthetic graft directly to a small infrapopliteal vessel may explain some of the differences between the results of grafting with PTFE and vein. Thin-walled flexible vein is better to handle and makes the anastomosis easier.

Anastomotic hyperplasia has been shown to be a cause of PTFE graft failure in approximately 20% of cases.[15,16] It has been suggested that the process is an abnormal response of the smooth muscle cells to endothelial injury with resultant proliferation and overgrowth.[21] Various terms have been used to describe the thickened fibrotic area found at PTFE-arterial anastomoses. Some authors describe this fibroblastic cell proliferation[22] in a PTFE graft as intimal hyperplasia, but because there is no true intima, others have used the more appropriate terms *neointimal*[23] or *pseudointimal*[24] hyperplasia to describe this phenomenon. Both distal and proximal anastomoses may be affected; the former six times more so than the latter.[18] The cells involved in the process include platelets, (releasing various factors including platelet-derived growth

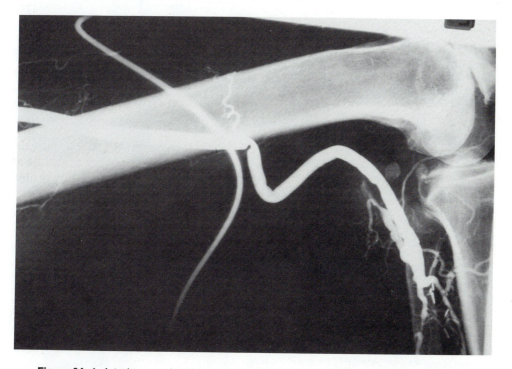

Figure 34–1. Arteriogram showing severe narrowing of an unsupported PTFE graft with the knee flexed.

factor, which are mitogenic and chemotactic), smooth muscle cells, endothelial cells and macrophages.[25–27] A complex interaction occurs in the presence of abnormal situations of different flow rates,[28,29] shear stresses[30–32] and compliance mismatch.[33] Graft porosity[34] and anastomotic angles[35] may also play a part in creating circumstances conducive to the development of intimal hyperplasia.

The heel and the roof of the anastomosis are the most frequently affected areas[15,22] (Fig. 34–2 and 34–3). Figure 34–2 shows an above-knee femoropopliteal graft that has been thrombolysed after occlusion. The cause of the occlusion is shown to be severe intimal hyperplasia just proximal to the distal anastomosis, occurring mainly at the heel and to a lesser extent at the roof of the anastomosis. An example of intimal hyperplasia occurring at the proximal anastomosis is shown in Figure 34–3; usually only the inlet of the graft is involved and not the donor artery.

ANASTOMOTIC VEIN PATCHES

Description and Technique

The incorporation of vein into vascular anastomoses has been employed since the 1970s. Linton, as discussed by Batson et al,[36] described the use of a vein patch onto which a vein or prosthetic graft was sutured to a longitudinal incision in the patch. He believed that this method facilitated anastomosis to a thick-walled diseased artery and avoided the risk of narrowing the inflow.

Venous cuffs also have been described. In 1984, Miller et al[37] reported their experience using the venous cuff. Siegman,[38] however, had initially described the same technique used in the Miller collar as a method of providing a "smooth transition between a thickened artery and relatively rigid prosthetic graft" (Fig. 34–4 top).

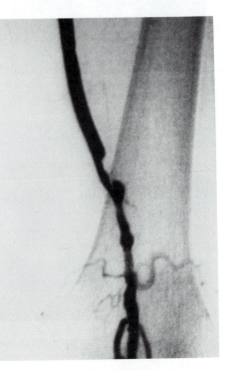

Figure 34–2. Arteriogram after thrombolysis of an occluded above-knee popliteal PTFE bypass showing distal anastomotic hyperplasia mainly at the heel of the graft and to a lesser extent at the roof.

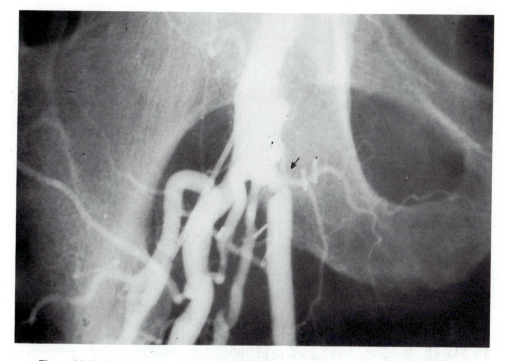

Figure 34–3. Arteriogram 6 months after PTFE femoropopliteal bypass showing narrowing at the mouth of the graft due to intimal hyperplasia.

Siegman also suggested that the anastomotic hemodynamics between graft and vein segments of a composite graft could be improved by providing a "gracefully tapered funnel connection" (Fig. 34–4 bottom). These techniques have been modified by Tyrrell and Wolfe[39] in an attempt to make the anastomosis less turbulent and more streamlined (Fig. 34–5).

The Taylor Vein Patch

In 1983, Taylor introduced a technique whereby a vein patch is incorporated into the PTFE-arterial anastomosis. This technique was based on the observation that in a small series of cases in which a vein extension had been directly anastomosed to PTFE, there was very little anastomotic hyperplasia. This section describes the operative technique.

The PTFE graft is first prepared by removing the external support over a length of 3 to 4 cm. A short (1 cm) U-shaped slit is cut, and an arteriotomy 3 to 4 cm long is made. The first six continuous heel stitches are inserted in a parachute manner and suturing is completed along each side (Fig. 34–6) using either 6–0 polypropylene or Gore-Tex sutures. The PTFE graft is then incised in line with the arteriotomy to a point 2 to 3 cm proximal to the heel of the anastomosis. The limit of this incision is also fashioned in a U shape and the surplus graft trimmed as shown by the dotted lines in Figure 34–6. This leaves a diamond-shaped area into which a vein patch is inserted. Placement of the patch begins distally using six to eight 6–0 or 7–0 interrupted sutures, all inserted before any are tied. The rest of the patch is then completed using a continuous suture.

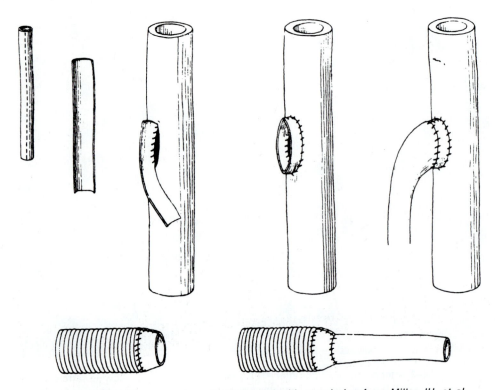

Figure 34–4. The Siegman vein cuff. (*Reprinted with permission from Miller JH, et al. Interposition vein cuff for anastomosis of prosthesis to small artery. Aust NZ J Surg. 1984;54:283–285.*)

Considerable care must be taken to avoid narrowing at the point representing the distal limit of the PTFE-arterial anastomosis, and the vein patch should be carefully placed so that the widest part overlies this area. Insertion of sutures in the vein at slightly wider intervals than on the artery or graft at this point prevents in drawing of the patch and allows for a more satisfactory appearance (Figs. 34–7 and 34–8).

The proximal vein patch measures about 3 cm and overlies the inlet to the graft (Fig. 34–9).

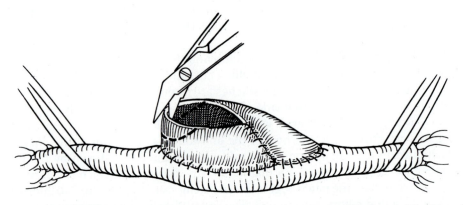

Figure 34–5. The St. Mary's boot. (*With permission from Wolfe JHN, Tyrrell MR. New prosthetic venous collar anastamotic technique combining with the best of other procedures. Br J Surg. 1991;78:1016–1017.*)

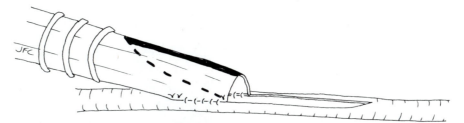

Figure 34–6. The heel of the graft has been inserted in a parachute manner, and suturing has been completed on each side. The graft is then incised over a length of 3 cm, and a U-shaped area is trimmed away, as shown by the dotted lines.

Clinical Results Using Anastomotic Vein Patches

The results of the use of these various interposition vein techniques are shown in Table 34–3. Miller et al[37] in 1984 reported on their experience with prosthetic grafting utilizing the interposition vein cuff in 114 bypasses over an 18-month period. Of these, 29 bypasses were to the tibial vessels, and 21 remained patent over a mean follow-up period of 8 months. Tyrrell et al,[40] using a similar technique in 30 cases, recorded a crude patency rate of 40% to infrapopliteal vessels at 1 year. Recently an improved 3-year patency rate of 52% has been reported by the same group in 55 PTFE bypass grafts to crural vessels.[14]

In 1992[3] we reported the results of 256 PTFE bypass grafts with the incorporation of the Taylor patch. Eighty-three of these were to an infrapopliteal vessel with a mean follow-up period of 3 years (range, 1 to 9 years); the indication for surgery was limb salvage in all cases. For these patients the maximum ankle arterial systolic pressure was below 50 mm Hg and the mean preoperative ankle–brachial index was 0.18 (excluding diabetics). Data were evaluated using Life Table analysis. The most significant improvement (compared to reported results) was seen in the infrapopliteal group, in which primary cumulative patency rates of 74%, 59%, and 54% were achieved after 1, 3, and 5 years, respectively. Comparable figures for grafts placed in the above-knee popliteal artery were 94%, 85%, and 77%, and for those placed in the below-knee popliteal artery were 88%, 77%, and 65%, respectively. Limb salvage rates for the surviving patients in the whole group were 96%, 88%, and 80% at 1, 5, and 8 years, respectively.

EXPERIMENTAL STUDY USING A SHEEP MODEL

The Sheep Model

Between 1990 and 1991, a new sheep model for the development of anastomotic hyperplasia in PTFE grafts with a reproducible high failure rate was developed. Such

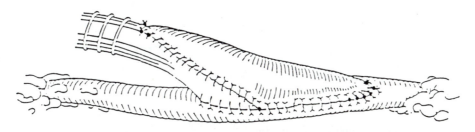

Figure 34–7. Final appearance of the completed vein patch.

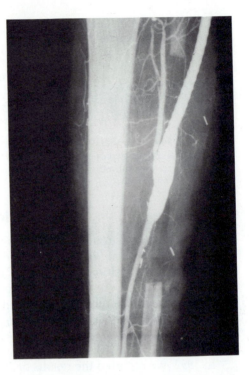

Figure 34–8. Operative arteriogram of the completed distal anatomosis with the Taylor vein patch incorporated.

a model has not been previously described, has no deleterious effect on the animal, and is less expensive than existing alternatives. It also allows comparisons of anastomotic configurations or different graft materials. Bilateral carotid bypass grafting was performed on 10 adult female sheep under general anesthesia. All procedures performed were in accordance with the guidelines of the Animals (Scientific Procedures) Act of 1986. A 15-cm length of 6-mm PTFE was inserted, end-to-side anastomoses were made, and the intervening native carotid artery was ligated. Grafts were monitored for patency with a handheld Doppler probe, and occluded grafts were removed soon after detection. Grafts that remained patent were harvested 8 weeks after insertion.

In this series, of the 18 grafts at risk, 13 failed. In five of these grafts severe anastomotic hyperplasia involving the roof and heel of the anastomosis was the cause (Fig. 34–10). In three of the six patent grafts this was also seen to a lesser extent. This distribution of neointimal hyperplasia corresponds almost exactly to that seen

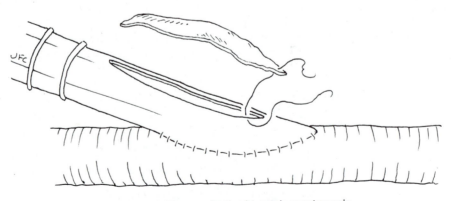

Figure 34–9. The proximal vein patch anastomosis.

TABLE 34–3. RESULTS OF INFRAPOPLITEAL PTFE BYPASS GRAFTING WITH ADJUNCTIVE VEIN CUFFS OR PATCHES

Author	Year	n	Method	Percentage cumulative patency (y) 1	3	5	Percentage of patients with critical limb ischemia
Miller et al[37]	1984	29	Miller cuff	72 [a](8 mo)	ND	ND	Not stated
Batson et al[36]	1984	68	Linton patch	74[b]	64[b]	ND	85
Tyrell et al[40]	1989	30	Miller cuff	40[a]	ND	ND	100
Wolfe & Tyrrell et al[14]	1991	55	Miller cuff	ND	52	ND	100
Taylor et al[3]	1992	83	Taylor patch	74	58	54	100

[a]Crude patency.
[b]Includes 48 below-knee popliteal grafts.
ND, no data.

in the human clinical situation. Histologic analyses showed the involved areas to comprise granulation tissue as well as fibroblasts, macrophages, and smooth muscle cells. Graft infection, technical failures, and anastomotic aneurysms were the causes of failure in the remaining grafts.

Experimental Study

Using the aforedescribed model, three main sets of experiments were performed. In the first group of 12 sheep, PTFE bypass grafting was performed with direct end-to-side anastomosis on one side and a vein-patched anastomosis on the other side

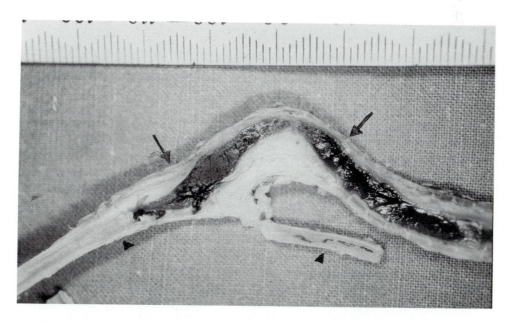

Figure 34–10. Longitudinal section of an occluded graft showing severe narrowing at the anastomoses. Arrows = PTFE graft, arrowhead = native artery.

(Fig. 34–11). The side from which the vein was taken to fashion the patch, the side that was vein-patched, and the order in which the anastomoses were constructed were prospectively randomized. Operative arteriograms were obtained and repeated at 6 weeks. Any occluded graft detected was removed immediately, and all grafts remaining patent were harvested 12 weeks after insertion. Aspirin was prescribed preoperatively and continued throughout the study period.

In this group, there were two (20%) occluded vein-patched grafts at the end of the study period compared with six (60%) non-patched grafts. Although the latter group occluded three times more than vein-patched grafts, this difference did not achieve statistical significance ($P = .085$, Fischer exact test). However, when each sheep was considered as its own control, non-patched grafts were more likely to occlude first compared with vein-patch grafts; this occurred in six of the 10 pairs ($P = .031$, sign test). In none of these sheep did the vein-patched grafts occlude earlier than the grafts on contralateral side.

When the duration of patency was analyzed, vein-patched grafts were patent longer than non-patched grafts (mean 10.2 weeks compared with 8.3 weeks, respectively, $t = 2.62$, $P .05$, 9 degress of freedom, paired t test).

To test whether these improved results could be attributed to the widening and streamlining of the anastomoses by the patch, in an addition 12 sheep vein-patched grafts were compared with grafts similarly patched with PTFE (Fig. 34–12). The study period was maintained at 12 weeks, and aspirin was stopped after 6 weeks in an attempt to stress the model to induce further failures.

In this group results were notably similar to those found in the first group. Three of the 12 (25%) vein-patched grafts occluded compared with seven (58%) PTFE-patched grafts at the end of the study period. Again, although there were more than twice the number of occlusions in the PTFE-patched group, this difference did not achieve statistical significance ($P = .106$, Fischer exact test). However, as seen in the previous group, occlusion of the PTFE-patched grafts developed significantly earlier in six of 10 sheep, with no sheep exhibiting the converse ($P = .031$, sign test). In one sheep both grafts were found to be occluded at the same time. As in the first group, vein-patched grafts were patent significantly longer than PTFE-patched grafts (mean 11.1 weeks compared with 8.2 weeks, $t = 2.69$, $P < .05$, 11 degrees of freedom).

In the final group of experiments, we tested the effect of decreasing the compliance of the vein patch. In this group, 12 vein-patched grafts were compared with grafts

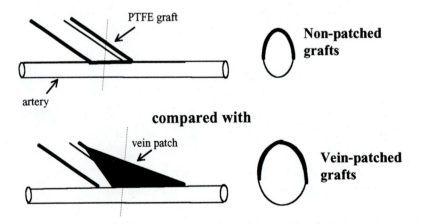

Figure 34–11. Vein-patched grafts compared to unpatched grafts.

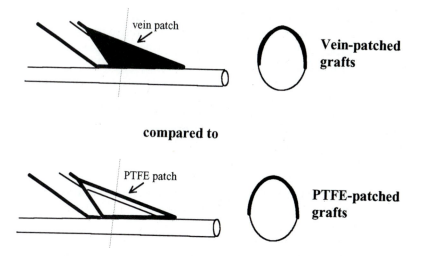

Figure 34–12. Vein-patched grafts compare with PTFE-patched grafts.

that were patched with vein and PTFE on the others side. The latter grafts had an additional PTFE patch on the outside. This gave the undersurface of the PTFE a lining of endothelium (Fig. 34–13) but also rendered the vein patch less compliant. Aspirin was not given at any time, and the study period remained at 12 weeks.

In this group, four of 12 vein-patched grafts (33%) occluded compared with seven in the test group. This difference was not significant ($P = .21$, Fischer exact test). Unlike in the previous two experiments, the test grafts (in this case, the grafts with PTFE patches lined with vein) did not occlude significantly earlier than vein-patched grafts.

Earlier occlusion occurred in three sheep only, and in one the vein-patched side occluded first ($P = .25$, sign test). In three sheep, occlusion of both sides was detected simultaneously. There was no significant difference between the groups either in

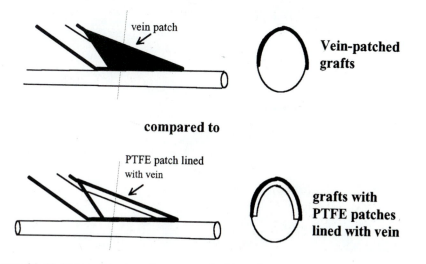

Figure 34–13. Vein-patched grafts compared with grafts patched with PTFE lined with vein.

terms of overall patency at the end of study period or in terms of one side occluding earlier than the other. Furthermore, there was no difference in the length of patency between the two groups. Vein-patched grafts had a mean patency period of 10.1 weeks compared with 9.8 weeks for the test group (t = 0.337, P > .05, 11 degrees of freedom).

In the majority of failures in all three groups the main cause was anastomotic hyperplasia. There were no significant differences in the thickness of hyperplasia in the distal anastomoses of patent grafts in all three groups. The proximal portions of these patent grafts were sectioned longitudinally to determine the extent of endothelial coverage. In the first group endothelial coverage was significantly greater in all vein-patched grafts when compared with the contralateral non-patched sides (t = 3.07, P < .05, 3 degrees of freedom). Similar findings were obtained in the second group, in which vein-patched grafts had significantly more endothelial coverage than the contralateral grafts, which were patched with PTFE (t = 4.42, P < .02 for 4 degrees of freedom) (Fig. 34–14). Unlike the findings in the first two groups, there were no significant differences in the amount of endothelial coverage in the patent pairs of grafts in last group. Both vein-patched grafts and grafts with PTFE patches lined with vein had an average of 25 mm of endothelial coverage.

DISCUSSION

Why Do Vein Patches Work?

The findings in the first experimental group reproduced clearly the improved results seen with vein patches in the human situation. Why the incorporation of such a vein

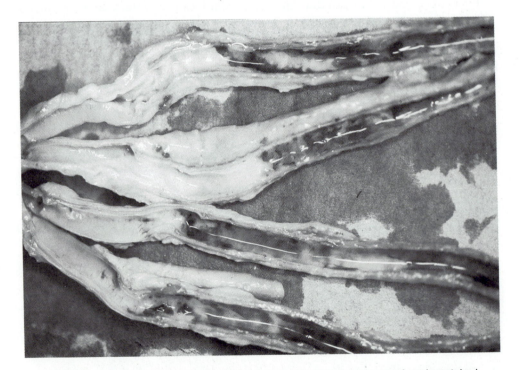

Figure 34–14. Longitudinal sections showing the proximal anastomoses of a vein-patched graft (top) and a PTFE-patched graft (bottom) with a greater amount of endothelial coverage in the former.

patch is beneficial is discussed in the following sections by exploring various possible theories.

Theory 1—The Vein Patch Makes the Anastomosis Technically Easier

Although it is probably true that it is easier to suture vein to a small or diseased artery compared with the much stiffer nonelastic PTFE, this would be unlikely to have affected long-term patency in this series because any technical defects were excluded by completion arteriography. Two other factors suggest that it may be more than just technical advantages that account for the improved patency. First, the learning curve in the first experiment is for the vein-patched group. Second, the use of interrupted sutures at the toe of the graft allows careful placement under direct vision at the most critical point of the anastomosis. This was performed in all grafts, is routine practice in human bypass grafting, and is, therefore, unlikely to be responsible for the improved patency.

Theory 2—The Vein Patch Improves Hemodynamics by Altering the Configuration at the Anatomosis: The Silt-Deposition-on-a-River Theory

This is an attractive theory whereby the angle of the anastomosis is made more streamlined by the vein patch. The alteration in configuration allows the boundary layer separation[41] phenomenon to be less evident with resulting changes in shear stresses.[42] This decrease in separation with normalization of shear stresses, however, was not related to any decrease in intimal hyperplasia found at the roof of vein-patched anastomoses.

Nevertheless, this theory may be supported by the distribution of anastomotic hyperplasia just proximal to the distal anastomosis in the non-patched grafts. It is in this area where the maximal kink occurs. The situation can be likened to the process of deposition of silt in a river bend; maximal silting occurs on the inner bends, where the flow is slowest. It would therefore be simple to postulate that the configuration of the end-to-side anastomosis (which is unnatural) with two kinks results in boundary layer separation and the resultant deposition of anastomotic hyperplasia at the heel and roof of the anastomosis (Fig. 34–10). The vein patch largely abolishes the kinks, rendering the anastomosis more streamlined.

Another way in which the vein patch modifies the configuration is by making the anastomosis closer to round. Comparing this configuration with that of a much more oval non-patched anastomosis (caused by compression of the artery by the inelastic PTFE), it is possible to postulate that this altered configuration has certain advantages. When the overall size is increased, any thickening is compensated for in vein-patched anastomoses. Furthermore, on the theoretic grounds, local turbulence is much greater in an oval than in a round vessel.

Against this theory are the results obtained in the second experiment. Here a similar patch made of PTFE did not lead to the expected improved results. In fact, the results of the PTFE-patched group were nearly identical to the non-patched grafts in the first group, showing no advantage conferred by the altered configuration.

Finally, if the configuration of the anastomosis was an important factor, there would not be any difference between PTFE and vein grafts clinically in the human clinical situation. In reality this is not the case, as already described. Anastomotic configuration may determine in part where deposition occurs but neither precipitates nor prevents the formation of anastomotic hyperplasia.

Theory 3—The Vein Patch Improves Compliance Mismatch

The results of the third set of experiments did not show any significant differences between the two groups, suggesting that the benefits of the vein patch are not due to improved compliance. Although the numbers are not large enough to reach a firm conclusion, this is supported by the fact there was a similar amount of endothelial coverage in both groups of grafts and is thought to be one of the reasons for the improved patency of the vein-patched grafts in the first two groups.

Theory 4—The Vein Patch Decreases Anastomotic Hyperplasia

Because the number of patent pairs of grafts was small, it was not possible to show that the vein patch significantly decreases anastomotic hyperplasia. Instead, it may be that it simply moves the deposition more proximally away from the critical areas of the distal anastomosis. Furthermore, if hyperplasia should occur at the anastomosis, the surface area afforded by the patch is much greater than in unpatched grafts. However, for the reasons stated earlier and when the results of the second group are taken into consideration, this is unlikely to be the mechanism. It is surprising that in terms of the number of the anastomotic stenoses, there seems to be little difference between patched and non-patched groups. As already mentioned, it is possible that the vein patch affords some protection from occlusion, despite the presence of anastomotic hyperplasia, by the increase in endothelial coverage. In the third group, the grafts patched with PTFE lined with vein endothelialized just as well. This may account for the slightly improved patency in this group. The increase in endothelial coverage (and coversely, decrease in areas without a smooth pseudointima) may allow the grafts to withstand thrombosis better in the presence of a distal stenotic lesion due to anastomotic hyperplasia.

Theory 5—The Vein Patch Increases Endothelial Coverage

Endothelial coverage of PTFE grafts has been studied extensively,[43,44] but as yet there have been no reports correlating this coverage to graft patency. It is possible that the sheep is a good model of anastomotic hyperplasia because endothelial coverage is as slow as in humans, unlike other species (dog, pig, baboon), in which coverage is complete within several weeks.[45] The results in all three groups suggest that endothelial coverage is an important factor in this model. Unlike anastomotic hyperplasia, the amount of graft covered by endothelium correlates well with graft patency.

Clinically, endothelial seeding of PTFE grafts has been shown experimentally to improve patency[46,47] but has yet to be sufficiently developed to allow any firm conclusions to be made in the human situation. The other flaw of this theory is the results obtained with composite grafting, which have not been consistently superior. Part of this variability may be related to how the PTFE is anastomosed to vein. It has already been seen that hyperplasia occurs at the PTFE-vein junction. It is possible that an anastomosis constructed in either a fish-shaped or oblique manner would do better than end-to-end anastomosis by moving the areas of thickening away from each other. This information is not available, nor are the causes of failure of composite grafts well documented. The role of proximal disease is probably even more relevant for composite grafts because the proximal ends do not have any interposed vein.

Theory 6—The Vein Patch Has Prostacyclin-like Activity

One unresolved theory is the possibility that the vein patch secretes prostacyclin-like substances that in turn decrease the formation of anastomotic hyperplasia. It is possible that no significant differences were observed in the last group because of this. Similarly the improved results of vein patches over PTFE patches in the second group could be due to a prostacyclin-secreting ability. At present there is no real evidence to support this theory, but further experiments could be performed to elucidate this.

CONCLUSION

Anastomotic vein patches have already been shown to improve the results of PTFE bypass grafting in the human situation, particularly in the infrapopliteal region. The experimental work attempts to elucidate some of the possible mechanisms of this improvement. It may be a combination of factors, each with a relative importance, rather than one factor alone. It is unlikely that the vein patch decreases anastomotic hyperplasia. Instead, it is more probable that the consequently increased endothelial coverage plays a part, offering the graft some sort of protection, even when a great deal of narrowing is present. We were not able to show conclusively that the improvement in compliance affects graft patency.

A fundamental difference between this simple technique and the somewhat more complicated vein cuffs relates to the fact that a short segment of PTFE is anastomosed directly to the host artery. We believe this factor to be important in stabilizing the anastomosis, although the value remains as yet unproven. Further modifications of the anastomotic techniques are being investigated, although it seems probable that advances will relate to the development of improved graft materials with increased compliance and reduced thrombogenicity or possibly to therapeutic drug manipulation.

REFERENCES

1. Kunlin J. Le traitement de l'arterite obliterante par la greffe veineuse. *Arch Mal Coeur.* 1949;42:371–372.
2. RJ McFarland, RS Taylor. Une amelioration technique d'anastomose des prostheses arterielles femoro-distales. *Phlebologie.* 1988;41:229–233.
3. Taylor RS, Loh A, McFarland RJ, et al. Improved technique for polytetrafluoroethylene bypass grafting: long term results using anastomotic vein patches. *Br J Surg.* 1992;79:348–354.
4. Brewster DC. Composite grafts. In: Rutherford RB, ed. *Vascular Surgery.* 3rd ed. Philadelphia: WB Saunders; 1989:481–486.
5. Cranley JJ, Haffner CD. Revascularization of the femoropopliteal arteries using saphenous vein, polytetrafluoroethylene, and umbilical vein grafts. *Arch Surg.* 1982;117:1543–1550.
6. Christenson JT, Broome A, Norgren L, Eklof B. Revascularization of popliteal and below-knee arteries with polytetrafluoroethylene. *Surgery.* 1985;97:141–149.
7. Hobson RW II, Lynch TG, Jamil Z, et al. Results of revascularization and amputation in severe lower extremity ischaemia: a five year clinical experience. *J Vasc Surg.* 1985;2:174–185.
8. Veith FJ, Gupta SK, Ascer E, et al. Six-year prospective multicenter randomized comparison of autologous saphenous vein and expanded polytetrafluoroethylene grafts in infrainguinal arterial reconstructions. *J Vasc Surg.* 1986;3:104–114.
9. Rafferty TD, Avellone JC, Farrell CJ, et al. A metropolitan experience with infrainguinal revascularization: operative risk and late results in northeastern Ohio. *J Vasc Surg.* 1987;6:365–371.
10. Flinn WR, Rohrer MJ, Yao JST, et al. Improved long-term patency of infragenicular polytetrafluoroethylene grafts. *J Vasc Surg* 1988;7:685–690.

11. Whittemore AD, Kent KC, Donaldson MC, et al. What is the proper role of polytetrafluoro-ethylene grafts in infrainguinal reconstruction? *J Vasc Surg.* 1989;10:299–305.

12. Johnson WC, Squires JW. Axillo-femoral (PTFE) and infrainguinal revascularization (PTFE and umbilical vein). *J Cardiovasc Surg.* 1991;32:344–349.

13. Londrey GL, Ramsey DE, Hodgson KJ, et al. Infrapopliteal bypass for severe ischemia: Comparison of autogenous vein, composite and prosthetic grafts. *J Vasc Surg.* 1991;13:631–636.

14. Wolfe JHN, Tyrrell MR. Justifying arterial reconstruction to crural vessels: even with a prosthetic graft. *Br J Surg.* 1991;78:897–899.

15. Taylor RS, McFarland RJ, Cox MI. An investigation into the causes of failure of PTFE grafts. *Eur J Vasc Surg.* 1987;1:335–343.

16. Veith FJ, Gupta SK, Daly V. Management of early and late thrombosis of expanded polytetra-fluoroethylene (PTFE) femoropopliteal bypass grafts: favorable prognosis with appropriate reoperation. *Surgery.* 1980;87:581–587.

17. O'Donnell TF, Mackey W, McCullough JL, et al. Correlation of operative findings with angiographic and non-invasive hemodynamic factors associated with failure of polytetra-fluoroethylene grafts. *J Vasc Surg.* 1984;1:136–146.

18. Sterpetti AV, Schultz RD, Feldhaus RJ, Peetz DJ Jr. Seven year experience with polytetraflu-oroethylene as above-knee femoropopliteal bypass graft: is it worthwhile to preserve the autologous saphenous vein? *J Vasc Surg.* 1985;2:907–912.

19. Ascer E, Collier P, Gupta SK, Veith FJ. Reoperation for polytetrafluoroethylene bypass failure: the importance of distal outflow site and operative failure in determining outcome. *J Vasc Surg.* 1987;5:298–310.

20. Quinones-Baldrich WJ, Prego A, Ucelay-Gomez R, et al. Failure of PTFE infrainguinal revascularization: patterns, management alternatives and outcome. *Ann Vasc Surg.* 1991;5:163–169.

21. De Weese JA, Green RM. Control of anastomotic neointimal fibrous hyperplasia in vascular grafts. In: Stanley JC, Burkel WE, Lindenauer SM, eds. *Biologic and Synthetic Vascular Prostheses.* Philadelphia: Grune & Stratton; 1982:653–659.

22. Echave V, Koornick AR, Haimof M, Jacobsen JH. Intimal hyperplasia as a complication of the use of the polytetrafluoroethylene graft for femoropopliteal bypass. *Surgery.* 1979;86:791–798.

23. Selman SH, Rhodes RS, Anderson JM, et al. Atheromatous changes in expanded PTFE grafts. *Surgery.* 1980;87:630–637.

24. Watase M, Kambayashi J, Itoh T, et al. Ultrastructural analysis of pseudo-intimal hyperplasia of polytetrafluoroethylene prostheses implanted into the venous and arterial systems. *Eur J Vasc Surg.* 1992;6:371–380.

25. Clowes AW, Reidy MA, Clowes MM. Mechanisms of stenosis after arterial injury. *Lab Invest.* 1983;49:208–215.

26. Clowes AW, Reidy MA, Clowes MM. Kinetics of cellular proliferation after arterial injury. I. Smooth muscle growth in the absence of endothelium. *Lab Invest.* 1983;49:327–333.

27. Clowes AW, Gown AM, Hanson SR, Reidy MA. Mechanisms of arterial graft failure. I. Role of cellular proliferation in early healing of PTFE prostheses. *Am J Pathol.* 1985;118:43–53.

28. Imparato AM, Baumann FG, Pearson J, et al. Electron microscopic studies of experimentally produced fibromuscular arterial lesions. *Surg Gynecol Obstet.* 1974;139:497–504.

29. Berguer R, Higgins RF, Reddy DJ. Intimal hyperplasia: an experimental study. *Arch Surg.* 1980;115:332–335.

30. Binns RL, Ku DN, Stewart MT, et al. Optimal graft diameter: effect of wall shear stress on vascular healing. *J Vasc Surg.* 1989;10:326–337.

31. Okadome K, Miyazaki T, Onohara T, et al. Hemodynamics and the development of anasto-motic intimal hyperplasia of the polytetrafluoroethylene graft in dogs. *Int Angiol.* 1991;10:238–243.

32. Zarins CK, Zatina MA, Giddens DP, et al. Shear stress regulation of artery lumen diameter in experimental atherogenesis. *J Vasc Surg.* 1987;5:413–420.

33. Abbott WM, Megerman J, Hasson JE, et al. Effect of compliance mismatch on vascular graft patency. *J Vasc Surg.* 1987;5:376–382.

34. Kusaba A, Fisher CR, Matulewsi TJ, Matsumoto T. Experimental study of the influence of porosity on development of neo-intima in Gore-Tex grafts: a method to increase long term patency rate. *Am Surg.* 1981;47:347–354.
35. Crawshaw HM, Quist WC, Serrallach E, et al. Flow disturbance at the distal end-to-side anastomosis: effect of patency of the proximal outflow segment and angle of anastomosis. *Arch Surg.* 1980;115:1280–1284.
36. Batson RC, Sottiurai VS, Craighead CC. Linton patch angioplasty; an adjunct to distal bypass with polytetrafluoroethylene grafts. *Ann Surg.* 1984;199:684–693.
37. Miller JH, Foreman RK, Ferguson L, Faris I. Interposition vein cuff for anastomosis of prosthesis to small artery. *Aust NZ J Surg.* 1984;54:283–285.
38. Siegman FA. Use of the venous cuff for graft anastomosis. *Surg Gynecol Obstet.* 1979;148:930.
39. Tyrrell MR, Wolfe JHN. New prosthetic venous collar anastomotic technique: combining the best of other procedures (Surgical Workshop). *Br J Surg.* 1991;78:1016–1017.
40. Tyrrell MR, Grigg MJ, Wolfe JHN. Is arterial reconstruction to the ankle worthwhile in the absence of autologous vein? *Eur J Vasc Surg.* 1989;3:429–434.
41. LoGerfo FW, Soncrant T, Teel T, Dewey CF. Boundary layer separation in models of side-to-end arterial anastomoses. *Arch Surg.* 1979;114:1369–1373.
42. Keynton RS, Rittgers SE, Shu MCS. The effect of angle and flow rate upon hemodynamics in distal vascular graft anastomoses: an in vitro model study. *J Biomech Eng.* 1991;113:458–463.
43. Clowes AW, Zacharias RK, Kirkman TR. Early endothelial coverage of synthetic arterial grafts: porosity revisited. *Am J Surg.* 1987;153:501–504.
44. Zacharias RK, Kirkman TR, Clowes AW. Mechanisms of healing in synthetic grafts. *J Vasc Surg.* 1987;6:429–436.
45. Sauvage LR, Berger KE, Wood SJ, et al. Interspecies healing of porous arterial prostheses: observations, 1960 to 1974. *Arch Surg.* 1974;109:698–705.
46. Campbell JB, Glover JL, Herring B. The influence of endothelial seeding and platelet inhibition on the patency of ePTFE grafts used to replace small arteries: an experimental study. *Eur J Vasc Surg.* 1988;2:365–370.
47. Hess F, Steeghs S, Jerusalem R, et al. Patency and morphology of fibrous polyurethane vascular prostheses implanted in the femoral artery of dogs after seeding with subcultivated endothelial cells. *Eur J Vasc Surg.* 1993;7:402–408.

35

The Role of Anticoagulation in Infrainguinal Bypass Surgery

Georg J. Kretschmer, MD, and Thomas Hölzenbein, MD

In the treatment of peripheral arterial occlusive disease, autologous saphenous vein is the vascular substitute of choice for infrainguinal bypass grafting. All the other methods of treatment have shown less than favorable results.[1] During the past decades many studies have evaluated the long-term outcome of bypass grafting and investigated problems and refinements in the technique.[2-5] The orthograde technique has gained popularity, handling the vein as a free transplant or leaving it *in situ*. Gradually the results have become more and more gratifying, but even considering a modern series of patients there seems to be considerable room for improvement.[2] Similar to postoperative surgical chemotherapy, several studies evaluated the potential of postoperative pharmacotherapy.[6,7] In peripheralarterial occlusive disease the drugs most discussed are antiaggregants (AGGs) and oral anticoagulants (ACs).[7-9] This chapter is devoted to the influence of anticoagulation treatment after infrainguinal vein bypass surgery. It discusses the results found in the literature and describes our experience, which we gained during a clinical trial conducted at our institution since the early 1980s.

Reconstructions of small-caliber arteries in general require conduits, which bridge a long gap and end in native arteries with limited and probably severely compromised outflow tracts; they are prone to thrombosis. Such conduits do not branch along their course, the flow is slow, and thrombosis due to stagnation may follow. Studies of flow rates immediately after bypass surgery have shown that critical flow rates exist below which the incidence of reocclusion raises markedly.[10] Two recent major investigations that assessed the value of surgery in symptomatic high-grade stenotic carotid lesions set the standard for clinical trials, rendering clinical recommendations of the highest possible standards feasible.[11,12]

Peripheral vascular surgery at the infrainguinal level is an excellent model to test antithrombotic therapy, because the primary end points are easy to define. Unlike in coronary artery bypass grafting, one anastomosis can be evaluated. The principal question of course is, Is the graft patent or reoccluded? Angiography may be a valuable adjunct, but it is by no means mandatory.[7]

As early as 1979 a prospective trial was carried out in Zurich, Switzerland, that tried to define whether AGGS or ACs is the superior option.[13] Because the primary question—whether a postoperative pharmacotherapy is beneficial at all—has not been answered, we embarked on a clinical trial, to try to answer that question.

PATIENTS AND METHODS

Beginning in 1979 a consecutive series of 175 patients not older than 75 years were evaluated for the study. All patients suffered chronic obliterative arterial disease at the femoropopliteal above-knee or below-knee level. Participants in the trial were operated on electively. The patients' conditions were staged according to the classification of Fontaine et al.[14] Stage I was asymptomatic disease; stage II, intermittent claudication; stage II/III very limited walking ability (disabling claudication); stage III, pain at rest; and stage IV, frank gangrene. Treating a patient with progressed stage III or IV disease meant operating for limb salvage. A standard reversed saphenous vein bypass was performed using the great saphenous vein. The proximal anastomosis was constructed at the common femoral level. The distal suture line was acceptable above or below the knee. The operative procedure was tested by means of on-table or postoperative arteriography.

During the second postoperative week 130 patients were assigned to either the therapy group ($n = 66$; treatment with phenprocoumon tablets to 3 mg) or the control group ($n = 64$; no oral AC or AGG). Adaptive randomization was used to allow optimum balancing of risk factors between groups, even for small random samples.[15] Prognostic factors taken into consideration were sex, age, diabetic metabolic state, blood pressure, and clinical status prior to surgery. Exclusion criteria were unwillingness to comply with the requirements of the trial, a history or a diagnosis of gastrointestinal ulcer confirmed with endoscopy, and need for or contraindications to AC or platelet inhibitory drugs. During the last years of the trial, it became increasingly difficult to recruit patients who had not been previously treated with AGG before femoropopliteal bypass surgery was considered.

After surgery, patients were scheduled for outpatient appointments at 3-month intervals during the first postoperative year and 6-month intervals thereafter; they were seen at shorter intervals if necessary. At these visits a clinical examination performed that included pulse palpation and Doppler ultrasound. Clinical deterioration, loss of previously palpable pulses, and/or drop of ankle–brachial index of 30% or more prompted follow-up arteriography.

Special attention was paid to compliance with pharmacotherapy and satisfactory anticoagulation by monitoring prothrombin time (using the Quick-Test-value) or results from the Hepatoquick test (Boehringer, Ingelheim, Germany) or the Thrombotest (Nycomed, Immuno AG, Vienna, Austria). The treatment was modified accordingly. The goals were 15% to 25% for the Quick-Test-value, 10% to 20% for Hepatoquick, and 5% to 12% for Thrombotest. In addition to the coagulation laboratory, which routinely monitored the anticoagulation status of the participants at each visit, the policy was to check the AC levels at each outpatient appointment. The staff in the outpatient department continuously followed up more than 350 vascular patients receiving oral AC, but they did not know who was participating in the trial.

STATISTICAL METHODS

We had access to the mainframe computer (4381 IBM) at the Faculty of Medicine in Vienna. Data were stored on-line and retrieved with Statistical Analysis System Software (SAS Inc, Cary, NC) and Biomedical Dixon Program (BMDP, Berkeley, Calif). Kaplan–Meier estimations were performed[16] and checked using the tests of Mantel[17] and Breslow.[18] Two-tailed P values $< .05$ were considered significant.

Patients were assigned to the two groups by adaptive randomization. In six patients ACs were discontinued for the following reasons: epistaxis in one, gastrointestinal hemorrhage in three, coronary artery surgery in one, unknown cause in one, and suspected cerebral stroke in one. Nevertheless, for evaluation these patients remained in the group to which they had been assigned originally (i.e., the intention-to-treat principle).

Accurate information about patient survival and the cause of death were possible because of Austria's Act on Reporting of Residency. This law requires residents to report their place of residence and all changes thereof to the local authorities or to the police. In addition, if a person dies in a hospital, the director of the clinic or the physician who performed the coroner's inquest is required to report to the local authorities the cause of death to enable the local authorities to relay that information to the Austrian Central Statistical Office (Osterreichisches Statistisches Zentralamt, Wien, Austria). This leads to an estimated postmortem examination frequency of 70% to 75%.

RESULTS

By the end of January 1989, the last of 130 patients was recruited for the trial. After the end of the recruitment phase, the patients were followed up for more than 5 years. The final evaluation was done by April 1994, allowing a follow-up period of 12 years, as compared to 10 years for the evaluation done in 1992.[19]

The treatment ($n = 66$) and control groups ($n = 64$) were reasonably well matched, as shown in Table 35–1. Fifteen patients in the treated group had primarily occluded grafts, as did 27 in the untreated control group. The median duration of graft function was more than 144 months for the treated group, whereas it was only 96 months for the untreated patients. The therapy group demonstrated a higher probability of primary graft function ($P < .011$ by Breslow test; $P < .017$ by Mantel test) (Fig. 35–1).

The runoff quality was evaluated according to the number of occluded crural vessels (0–1; 2; 3). With 53/11/2 versus 49/12/3, the groups were well matched. Four patients in the therapy group lost a limb, as did 13 in the control group; the difference reached statistical significance ($P < .012$ Breslow test; $P < .009$ Mantel test).

Sixty-eight patients died: 29 in the treated and 39 in the untreated group. The probability of survival was in favor of patients who were treated ($P < .029$ by Breslow test; $P < .028$ by Mantel test) (Fig. 35–2). Causes of death were malignant disease in eight patients (four in each group); gastrointestinal hemorrhage due to AC in one patient (after 68 months of treatment); cerebrovascular disease in 10 patients (two in the treated and eight in the control group); and various causes (pulmonary infections, trauma) in eight patients (three in the treated and five in the untreated group). In three patients the causes of death remained unclear (one in the therapy and two in the control group). The remaining patients died of underlying cardiovascular disease. Only one serious drug-related complication was observed.

Altogether, 1,432 single prothrombin time estimations were carried out. Over the years, 75% to 81% of the estimations were safe within therapeutic limits. Three percent to 5% were below the margin of safety; the remaining estimations were above the level of safety. Estimations outside the therapeutic limits were dealt with by adjustment of

TABLE 35–1. BALANCING OF RISK FACTORS IN THE TREATMENT GROUP VERSUS THE CONTROL GROUP

Variable	Treatment Group	Controls
$N = 130$	66	64
Sex		
Male ($N = 102$)	52	50
Female ($N = 28$)	14	14
Age (y)		
mean ± SEM	62.5 ± 8.3	62.3 ± 8.9
<55	12	13
55–65	27	23
>65	27	28
Diabetic state		
None	43	41
Diabetes mellitus	19	17
Insulin-dependent diabetes	4	6
Blood pressure (mm Hg)		
<160/90	48	47
>160/90	18	17
Cardiac pathology		
None	38	38
Ischaemic myocardiopathy	3	3
History of myocardial infarction	14	13
Arrhythmia	11	10
Smoking habits (No. of cigarettes per day)		
Nonsmoker	12	14
<10	7	5
10–20	23	19
>20	24	26
Clinical Stage prior to surgery[a]		
II, II–III	32	30
III, IV	34	34
Distal anastomotic site		
Above knee	28	28
Below knee	38	36
Ankle–brachial pressure Index		
<0.3	21	24
0.3–0.4	17	13
0.4–0.5	13	20
>0.5	15	7

[a] According to the Fontaine classification.

the phenprocoumon dosage. It seemed possible to train patients to take AC reliably, because the longer a patient took AC the more estimations were found in therapeutic limits.

Twenty-two arteriograms were obtained in the therapy group. They showed 13 reocclusions. For the untreated group 36 angiograms confirmed 23 graft losses. Five graft stenoses were detected and repaired by transluminal angioplasty (two patients)

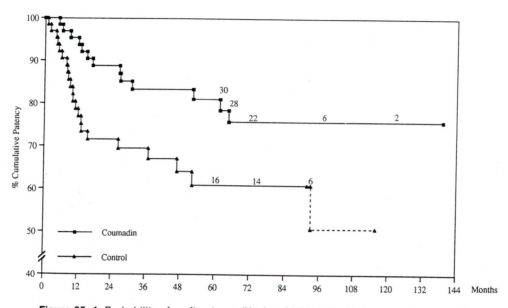

Figure 35–1. Probability of graft patency (Kaplan–Meier estimates); treatment group (■) versus control group (▲). Numbers above the curve indicate grafts at risk. Dashed line indicates when the standard error exceeds 10%.

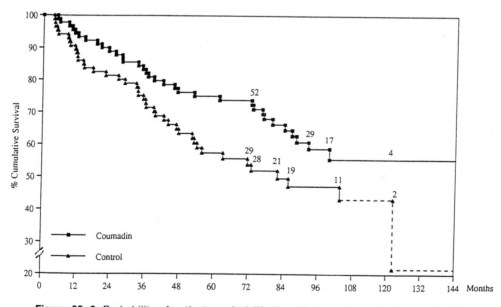

Figure 35–2. Probability of patient survival (Kaplan–Meier estimates); treatment group (■) versus control group (▲). Numbers above the curve indicate patients at risk. Numbers below the curve indicate the cumulative proportion who survived. Dashed line indicates the interval when the standard error exceeds 10%.

or reoperations (three patients). Only occluded grafts were recorded to be failures, whereas bypasses with successfully treated stenoses remained in the "patent" group.

CONCLUSION

In an analysis of the clinical series the hypothesis emerged that treatment with AC might improve vein graft performance at the infrainguinal level.[20] The results were reproduced in a prospective clinical trial, which was continued for 12 years.

Although restricted by the number of patients involved, this single-center trial comprised a group of patients that was uniformly assessed, treated, and followed up. The trial was randomized but not placebo controlled, because it was found difficult to argue for regular blood sampling with adjustment of placebo through many years and to distribute "blinded" anticoagulant charts, which patients were supposed to carry and produce in the event of a medical emergency. These difficulties are such an obstacle that only a few placebo-controlled trials have administered oral AC and have been continued over a long period of time.

Active anticoagulation was maintained in a high percentage of patients. The incidence of severe complications was acceptable; one severe drug-related complication was observed. Of course the reliability of the trial depended heavily on the fact that the patients in both groups were seen with equal frequency. The BMDP program helped ensure that more medical care was not being given to patients in the therapy group.

Two other trials similar in size to ours (one in Switzerland[13] the other in the Netherlands[21]) demonstrated a beneficial effect of treatment with AC in peripheral arterial occlusive disease and an improvement following vascular repair. The Dutch trial is one of the very rare double-blind and placebo-controlled studies. In a Scandinavian trial, the authors were unable to confirm that ACs are of any value, but drug-related complications seemed to be a problem.[22]

In our trial, therapy was continued until the death of a patient, irrespective of graft or limb loss. The most remarkable difference between the two groups became obvious during the first 2 years following surgery. The medication could be discontinued after 2 years, but cancellation of AC has been known to induce adverse cardiac effects, at least in patients older than 60 years with a history of coronary artery disease.[23] We produced evidence that AC might prolong the life of patients with vascular disease, even though only the subgroup of patients with patent grafts was analyzed.[24]

For data from large, multicenter investigations that enrolled several hundreds of patients, one has to rely on various trials carried out in coronary artery bypass surgery. It is difficult, however, to translocate the results of aortocoronary bypass surgery to femoral–distal arterial repair.[7,25,26] Preoperative start of medication seemed of particular importance, although low doses of AGG were sufficient to demonstrate a clinically relevant effect. A variety of changes are responsible for vein graft failure, such as intimal hyperplasia, suture line stenosis, obliterating changes at valvular remnants, and progression of the underlying arterial disease. Taking into consideration the mode of action of AGG their prescription is reasonable to prevent bypass reocclusion and vascular events in general.[6] In most trials AGG were prescribed, which is not surprising, because it might be difficult to perform open heart surgery on patients already taking oral AC prior to surgery. The various prescribed aspirin dosages were similarly effective, although there was a relation between the size of the administered doses and the incidence of unwanted side effects.[7]

AC and AGG were similiarily effective, but AC were cumbersome to use.[26] Patients with vascular disease are often elderly and cannot be relied upon to take medication regularly.[27] (More than 40% of the participants in the trial were older than 65 years of age.) To ensure that the benefits outweigh the risks, exact monitoring of the treatment is mandatory by checking the coagulation parameters for each patient whenever needed. In central Europe (the Netherlands, Germany, Switzerland, Austria) the "art" of treatment with AC has been developed, and vascular surgeons are inclined to use AC liberally. In other parts of the world, the fear of potentially lethal complications restricts the use of AC.

Much of the current enthusiasm for using AGG originates from the classic study by Chesebro et al[25] and a recent multicenter trial conducted in Great Britain, which seemed to be in favor of the AGG.[28,29] In a further evaluation of the trial, patients' compliance with therapy as well as the mode of evaluating the results (intention-to-treat versus treatment analysis) turned out to be a major issue.[30]

Alloplastic grafts take up labeled platelets. Aspirin reduces the platelet consumption of such grafts, and therefore treatment with AGG is reasonably well established to improve the performance of such grafts. The adjunctive prescription of dipyridamole to protect alloplastic grafts from reocclusion is probably supported by experimental data.[7]

The question, which drugs are best to use for postoperative reocclusion prophylaxis—AGG or AC, is still unanswered. A trial has been proposed with the running title "Antithrombotic Therapy for Lower Extremity Bypass." This study should arrive at an answer and allow a clinical recommendation with high reliability.[31] Since it has been shown that low doses of AGG are of clinical value and low-dose AC seem to be effective in preventing embolic events in patients with atrial fibrillation,[32] the combination of low-dose AGG and AC might be a promising alternative.[7] In addition, different types of antiplatelet drugs prescribed as a combined therapeutic regimen might become reality because their mode of action is entirely different.

REFERENCES

1. Veith FJ, Gupta SK, Ascer E. Six years prospective multicentre, randomized comparison of autologous saphenous vein and expanded polytetrafluoroethylene grafts in infrainguinal arterial reconstructions. *J Vasc Surg* 1986;3:104–113.
2. Calligaro RD, Friedell ML, Rollins DL, et al. A comparative review on in situ versus reversed vein grafts in the 1980s. Collective review. *Surg Gynecol Obstet*. 1991;172:247–252.
3. DeWeese JA, Rob CG. Autologous venous bypass grafts five years later. *Ann Surg*. 1971;174:346–365.
4. DeWeese JA, Rob CG. Autogenous venous grafts ten years later. *Surgery*. 1977;82:775–784.
5. Kretschmer G, Huk I, Polterauer P, et al. Der autologe Venenbypass in der Therapie der arteriellen Verschlusskrankheit der femoro-poplitealen Etage: Langzeitresultate. *Wien Klin Wochenschr*. 1986;98:830–838.
6. Gloviczki P, Hollier, LH. Can graft occlusion be prevented by drugs? In: Greenhalgh RM, Jamieson CW, Nicolaides AW, eds. *Vascular Surgery: Issues in Current Practice*. London, England: Grune & Stratton; 1986:37–41.
7. Clagett PG, Graor RA, Salzman EW: Antithrombotic therapy in peripheral arterial occlusive disease. *Chest*. 1992;102:516S–528S.
8. Van Urk H, Kretschmer G. What is the role of oral anticoagulants and platelet inhibitors in peripheral vascular surgery? *Eur J Vasc Surg*. 1990;4:553–555.

9. Dorrmandy J. Surgical pharmacotherapy. *Eur J Vasc Surg.* 1989;3:379–380.
10. Grimley RP, Obeid ML, Ashton F, Slaney G. Long term results of autogenous vein bypass grafts in femoro-popliteal occlusion. *Br J Surg.* 1971;174:346–365.
11. North American Symptomatic Carotid Endarterectomy Trial Collaborators. Beneficial effect of carotid endarterectomy in symptomatic patients with high-grade carotid stenosis. *N Engl J Med.* 1991;325:445–453.
12. European Carotid Surgery Trialists' Collaborative Group. MRC European carotid surgery trial: interim results for symptomatic patients with severe (70–99%) or with mild (0–29%) carotid stenosis. *Lancet.* 1991;337:15–1243.
13. Schneider E, Brunner U, Bollinger A. Medikamentöse Rezidivprophylaxe nach femoro-poplitealen Arterienrekonstruktionen. *Angiologia.* 1979;2:73–77.
14. Fontaine R, Klm M, Kieny R. Die chirurgische behandlung der peripheren Durchblutungsstörungen. *Helv Chir Acta.* 1954;21:499–533.
15. Pocock SJ, Simon R. Sequential treatment assignment with balancing for prognostic factors in the controlled clinical trial. *Biometrics.* 1975;31:103–115.
16. Kaplan EL, Meier P. Nonparametric estimation from incomplete observations. *J Am Stat Assoc.* 1958;53:457–481.
17. Mantel N. Evaluation of survival data and two new rank order statistics arising in its consideration. *Cancer Chemother Rep.* 1966;50:163–165.
18. Breslow N. A generalized Kruskal-Wallis test for comparing K-samples subject to unequal patterns of censorship. *Biometrika* 1970;57:579–582.
19. Kretschmer G, Herbst F, Prager M, et al. A decade of oral anticoagulant treatment to maintain autologous vein grafts for femoro-popliteal atherosclerosis. *Arch Surg.* 1992;127:1112–1115.
20. Herbst F, Berlakovich G, Steger G, et al. Langzeitresultate des femoro-poplitealen und femoro-cruralen Saphenabypass: eine multivariate logistische Regressionsanalyse. *Angiologia.* 1991;13:161–168.
21. De Smit P, van Urk H. The effects of long term treatment with oral anticoagulants in patients with peripheral vascular disease. *Acta Chir Austriaca.* 1992;24:5–7.
22. Arfvidsson B, Lundgren F, Drott Ch, et al. Influence of coumarin treatment on patency and limb salvage after peripheral arterial reconstructive surgery. *Am J Surg.* 1990;159:556–560.
23. Sixty-plus Reinfarction Study Research Group. A double blind trial to assess long term anticoagulation therapy in elderly patients after myocardial infarction. *Lancet.* 1980; 2:989–993.
24. Kretschmer G, Wenzl E, Schemper M, et al. Influence of postoperative anticoagulant treatment on patient survival after femoropopliteal vein bypass surgery. *Lancet.* 1988;1:797–799.
25. Chesebro JH, Fuster V, Elvenback LR, et al. Effect of dipyridamole and aspirin on late vein grafts patency after coronary bypass operations. *N Engl J Med.* 1984;310:209–214.
26. Pfisterer M, Burkart F, Jockers G, et al. Trial of low dose aspirin plus dipirydamole versus anticoagulants for prevention of aortocoronary vein graft occlusion. *Lancet.* 1989;2:1–7.
27. Scott PJW. Anticoagulant drugs in the elderly: the risk usually outweighs the benefit. *Br Med J.* 1988;297:1261–1263.
28. Mc Collum CH, Alexander C, Kenchington G, et al. Antiplatelet drugs in femoro-popliteal vein bypass; a multicentre trial. *J Vasc Surg.* 1992;13:150–162.
29. Mc Collum CH, Kenchington G, Alexander C, and the femoro-popliteal trial participants. PTFE or HUV for femoro-popliteal bypass: a multicentre trial. *Eur J Vasc Surg.* 1991; 5:435–443.
30. Franks PJ, Sian M, Kenchington L. Aspirin usage and its influence on femoropopliteal vein graft patency. *Eur J Surg.* 1992;6:185–188.
31. Clagett PG. Antithrombotic therapy for lower extremity bypass. *J Vasc Surg.* 1992; 15:873–875.
32. The Boston Area Anticoagulation Trial for Atrial Fibrillation Investigators. The effect of low dose warfarin on the risk of stroke in patients with nonrheumatic atrial fibrillation. *N Engl J Med.* 1990;323:1505–1511.

36

Influence of Surveillance
Programs on Femoral–Distal
Bypass Graft Patency

David S. Sumner, MD, and Mark A. Mattos, MD

Failure of a femoral–distal bypass graft may have devastating consequences. Because a large portion of these operations are performed for critical ischemia, graft occlusion may jeopardize limb survival. The results of thrombectomy or thrombolysis with or without graft revision are poor, 5-year cumulative patencies ranging from 5% to 32%.[1-4] If the graft cannot be salvaged by these measures and the leg remains ischemic, a new graft will be needed to avoid major amputation. "Redo" procedures are often difficult and may be impossible when there are no suitable recipient arteries. With each subsequent revascularization, the distal anastomotic site may have to be moved farther down the leg. Prosthetic grafts must be used when, after multiple operations, the supply of greater and lesser saphenous veins and arm veins has been exhausted. Although the 5-year patency rate of secondary autogenous vein bypasses is reasonably good (50% to 77%), the results with prosthetic grafts have generally been disappointing (18% to 37%).[5-10] Even when secondary bypasses are successful, they subject the patient to the anxiety, expense, discomfort, and trauma associated with major surgery. These are all important reasons for making every effort to prevent graft failure.

Donaldson et al, in a careful review of 70 occluded *in situ* vein grafts and 20 with preocclusive lesions, attributed most (63%) of the failures to lesions intrinsic to the graft itself and another 20% to stenoses in the inflow and outflow arteries.[11] Only 8% of the failures were unexplained. Others have arrived at similar conclusions.[12] Thus, the vast majority of lesions responsible for graft failure are potentially detectable and should be correctable by relatively simple interventional procedures. It seems logical, therefore, that the long-term care of patients who have undergone a femoral–distal bypass should incorporate a program of graft surveillance. Surveillance, however, detects some stenoses that remain stable and do not lead to graft thrombosis and inevitably misses other problems that may adversely affect graft survival. Revision of the former is unnecessary, whereas failure to treat the latter undermines the usefulness of surveillance. At present, there are no universally accepted criteria for identifying which lesions can be followed safely without treatment. To determine the usefulness and cost-effectiveness of surveillance, we need to know the natural history of untreated recurrent lesions and the influence of revision of the graft to correct these problems on graft survival.

SURVEILLANCE METHODS

Methods used for graft surveillance should have a high positive and negative predictive value and be able to identify, locate, and assess the severity of recurrent lesions.[13] Ideally, the method (or combination of methods) should be noninvasive, safe, universally applicable, easily performed, and inexpensive. The method should also be able to predict which lesions place the grafts at risk for sudden thrombosis and which do not.[14] No technique currently available satisfies all of these requirements, but color-flow duplex ultrasonic (US) scanning comes the closest.

Clinical Examination

Clinical follow-up alone is inadequate and far too insensitive to detect early lesions. Although return of symptoms in a patient who has had no symptoms after bypass grafting is an important warning sign, symptoms often re-appear only after the graft has thrombosed.[15,16] Because most isolated stenoses do not seriously impair blood flow, about 60% to 90% of patients with graft-threatening lesions continue to have no symptoms.[14,15,17–22] This is especially true in elderly and debilitated patients, who, because of their relatively sedentary habits, put little stress on their limb circulation. Likewise, loss or diminution of palpable pedal pulses that had been present after revascularization is indicative of an obstructive lesion somewhere along the graft-arterial system, but again, these changes are absent in about half of limbs with graft stenoses[4] and may become evident only after graft failure.[15,16] Moreover, assessment of pulses is highly subjective, and interobserver agreement is poor. Some patients, such as those in whom the distal anastomoses are to "blind" popliteal segments or to peroneal arteries, rarely regain pedal pulses even after successful bypass grafting. The presence of a palpable graft pulse also may be misleading, because pulsations may be strong even in the presence of a severe distal stenosis.

Ankle Pressure Measurement

The ankle–brachial pressure index (ABI), obtained by dividing the Doppler-derived systolic pressure in the pedal arteries by that in the arm with the higher pressure, is an essential part of the follow-up protocol. ABIs provide a measure of the initial physiologic success of arterial reconstruction. Any subsequent deterioration of the ABI is indicative of a hemodynamically significant obstruction at one or more locations in the graft-arterial complex. ABIs, however, are sensitive only to stenoses that narrow the diameter of the vascular lumen by at least 50% (75% cross-sectional area reduction) and, therefore, fail to detect lesions of less severity. In addition, even in the absence of structural changes, ABIs measured by different observers or by the same observer on different occasions vary considerably. A 95% confidence limit of ±0.15 is generally accepted for serial measurements.[23] On the basis of this figure, a drop of 0.15 or more in the ABI is required by most investigators before the change is considered significant. Others use 0.20 or 0.10 as the critical figure, but the former is apt to miss many hemodynamically significant lesions and the latter is likely to produce a large number of false-positive results. Although an ABI greater than 0.90 is compatible with a "normal" circulatory status, patients with a patent graft who have pre-existing arterial disease distal to the lower anastomosis have ABIs less than this value; so an absolute lower limit cannot be specified.

Once a stenosis exceeds 50%, further narrowing of the lumen causes a precipitous drop in the ankle pressure. Sudden thrombosis is often the final event. Consequently, a gradually declining ankle pressure is seldom observed; a significant fall in the ABI occurring in the interval between the last measurement and graft thrombosis is likely to be missed; and the stenosis responsible for the hemodynamic deterioration may be detected only after thrombosis occurs.

Other problems exist that detract from the usefulness of the ABI. Calcification may restrict compressibility of arteries at the ankle level, leading to falsely elevated values. Because calcification is common in diabetic patients, up to 20% of ABIs may be uninterpretable. Ankle pressures measured in limbs with grafts that terminate in the pedal arteries are meaningless. Compression of the graft during inflation of a pneumatic cuff placed at ankle level produces a static column of blood that extends to the proximal anastomosis. Thus, measurements obtained in this way are analogous to carotid stump pressures and reflect the pressure in the inflow artery rather than that which would be found at the ankle if blood were flowing. Even if a clinically significant stenosis were present in the graft, it would not be detected. Although toe pressure can be substituted for ABIs in situations in which the ankle pressure is unreliable, they are even more variable and may reflect disease progression in the pedal or digital arteries rather than in the graft itself.

An important study by Barnes et al highlighted the deficiencies of the ABI as a method of graft surveillance.[24] They found that the 5-year cumulative primary patency rate of grafts in limbs with a 0.20 or greater drop in the ABI was almost identical to that in limbs with stable ABIs (62% and 60%, respectively). Similarly, Mattos et al noted interval drops in the ABI of 0.20 or more in 20% of limbs with grafts that subsequently occluded and in 25% of limbs with grafts that remained patent.[25] Other investigators also have concluded that the ABI lacks sufficient sensitivity or specificity to be a reliable screening test for graft stenoses.[13,21,22,26-31] The experience of Green et al has been somewhat more positive.[14] In their series, 11 of 26 grafts in legs with persistent drops of 10% or greater in the ABI occluded, and eight others required revision because of symptoms, but transient drops of a similar magnitude in 42 limbs did not predict graft failure. Serial falls of more than 0.10 in the ABI identified all 12 grafts at risk in a prospective study of 43 infrainguinal bypass grafts reported by Stierli et al, prompting them to conclude that the ABI is an effective screening method provided that the ankle arteries are compressible and that the graft terminates well above the site of measurement.[20] The specificity, however, was only about 70%.

Because of its deficits, the ABI alone does not satisfy the requirements of an effective surveillance program. Nonetheless, there is general agreement that a decrease in the ABI is always a matter of concern and should prompt further investigation.

Other Physiologic Tests

Air plethysmography has been employed as a surveillance method, but experience with this technique is limited.[4] Studies obtained at the foot or toe levels are of some value in cases in which the ankle pressure is unreliable. Impedance analysis, a techique that combines plethysmography and Doppler waveform recordings, is reasonably accurate but apparently somewhat less sensitive and specific than color duplex US scanning for detecting and ruling out graft stenoses.[32,33] This method, however, requires the use of a computer and has the disadvantage of being unable to locate the offending lesion.

Arteriography

Although conventional arteriography is highly sensitive and specific for identifying problems that threaten graft survival, it is invasive, far too expensive, and too risky to be employed for routine surveillance. Arteriograms, however, may be necessary to confirm noninvasive findings. A few investigators have used intravenous digital subtraction angiography for graft surveillance.[16,27] Although IVDSA is minimally invasive, it subjects the patient to the risk of contrast agents and radiation and may not have the resolution required to identify or grade some lesions (such as web-like stenoses) that threaten graft survival. Turnipseed and Sproat have investigated the use of magnetic resonance angiography in graft surveillance.[34] In their preliminary study of 20 infrainguinal bypass grafts thought to be at risk for occlusion on the basis of noninvasive tests or recurrent symptoms, magnetic resonance angiograms and intra-arterial DSA agreed in 15 cases. Four magnetic resonance angiograms were falsely positive and one was falsely negative. The role of this currently expensive technique remains to be established. At present, it appears to have no discernable advantage over duplexus imaging.

Duplex and Color-Flow Ultrasonic Scanning

The advent of duplex US scanning made it possible to survey the entire length of the graft, the proximal and distal anastomoses, and the adjacent inflow and outflow arteries. Unlike other noninvasive methods, duplex scans provide both anatomic and functional information—information that allows stenoses to be localized and their severity estimated.

Conventional duplex US scanning, however, proved to be a time-consuming, tedious exercise and was not widely accepted.[19] Color-flow scanning, which superimposes a color-coded flow-map on the B-mode image, greatly simplified the scanning process and was the development responsible for making surveillance feasible. Color expedites the study by depicting flow over an extended segment of the graft and by immediately highlighting areas of increased velocity and turbulence.[13] These features facilitate longitudinal scanning, obviating the need for frequent cross-sectional studies; focus attention on regions that require Doppler spectral analysis, making random or centimeter by centimeter flow sampling unnecessary; and help locate grafts or arteries that are deeply situated in the leg.[26,35,36] With color, proximal anastomoses are always seen and distal anastomoses are visualized in about 90% of the studies.[37] Arteriovenous fistulas, hematomas, fluid collections, false aneurysms, kinks, and other defects related to bypass grafting are readily identified. A complete scan usually requires about 20 minutes—no more than a carotid study.[36,38,39]

Normal segments of bypass grafts have a smooth contour on the B-mode scan, and the outline and color of the flow image is uniform.[13] A red color is assigned to flow down the leg (arterial direction) and a blue color to flow up the leg (venous direction). Color saturation is determined by the Doppler frequency shift, which in turn is proportional to the velocity of flow and the angle that the flow vectors make with the ultrasonic sound beam. Deeper colors correspond to low velocities and lighter colors, to high velocities (or to a more acute angle of insonation). Because stenoses are associated with increased flow velocities, a localized change in color from red to white (or light blue if aliasing occurs) is a sensitive indicator of the presence of a stenosis.[19,35,38] Narrowing of the flow image and a decrease in lumen diameter on the B-mode scan are usually seen as well (Fig. 36–1).[25,35,40] A totally black image indicates graft thrombosis or flow vectors at right angles to the direction of the sound beam. Color changes, however, must be interpreted cautiously at anastomoses, where the direction of flow and the diameter of the blood conduit may change abruptly.

Once a lesion is identified, it is necessary to evaluate the Doppler flow spectrum to determine the degree of stenosis. Peak systolic velocities (PSVs) are measured at the proximal and distal ends of the graft, in the inflow and outflow arteries, at sites of suspected stenosis, and in "normal" segments of graft a few centimeters above or below the area of concern. Velocity ratios, calculated by dividing the PSV obtained at the stenotic site by the PSV in the adjacent "normal" segment, correlate well with the degree of stenosis.[38,40,41] Criteria vary from one laboratory to the next, but in general a velocity ratio greater than 2.0 is predictive of a 50% diameter–reducing lesion.[21,38,39,42] Higher ratios are indicative of more severe diameter reductions.[36,38,41]

A PSV greater than 150 to 180 cm/sec is also indicative of a greater than 50% diameter reduction.[43] High-grade stenoses (>70% or 80% diameter reduction) are usually associated with PSVs exceeding 170 to 300 cm/sec[36,40] and end-diastolic velocities of 20 to 100 cm/sec or more.[21,40] In our experience, 83% of grafts with velocity ratios exceeding 2.0 had PSVs greater than 150 cm/sec at the stenotic site.[35] PSVs over 300 cm/sec were recorded in 21% of the grafts.

Additional information may be obtained from the Doppler frequency spectrum. Loss of the reversed flow component (typically seen during early diastole in normal grafts after the initial postoperative hyperemia has subsided) and a change from a triphasic to a monophasic flow pattern suggest the presence of a greater than 50% diameter stenosis at or above the recording site.[21,44] Normal velocity spectra are charac-

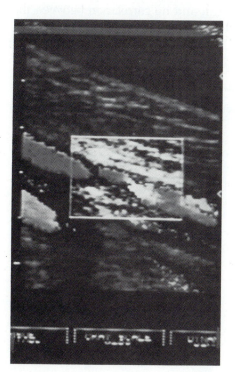

Figure 36–1. Color duplex image of a high-grade stenosis in an *in situ* vein graft. Red to white shift indicates increased flow velocity. Narrowing of the flow image and encroachment of the B-mode echoes on the lumen also delineate the site of the lesion but are not reliable for estimating the degree of stenosis.

terized by a narrow band of frequencies. When the laminar flow pattern is disturbed or turbulence develops, spectral broadening occurs. Even low-grade stenosis may produce some spectral broadening, but the effect becomes more pronounced as the stenosis becomes more severe.[21] These findings, however, are more subjective and consequently less useful than velocity measurements.

Bandyk et al observed an increased incidence of graft occlusion when the PSV measured at the narrowest segment of a graft (usually the upper end of a reversed graft or the lower end of an *in situ* graft) was less than 45 cm/sec.[45] Although a low PSV may indicate the presence of a problem somewhere in the graft–host artery complex and should prompt a careful duplex US study to search for a lesion, it is not highly sensitive for identifying hemodynamically significant lesions or specific for predicting graft thrombosis.[25,28,33,36,40,46] Because PSVs depend on the diameter of the graft and the outflow resistance, the measurement site and the location of the distal anastomosis should be considered in evaluating the results of this test.[47] In general, PSVs are higher in grafts anastomosed to the popliteal artery than they are in grafts terminating at the pedal level, owing to the different capacities of the outflow beds.[28,36,37]

RESULTS OF SURVEILLANCE

Routine surveillance reveals that hemodynamically significant stenoses (>50% diameter reduction) develop in 10% to 34% of infrainguinal grafts,[12,20,22–25,26,29,31,33,36,39,48–51] and that about two-thirds to four-fifths of these appear within the first year after operation (Table 36–1 and Fig. 36–2).[12,22,25,50,52,53] Only 5% to 10% develop after 2 years. Approximately 50% to 60% involve the graft itself.[22,25,36,50,53,54] Retained valve leaflets, valve-site stenoses, diffuse intimal thickening, fibrotic strictures, atherosclerotic lesions, muscular entrapment, and torsion are among the multiple causes that have been identified.[11,54,55] Moody et al, however, found no correlation between the location of postoperative strictures and valve sites, retained valve cusps, tributaries,

TABLE 36–1. INCIDENCE OF STENOSIS IN INFRAINGUINAL BYPASS GRAFTS

Author	Year	Grafts at Risk (n)	Stenoses (n)	Incidence (%)
Sladen[36]	1989	173	33	19
Moody[49]	1990	63	15	24
Mills[29]	1990	379	48	13
Taylor[50]	1990	412	42	10
Bandyk[51]	1991	372	83	22
Taylor[39]	1992	74	19	26
Stierli[20]	1992	43	10	23
Laborde[26]	1992	124	21	17
Harris[31]	1992	200	53	27
Mattos[25]	1993	170	57	34
Idu[22]	1993	160	52	33
Mills[12]	1993	227	29	13
Green[48]	1994	79	26	33
Davies[33]	1994	88	20	23
Total		2,564	508	20

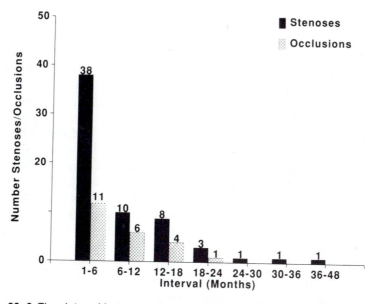

Figure 36–2. Time interval between primary operation and identification of stenoses and occlusions in 170 infrainguinal vein grafts. Forty-eight (77%) of the 62 stenoses and 17 (77%) of the 22 occlusions developed in the first 12 months. By 18 months, 90% of the stenoses and 95% of the occlusions had occurred. (*Reproduced with permission from Mattos MA, van Bemmelen PS, Hodgson KJ, et al. Does correction of stenoses identified with color duplex scanning improve infrainguinal graft patency? J Vasc Surg. 1993; 17:54–66.*)

or clamp sites that were marked with surgical clips at the time of the initial procedure.[56] Histologically, most of the early lesions are due to myointimal hyperplasia, and there is increasing evidence that pre-existing microscopic or macroscopic disease of the vein wall may be responsible for the majority of stenoses.[57,58] Stenoses that occur after the first year are more likely to be atherosclerotic and involve the inflow and outflow arteries with increasing frequency.[59] Late lesions appear to be particularly common at sites of previous revision.[59]

Residual arteriovenous fistulas have been reported in 22% to 37% of *in situ* bypass grafts.[19,35,36] Most of these fistulas are of little consequence and close with time.[46,60] A rare fistula, however, may be detrimental to graft function.[61] Some are even associated with reversed flow in the distal graft.[62]

GRAFT SURVIVAL

Interpreting the already voluminous literature on graft survival and its relationship to stenotic lesions that develop within the graft–host artery complex is somewhat difficult owing to inconsistencies in the terminology used by various investigators. For example, *failed* grafts and *failing* grafts are not always clearly distinguished, and terms such as *pseudo-occlusion* and *hemodynamic failure* may have different implications from one report to the next. Moreover, stenoses may be classified as *mild, moderate, and severe* or *insignificant and significant,* terms that are used differently by individual authors to designate varying degrees of diameter reduction.

In an effort to standardize reporting practices, the Ad Hoc Committee on Reporting Standards of the Society for Vascular Surgery and the North American Chapter of the International Society for Cardiovascular Surgery formulated guidelines to distinguish between *primary* and *secondary* graft patency.[63] According to the committee's original definition, primary patency ceases with graft occlusion or whenever any procedure, major or minor, is performed on a patent graft, the anastomoses, or adjacent inflow vessels. Therefore, operations that have little effect on graft survival, such as ligation of a missed arteriovenous fistula, count against primary patency.[64] Once there has been any intervention, however minor, the graft is placed in the secondary patency category. Because the long-term survival of grafts that are revised before they occlude is markedly superior to that of occluded grafts that are revised after thrombectomy or thrombolytic therapy, this classification tends to improve the apparent secondary patency rate and detract from the primary patency rate. To circumvent this problem, Rutherford proposed the term *assisted primary patency* to designate survival data derived from populations that include grafts that remain patent at the time of intervention.[65]

Unfortunately, Rutherford's suggestion does not eliminate the problem entirely. Because the definition of primary patency remains unaltered, primary patency rates continue to convey misleading information—at least in regard to the beneficial effects of revision of patent grafts. As Green et al emphasized, it is fallacious to compare assisted primary patency rates and primary patency rates, since inevitably the latter must be lower than the former.[14] The comparison would be valid only if it were assumed that all nonrevised stenotic grafts would eventually fail, and we know this is not the case.

To evaluate the contribution of revision to graft survival, the natural history of nonrevised stenotic grafts must be compared with the assisted primary patency rate of revised grafts that have never occluded. To determine the effect of surveillance on graft survival, secondary patency rates in limbs followed clinically should be compared with secondary patency rates in limbs followed with a surveillance protocol. Ideally, studies designed to answer these questions should be prospective and randomized. None has been performed, and, for ethical reasons, it is unlikely that any will be performed.[49] Although most surgeons would agree to follow low-grade stenoses, they would be hesitant to randomize grafts with high-grade stenoses to the nonoperative arm. Too much is at stake if the graft were to fail. Nonetheless, there are abundant data in the literature that allow one to estimate the effect of surveillance and revision on graft survival.

Natural History of Graft Stenoses

The concept that infrainguinal graft stenoses are responsible for thrombosis is intellectually appealing and widely accepted, but the evidence for a direct cause-and-effect relationship is remarkably scant. Before the introduction of surveillance techniques, most stenoses went unrecognized until the graft occluded. That stenoses involving the graft, its anastomoses, or the adjacent inflow or outflow arteries are found in 80% to 95% of cases after thrombectomy or thrombolytic therapy implicates these lesions by association.[11,12] Moreover, surveillance studies have consistently shown that the incidence of graft occlusion parallels the development of stenoses (Fig. 36–2).[5,25,53] Thus, the indirect evidence that links thrombosis to stenotic lesions is strong. Such studies, however, do not tell us what proportion of the lesions or even which lesions are most likely to eventuate in thrombosis.

Szilagyi et al, in a classic investigation that is unlikely ever to be repeated, followed 260 autogenous vein grafts with serial arteriograms for 1 to 10 years.[55] Structural defects were detected in 85 (33%) of these grafts. During the period of observation, 77% of the lesions progressed and 38% of the grafts with lesions thrombosed. Moody et al, in what is perhaps the only truly prospective study of the natural history of graft stenoses, used IVDSA to follow 80 autogenous femoropopliteal vein grafts in 69 patients.[16] The unique feature of their investigation was the decision to adopt "a deliberate policy of nonintervention" when an asymptomatic stenosis was detected. At the first examination, strictures were found in 22 (28%) of the grafts. Five (23%) of these grafts occluded at a median interval of 13 months. In contrast, occlusions occurred in only four (7%) of 58 angiographically normal grafts. Thus, the presence of a stenosis was associated with a threefold increase in the risk of graft failure. Occlusions were more frequent (30%) in grafts with stenoses that reduced the lumen diameter by more than 66% than they were in grafts with a 33% to 66% diameter–reducing lesion (11%). Only 6% of grafts with mild stenoses (less than 33% diameter reduction) thrombosed.

Grigg et al identified "mild to moderate" stenoses (<33% to 67% diameter reduction) in 19 of 75 femoral–distal vein bypass grafts within 12 months of the initial operation.[41] Only one of the stenoses was associated with a greater than 0.2 fall in ABI. During a follow-up period of 3 to 18 months, five stenoses progressed to the severe category (>67% diameter reduction). After revision, all five of these grafts remained patent. Occlusion, however, occurred without warning in three (21%) of the 14 grafts with "hemodynamically insignificant" stenoses.

In our most recent series, 38 grafts with asymptomatic stenoses identified by color-flow duplex US scanning were followed without revision.[25] The decision not to intervene was influenced by a normal or unchanged ABI, unwillingness of the patient to undergo a second procedure, and reluctance on the part of the surgeon to subject a patient without symptoms to operation. Ten (30%) of 33 grafts with nonrevised stenoses that had velocity ratios exceeding 2.0 occluded during follow-up. Five grafts with low-grade stenoses (velocity ratios less than 2.0) remained patent. Only 10 (9%) of 108 grafts with no detectable stenosis thrombosed. Measured from the time of operation, the 2-year cumulative patency rate of grafts with velocity ratios greater than 2.0 was 57% (Fig. 36–3). The cumulative patency rate 2 years after the stenoses were first detected was only 33% (Fig. 36–4). These data contrast with the 83% 2-year patency rate of grafts in which there was no identifiable stenosis (Fig. 36–3).

Similarly, Idu et al reported a 39% incidence of occlusion in nonrevised grafts with stenoses identified by color-flow scanning.[22] Although none of the eight grafts with stenoses in the 30% to 49% diameter reduction category thrombosed, 57% (4 of 7) in the 50% to 69% category and 100% (3 of 3) in the 70% to 99% category occluded.

Despite the high number of occlusions that occur in vein bypasses with stenotic lesions, between one-third and two-thirds of strictured grafts remain patent for 1 to 2 years (Table 36–2). As expected, the prognosis appears to be related to the severity of the stenosis.

Patency Rates of Revised Grafts with Stenotic Lesions

The assisted primary patency rates achieved by revision of nonoccluded grafts with stenotic lesions closely approximate those of grafts with no identifiable structural problem (Table 36–3). In other words, a timely operation restores the potential for long-term survival (Table 36–2). Idu et al reported that only four (10%) of 40 revised grafts with 50% to 99% stenoses occluded during follow-up.[22] In our series, occlusions

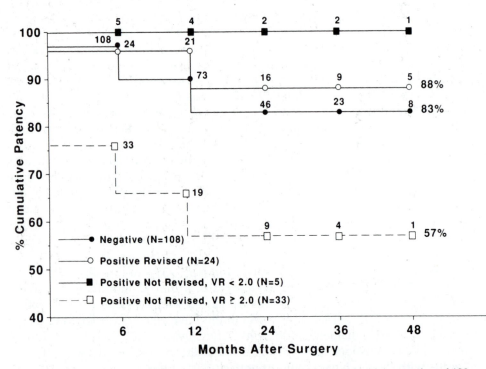

Figure 36–3. Cumulative patency rates measured from the time of initial operation of 108 vein grafts with no detectable stenosis (negative), 24 vein grafts with revised stenoses (positive revised), 33 vein grafts with unrevised stenoses having velocity ratios (VRs) greater than 2.0 (positive not revised, VR ≥ 2.0), and five vein grafts with unrevised stenoses having VRs less than 2.0 (positive not revised, VR < 2.0). (*Modified from Mattos MA, van Bemmelen PS, Hodgson KJ, et al. Does correction of stenoses identified with color duplex scanning improve infrainguinal graft patency? J Vasc Surg. 1993;17:54–66.*)

occurred after revision in only two (8%) of 24 patent but stenotic infrainguinal vein bypass grafts.[25] All stenoses were identified by color-flow US surveillance and all were associated with velocity ratios of 2.0 of more. The cumulative patency rate at 2 to 4 years after the initial operation was 88% (Fig. 36–3). Ninety percent of the grafts were patent 1 to 3 years after the stenoses were first detected (Fig. 36–4). These survival figures compare favorably with the 83% cumulative patency rate of nonstenotic nonrevised grafts and are far superior to the patency rate of stenotic grafts not treated surgically, as mentioned earlier.

Effect of Surveillance and Graft Revision

In any series of grafts subjected to postoperative surveillance, most remain negative for stenosis throughout the follow-up period, some develop stenoses of which a portion will be revised, and others thrombose before a stenosis is detected. The overall benefit of surveillance can be determined only by considering the entire population of surveyed grafts. To study the impact of surveillance on graft survival, a number of investigators have compared "secondary" and "primary" patency rates calculated on the same group of infrainguinal bypass grafts (Table 36–4). These studies report 5-year "secondary" patency rates of 76% to 88% that are 5 to 22 percentage points better than "primary" patency rates.[11,14,20,22,25,26,33,52,60,66,67] As mentioned earlier, this

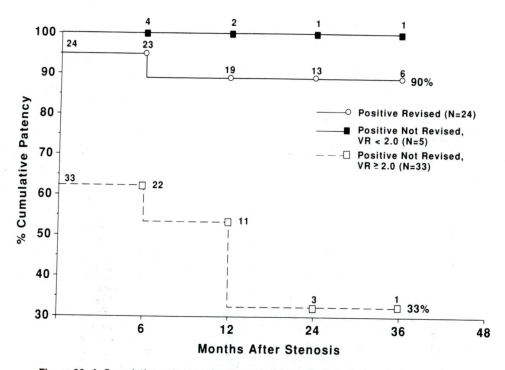

Figure 36–4. Cumulative patency rates measured from the time that graft stenoses were first detected. (See Key Fig. 36–2). (*Modified from Mattos MA, van Bemmelen PS, Hodgson KJ, et al: Does correction of stenoses identified with color duplex scanning improve infrainguinal graft patency? J Vasc Surg 17:54–66, 1993.*)

type of comparison is simply not valid because the Life Tables, from which the two patency rates are estimated, are based on an identical cohort of grafts, the only difference being that revisions are classified as failures in the "primary patency" table.[14] Thus, this method of analysis artificially assures the superiority of the "secondary" patency rate (which in many reports is actually an amalgam of assisted primary patency rates and secondary patency rates). Nonetheless, the "secondary" patency

TABLE 36–2. INCIDENCE OF OCCLUSION DURING FOLLOW-UP

Author	Year	Stenotic Grafts Not Revised Occluded/Total (%)	Stenotic Grafts Revised Occluded/Total (%)	Grafts Without Detectable Stenoses Occluded/Total (%)
Grigg[41]	1988	3/14 (21)[a]	0/5 (0)	4/56 (7)
Moody[16]	1989	5/22 (28)	ND	4/78 (7)
Idu[22]	1993	7/10 (70)[b]	4/40 (10)	ND
Mattos[25]	1993	10/33 (30)[c]	2/24 (8)	10/108 (9)
Nielsen[61]	1993	10/18 (56)[d]	4/13 (31)	1/76 (1)

[a] Non–hemodynamically significant stenoses.
[b] Diameter reduction greater than 50%.
[c] Velocity ratio 2.0 or greater.
[d] Stenoses not considered a threat to a graft survival.
ND, no data.

TABLE 36–3. RESULTS OF REVISION OF STENOTIC BUT PATENT GRAFTS

Author	Year	Grafts At Risk (n)	Follow-Up Duration (y)	Cumulative Patency[a] (%)
Donaldson[11]	1992	22	2	95
Bergamini[67]	1991	72	3	93
Mattos[25]	1993	24	4	88
Sladen[52]	1981	33	5	76
Berkowitz[4]	1992	72	5	61

[a] Includes only grafts that were revised for stenosis.

rate is a valid representation of the contribution that surveillance makes to graft survival.

In a recent prospective study reported by Lundell *et al*, infrainguinal bypass grafts were randomized to a "surveillance" group, in which all limbs underwent serial ABIs and duplex US scans, and to a "normal" clinical follow-up group.[68] Two and three years after the initial operation, the cumulative patency rate of autogenous vein grafts in the surveillance group was 78%, 25 percentage points higher than the 53% patency rate in grafts that were followed clinically without surveillance. This, apparently, is the only prospective, randomized study that compares the results achieved with surveillance with those obtained by clinical follow-up alone.

Idu et al compared the assisted primary patency rate of infrainguinal vein grafts in 160 patients who underwent routine surveillance with color-flow duplex US scans with that of 41 patients who were followed-up clinically.[22] The two groups were concomitant and were drawn from the same population but were not randomized. Stenoses were detected in 52 (32.5%) of the surveillance group and in three (7%) of the clinical group. Forty graft stenoses in the surveillance group and all three in the clinical group were revised. Three years after the original operation, the cumulative survival rate of grafts in the surveillance group (91%) was significantly ($P = .004$) higher than that of grafts in the clinical follow-up group (78%).

Other authors using historical controls have arrived at similar conclusions. These comparisons, however, are always somewhat suspect because the populations in-

TABLE 36–4. CUMULATIVE PATENCY RATES OF INFRAINGUINAL GRAFTS: COMPARISON OF PRIMARY AND SECONDARY PATENCY RATES

Author	Year	Follow-Up Duration (y)	Secondary Patency (%)	Primary Patency (%)	Difference (%)
Sladen[52]	1981	5	80	64	16
Leather[60]	1988	5	76	59	17
Taylor[66]	1990	5	80	75	5
Green[14]	1990	5	80	66	14
Bergamini[67]	1991	5	81	63	18
Donaldson[11]	1992	5	79	70	9
Idu[22]	1993	5	88	66	22
Mattos[25]	1993	4	79	60	19
Laborde[26]	1992	3	87	62	25
Stierli[20]	1992	1	88	54	34
Davies[33]	1994	1	85	55	30

cluded in the surveillance and the historically based clinical follow-up groups may not be well-matched. In addition, improvements in surgical techniques tend to favor the surveillance group. The results reported by Green et al are typical.[48] Whereas the 5-year cumulative secondary patency rate of 125 vein grafts performed between 1982 and 1986 was 79%, the 5-year assisted primary patency rate of 79 grafts inserted between 1987 and 1992 was 93%. The first group was followed clinically; the second group was followed with serial ABIs and duplex US scans. Surveillance identified 26 grafts with preocclusive lesions. Of these, 17 underwent successful revision, but three occluded before revision could be accomplishd. Six other limbs could not be operated on because of inadequate outflow. In three of these, the graft thrombosed and amputation was required.

In another historical control study, Moody et al found a 2% failure rate over a 12-month period in a series of grafts subjected to surveillance and a 13% failure rate in a similar group of grafts that were not screened for stenoses.[49]

In the aggregate, this information, though flawed, suggests that surveillance of all infrainguinal bypass grafts coupled with revision of graft stenoses improves the survival rate of vein bypass graft by about 10% to 25% over that obtained in grafts followed clinically.[22,25,48,49,68]

INDICATIONS FOR INTERVENTION

The incidence of revision of patent stenotic grafts is much higher when surveillance is used than it is when the decision to intervene is made on the basis of clinical observations. In the series reported by Idu et al, 21% of surveyed grafts were revised compared with only 3% of those followed clinically.[22] Reported revision rates vary from 7% to 26% (accumulated mean, 16%; 365/2357).[4,22,25,29,33,48,50,61,67,68] Although 42% to 100% (accumulated mean, 78%) of stenoses detected by surveillance have been revised,[22,25,29,33,48,50,67] a large fraction of these lesions probably did not constitute an immediate threat to limb survival and could have been followed without treatment (Table 36–2).[14,16,22] Unfortunately, there is no certain way of differentiating lesions that require revision from those that do not.

In our study, stenoses involving the graft itself appeared to have a worse prognosis than those developing at the anastomoses or in the inflow or outflow arteries, but the numbers were too low to achieve statistical significance (Fig. 36–5).[25] It is well known, however, that vein grafts may remain patent despite the presence of significant stenoses or occlusions of the inflow arteries.[12] Also, progression of disease in outflow arteries may be compatible with continued patency, provided sufficient collaterals exit the artery in the segment between the distal anastomosis and the occlusion. Therefore, lesions remote from the graft or its anastomoses can be regarded with somewhat less urgency than lesions intrinsic to the graft.

Several studies suggest that stenoses that narrow the graft lumen by less than 50% can be followed safely.[22,46] This coincides with our finding that none of the five grafts in our series with stenoses having velocity ratios less than 2.0 occluded during the period of observation.[25] On the other hand, grafts with higher-grade lesions, especially those that narrow the lumen by 70% to 80% or more, are prone to thrombosis and should be revised.[22] Stenoses of this severity are associated with velocity ratios of 2.0 or more (Fig. 36–6). Although we could not confirm a direct relationship between increasing velocity ratios and an increased incidence of graft occlusion, it seems logical that this should be the case.[25] Others rely on absolute elevations of the peak systolic

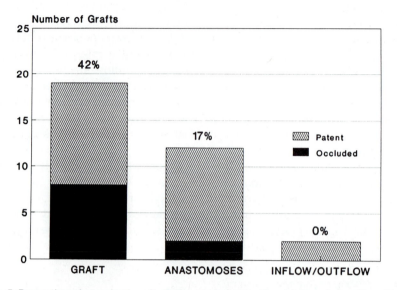

Figure 36–5. Proportion of unrevised grafts that occluded according to stenosis location. (*Reproduced with permission from Sumner DS. When is correction of vein graft stenosis detected by duplex necessary to maintain patency and when is it not. In: Veith FJ, ed.* Current Critical Problems in Vascular Surgery. *Vol. 6. St. Louis, Mo: Quality Medical Publishing, 1995, p. 80.*)

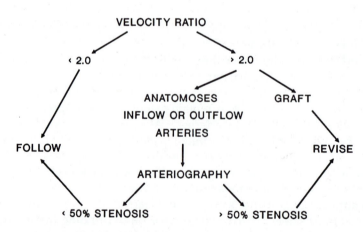

Figure 36–6. A simple algorithm for management of graft stenoses detected by duplex scanning. Decisions are based solely on velocity ratios, arteriography, and stenosis location. Return of clinical symptoms, low or falling ankle–brachial indices, or peak systolic velocities <45 cm/sec support the decision to intervene. Absence of these findings in limbs with velocity ratios exceeding 2.0 should not alter the decision to revise the graft. (*Reproduced with permission from Sumner DS. When is correction of vein graft stenosis detected by duplex necessary to maintain patency and when is it not. In: Veith FJ, ed.* Current Critical Problems in Vascular Surgery. *Vol. 6. St. Louis, Mo: Quality Medical Publishing, 1995, p. 80.*)

velocity to identify high-grade lesions that jeopardize graft survival. Systolic velocities greater than 250 cm/sec and end-diastolic velocities greater than 100 cm/sec are particularly ominous when they are found in the vicinity of a stenosis.[43]

Not all increases in velocity are due to stenoses. Any disparity in the diameter of the flow conduit or abrupt change in the direction of flow can be responsible for real or apparent velocity changes, which may be misinterpreted as indicating a stenosis when in fact there is none (pseudostenosis). Potentially confusing velocity changes can occur in composite grafts in which the diameter of the anastomosed conduits differ, in normal vein grafts in which large side branches have been ligated, at the proximal anastomosis when the host artery is usually considerably larger than the graft, and at the distal anastomosis when the diameter of the vein graft exceeds that of the recipient artery. Because of the inverted taper of reversed vein grafts, these size discrepancies are more pronounced in reversed vein grafts than they are in *in situ* or nonreversed translocated vein grafts. At the proximal side-to-end and the distal end-to-side anastomoses, the orientation of the graft and host artery differ in respect to the ultrasonic sound beam. Despite angle corrections made on the basis of the B-mode or color-flow US scan, velocity measurements and velocity ratios made in these areas are apt to be misleading and should be interpreted cautiously.

When a severe stenosis is detected in the graft itself, arteriography is often unnecessary and revision can be planned based on duplex US findings alone.[25] Even if the graft fails before prophylactic intervention, knowledge of the precise location of the responsible lesion simplifies the approach to thrombectomy. On the other hand, apparent stenoses at the anastomoses or in the immediately adjacent host artery should be confirmed with arteriography. If the arteriogram verifies the presence of a 50% diameter or greater stenosis, revision is indicated (Fig. 36–6).

Duplex US scans usually identify the source of the problem in limbs with recurrent symptoms or a decreasing ABI. A negative duplex US scan of the graft, anastomoses, and adjacent arteries implicates advancing disease in vessels remote from the graft (in the aorta or iliac arteries or in the distal tibial or pedal arteries).[30] Although the Doppler spectrum or more extensive duplex US scanning may locate the offending lesion (or lesions), arteriography is often required, especially when an operation is contemplated. Most authors (ourselves included) agree that all stenoses responsible for recurrent symptoms or a persistent fall in the ankle pressure should be considered for revision.[16,18,20] The observations of Green et al strongly support this stance.[14] In their series, 66% of grafts with both a decreased ABI and an abnormal duplex US scan either thrombosed or caused symptoms before the next follow-up visit. In contrast, only 4% of grafts with a abnormal duplex scans and normal ABIs suffered a similar fate. Our experience differs in that lesions with high velocity ratios (exceeding 2.0 or 3.0) had a very poor prognosis regardless of the ABI or the presence or absence of symptoms.[25] Therefore, we continue to believe that intervention should be considered in all limbs with severe graft stenoses even when the hemodynamic status remains stable (Fig. 36–6). Although this aggressive policy will lead to some unnecessary revisions, the alternative (a high incidence of graft thrombosis) is unacceptable.

A PSV less than 45 cm/sec measured at the widest portion of the graft is a matter of some concern, especially when the low flow rate can be attributed to occlusion in the outflow bed.[43] In this event, anticoagulation or jump grafting to a more distal arterial segment may be necessary to preserve patency. Many "unexplained" failures may be due to hypercoagulable states, including protein C and S and antithrombin III deficiencies, or to the presence of lupus anticoagulant or anticardiolipin antibodies.[9,69] When any of these abnormalities is identified, graft survival may be enhanced by long-term anticoagulation.

Because about three-quarters of graft-threatening stenoses develop within 12 months of the initial operation, surveillance should be relatively frequent during this period.[20,29,40,53] Unfortunately, no matter how often scans are obtained, stenoses may develop and thrombose during the interval. Schedules vary, but most include a baseline duplex US scan obtained within a few weeks of operation and subsequent follow-up scans every 3 months during the first year. As a cost-saving measure, some authors recommend that surveillance be discontinued after the first year;[50] others, however, advocate continued scanning at 6- or 12-month intervals to detect late atherosclerotic progression.[22,59,70] When a low-grade stricture or other problem that does not require immediate intervention is identified, the interval between scans should be decreased until the stability of the lesion is established. Although a few stenoses seem to disappear, an appreciable number progress, and these must be regarded with special concern.

The role of surveillance in the long-term management of infrainguinal prosthetic grafts has not been clearly established.[50] Because most failures appear to be due to progression of atherosclerotic disease in the inflow or outflow arteries, surveillance of these areas coupled with hemodynamic studies may help preserve graft patency.[71]

COST-EFFECTIVENESS

The cost of routine surveillance and elective revision of a relatively large number of stenotic grafts must be balanced against the cost of restricting secondary operations to a smaller number of patients with symptomatic failed grafts. Although the cost of graft revision is relatively low and hospital stays are short, the cost of thrombectomy, thrombolysis, and "redo" procedures may be quite high. Whereas graft revisions are ordinarily relatively simple procedures with little associated morbidity, operations to restore graft patency are often complicated, require prolonged hospitalization, and subject the patient to considerable pain, anxiety, and the threat of limb loss. If patency cannot be restored, amputation may be required, an eventuality that contributes additional expenses, including those of physical therapy, prosthesis fitting, disability, and possible institutional care. Therefore, even if precise data concerning the natural history of graft stenoses and the effect of surveillance on graft survival were available and the imponderables mentioned above could be discounted, estimation of the cost-effectiveness of surveillance would be extraordinarily difficult.

CONCLUSION

Color duplex US scanning has been established as an accurate and clinically feasible method for surveillance of infrainguinal vein bypass grafts. During follow-up, this technique detects 50% or greater diameter–reducing stenoses in about 20% of grafts. Most of these lesions develop in the first year after operation. The natural history of graft stenoses is distinctly unfavorable; without treatment, 20% to 70% of stenotic grafts thrombose. Although it is well established that the risk of occlusion is greater when stenoses are severe, no definite criteria have been proposed for identifying grafts with lower-grade lesions that may remain patent and do not require intervention. Revision, however, is seldom complicated and is associated with long-term patency rates comparable with those achieved in grafts without stenoses. Secondary patency rates of grafts in limbs subjected to routine surveillance are 10 to 25 percentage points better than they are in grafts that have been followed clinically. Despite the added expense of repeated duplex US scans and an increased incidence of revision, routine graft surveillance is probably cost-effective and should be considered as essential to the follow-up of patients with infrainguinal bypass grafts.

REFERENCES

1. Whittemore, AD, Clowes AW, Couch NP, Mannick JA. Secondary femoropopliteal reconstruction. *Ann Surg.* 1981;193:35–42.
2. Green RM, Ouriel K, Ricotta JJ, DeWeese JA. Revision of failed infrainguinal bypass graft: principles of management. *Surgery.* 1986;100:646–653.
3. Cohen JR, Mannick JA, Couch NP, Whittemore AD. Recognition and management of impending vein-graft failure: importance for long-term patency. *Arch Surg.* 1986;121:758–759.
4. Berkowitz HD, Fox AD, Deaton DH: Reversed vein graft stenosis: early diagnosis and management. *J Vasc Surg.* 1992;15:130–142.
5. Brewster DC, LaSalle AJ, Robison JG. Femoropopliteal graft failures: clinical consequences and success of secondary reconsructions. *Arch Surg.* 1983;118:1043–1047.
6. Bartlett ST, Olinde AJ, Flinn WR. The reoperative potential of infrainguinal bypass: long-term limb and patient survival. *J Vasc Surg.* 1987;5:170–179.
7. Dennis JW, Litooy FN, Greisler HP, Baker WH. Secondary vascular procedures with polytetrafluoroethylene grafts for low extremity ischemia in a male veteran population. *J Vasc Surg.* 1988;8:137–142.
8. Edwards JE, Taylor LM Jr, Porter JM. Treatment of failed lower extremity bypass grafts with new autogenous vein bypass grafting. *J Vasc Surg.* 1990;11:136–145.
9. DeFrang RD, Edwards JM, Moneta GL, et al. Repeat leg bypass after multiple prior bypass failures. *J Vasc Surg.* 1994;19:268–77.
10. Belkin M, Conte MS, Whittemore AD, et al. Preferred strategies for secondary infrainguinal bypass surgery: lessons learned from 300 consecutive re-operations. Presented at the 48th Annual Meeting of the Society for Vascular Surgery, Seattle, Washington, June 7–8, 1994.
11. Donaldson MC, Mannick JA, Whittemore AD. Causes of primary graft failure after in situ saphenous vein bypass grafting. *J Vasc Surg.* 1992;15:113–120.
12. Mills JL, Fujitani RM, Taylor SM. The characteristics and anatomic distribution of lesions that cause reversed vein graft failure: a five-year prospective study. *J Vasc Surg.* 1993;17:195–206.
13. Sumner DS, Mattos MA, Hodgson KJ. Surveillance program for vascular reconstructive procedures. In: Yao JST, Pearce WH, eds. *Long-Term Results in Vascular Surgery.* Norwalk, Conn: Appleton & Lange; 1993:33–59.
14. Green RM, McNamara J, Ouriel K, DeWeese JA. Comparison of infrainguinal graft surveillance techniques. *J Vasc Surg.* 1990;11:207–215.
15. Blackshear WM, Thiele BL, Strandness DE: Natural history of above and below-knee femoropopliteal grafts. *Am J Surg.* 1980;140:234–241.
16. Moody P, de Cossart LM, Douglas HM, Harris PL. Asymptomatic strictures in femoropopliteal vein grafts. *Eur J Vasc Surg.* 1989;3:389–392.
17. Berkowitz HD, Hobbs CL, Roberts B, et al. Value of routine vascular laboratory studies to identify vein graft stenosis. *Surgery.* 1981;90:971–978.

18. McShane MD, Gazzard VM, Clifford PC, et al. Duplex ultrasound monitoring of arterial grafts: prospective evaluation in conjunction with ankle pressure indices after femorodistal bypass. *Eur J Vasc Surg.* 1987;1:385–390.

19. Disselhoff B, Buth J, Jakimowicz J. Early detection of stenosis of femoro-distal grafts: a surveillance study using colour-duplex scanning. *Eur J Vasc Surg.* 1989;3:43–48.

20. Stierli P, Aeberhard P, Livers M. The role of colour duplex screening in infra-inguinal vein grafts. *Eur J Vasc Surg.* 1992;6:293–298.

21. Bandyk DF, Seabrook GR, Moldenhauer P, et al. Hemodynamics of vein graft stenosis. *J Vasc Surg.* 1988;8:688–695.

22. Idu MM, Blankenstein JD, de Gier P, et al. Impact of a color-flow duplex surveillance program on infrainguinal vein graft patency: a five-year experience. *J Vasc Surg.* 1993;17:42–53.

23. Baker DJ, Dix D. Variability of Doppler ankle pressure with arterial occlusive disease: an evaluation of ankle index and brachial-ankle pressure gradient. *Surgery.* 1981;89:134–137.

24. Barnes RW, Thompson BW, MacDonald CM, et al. Serial noninvasive studies do not herald postoperative failure of femoropopliteal or femorotibial bypass grafts. *Ann Surg.* 1989;210:486–494.

25. Mattos MA, van Bemmelen PS, Hodgson KJ, et al. Does correction of stenoses identified with color duplex scanning improve infrainguinal graft patency? *J Vasc Surg.* 1993;17:54–66.

26. Laborde AL, Synn AY, Worsey J, et al. A prospective comparison of ankle/brachial indices and color duplex imaging in surveillance of the in situ saphenous vein bypass. *J Cardiovasc Surg.* 1992;33:420–425.

27. Wolfe JHN, Lea Thomas M, Jamieson CW, et al. Early diagnosis of femorodistal graft stenoses. *Br J Surg.* 1987;74:268–270.

28. Robison JG, Elliott BM. Does postoperative surveillance with duplex scanning identify the failing distal bypass? *Ann Vasc Surg.* 1991;5:182–185.

29. Mills JL, Harris EJ, Taylor LM Jr, et al. The importance of routine surveillance of distal bypass grafts with duplex scanning: a study of 379 reversed vein grafts. *J Vasc Surg.* 1990;12:379–389.

30. McShane MD, Gazzard VM, Clifford PC, et al. Duplex ultrasound assessment of femorodistal grafts: correlation with angiography. *Eur J Vasc Surg.* 1987;1:409–414.

31. Harris JP, Kidd JF, Waugh RC, et al. Color-enhanced duplex detection of vein graft stenoses after lower extremity arterial reconstruction. *J Vasc Technol.* 1992;16:129–132.

32. Wyatt MG, Muir RM, Tennant WG, et al. Impedance analysis to identify the at risk femorodistal graft. *J Vasc Surg.* 1991;13:284–293.

33. Davies AH, Magee TR, Tennant SGW, et al. Criteria for identification of the "at-risk" infrainguinal bypass graft. *Eur J Vasc Surg.* 1984;8:315–319.

34. Turnipseed WD, Sproat IA. A preliminary experience with use of magnetic resonance angiography in assessment of failing lower extremity bypass grafts. *Surgery.* 1992;112:664–669.

35. Londrey GL, Hodgson KJ, Spadone DP, et al. Initial experience with color-flow duplex scanning of infrainguinal bypass grafts. *J Vasc Surg.* 1990;12:284–290.

36. Sladen JG, Reid JDS, Cooperberg PL, et al. Color-flow duplex screening of infrainguinal grafts combining low and high-velocity criteria. *Am J Surg.* 1989;158:107–112.

37. Bartlett ST, Killewich LA, Fisher C, Ward RE. Duplex imaging of in situ saphenous vein bypass grafts and late failure reduction. *Am J Surg.* 1988;156:484–487.

38. Polak JF, Donaldson MC, Dobkin GR, et al. Early detection of saphenous vein arterial bypass graft stenosis by color-assisted duplex sonography: a prospective study. *AJR.* 1990;154:857–861.

39. Taylor PR, Tyrrell MR, Crofton M, et al. Colour flow imaging in the detection of femorodistal graft and native artery stenosis: improved criteria. *Eur J Vasc Surg.* 1992;6:232–236.

40. Buth J, Disselhoff B, Sommeling C, Stam L. Color-flow duplex criteria for grading stenosis in infrainguinal vein grafts. *J Vasc Surg.* 1991;14:716–728.

41. Grigg MJ, Nicolaides AN, Wolfe JHN. Detection and grading of femoro-distal vein graft stenoses: duplex velocity measurements compared with angiography. *J Vasc Surg.* 1988;8:661–666.

42. Jager KA, Phillips DJ, Martin RL, et al. Noninvasive mapping of lower limb arterial lesions. *Ultrasound Med Biol.* 1985;11:515–521.
43. Bandyk DF. Monitoring during and after distal arterial reconstruction. In: Bernstein EF, ed. *Vascular Diagnosis.* 4th ed. St. Louis, Mo: Mosby: 1993:579–587.
44. Bandyk DF, Kaebnick HW, Bergamini TM, et al. Hemodynamics of in situ saphenous vein arterial bypass. *Arch Surg.* 1988;123:477–482.
45. Bandyk DF, Cato RF, Towne JB. A low flow velocity predicts failure of femoropopliteal and femorotibial bypass grafts. *Surgery.* 1985;98:799–809.
46. Chang BB, Leather RP, Kaufman JL, et al. Hemodynamic characteristics of failing infrainguinal in situ vein bypass. *J Vasc Surg.* 1990;12:596–600.
47. Belkin M, Raftery KB, Mackey WC, et al. A prospective study of the determinants of vein graft flow velocity: implications for graft surveillance. *J Vasc Surg.* 1994;19:259–267.
48. Green RM, Eagleton M, DeWeese JA. The impact of a graft surveillance program on long-term patency of saphenous vein bypass grafts. Poster at the 48th Annual Meeting of the Society for Vascular Surgery, Seattle, Washington, June 7–8, 1994.
49. Moody P, Gould DA, Harris PL. Vein graft surveillance improves patency in femoro-popliteal bypass. *Eur J Vasc Surg.* 1990;4:117–121.
50. Taylor PR, Wolfe JHN, Tyrrell MR, et al. Graft stenosis: justification for 1-year surveillance. *Br J Surg.* 1990;77:1125–1128.
51. Bandyk DF, Bergamini TM, Towne JB, et al. Durability of vein graft revision: the outcome of secondary procedures. *J Vasc Surg.* 1991;13:200–210.
52. Sladen JG, Gilmour JL. Vein graft stenosis: characteristics and effect of treatment. *Am J Surg.* 1981;141:549–563.
53. Berkowitz HD, Greenstein S, Barker CF, Perloff LJ. Late failure of reversed vein bypass grafts. *Ann Surg.* 1989;210:782–786.
54. Bandyk DF, Schmitt DD, Seabrook GR, et al. Monitoring functional patency of in situ saphenous vein bypasses: the impact of a surveillance protocol and elective revision. *J Vasc Surg.* 1989;9:284–296.
55. Szilagyi DE, Elliott JP, Hageman JH, et al. Biologic fate of autogenous vein implants as arterial substitutes: clinical, angiographic and histopathologic observations in femoro-popliteal operations for atherosclerosis. *Ann Surg.* 1973;178:232–246.
56. Moody AP, Edwards PR, Harris PL. The aetiology of vein graft strictures: a prospective marker study. *Eur J Vasc Surg.* 1992;6:509–511.
57. Marin ML, Veith FJ, Panetta TF, et al. Saphenous vein biopsy: a predictor of vein graft failure. *J Vasc Surg.* 1993;18:407–415.
58. Panetta TF, Marin ML, Veith FJ, et al. Unsuspected preexisting saphenous vein disease: an unrecognized cause of vein bypass failure. *J Vasc Surg.* 1992;15:102–112.
59. Reifsnyder T, Towne JB, Seabrook GR, et al. Biologic characteristics of long-term autogenous vein grafts: a dynamic evolution. *J Vasc Surg.* 1993;17:207–217.
60. Leather RP, Shah DJ, Chang BB, Kaufman JL. Resurrection of the in situ saphenous vein bypass: 1000 cases later. *Ann Surg.* 1988;208:435–442.
61. Nielsen T, von Jessen F, Sillesen H, Schroeder TV. Doppler spectral characteristics of infrainguinal vein bypasses. *Eur J Vasc Surg.* 1993;7:610–615.
62. Kupinski AM, Khan AM, Evans SM, et al. Retrograde flow in infrainguinal arterial bypasses. *J Vasc Technol.* 1992;16:281–283.
63. Ad Hoc Committee on Reporting Standards, Society for Vascular Surgery/North American Chapter, International Society for Cardiovascular Surgery. Suggested standards for reports dealing with lower extremity ischemia. *J Vasc Surg.* 1986;4:80–94.
64. Testart J, Watelet J. Suggested standards for reports dealing with lower extremity ischemia. (Letter to the Editors.) *J Vasc Surg.* 1988;7:717.
65. Rutherford RB. "Reply." (Letter to the Editors.) *J Vasc Surg.* 1988;7:718.
66. Taylor LM Jr, Edwards JM, Porter JM. Present status of reversed vein bypass grafting: five-year results of a modern series. *J Vasc Surg.* 1990;11:193–206.
67. Bergamini TM, Towne JB, Bandyk DF, et al. Experience with in situ saphenous vein bypasses during 1981 to 1989: determinant factors of long-term patency. *J Vasc Surg.* 1991;13:137–149.

68. Lundell AJB, Lindblad B, Hansen F, Bergqvist D. Femoropopliteo-crural graft patency is improved by an intensive surveillance program: a prospective randomized study. Presented at the 48th Annual Meeting of the Society for Vascular Surgery, Seattle, Washington, June 7–8, 1994.

69. Donaldson MC, Weinberg DS, Belkin M, et al. Screening for hypercoagulable states in vascular surgical practice: a preliminary study. *J Vasc Surg.* 1990;11:825–831.

70. Sanchez LA, Gupta SK, Veith FJ, et al. A ten-year experience with one hundred fifty failing or threatened vein and polytetrafluoroethylene arterial bypass grafts. *J Vasc Surg.* 1991;14:729–738.

71. Sanchez LA, Suggs WD, Veith FJ, et al. Is surveillance to detect failing polytetrafluoroethylene bypasses worthwhile?: Twelve-year experience with ninety-one grafts. *J Vasc Surg.* 1993;18:981–990.

IX

Redo Operation for Failed Infrainguinal Bypass

37

The Use of Rotational Muscle Flaps in the Management of Graft Infection

Bruce A. Perler, MD

Although infection complicates less than 3% of peripheral arterial bypass grafts in most large series[1-4], in view of the growth in the performance of arterial reconstructions in recent years, it has been estimated that currently as many as 10,000 patients per year in the United States are treated for prosthetic graft infection.[5] Furthermore, this complication continues to represent a substantial challenge for the surgeon and a potentially devastating complication for the patient. The mortality associated with prosthetic graft infection has ranged from 25% to 75%, and serious morbidity, including limb loss, has been reported among 30% to 75% of patients.[1,2,6-9]

Because it is axiomatic that infection involving a foreign body can be eradicated only by complete removal of that foreign body, the conventional management of synthetic graft infection has included complete excision of the graft and revascularization, if necessary, through uninvolved and usually extra-anatomic tissue planes. Although theoretically appealing, in the past this approach has been associated with some of the highest rates of morbidity and mortality for several reasons. First, in most cases reoperation to remove the infected prosthesis is technically demanding and physiologically stressful for the patient. Second, graft excision typically requires repair of the original anastomotic sites in infected fields, so that native arterial sutures lines are at risk of late rupture due to indolent residual infection. In addition, in many patients distal extremity arterial perfusion becomes dependent on extra-anatomic bypass grafts that are vulnerable to recurrent thrombosis, thus jeopardizing limb viability. In view of this, a number of alternative approaches to the problem of graft infection have been explored over the years. The most appropriate treatment of many of these patients remains somewhat controversial. For example, some authors have advocated graft excision and *in situ* replacement with autogenous arteries or veins.[10,11] At other centers, cadaveric homograft veins[12] or arteries[13] have been placed *in situ* at the time of graft removal. Perhaps one of the earliest unconventional approaches to an infected prosthetic graft, and clearly one of the most controversial, is aggressive local wound care with attempted preservation of all, or most, of the original graft.

Although contrary to conventional dogma, several previous reports have suggested that in selected cases, infected synthetic bypass grafts may be salvaged with repeated soft-tissue debridements, performance of frequent dressing changes, and the administration of antibiotics both systemically and topically. For example, Carter et al reported the successful treatment of six (86%) of seven infected Dacron bypass grafts in this manner more than 30 years ago.[14] Other workers more recently have reported success with this approach in limited numbers of cases.[15–17] This experience suggests that aggressive local care may sterilize these wounds and allow healing to occur by secondary intention.

The obvious appeal of this approach includes avoiding the potential morbidity associated with removing the original graft as well as obviating the need for an extra-anatomic bypass and its susceptibility to recurrent thrombosis. On the other hand, the local management of graft infection conveys other disadvantages. For example, the patient is usually committed to a prolonged period of hospitalization and its attendant financial cost. Second, and perhaps more important, while awaiting healing by secondary intention, the graft is vulnerable to other secondary complications, such as thrombosis, anastomotic hemorrhage, and superinfection by more virulent organisms. I believe that coverage of the graft with a rotational muscle flap (RMF) addresses these limitations and represents a logical and important advance in the local management of prosthetic graft infection. In fact, the use of RMFs to treat arterial graft infection is an extension of a growing experience with this approach in the management of serious infectious complications in nonvascular surgical disciplines. It is supported by a solid background of basic laboratory investigation.

NONVASCULAR CLINICAL EXPERIENCE

Over the past 20 years, well-vascularized muscle tissue has been used to fill soft-tissue defects and promote healing of difficult wounds resulting from radiation injury, trauma, tumor excision, and other causes.[18,19] Recently muscle flaps have been utilized in the management of infectious wound complications in the areas of cardiothoracic and orthopedic surgery.

Cardiothoracic Surgery

A growing clinical experience has demonstrated the potential of muscle flaps to promote eradication of infection and expedite the healing of difficult wounds following major thoracic surgery.[20–22] In one series, for example, 87 consecutive patients, including 65 with active infection, underwent muscle transposition to close chest wounds after esophageal or pulmonary surgery. Healing was reported in 65 (75%) with a mean follow-up period of just over 2 years.[21]

Perhaps more relevant to the issue of arterial graft infection has been the experience with muscle flaps in treating infectious complications after cardiac surgery. For example, the treatment of mediastinal infection has traditionally consisted of repeated sternal debridements, antibiotic irrigations and systemic administration, repeated dressing changes, and delayed secondary closure. Like the local treatment of graft infection, however, this approach mandated a prolonged period of hospitalization and considerable associated morbidity. The use of RMFs as part of the overall management strategy has substantially improved the outcome among patients with this potentially life-threatening cardiac surgical complication.[23–26] In one report, for example, six patients whom conventional management had failed achieved healing after RMF closure with an average hospitalization of only 19 days after the flap was performed.[28] Other larger series have documented successful healing in approximately 90% of patients with mediastinal infection after muscle flap closure.[24-26] In another report, an infected left ventricular aneurysm was resected through the septic field, and the repair was covered with a pectoralis major muscle flap with complete healing.[27]

Orthopedic Surgery

Chronic osteomyelitis is another clinical problem that has been treated locally with repeated bone debridements and antibiotics. Muscle flaps have been utilized to cover the debrided bone with impressive results. In one series, for example, 84% of wounds closed with muscle flaps remained healed versus only 43% of wounds treated without muscle flaps.[28] In another report, 17 patients with chronic osteomyelitis were successfully treated with debridement and muscle flap closure.[29] Mathes et al,[30] have treated 11 patients with lower extremity chronic osteomyelitis of 14 years' average duration with local muscle transfer, and all patients' wounds remained healed with a mean follow-up period of nearly 2 years.

Perhaps even more germane to a discussion of arterial prosthetic bypass graft infection is infection involving an orthopedic joint endoprosthesis, since the conventional management has required removal of the prosthesis. Four patients with exposed and infected joint prostheses, including two in the arm and two in the leg, were successfully treated by local debridement and coverage with RMFs.[31]

ROTATIONAL MUSCLE FLAPS: EXPERIMENTAL FOUNDATION

Hypoxia appears to be an important factor in the development of wound infection and also may retard its eradication through inhibition of leukocyte function.[32] It has been postulated that the acellular and relatively avascular capsule that typically forms around an implanted prosthetic graft as a component of the normal healing process impedes eradication of infection, at least in part, by creating a hypoxic environment.[33,34] The rationale for using muscle flaps in the management of prosthetic graft infection is based on the capability of well-vascularized tissue to increase oxygen delivery to, and thus increase the oxygen tension within, the infection site.[34] The potential of muscle flaps to effectively treat invasive infection has been studied in a number of laboratory models both with and without inclusion of synthetic bypass grafts.

In one study, for example, deep-space *Staphylococcus aureus* infections were produced in dogs, and the wounds were closed with either rectus abdominis musculocutaneous or random-pattern flaps.[35] Significantly reduced bacterial counts, and less tissue necrosis, were noted in the wounds closed with muscle flaps, and the apparent benefit of muscle flap closure was specifically attributed to the higher oxygen tension noted within those wounds.[35] Similar findings were reported in another study in which musculocutaneous flaps were compared with fasciocutaneous flaps.[36] Calderon et al[36] created paired musculocutaneous and fasciocutaneous flaps over staphylococcal deep-space infections in dogs. Significantly reduced bacterial counts were observed on days 1, 3, and 6 in the wounds closed with muscle flaps ($P < .001$).[36,37] The reduction in bacterial counts among these dogs was most pronounced within the first day after wound closure and, on the basis of radionuclide microsphere flow data, was attributed to a marked increase in arterial blood flow that occurred in the wounds closed with musculocutaneous flaps.[37]

Other studies have specifically investigated the efficacy of muscle flaps in treating wound infection involving synthetic graft material. In one experimental model, the carotid arteries of dogs were replaced with polytetrafluoroethylene (PTFE) grafts and infected with *Staphylococcus aureus*. Three days later the wounds were drained, debrided, and randomized to primary closure and antibiotic administration; closure with a sternocephalicus muscle flap and no antibiotics; or muscle flap closure and antibiotic administration. The dogs were observed for 60 days or until anastomotic disruption occurred. When the dogs were killed quantitative wound cultures were obtained. Only 20% of the dogs in the third group experienced anastomotic rupture compared with a 100% incidence of anastomotic rupture in the former two groups ($P < .05$). When the dogs were killed, significantly lower bacterial counts were noted in the neck wounds of the dogs treated with a muscle flap and antibiotics than in the other two groups ($P < .05$).[38]

Other workers replaced the abdominal aorta of a pig with PTFE grafts and inoculated them with *Staphylococcus aureus*. Seven days later the pigs were randomized to one of six treatments as follows: (1) debridement only; (2) debridement and placement of a new graft; (3) rectus abdominis coverage of the original graft; (4) coverage of the graft with the seromuscular layer of jejunum; (5) placement of a new graft and coverage with rectus abdominis; or (6) placement of a new graft and coverage with a seromuscular layer of jejunum. The pigs were re-explored 2 weeks after treatment, and bacterial cultures were obtained. Graft infection was confirmed in none of 10 group 5 ($P < .01$) and 1 of 10 group 6 ($P < .02$) pigs compared with seven of 10 group 1 pigs. Furthermore, all of the group 1 grafts were thrombosed compared with only two of the 10 group 5 and one of the 10 group 6 grafts ($P < .01$). In addition, although infection was documented in only one of six group 3 and two of six group 4 pigs, all these grafts were thrombosed at 2 weeks.[34]

Although these studies have provided objective evidence to support the hypothesis that well-vascularized muscle tissue may control or help promote eradication of infection, other studies have emphasized that this benefit may be limited by the degree of bacterial contamination. In one investigation, for example, the femoral arteries of 20 dogs were replaced with PTFE interposition grafts and inoculated with 1×10^4 or 1×10^5 *Staphylococcus aureus* organisms per milliliter. The wounds were closed in layers, although in 10 dogs the graft was also covered with a sartorius muscle flap, and the dogs were killed 1 month later. Among the dogs inoculated with 1×10^4 organisms per milliliter, positive wound cultures were obtained from none of 10 dogs treated with the muscle flap versus five of 10 closed without the sartorius flap ($P < .05$). Among the dogs inoculated with the greater concentration of organisms, however, positive cultures were obtained from six of 10 dogs closed with a sartorius flap compared with 9 of 10 in which a flap was not performed. This difference was not statistically significant.[39]

MUSCLE FLAPS FOR GRAFT INFECTION

The most obvious benefit of performing a muscle flap procedure on a patient with a graft infection is a mechanical one; that is, the flap can cover the graft and fill the defect. Well-vascularized muscle tissue provides an excellent bed upon which a split-thickness skin graft can be placed to complete closure. However, if the muscle is rotated with its overlying skin as a musculocutaneous flap, immediate closure is achieved. Expediting graft coverage should reduce the duration of hospitalization and reduce the risk for secondary complications.

In essence, two types of muscle flap procedures have been performed to treat arterial graft infection, namely, local muscle transfer or a formal RMF procedure whereby a muscle bundle is mobilized from a site separate from the focus of infection and based on a pedicled blood supply. For a number of reasons, I favor the former approach. Because most graft infections occur in the groin, it is not surprising that local transfer of the sartorius muscle has been one of the more frequently performed muscle flap procedures in this clinical setting.

Local Sartorius Transfer

Technical Considerations

Local transfer of the sartorius to cover an infected graft in the groin is very appealing for several reasons (Table 37–1). The sartorius, which originates from the anterior superior iliac spine and inserts on the medial upper shaft of the tibia, is the longest muscle in the body. Although the most cephalad portion is perfused by branches of the lateral femoral circumflex artery, and the portion distal to the adductor canal is supplied by geniculate branches of the popliteal artery, most of the muscle receives its arterial supply from eight to 11 segmental branches of the superficial femoral artery. Therefore, the muscle may be detached proximally, distally, or along its midportion to provide graft coverage anywhere from the groin to the knee.[40] From a technical standpoint, this is a relatively simple procedure that does not leave the patient with any residual functional deficit (Table 37–1).

However, there may be limitations of local sartorius transfer when compared with a formal RMF procedure (Table 37–1). Because many patients who have undergone peripheral arterial reconstructive surgery have arteriosclerotic occlusive disease within the superficial femoral artery, one must assume that the vascularity of the muscle is less than optimal in these patients. Second, it has been demonstrated that interruption of three or more of the segmental branches of the superficial femoral artery that perfuse the sartorius can lead to ischemia and muscle necrosis.[41] In addition, because the muscle borders the infected graft, one must assume there is some element of bacterial contamination even before its translocation. Nevertheless, local sartorius transfer has been a useful adjunct in the treatment of selected patients with arterial graft infection.

Clinical Experience

Local sartorius transfer has been performed to manage infection involving native arteries, autogenous vein, and synthetic bypass grafts. In one series, for example, local sartorius transfer was performed to cover exposed saphenous vein grafts in eight patients with infected groin wounds. The wounds remained healed without evidence of recurrent infection with a mean follow-up period of 16 months.[42] In another report,

TABLE 37–1. LOCAL SARTORIUS TRANSFER

Advantages	Disadvantages
Coverage groin to knee	Suboptimal perfusion
Easy procedure	Compromise of superficial femoral artery branches
No functional deficit	Bacterial contamination

eight groin wounds that involved four native arterial and four saphenous graft infections were successfully treated with local sartorius transfer.[40]

On the other hand, eradication of infection involving a foreign body, such as a prosthetic bypass graft, is a different and somewhat more difficult clinical problem. Therefore, it is in the management of prosthetic bypass graft infection that the limitations of local sartorius transfer may become more apparent. For example, Cherry et al performed local sartorius transfer to cover infected PTFE-saphenous vein composite femoral–distal bypass grafts in the groin in two patients.[43] One wound healed and remained intact for 62 months, but the other wound broke down because of necrosis of the sartorius muscle. However, the graft in the latter case was salvaged with performance of a rectus femoris RMF, and the wound remained healed after 25 months of follow-up.[43] In another series, eight patients with infected Dacron prostheses in the groin underwent *in situ* replacement with PTFE grafts and coverage with local sartorius transfer. All wounds healed, and only one patient had a lymphocele after 5 months of follow-up.[44] However, the responsible organism in all of these cases was *Staphylococcus epidermidis*, a relatively low-virulence species.[44] Clearly, reported clinical experience to date is too limited to draw any firm conclusions with respect to the efficacy of local sartorius transfer in managing prosthetic graft infections that involve more virulent organisms. Furthermore, others have expressed concern about covering a graft with sartorius muscle when there is anastomotic exposure.

Rotational Muscle Flaps

Technical Considerations

It must be emphasized that the rotational muscle flap is a treatment appropriate only for localized infection that involves a patent graft. Ultrasound, computed tomography, sinography, and radionuclide scans can provide useful information, which when combined with the findings at exploration of the graft can solidify the surgeon's impression of the extent of the infectious process. Second, aggressive and wide soft-tissue debridement is an essential component of this approach to graft infection. In fact, inadequate debridement may be one of the more important causes of an unsuccessful outcome. Although it has been suggested by some that involvement, or exposure, of an anastomosis is a relative contraindication to the local management of graft infection and thus performance of a RMF,[45] my experience does not support this reservation.[46,47] If the anastomosis can be adequately repaired primarily, or by placement of a new interposition graft segment, coverage with a RMF is appropriate and likely to be successful.[46,47] Therefore, one should not limit the extent of soft-tissue debridement for fear of exposing an anastomosis that is not apparently involved in the presenting wound. Furthermore, one should not be concerned about the size of the soft-tissue defect that is created.

A variety of muscles can be rotated to cover exposed grafts and fill soft-tissue defects in the groin, as well as at other anatomic sites throughout the body (Table 37–2).[48] In some cases more than one muscle may be required to complete the wound closure. The specific muscle or muscles selected depend on the size of the wound to be closed, and the blood supply of the respective muscles in the patient being treated. For example, the rectus abdominis muscle is frequently used to treat prosthetic graft infection in the groin. It is fairly long, bulky, and therefore can be wrapped circumferentially around an extended length of exposed graft (Fig. 37–1). It has a long arc of rotation, and division of the inguinal ligament allows the muscle to be translocated to an infrainguinal location fairly easily. In some patients rotation of this muscle

TABLE 37–2. ROTATIONAL MUSCLE FLAPS: MOST FREQUENTLY USED MUSCLES

Site	Muscles
Groin	Rectus abdominis
	Rectus femoris
	Tensor fasciae latae
	Gracilis
Knee	Medial gastrocnemius
	Lateral gastrocnemius
	Soleus
Neck	Pectoralis major
	Sternocleidomastoid
	Latissimus dorsi
Axilla	Pectoralis major
	Latissimus dorsi
Forearm	Latissimus dorsi
	Flexor digitorum sublimis
Chest	Pectoralis major
	Rectus abdominis
	Latissimus dorsi

results in abdominal wall laxity, or hernia formation, although generally without functional disability.

Other frequently used muscles for graft coverage in the groin include the rectus femoris, tensor fasciae latae, and gracilis. The rectus femoris has a wide arc of rotation and reasonable size. However, in some patients rotation of this muscle has resulted

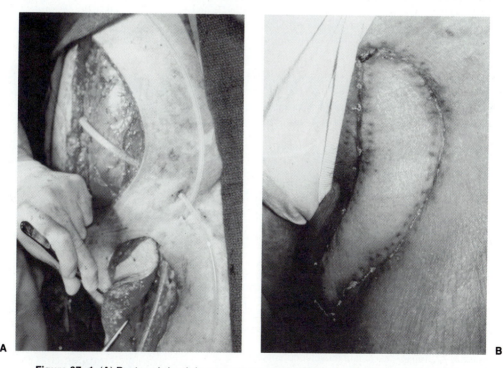

Figure 37–1. (A) Rectus abdominis musculocutaneous flap being mobilized to close groin wound. **(B)** Healed groin wound 1 week later. (*Reproduced with permission from Perler BA. Muscle flaps for graft infection. In: Bunt TJ, ed, Vascular Graft Infections. Armonk, NY: Futura Inc, 1994, 235.*)

in loss of terminal knee extension. Furthermore, because the muscle is perfused by the descending branch of the lateral femoral circumflex artery, occlusive disease in the profunda femoris (deep femoral) artery may compromise flap perfusion. The tensor fasciae latae is a long and flat muscle that can fill sizeable defects (Fig. 37–2). Furthermore, because the tensor fasciae latae is a relatively thin muscle, the donor site often can be closed primarily. Although this muscle normally contributes to abduction and medial rotation of the thigh, its mobilization for graft coverage usually does not leave a substantial functional deficit.[18] Although the relatively small size of the gracilis muscle has limited its usefulness for graft coverage, in the occasional patient with a relatively small wound, it can provide adequate graft coverage without leaving the patient with functional impairment.[18]

In addition to allowing selection of a muscle that is most anatomically appropriate for the wound that is being treated, a formal RMF conveys other advantages when compared with local sartorius transfer in the groin. Because the selection of the muscle depends on its anticipated blood supply, and because in most cases the arterial supply of the muscle selected is independent of the site of infection, one can ensure coverage of the graft with a maximally vascularized flap. Furthermore, because the muscle will be translocated from a site that is at least somewhat remote from the infected graft, unlike the sartorius, one can assume that the RMF is sterile at the time of graft coverage.

The timing of RMF coverage of the graft is problematic and largely a clinical judgment. Although a period of dressing changes after the initial wound debridement is required in some cases to optimally prepare the site for muscle flap closure, if adequate wound debridement can be accomplished at the original wound exploration, definitive closure at that time with an RMF has an excellent chance of securing heal-

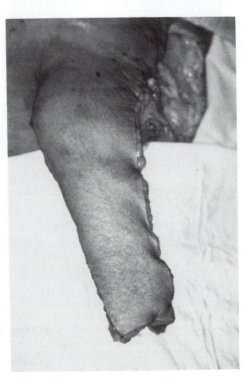

Figure 37–2. Tensor fascia lata musculocutaneous flap mobilized to close a large groin wound. (*Reproduced with permission from Perler BA. Muscle flaps for graft infection. In: Bunt TJ, ed, Vascular Graft Infections. Armonk, NY: Futura Inc, 1994, 235.*)

ing.[46,47] In addition to reducing the length of hospitalization, this may reduce the incidence of secondary complications such as graft thrombosis, hemorrhage, or contamination with more virulent organisms.

Clinical Experience

Reported clinical experience utilizing RMFs to treat arterial infection is somewhat limited when compared with the experience in cardiothoracic surgery, but the results to date are quite encouraging. In an early report, a brachial artery suture line exposed in a septic wound was covered and the wound successfully closed with a brachioradialis muscle flap and split-thickness skin graft.[49] RMF coverage of an exposed synthetic conduit was first reported in 1982, when a sublimis musculocutaneous flap was utilized to cover a PTFE dialysis shunt.[50] In a more recent report, three infected groin wounds involving two Dacron and one PTFE graft were closed with tensor fasciae latae musculocutaneous flaps, and all three wounds remained healed in a follow-up period ranging from 31 to 68 months.[51] In a series of infected femoral–distal bypass grafts, two patients underwent prosthetic graft coverage with rectus femoris flaps, and the wounds healed, although one patient died 3 months after treatment with a patent graft. In another patient in this series, a synthetic graft was salvaged by coverage with a rectus femoris RMF after a previous sartorius flap became necrotic and the wound broke down.[43] Mixter et al performed RMF procedures on 20 patients with infected prosthetic grafts, including 14 Dacron and seven PTFE conduits. Healing was achieved in 19 (95%) cases, and there was no evidence of recurrent infection in any cases in a mean follow-up period of 36 months.[45] None of the patients had experienced anastomotic disruption, however, which the workers consider a contraindication to this approach to synthetic graft infection.[45]

Johns Hopkins Experience

My experience suggests that anastomotic involvement is not an absolute contraindication to performing a RMF procedure for prosthetic graft infection.[47] Over the past 7 years, RMF procedures have been performed to close 19 wounds involving 21 exposed, infected prosthetic grafts in 18 patients, with a mean age of 63.7 (range, 39 to 79) years. All of the infections presented in the groin, with the exception of two in the neck and one in the chest (Table 37–3). One patient with an aortofemoral graft underwent metachronous groin procedures. A single graft was exposed in 17 wounds, and in the other two patients, aortofemoral–femoropopliteal and femorofemoral–femoropopliteal grafts were exposed, respectively (Table 37–3). Fever or leukocytosis was noted at the time of presentation for closure of 18 (95%) of the 19 wounds. Positive

TABLE 37–3. JOHNS HOPKINS ROTATIONAL MUSCLE FLAP SERIES: GRAFTS

Bypass	Location	Conduit	n
Aortofemoral	Groin	Dacron	9
Femoropopliteal	Groin	PTFE[a]	4
Femorofemoral	Groin	PTFE	2
		Dacron	1
Ascending aorta	Chest	Dacron	1
Subclavian–carotid–carotid	Neck	Darcon	1
Common–internal carotid	Neck	Darcon	1
Axillofemoral	Groin	PTFE	2

[a] PTFE, polytetrafluorethylene.

bacterial cultures were obtained from each wound closed with a RMF in this series, including a total of 30 organisms in these 19 wounds (Table 37–4). One bacterial species was cultured from 12 wounds, including eight gram-positive and four gram-negative organisms; two species, including one gram-positive and one gram-negative organism, were cultured from five wounds; and four organisms, including both gram-positive and gram-negative species, were cultured from two wounds (Table 37–4). The clinical presentations included wound abscess or purulent drainage from a sinus tract in 14 (74%) wounds, an infected pseudoaneurysm in two (11%), and acute hemorrhage in three (16%) wounds. Twelve (63%) infections were diagnosed less than 30 days after graft placement (acute); two were diagnosed 2 and 3 months, respectively, after graft placement (subacute); and five were diagnosed 29, 32, 36, 39, and 168 months, respectively, after graft placement (chronic).

The RMF closure was performed on 12 (63%) of these patients at the time of the initial wound debridement, including three patients who had undergone limited incision and drainage procedures weeks or months previously. Fourteen operative RMF procedures were carried out to close these 12 wounds, including a procedure on one patient with an exposed ascending aortic graft in the chest who required mobilization of four separate muscles during two operative procedures to achieve complete closure. Another patient in this group underwent RMF coverage of a subclavian–carotid–carotid graft in the neck. The wound healed, but the patient returned with recurrent infection 19 months later and was successfully treated with a secondary RMF procedure. In four (21%) cases the wounds were treated with dressing changes after the initial debridement procedure, and definitive RMF closure was performed 4 to 30 days later. In one of these patients two separate muscles were rotated to achieve complete wound closure. Similar to the experience of Cherry et al,[43] three (16%) wounds were closed with RMF procedures 1 to 26 days after previous attempts to cover the grafts with local sartorius transfer had failed. One of these patients underwent two RMF operations, each utilizing a single muscle, to achieve complete wound closure. In total, 22 RMF operations were performed utilizing 25 muscles to close the 19 wounds in this series, including one procedure that was performed for recurrent infection 19 months after the original RMF operation (Table 37–5).

These procedures were well tolerated by this generally elderly patient population with multiple arteriosclerotic risk factors. One patient suffered a fatal myocardial infarction on the sixth postoperative day, yielding an operative mortality of 5.6%.

TABLE 37–4. JOHNS HOPKINS ROTATIONAL MUSCLE FLAP EXPERIENCE: CULTURE DATA

Organism	No. of Cultures
Staphylococcus aureus	3
Staphylococcus epidermidis	6
Streptococcus B	2
Enterococcus	5
Pseudomonas aeroginosa	6
Escherichia coli	2
Enterobacter cloacae	1
Proteus Mirabilis	2
Corynebacterium spp	1
Bacteroides spp	2

TABLE 37–5. JOHNS HOPKINS ROTATIONAL MUSCLE FLAP EXPERIENCE: MUSCLE FLAPS

Muscle	Wound Location	*n*
Rectus abdominis	Groin	10
Rectus femoris	Groin	5
Gracilis	Groin	2
Tensor fasciae latae	Groin	1
Pectoralis major	Neck, chest	4
Sternocleidomastoid	Neck	1
Latissimus dorsi	Chest	1
Serratus	Chest	1

The 18 wounds in the 17 survivors of the operations healed. Recurrent infection developed in only three (15.8%) patients 12 to 22 (mean, 18) months after the original RMF procedure. One patient presented 12 months after rectus abdominis coverage of a femorofemoral graft in the groin with recurrent infection. Because at that time the graft was noted to be occluded, it was excised without sequelae. As noted earlier, one patient re-presented with recurrent infection 19 months after coverage of a graft in the neck and underwent a secondary RMF procedure with salvage of the graft. The third patient had undergone metachronous muscle flaps 6 months apart for bilateral groin infections involving the limbs of an aortofemoral graft. Although before each of the original muscle flap procedures the work-up suggested the infection was localized to the groin, this patient re-presented 16 months after the most recent groin procedure with infection that involved the entire graft. The patient underwent graft excision and axillofemoral bypass but died of multiple organ system failure. This was the only death in this series due to persistent or recurrent graft infection. Four other patients died, during follow-up, of causes unrelated to their graft infections and with intact grafts. Eleven (92%) of the 12 long-term survivors had healed wounds and intact grafts after a mean follow-up time of 39 (range, 8 to 83) months. Furthermore, wounds of 15 (88%) of the 17 original operative survivors remained healed with intact grafts at the time of the last follow-up visit or death with a mean follow-up period of 30 months.

Several findings in this series deserve emphasis. For example, all 12 patients with acute infections experienced wound healing, whereas wounds of only three (60%) of the five patients with subacute or chronic infections healed successfully. These observations may reflect minimal bacterial invasion of the synthetic conduit during the short period of time that they were implanted. On the other hand, the timing of wound closure was not predictive of outcome. In fact, nine (90%) of 10 patients who underwent RMF closure at the original debridement operation had a successful outcome. It is noteworthy that wounds of all three patients who underwent RMF closure of their groin wounds after previous attempts to achieve healing with local sartorius transfer failed remained healed. This confirms my prejudice with respect to the theoretic advantages of formal RMF procedures in this setting. While the number of cases in this series is too small to draw firm statistical conclusions, the available data suggest that graft material and anatomic location of the wound are not predictive of outcome and therefore should not influence one's decision to attempt an RMF procedure in any particular patient. Finally, although there is a consensus that gram-negative graft infection is a more formidable problem, all 11 patients in the Johns Hopkins series with gram-negative or mixed infections had a successful outcome in contrast to only two-thirds of those with purely gram-positive infection. Although this observation may reflect in part the limited number of patients in this series, it clearly suggests that gram-negative infection should not be considered a contraindication to an attempt at graft salvage with a RMF procedure if the infection is truly localized.

CONCLUSION

Despite improvements in anesthetic and perioperative surgical care, the potential morbidity associated with excision of an infected arterial graft and extra-anatomic reconstruction remains considerable. To justify any particular unconventional approach to this clinical problem, it must be demonstrated that the alternative treatment has a reasonable chance of being successful and that it is associated with less morbidity than the conventional approach. The goal of treatment in these cases is to eradicate all signs of infection and to preserve limb viability with minimal risk to life. While reported clinical experience to date is limited, the preponderance of available evidence strongly suggests that the local treatment of arterial graft infection and closure with an RMF clearly satisfies these requirements.

It cannot be overemphasized that the RMF is a treatment suitable only for localized infection involving a patent graft. Although exposure or involvement of an anastomosis has been suggested by some to be a contraindication to the local treatment of graft infection, a growing body of evidence suggests that if the anastomosis can be repaired, or redone with a new interposition segment *in situ*, RMF closure may still be appropriate and have a reasonable chance of being successful.[46,47] This clinical experience also suggests that performance of a RMF flap based on a pedicled blood supply independent of the site of infection is a superior method of graft coverage and wound closure than local muscle transfer, such as sartorius transfer in the groin. Furthermore, performance of an RMF procedure does not "burn any bridges." If recurrent graft infection develops, or if persistent graft infection becomes clinically apparent, it usually does so at the original site of presentation. In this situation, further local debridement may allow a new RMF procedure to be performed, or, if necessary, the graft may be excised and extra-anatomic reconstruction performed, according to conventional dogma.

REFERENCES

1. Bunt TJ. Synthetic vascular graft infections. I. Graft infections. *Surgery*. 1983;93:733–746.
2. Szilagyi DE, Smith RF, Elliott JP, Vrandecic MP. Infection in arterial reconstruction with synthetic grafts. *Ann Surg*. 1972;176:321–333.
3. Edwards WH Jr, Martin RS III, Jenkins JM, et al. Primary graft infections. *J Vasc Surg*. 1987;6:235–239.
4. Johnson JA, Cogbill TA, Strutt PJ, Gunderson AL. Wound complications after infrainguinal bypass: classification, predisposing factors, and management. *Arch Surg*. 1988;123:859–862.
5. Greco RS. Utilizing vascular prostheses for drug delivery. *J Vasc Surg*. 1991;5:753–755.
6. Lindenauer SM, Fry WS, Schaub G, Wild D. The use of antibiotics in the prevention of vascular graft infections. *Surgery*. 1967;62:487–492.
7. Goldstone J, Moore WS. Infection in vascular prostheses. *Am J Surg*. 1974;128:225–233.
8. Jamieson GG, DeWeese JA, Rob CG. Infected arterial grafts. *Ann Surg*. 1975;181:850–852.
9. Yashar JJ, Weyman AK, Burnard RD, Yashar J. Survival and limb salvage in patients with infected arterial prostheses. *Am J Surg*. 1978;135:499–504.

10. Seeger JM, Wheeler JR, Gregory RT, et al. Autogenous graft replacement of infected prosthetic grafts in the femoral position. *Surgery.* 1983;93:39–45.
11. Claggett GP, Bowers BL, Lopez-Viego M, et al. Creation of a neo-aorto-iliac system from lower extremity deep and superficial veins. *Ann Surg.* 1993;218:239–249.
12. Snyder SO, Wheeler JR, Gregory RT, et al. Freshly harvested cadaveric venous homografts as arterial conduits in infected fields. *Surgery.* 1987;101:283–291.
13. Kieffer E, Bahnini A, Koskas F, et al. In situ allograft replacement of infected infrarenal aortic prosthetic grafts: results in forty-three patients. *J Vasc Surg.* 1993;17:349–356.
14. Carter SC, Cohen A, Whelan TJ. Clinical experience with management of the infected Dacron graft. *Ann Surg.* 1963;158:249–255.
15. Knight CD Jr, Farness MB, Hollier LA. Treatment of aortic graft infection with providone-iodine irrigation. *Mayo Clin Proc* 1983;58:472–475.
16. Kwann JHM, Connelly JE. Successful management of prosthetic graft infection with continuous povidone iodine irrigation. *Arch Surg.* 1981;116:716–720.
17. Poporsky J, Singer S. Infected prosthetic grafts: local therapy with preservation. *Arch Surg.* 1980;115:203–205.
18. Mathes SJ, McCraw JB, Vasconez LO. Muscle transposition flaps for coverage of lower extremity defects: anatomic considerations. *Surg Clin North Am.* 1974;54:1337–1354.
19. Mathes SJ, Vasconez LO, Jurkiewicz MJ. Extension and further applications of muscle flap transposition. *Plast Reconstr Surg.* 1977;60:6–13.
20. Pairolero PC, Arnold PG. Bronchopleural fistula: treatment by transposition of pectoralis major muscle. *J Thorac Cardiovasc Surg.* 1980;79:142–145.
21. Arnold PG, Pairolero PC. Intrathoracic muscle flaps: a 10-year eperience in the management of life-threatening infection. *Plast Reconst Surg.* 1989;84:92–98.
22. Arnold PG, Pairolero PC, Waldorf JC. The serratus anterior muscle: intrathoracic and extrathoracic utilization. *Plast Reconstr Surg.* 1984;73:240–248.
23. Jurkiewicz MJ, Bostwick J III, Hester TR, et al. Infected mediastinal wound. Successful treatment by muscle flaps. *Ann Surg.* 1980;191:737–744.
24. Pairolero PC, Arnold PG, Harris JB. Long-term results of pectoralis major muscle transposition for infected sternotomy wounds. *Ann Surg.* 1991;213:583–590.
25. Miller JI, Nahai F. Repair of the dehisced median sternotomy incision. *Surg Clin North Am.* 1989;69:1091–1102.
26. Kohman LJ, Auchincloss JH, Gilbert R, Beshara M. Functional results of muscle flap closure for sternal infection. *Ann Thorac Surg.* 1991;52:102–106.
27. Schaff HV, Arnold PG, Reeders GS. Late mediastinal infection and pseudoaneurysm following left ventricular aneurysmectomy; repair utilizing a pectoralis major muscle flap. *J Thorac Cardiovasc Surg.* 1982;84:912–916.
28. Stark WJ. The use of pedicled muscle flaps in the surgical treatment of chronic osteomyelitis resulting from compound fractures. *J Bone Joint Surg.* 1946;28:343–350.
29. Ger R. Muscle transposition for treatment of chronic posttraumatic osteomyelitis of the tibia. *J Bone Joint Surg.* 1977;59A:784–791.
30. Mathes SJ, Alpert BS, Chang N. Use of muscle flaps in chronic osteomyelitis: experimental and clinical correlation. *Plast Reconstr Surg.* 1982;69:815–828.
31. Lesavoy MA, Dubrow TJ, Wackym PA, Eckardt JJ. Muscle flap coverage of exposed endoprostheses. *Plast Reconstr Surg.* 1989;83:90–96.
32. Hahn DC, MacKay RD, Holliday B, Hunt TK. Effects of O_2 tension on microbial function of leukocytes in wounds and in vitro. *Surg Forum.* 1976;27:18–20.
33. Sauvage LR, Berger DE, Wood SJ, et al. Interspecies healing of porous arterial prostheses. *Arch Surg.* 1974;109:698–705.
34. Mehran RJ, Graham AM, Ricci MA, Symes JF. Evaluation of muscle flaps in the treatment of infected aortic grafts. *J Vasc Surg.* 1992;15:487–494.
35. Chang N, Mathes SJ. Comparison of the effect of bacterial inoculation in musculocutaneous and fasciocutaneous flaps. *Plast Reconstr Surg.* 1982;70:1–9.
36. Calderon W, Chang N, Mathes SJ. Comparison of the effect of bacterial inoculation in musculocutaneous and fasciocutaneous flaps. *Plast Reconstr Surg.* 1986;77:785–782.

37. Grosain A, Chang N, Mathes S, et al. A study of the relationship between blood flow and bacterial inoculation in musculocutaneous and fasciocutaneous flaps. *Plast Reconstr Surg.* 1990;86:1152–1162.

38. Dacey LJ, Miett TOC, Huntsman WT, et al. Efficacy of muscle flaps in the treatment of prosthetic vascular graft infections. *J Surg Res.* 1988;44:566–572.

39. Cruz NI, Canario QM. Muscle flaps in the management of vascular grafts in contaminated wounds: an experimental study in dogs. *Plast Reconstr Surg.* 1988;82:480–483.

40. Kaufman JL, Shah DM, Corson JD, et al. Sartorius muscle coverage for the treatment of complicated vascular surgical wounds. *J Cardiovasc Surg.* 1989;30:475–483.

41. Kaiser E, Genz KA, Habermeyer P, Mandelkow H. Die arterielle versorgung des musculus sartorius. *Chirurg.* 1984;35:731–732.

42. Meyer JP, Durham JR, Schwartz TH, et al. The use of sartorius muscle rotation-transfer in the management of wound complications after infra-inguinal vien bypass: a report of eight cases and description of the technique. *J Vasc Surg.* 1989;9:731–735.

43. Cherry KJ, Roland CF, Pairolero PC, et al. Infected femorodistal bypass: is graft removal mandatory? *J Vasc Surg.* 1992;15:295–305.

44. Bandyk DF, Bergamini TM, Kinney EV, et al. In situ replacement of vascular prostheses infected by bacterial biofilms. *J Vasc Surg.* 1991;13:575–583.

45. Mixter RC, Turnipseed WD, Smith DJ Jr, et al. Rotational muscle flaps: a new technique for covering infected vascular grafts. *J Vasc Surg.* 1989;9:472–478.

46. Perler BA, Vander Kolk CA, et al. Can infected prosthetic grafts be salvaged with rotational muscle flaps? *Surgery.* 1991;110:30–34.

47. Perler BA, Vander Kolk CA, Manson PW, Williams GM. Rotational muscle flaps to treat prosthetic graft infection: long-term follow-up. *J Vasc Surg.* 1993;18:358–365.

48. Budny PG, Fix RJ. Salvage of prosthetic grafts and joints in the lower extremity. *Clin Plast Surg.* 1991;18:583–591.

49. Ger R. The coverage of vascular repairs by muscle transposition. *J Trauma.* 1976;16:974–978.

50. Hodgkinson DJ, Shepard GTT. Coverage of exposed Gore-Tex dialysis access graft with local sublimis myocutaneous flap. *Plast Reconstr Surg.* 1982;69:1010–1012.

51. Ammar AD, Turrentine MW. Exposed synthetic vascular grafts of the groin; graft preservation by means of a tensor fasciae latae flap. *J Vasc Surg.* 1989;10:202–204.

38

The Use of a Lateral Routed Bypass for Treatment of an Infected Femoropopliteal-Tibial Bypass Graft

John D. Corson, MB, ChB, FRCS (Engl), FACS,
Jamal T. Hoballah, MD, William J. Sharp, MD,
and Timothy F. Kresowik, MD

The current results of lower extremity femoropopliteal-tibial artery revascularization are generally very gratifying.[1–7] Few ischemic limbs cannot now be successfully salvaged by an aggressive surgical approach that obviates the need for a major amputation. In addition, selected patients with claudication with infrainguinal arterial disease can obtain long-term symptom relief with modern revascularization techniques.[8] Despite these successes, a small number of patients who undergo a femoropopliteal-tibial bypass develop have serious complications due to infection, which may result in limb loss or even death.[9–12]

A variety of surgical philosophies abound as to the appropriate management of an infected infrainguinal bypass graft. The standard surgical dogma to completely remove the infected graft has been questioned by various authors.[13–16] The treatment options range from conservative local treatment to total graft excision. The options depend on a variety of factors, including the pathogenicity of the responsible organisms, the functional status and type of original bypass conduit, the extent and site of infection, the degree of ischemia of the extremity, availability of autogenous vein for bypass, and revascularization options.

General principles in the management of infrainguinal bypass graft infections and the indications for removal of an infected infrainguinal bypass graft are reviewed herein. Anatomic details and technical points for successful revascularization of these patients are discussed.

PRINCIPLES OF TREATMENT

It is of critical importance, before embarking on a prolonged course of surgical therapy for treatment of lower extremity graft infection and/or limb sepsis, to determine if the limb is salvageable. The goal is to maintain a functional limb for ambulation. The presence of extensive infection and/or tissue necrosis of the foot, heel, and ankle area that would not leave an adequate, healed stump for weight bearing would contraindicate an attempt at limb salvage. Also, hemodynamic instability due to septicemia or extremity ischemia associated with irreversible neuromuscular damage would be contraindications to an attempt at limb salvage.

Unless severe bleeding is the initial presenting symptom, there is usually adequate time for a comprehensive evaluation and an expedient work-up. When assessing treatment options in the management of an infected femoropopliteal-tibial bypass graft, it is important to ascertain the exact sites and levels of inflow and outflow and to determine the nature of the original bypass conduit. Details of all prior revascularization procedures must be carefully reviewed as must the most recent arteriogram. Immediate revascularization may be required for selected patients if a functioning infected bypass graft is excised. A new arteriogram is usually required only when limb revascularization is contemplated in the case of late graft infection or when an endovascular approach for revascularization is a possibility. An arteriogram helps identify the current status of the bypass and demonstrate the arterial inflow and distal runoff. Duplex ultrasound evaluation is useful in determining the functional status of a bypass, the presence of a false aneurysm, and/or evidence of a perigraft fluid collection. In addition, simultaneous vein mapping can be done to assess the availability of vein for use as an autogenous bypass conduit. The short saphenous and arm veins should be evaluated if there is a limited supply of autogenous long saphenous vein suitable for use as a bypass conduit. Computed tomography is of value in assessing the extent of infection. A perigraft fluid collection can be aspirated under computed tomographic or ultrasonographically guided control to obtain fluid for bacteriologic culture.

Systemic intravenous broad-spectrum antibiotics are begun after cultures are obtained. These may be modified later depending on the culture and sensitivity results. It is appropriate to drain an abscess once the differential diagnosis of an infected false aneurysm has been excluded. Incisions should be carefully placed to avoid compromising further reconstructive attempts. Such surgical procedures, which may involve exposure of the infected graft, should be performed in an operating suite under the guidance of an experienced surgeon who can then determine the optimal treatment plan.

A review of the literature suggests that preservation of a functioning infected infrainguinal bypass graft should be attempted except when the patient has anastomotic bleeding, systemic sepsis, or when certain dangerous bacterial pathogens such as *Pseudomonas*, *Enterobacter*, or *Clostridium* species are cultured.[14–17] In the face of a functioning infected bypass graft, it is always difficult to determine the degree of ischemia that will occur if the bypass graft must be removed. A general guide is that the patient usually returns to the pre-bypass ischemic status. Hence, the limbs of a patient operated on for claudication are not threatened after removal of a functioning bypass graft. In such a patient a later elective vascular reconstruction could be considered if symptoms of chronic ischemia persist after removal of the infected graft, after subsequent healing and resolution of the infective process. In contrast, limb loss would likely occur in a patient who was initially operated on for critical limb ischemia if a functioning infected graft were to be removed and no revascularization procedure were performed.

A variety of alternatives for revascularization may be available and should be carefully considered. These alternatives depend on the anatomic situation and may include the use of an endovascular procedure, profundaplasty, localized endarterectomy, or a distal bypass. When a new infrainguinal bypass is required for revascularization, we use an autogenous venous conduit. Our preference for autogenous vein relates to the fact that when a bypass extends across the knee joint, there appears to be a clear superiority in patency for an autogenous vein over a prosthetic bypass conduit.[1-7,18,19] In addition, the potential of seeding an autogenous vein graft in a patient with sepsis is thought to be less than with a prosthetic graft.[20-22] If a new bypass is required, we prefer to avoid the contaminated field altogether by routing the bypass through clean tissue planes. When the initial bypass graft has been placed from a conventional medial approach, a lateral subcutaneous bypass can be safely placed, thus avoiding contamination of the graft from the infected graft bed or wounds (Fig. 38–1). This procedure is done just before removal of the infected graft to limit the period of acute ischemia. However, if bleeding is the presenting symptom the infected graft is dealt with initially.

The need for revascularization in our patients is usually based on a clinical evaluation. We have not found the use of intraoperative Doppler studies to be especially helpful in making the decision for revascularization, although other authors have suggested its value, especially when distal Doppler signals are initially absent after removal of the infected bypass graft.[23]

When revascularization of the extremity can be done as the first procedure, the fresh lateral incisions are closed primarily and excluded from the surgical field with an impervious plastic dressing. The infected graft is then excised through the original medial incisions. If there is only minimal arterial anastomotic involvement, the artery is debrided and the arteriotomy patched with autogenous vein. These areas are then covered with a well-vascularized muscle flap. When there is considerable arterial anastomotic infection, the involved anastomotic sites are best oversewn with a monofilament suture through uninvolved artery after radical debridement of the infected artery. We remove the entire extent of the infected portion of the graft rather than perform subtotal graft excision, which leaves possibly infected graft remnants at the anastomoses.

The use of biologic tissue such as autogenous vein patch angioplasty of a debrided anastomosis has been very satisfactory in our experience. Appropriate patient selection, arterial debridement, and muscle coverage may be important factors in the success of this technique. Any residual infected or necrotic material in the field is aggressively debrided. The involved area is routinely drained and the wounds are allowed to heal by secondary intention, or occasionally delayed split-thickness grafting is done over a large well-granulating defect.

LATERAL BYPASS

It is important to differentiate between procedures in which the vessels are accessed through a lateral approach and those in which not only are the vessels approached laterally but also a bypass is routed laterally.[23-26] When the conventional medial approach is considered unsafe or contraindicated because of graft infection or the presence of contaminated or infected wounds on the medial side of the thigh or leg, a lateral routed graft provides a satisfactory bypass option. The appropriate utilization and routing of a lateral bypass for the treatment of an infrainguinal graft infection depends on the site and extent of the infective process.

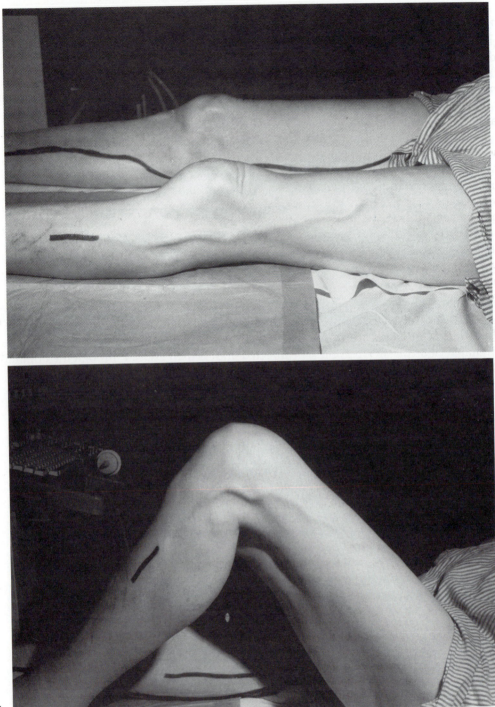

Figure 38–1. (**A**) The lateral routed subcutaneous vein graft to the anterior tibial artery utilized the contralateral long saphenous vein. The subcutaneous position of the bypass facilitates duplex ultrasonic surveillance. (**B**) There is no acute kinking of the bypass when the knee is flexed.

The classic text *Extensile Exposure* by A. K. Henry, which was first published in 1947, exquisitely details various approaches to important arteries[27] (Fig. 38–2). Medial, posterior, and lateral approaches to the arteries in the lower extremity are carefully described and clearly diagrammed. Traditionally most infrainguinal bypass procedures have been performed with a standardized medial approach.[7] This is appropriate for most patients, especially when the ipsilateral saphenous vein is used as the bypass conduit. More rarely, especially for short interposition popliteal bypasses, a posterior approach is used.[28] In contrast, lateral bypass procedures, although described, are rarely used by most vascular surgeons. A lateral bypass may be a suitable alternative when bypassing to the mid or distal portion of the anterior tibial artery or the peroneal artery, especially when ipsilateral saphenous vein is not available and a free vein graft is harvested or another conduit is used (Fig. 38–3). The vessel lies directly in line with a lateral routed bypass conduit, which simplifies the construction of the distal anastomosis. When the conventional medial route is used, the bypass must be tunneled either subcutaneously over the tibia or through the interosseous membrane. A lateral routed bypass can be done often with a limited length of autogenous vein because the distal profunda femoris (deep femoral) artery may frequently be used as an inflow source, and the lateral route is shorter compared to a conventional medial route.

The location of the peroneal artery lends itself to facilitating the placement of a lateral bypass graft. This artery is easily exposed from the lateral aspect after resection

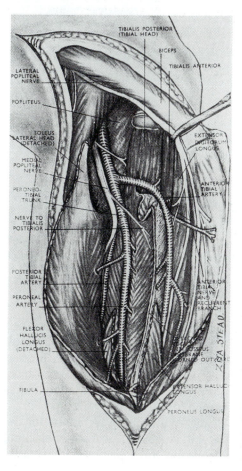

Figure 38–2. Resection of the proximal portion of the fibula allows exposure of the distal popliteal artery and the trifurcation vessels. (*Reprinted with permission from Henry AK.* Extensile Exposure. *London, England: Churchill-Livingstone; 1947:218–223.*)

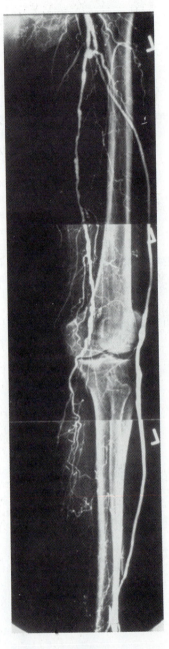

Figure 38–3. Arteriogram shows a superficial femoral–to–distal peroneal reversed vein bypass routed laterally.

of a small segment of the fibula.[24,26] In many diabetic patients the peroneal artery is the last and least diseased of the tibial vessels.[29] A satisfactory hemodynamic result can be achieved by peroneal bypass in most patients.[6,30] In the treatment of an infected infrainguinal bypass graft when a new bypass is required, although other authors have suggested the value of *in situ* biologic grafting, our preference and recommendation is to route the new bypass through clean tissue planes.[20–22,31,32]

Danese and Singer in 1967 described the details of a surgical technique for the exposure of the popliteal trifurcation using a lateral approach.[33] After undertaking some cadaveric dissections they used this approach on three patients whose arteriograms demonstrated severe disease at the popliteal trifurcation. In each case the area most suitable for the distal anastomosis was at or below the origin of the anterior tibial artery. Perry in 1979 described the use of a lateral bypass graft in four patients.[34] These procedures were used to treat patients with infected popliteal artery false aneurysms. Two false aneurysms were associated with distal bypass anastomoses and two were secondary to prior trauma. The use of a lateral approach satisfactorily avoided the need to place a fresh bypass in a contaminated field. Trout and Smith described an alternative lateral approach in the successful treatment of a patient with graft sepsis at the femoral level.[35] They placed an iliopopliteal graft to revascularize an ischemic limb. The bypass entered the proximal thigh laterally and then curved medially across the quadriceps tendon to utilize the conventional medial approach to the popliteal artery. Leather and Karmody and Narayansingh et al described lateral approaches to the superficial femoral artery and profunda femoris artery, respectively.[36,37] These two approaches are especially valuable when infection involves the common femoral artery and inflow is required for a distal bypass.

The various lateral approaches to the profunda femoris artery were reviewed by Veith et al.[38] These include an anteromedial approach along the medial border of the sartorius muscle to access the proximal portion of the mid third of the profunda femoris artery and an anterior approach lateral to the sartorius muscle to access the more distal portion of the profunda femoris artery. Veith et al also described a favorable experience with lateral access to lower extremity arteries as well as lateral routed bypass grafts.[39] Padberg performed anatomic dissections of six cadaveric limbs to delineate the technical limitations of a lateral approach to the popliteal artery and described the successful use of a lateral approach in three patients.[40]

TECHNICAL POINTS

Exposure of the most proximal portion of the popliteal artery and the distal superficial femoral artery is easily obtained via a lateral approach by using an incision placed between the iliotibial tract and the biceps tendon. Division of the biceps tendon as suggested by Kofsky et al is unnecessary.[41] Esses and Johnson recently described details of the exposure of the proximal popliteal artery from the lateral aspect in an article describing a lateral approach to the proximal popliteal artery for popliteal–to–anterior tibial artery bypass.[42] The mid-popliteal artery is exposed from an approach posterior to the biceps tendon. To approach the distal popliteal artery and trifurcation a segment of the fibula just below its head must be resected as described by Henry[27] and Elkin and Kelly.[43] The common peroneal nerve is in jeopardy at this level and must be carefully identified and gently mobilized. Injury to this nerve may be quite disabling. Hence, because of this risk, we have preferred to bypass more distally to a tibial vessel if such a suitable outflow artery is available and there is an adequate length of autogenous vein to reach it.

A modified operative description of the distal popliteal exposure by Danese and Singer is as follows.[33] The leg is positioned semiflexed and slightly medially rotated. The incision begins over the lower part of the biceps tendon and is carried distally below the knee over the upper end of the fibula for a total length of approximately 12 cm. The fascial plane between peroneus longus muscle anteriorly and the soleus muscle posteriorly is opened. Care is taken to avoid injury to the common peroneal nerve in the upper corner of the incision. This structure should be carefully identified and retracted on a vessel loop. The upper segment of the fibula is next identified and its upper 8 to 10 cm, including the lower part of the fibular head, is isolated subperiosteally and resected with the use of a microsagittal saw. The medial aspect of the periosteum is now incised and the lowest popliteal segment and the trifurcation are identified immediately deep to the periosteum and surrounding fascia.

Grafts that originate from the external iliac or common femoral artery can be safely routed subcutaneously over the sartorius muscle[25] (Fig. 38–4). However, grafts originating from the superficial or deep femoral arteries are routed deep to the sartorius muscle to avoid acute angulation of the proximal portion of the conduit (Fig. 38–5). If this point is appreciated, it is not necessary to divide the sartorious muscle, as was suggested by Kofksy et al.[41] The bypass graft is tunneled subcutaneously and passes directly over the center of the lateral hinge point of the knee joint lateral to the patella in the groove between the femoral condyle and the patella.

EXCISION OF INFECTED PROSTHETIC GRAFTS

Liekweg and Greenfield reviewed the literature on vascular prosthetic graft infections through 1974.[9] This review included an analysis of 164 suitable articles. They compared differences in morbidity and mortality for aortofemoral and femoropopliteal graft infections. The mortality for femoropopliteal graft infections was 9.9% with an amputation rate of 36.1%. This compared with a mortality of 47.9% and an amputation rate of 23% for infected aortofemoral grafts. These authors suggested that in the femoropopliteal region nonoperative treatment was acceptable if the bypass graft was patent. They emphasized, however, that any hemorrhage from a suture line was an absolute contraindication to nonoperative management.

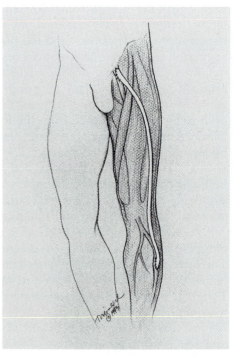

Figure 38–4. Lateral routed bypasses originating proximally from the common femoral artery can safely be routed superficial to the sartorius muscle. (*Reprinted with permission from Hoballah JJ, Chalmers RTA, Sharp WJ, et al. Lateral approach to the popliteal crural vessels for limb salvage.* J Cardiovasc Surg. *[In press].*)

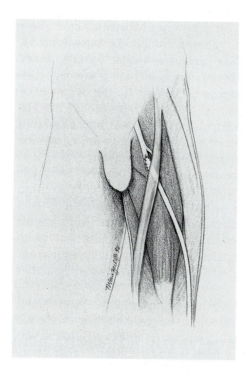

Figure 38–5. When the upper end of the lateral routed bypass originates below the common femoral artery, it is routed below the sartorius muscle to avoid any compression or kinking. (*Reprinted with permission from Hoballah JJ, Chalmers RTA, Sharp WJ, et al. Lateral approach to the popliteal crural vessels for limb salvage. J Cardiovasc Surg. [In press].*)

Carter et al[44] and several other authors have suggested that not excising infected prosthetic grafts is appropriate therapy in selected cases.[9,13–16,44–51] The Montefiore group developed a useful classification of graft infection by modifying the original graft infection classification of Szilagyi et al.[13,15] This modified classification was developed to aid in the planning of appropriate therapy. Samson et al classified prosthetic graft infections into five groups.[15] Groups I and II were classified as minor infections and groups III through V were classified as major infections. Group I were defined as infections (purulence and bacteria) extending no deeper than the dermis. Group II were defined as infections involving the subcutaneous tissue but not in grossly observable contact with the graft. Group III were defined as infections involving the body of the graft but not an anastomosis. Group IV were defined as infections surrounding an exposed anastomosis but in which bacteremia or anastomotic bleeding had not occurred. Group V were defined as infections involving a graft-arterial anastomosis and were associated with septicemia and/or anastomotic bleeding at the time of presentation. Minor infections were well treated by wound excision, antibiotics, local wound care with providone-iodine solution dressings, and subcutaneous wound closure by secondary intention or, rarely, skin grafting. The authors concluded from their experience with five patients that group III infections can be successfully treated without graft removal. Group IV infections in this series were treated by either total graft salvage, partial graft removal, or total graft removal. The graft salvage approach to grade IV infections was locally successful in 18 of 25 instances (72%) in which it was attempted. Despite successful treatment of functioning grafts with grade IV infection, partial graft removal was not uniformly successful in managing group IV graft infections with thrombosed grafts. Group V infections were all treated by total graft removal. In this series only 11 of 34 major graft infections ultimately required total graft removal.

Cherry et al also addressed the issue of the need to remove an infected femoral–distal bypass graft in a recent report based on experience with 39 infected lower extremity bypasses treated over a 10-year period.[14] These included 33 prosthetic grafts, four vein grafts, and two composite grafts. Their conclusions were that aggressive local treatment of an infected lower extremity bypass graft, including drainage, debridement, and muscle transposition for coverage, was suitable for the treatment of selected patients without the need for graft removal and with rates of limb salvage superior to those obtained with excisional therapy. Eleven patent bypasses were treated without graft excision, and eight remained patent on follow-up. Only nine new grafts were placed for revascularization in this series of 39 infected grafts.

Calligaro et al suggested the following treatment plan for infected prosthetic grafts after a review of their experience with a group of 28 patients with 33 groin infections involving a common femoral artery anastomosis of a prosthetic arterial graft.[16] Complete graft preservation should be attempted for patent infected prosthetic grafts. Subtotal excision should be performed for occluded infected grafts (leaving an oversewn 2- to 3-mm graft remnant attached to a patent artery critical for limb survival). Total graft excision should be performed along with arterial oversewing or ligation if there is anastomotic bleeding.

Another article on this subject by Calligaro et al questioned whether the presence of gram-negative bacteria was a contraindication to selective preservation of an infected prosthetic arterial graft.[17] Excluding *Pseudomonas* organisms, a successful outcome was accomplished in 92% (12/13) of their patients whose wounds cultured other gram-negative bacteria. When *Pseudomonas aeruginosa* was cultured from the wounds, successful graft preservation was accomplished in only 44% (4/9). On the basis of their experience the authors recommended complete graft preservation in the following circumstances: (a) if the graft is patent; (b) if the anastomoses are intact; (c) if the patient does not have systemic sepsis and cultures of the wound yield gram-positive bacteria or gram-negative bacteria other than *Pseudomonas* organisms. If the infected graft is occluded, the anastomoses are disrupted, or the patient has systemic sepsis, partial or total graft excision is routinely indicated. If *Pseudomonas* organisms are cultured from the wound, graft excision is generally recommended in most patients. In the discussion of this paper Mannick pointed out the potential for severe infection from gram-positive organisms such as *Clostridium* spp and also gram-negative bacteria such as *Enterobacter* spp.[17] Clearly the virulence and pathogenicity of any organisms cultured must be taken into account before determining optimal therapy. The more benign course of *Staphylococcus epidermis* graft infections as reported by other authors is an example of the opposite end of the spectrum of graft infection. It appears that most of these infections can be safely treated by conservative measures. Hence it is important to carefully identify the involved organism in all instances of suspected graft infection.

VEIN GRAFT INFECTION

Infected vein grafts tend to present with bleeding at the site of the graft infection.[52] Subcutaneous bypasses are at particular risk if there are local wound complications.[53,54] Unless a vein graft is adequately covered with vascularized tissue, it dries quickly and disrupts. Vein grafts are often infected over focal areas. Hence, short interposition vein grafts can be used to bypass an infected vein bypass segment. These bypasses are routed through clean tissue planes. The ends of the graft are oversewn after debridement and after the involved infected vein bypass segment is excised.

CONCLUSION

Various authors have supported the principle of the use of a biologic conduit in an infected field.[20-22,32] We prefer to place a new bypass with autogenous vein routed through clean tissue planes to obviate any potential for infection of the new bypass conduit. Fujitani et al have even suggested the use of a cryopreserved saphenous vein allogenic homograft as a bypass conduit in preference to a prosthetic graft when an adequate autogenous conduit is unavailable.[55] Their experience with ten reconstructed limbs after a mean follow-up period of 9.5 months (range, 6.0 to 14 months) resulted in seven primarily functioning allografts without obvious infection despite being placed in a contaminated field. Further data to support this approach are awaited.

In a recent review, Baxter et al reported their experience with nine laterally routed bypasses performed because of perigeniculate infections.[23] These bypasses were placed for problems relating to infection that prohibited the usual type of medial approach to revascularization. They achieved a primary and secondary graft patency of 66% and 78%, respectively. The limb salvage rate was 66%. The mean follow-up time was 19 months (range, 3 to 57 months). In our own reported experience with 24 lateral routed bypasses over a 7-year period, the primary patency rate was 61% (SE = 10.6) and the secondary patency rate was 86% (SE = 8.1) at 1 year. The subcutaneous position of the bypass facilitates duplex ultrasonic graft surveillance. Eight stenotic lesions in six bypasses were identified in this small series.

Patency data on lateral routed bypass grafts are limited. The available data suggest that the performance of such bypasses is similar to those placed using a conventional medial approach. The quality of the conduit rather than the route of the conduit should determine the longevity of the bypass. Appropriate revascularization and selective, conservative management of infected infrainguinal bypass grafts should reduce the previously reported high amputation rate in this group of patients.

REFERENCES

1. Corson JD, Hoballah JJ, Kresowik TF, et al. Technical aspects and results of the open in situ saphenous vein bypass technique. *Int Angiol.* 1993;12:162–163.
2. Leather RP, Shah DM, Chang BB, Kaufman JL. Resurrection of the in situ saphenous vein bypass: 1000 cases later. *Ann Surg.* 1988;208:435–442.
3. Berganini TM, Town JB, Bandyk DF, et al. Experience with in situ saphenous vein bypass during 1981 to 1989: determinant factors of core term patency. *J Vasc Surg.* 1991;13:137–149.
4. Taylor LM Jr, Edwards JM, Porter JM. Present status of reversed vein bypass grafting: five-year results of a modern series. *J Vasc Surg.* 1990;11:193–206.
5. Chalmers RTA, Hoballah JJ, Kresowik TF, et al. The impact of color duplex surveillance on the outcome of lower limb bypass with arm veins. *J Vasc Surg.* 1994;19:279–288.
6. Synn AY, Hoballah JJ, Sharp WJ, et al. Are there angiographic predictors of success for vein bypass to the peroneal artery? *Am J Surg.* 1992;164:276–280.
7. Kent KC, Whittemore AD, Mannick JA. Short-term and mid-term results of an all autogenous tissue policy for infrainguinal reconstruction. *J Vasc Surg.* 1989;9:107–114.
8. Kent KC, Donaldson MC, Attinger CE, et al. Femoropopliteal reconstruction for claudication. *Arch Surg.* 1988;123:1196–1198.

9. Liekweg WG, Greenfield LJ. Vascular prosthetic infections: collected experience and results of treatment. *Surgery.* 1977;81:335–342.

10. Kikta MJ, Goodson SF, Bishara RA, et al. Mortality and limb loss with infected infrainguinal bypass grafts. *J Vasc Surg.* 1987;5:566–571.

11. Bandyk DF. Graft infection: a dreadful challenge. *Semin Vasc Surg.* 1990;3:77–87.

12. Edwards WH Jr, Martin RS, Jenkins JM, et al. Primary graft infections. *J Vasc Surg.* 1987;6:235–239.

13. Szilagyi DE, Smith RF, Elliot JP, Brandecic MP. Infection in arterial reconstruction with synthetic grafts. *Ann Surg.* 1972;176:321–333.

14. Cherry KJ, Roland CF, Pariolero PC, et al. Infected femorodistal bypass: Is graft removal mandatory? *J Vasc Surg.* 1992;15:295–305.

15. Samson RH, Veith FJ, Janko GS, et al. A modified classification and approach to the management of infections involving peripheral arterial prosthetic grafts. *J Vasc Surg.* 1988;8:147–153.

16. Calligaro KD, Veith FJ, Gupta SK, et al. A modified method for management of prosthetic graft infections involving an anastomosis to the common femoral artery. *J Vasc Surg.* 1990;11:485–492.

17. Calligaro KD, Veith FJ, Schwartz ML, et al. Are gram-negative bacteria a contraindication to selective preservation of prosthetic arterial grafts? *J Vasc Surg.* 1992;16:337–345.

18. Franks PF, Greenhalgh RM, McCollum CN. Comparison of vein and prosthetic grafts in the femoropopliteal position and other results of the British multicenter trial. In: Veith F, ed. Current Critical Problems in Vascular Surgery. St Louis, MO: *Quality Medical.* 1993:47–49.

19. Veith FJ, Gupta SK, Ascer E, et al. Six-year prospective multicenter randomized comparison of autologous saphenous vein and expanded polytetrafluoroethylene grafts in infrainguinal arterial reconstructions. *J Vasc Surg.* 1986;3:104–116.

20. Ehrenfeld WK, Wilbur BG, Olcott CN, et al. Autogenous tissue reconstruction in the management of infected prosthetic grafts. *Surgery.* 1979;85:82–92.

21. Seeger JM, Wheeler JR, Gregory RT, et al. Autogenous graft replacement of infected prosthetic grafts in the femoral position. *Surgery.* 1983;93:39–45.

22. Fowl RJ, Martin KD, Sax HL, et al. Use of autologous spiral vein grafts for vascular reconstruction in contraindicated fields. *J Vasc Surg.* 1988;8:442–446.

23. Baxter BT, Mesh CL, McGee GS. Limb-threatening ischemia complicated by perigenicular infection. *J Surg Res.* 1993;54:163–167.

24. Dardik H, Dardik I, Veith FJ. Exposure of the tibial-peroneal arteries by a single lateral approach. *Surgery.* 1974;75:377–382.

25. Hoballah JJ, Chalmers RTA, Sharp WJ, et al. Lateral approach to the popliteal crural vessels for limb salvage. *J Cardiovasc Surg.* [In press].

26. Dardik H, Ibrahim IM, Dardik I. Femoral tibial-peroneal bypass: the lateral approach and use of glutaraldehyde-tanned umbilical vein. *Am J Surg.* 1977;134:199–201.

27. Henry AK. *Extensile Exposure.* London, England: Churchill-Livingstone; 1947:218–223.

28. Ouriel K. The posterior approach to popliteal-crural bypass. *J Vasc Surg.* 1994;19:74–80.

29. Karmody AM, Leather RP, Shah DM, et al. Peroneal artery bypass: a reappraisal of its value in limb salvage. *J Vasc Surg.* 1984;1:809–816.

30. Raftery KB, Belkin M, Mackey WC, O'Donnel TF. Are peroneal artery bypass grafts hemodynamically inferior to other tibial artery bypass grafts? *J Vasc Surg.* 1994;19:964–969.

31. Bandyk DR, Bergamini TM, Kinner EV, et al. In situ replacement of vascular prostheses infected by bacterial biofilms. *J Vasc Surg.* 1991;13:575–583.

32. Moore WS, Swanson RJ, Campagna G, Bean B. The use of fresh tissue arterial substitutes in infected fields. *J Surg Res.* 1975;18:229–233.

33. Danese CA, Singer A. Lateral approach to the popliteal artery trifurcation. *Surgery.* 1968;63:588–590.

34. Perry MO. Remote bypass grafts for managing infected popliteal artery lesions. *Arch Surg.* 1979;114:605–607.

35. Trout HH, Smith CA. Lateral ilopopliteal arterial bypass as an alternative to obturator bypass. *Ann Surg.* 1982;48:63–64.

36. Leather RP, Karmody AM. A lateral route for extra-anatomical bypass of the femoral artery. *Surgery*. 1977;81:307–309.
37. Naraynsingh VJ, Karmody AM, Leather RP, Corson JD. Lateral approach to the profunda femoris artery. *Am J Surg*. 1984;147:813–814.
38. Veith FJ, Ascer E, Wengerter KR, et al. Direct exposure of the mid and distal portions of the deep femoral artery. *Semin Vasc Surg*. 1989;2:223–226.
39. Veith FJ, Ascer E, Rivers SP, Gupta SK. Lateral exposure of the popliteal artery above and below the knee. *Semin Vasc Surg*. 1989;2:227–230.
40. Padberg FT. Lateral approach to the popliteal artery. *Ann Vasc Surg*. 1988;2:397–401.
41. Kofsky PM, Carroll SF, Morris MC. The lateral approach to the above knee femoropopliteal bypass. *Surg Gynecol Obstet*. 1988;166:67–68.
42. Esses GE, Johnson WC. The lateral approach to the proximal popliteal artery for popliteal to anterior tibial artery bypass. *J Am Coll Surg*. 1994;178:76–78.
43. Elkin DC, Kelly RP. Arteriovenous aneurysm: exposure of the tibial and peroneal vessels by resection of the fibula. *Ann Surg*. 1945;122:529–545.
44. Carter SL, Cohen A, Whelan TJ. Clinical experience with management of the infected Dacron graft. *Ann Surg*. 1963;158:249–255.
45. Kiwaan JHM, Connolly JE. Successful management of prosthetic graft infection with continuous povidone-iodine irrigation. *Arch Surg*. 1981;116:716–720.
46. Popovsky J, Singer S. Infected prosthetic grafts: local therapy with graft preservative. *Arch Surg*. 1980;115:203–205.
47. Johansen H, Hipp R. Healing of exposed prosthetic vascular grafts by vigorous wound care and povidone-iodine. *Vasc Surg*. 1981;15:421–424.
48. Schaberg FJ, Wong R, Phillips MR, et al. Management of draining wounds in vascular surgery. *Vasc Surg*. 1982;16:213–218.
49. Casali RE, Tucker WE, Thompson BW, Read RC. Infected prosthetic grafts. *Arch Surg*. 1980;115:577–580.
50. Hepp W, Schulze T. The management of infected grafts in reconstructive vascular surgery. *Thorac Cardiovasc Surg*. 1986;34:265–268.
51. Sweeney TF, Piorkowski R, Ariyan S, Kerstein N. An alternative in the management of the infected vascular prosthesis. *Vasc Surg*. 1983;17:195–198.
52. Folsom D, Rubin JR. The management of lower extremity graft infections. *Semin Vasc Surg*. 1990;3:114–121.
53. Johnson JA, Cogbill TH, Strutt PJ, Gundersen AL. Wound complications after infrainguinal bypass: classification predisposing factors and management. *Arch Surg*. 1982;48:63–64.
54. Wengnovitz M, Atnip RG, Gifford RN, et al. Wound complications of autogenous subcutaneous infrainguinal arterial bypass surgery predisposing factors and management. *J Vasc Surg*. 1990;11:156–163.
55. Fujitani RM, Bassiouny HS, Gewertz BL, et al. Cryopreserved saphenous vein allogenic homografts: an alternative conduit in lower extremity arterial reconstruction in infected fields. *J Vasc Surg*. 1992;153:519–525.

39

Repeat Leg Bypass:

How Much Is Enough?

Robert D. De Frang, MD, Lloyd M. Taylor, Jr, MD, and John M. Porter, MD

Even though prolonged patency and excellent limb salvage with leg bypass have become standard,[1,2] virtually all vascular surgeons are encountering increasing numbers of patients with recurrent limb ischemia after graft failure, in large measure related to the increasing number of leg bypasses performed on our aging population. Patient outcome after a second ipsilateral leg bypass following graft failure has been described in several older publications, all describing poor primary patency and limb salvage rates of 30% to 52% at 3 to 5 years.[3-10] In 1990, we reported our experience with first time redo leg bypass in 87 patients following a single graft occlusion.[11] While satisfactory, patency was significantly lower than the primary patency observed in the remainder of our patients undergoing leg bypass. However, these results were distinctly better than first time redo results reported by others,[4-8] an improvement we ascribed to our all autogenous leg bypass policy. More recently, we reported 85 redo bypasses in 81 patients after failure of two or more prior infrainguinal bypasses in the same leg.[12] On the basis of results from first time redo patients we hypothesized the multiple redo's would fare progressively worse. Much to our surprise this was not the case. Our results with both first-time and multiple redo leg bypasses form the basis for this chapter.

PATIENT SELECTION

The clinical manifestations of a failed leg bypass typically fall into a narrow range between severe, life-altering claudication and rest pain with or without tissue loss. The predominate indication (>90%) for leg bypass surgery in our entire redo leg bypass series has been limb salvage as defined by the Society for Vascular Surgery/International Society for Cardiovascular Surgery reporting standards. These standards include rest pain and/or ulceration or gangrene together with an ankle–brachial index (ABI) of less than 0.4. Limb salvage patients typically have multilevel occlusive disease associated with advanced ischemia. Significant co-morbid illness are not regarded by us as a contraindication to necessary leg bypass. The only patients not considered for limb salvage are patients with severe neurological disorders who cannot leave their beds and have no prospect for ambulation.

Patients determined to have a failing graft by postoperative duplex ultrasonic graft flow and ABI surveillance methods undergo arteriography and graft repair of a stenosis of more than 60% of the vessel diameter when found. Those patients are considered as having a new bypass in accordance with SVS/ISCVS reporting standards. Surveillance-detected failing grafts include those with a flow velocity less than 45 cm/sec, isolated stenoses with a flow velocity greater than 200 cm/sec, or an ABI decrease greater than 0.15 from initial postoperative values.

DEMOGRAPHICS

Our patients with a single failed leg bypass as well as those with multiple leg bypass failures have typical atherosclerotic risk factors (Table 39–1). The notable exceptions are in the categories of diabetes and renal failure. No patients with two or more ipsilateral leg bypass failures have had renal insufficiency or failure and only 20% had diabetes.

REOPERATIONS

Second Operation

Between January 1, 1980, and December 15, 1988, we performed first-time redo leg bypasses on 111 limbs in 87 patients following a single prior failed bypass.[11] Autogenous reversed vein was placed in 103 of these limbs. The distal anastomosis of the repeat bypass was to the above-knee popliteal artery in 10 limbs, the below-knee popliteal artery in 26 limbs, the infrapopliteal arteries in 54 limbs, and the pedal arteries in seven limbs. In the remaining limbs the graft was found to be patent with either outflow occlusion or high-grade stenoses, and a new bypass was constructed from the previously placed graft. Grafts were constructed of ipsilateral greater saphenous vein in 22 limbs, contralateral greater saphenous vein in 32 limbs, portions of remaining ipsilateral greater saphenous vein in 14 limbs, arm vein in 31 limbs, lesser saphenous vein in 17 limbs, or some combination of the above. At least one venovenostomy was required in 31 bypasses.

TABLE 39–1. PATIENT DEMOGRAPHICS*

Characteristic	2nd Operation	3rd, 4th, or 5th Operation
Age (mean, y)	68	68
Sex (M/F %)	68/32	64/36
History of smoking (%)	90	83
Diabetes (%)	39	19.75
Renal insufficiency (%)	NA	0

* NA, not applicable.

Third, Fourth, or Fifth Operation

In 1993 we reported on 81 patients who underwent 85 lower-extremity bypasses after two or more failed prior revascularizations in the same leg.[12] Over the period of review, 1980–1992, this subgroup represented 8.8% of all infrainguinal bypasses performed at our institution. Seventy-two operations were the third redo procedure. Six were the fourth redo, and seven were the fifth redo.

The distal anastomosis was to the popliteal artery in 22% and infrapopliteal arteries in 78% of the patients. Autogenous reconstruction was used in 67 of 85 limbs (79%), and prosthetic was used in the remaining 18 limbs (21%), in each case only after a vigorous unsuccessful search for autogenous vein. Arm veins were used in 31% of this group, while another 31% required autogenous vein other than a continuous piece of arm vein or greater saphenous vein. Only two patients had ipsilateral greater saphenous vein available for bypass. Distal anastomosis was to an infrapopliteal artery in 68 of the 85 limbs. Twenty-six of the 85 operations consisted of repair of a failing graft.

RESULTS

Second Operation

The indication for the first redo bypass was limb salvage in 90% of patients and short distance claudication in the remaining 10%. The mean follow-up period for this patient group was 20.5 months. Primary patency at 5 years was 57%, as seen in Table 39–2 and Figure 39–1. At 5 years, the limb salvage rate was 90% (Table 39–3, Fig. 39–2), and the Life Table patient survival rate was a dismal 12%, as seen in Table 39–4 and Figure 39–3. Infrapopliteal artery bypass grafts had a 5-year primary patency rate of 59%, no different from that for popliteal bypasses.

Third, Fourth, and Fifth Operation

The mean follow-up period after the most recent operation was 17 months. Indications for reoperation were limb salvage in 60% instances, severe claudication in 6%, and surveillance-detected graft abnormalities in 34%. Claudication was the indication for the first leg bypass in 67% of limbs and 23% for the first redo operation. The primary patency rate for all multiple redo grafts was 80% at 1, 2, 3, and 4 years. The limb salvage rate at 4 years was 69.6%, and the Life Table patient survival rate after the

TABLE 39–2. PRIMARY PATENCY AFTER FIRST REDO GRAFT*

Interval (mo)	No. at Risk	No. Occluded	No. Withdrawn	Interval Patency Rate	Cumulative Patency Rate	SE
0	103	4	3	0.96	0.96	0.019
6	96	13	20	0.85	0.82	0.041
12	63	2	14	0.96	0.79	0.044
24	47	4	11	0.90	0.71	0.054
36	32	3	16	0.88	0.62	0.067
48	13	1	4	0.91	0.57	0.081
60	8	0	4	1.0	0.57	0.081

* SE, standard error.

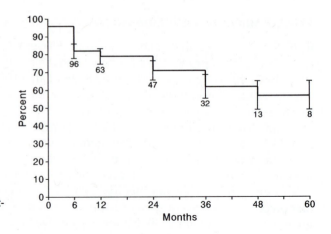

Figure 39–1. Life Table primary patency of the first redo graft.

TABLE 39–3. LIMB SALVAGE RATE AFTER FIRST REDO GRAFT

Interval (mo)	No. at Risk	No. Amputated	No. Withdrawn	Interval Salvage Rate	Cumulative Salvage Rate	SE*
0	90	0	4	1.0	1.0	0.0
6	83	4	24	0.94	0.94	0.027
12	55	0	13	1.0	0.94	0.027
24	42	0	13	1.0	0.94	0.027
36	29	1	17	0.95	0.90	0.052
48	11	0	5	1.0	0.90	0.052
60	6	0	2	1.0	0.90	0.052

* SE, standard error.

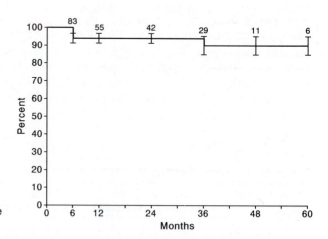

Figure 39–2. Life Table limb salvage following the first redo graft.

most recent operation was 68% at 4 years (see Tables 39–5 through 39–7; Fig. 39–4 through 39–6). The primary patency rate for infrapopliteal bypass grafts was 81% at 4 years, no different from popliteal patency. Three deaths occurred within 30 days of operation. Twenty-one other postoperative complications were recognized, including superficial wound infection in seven instances (8%) and bleeding requiring reoperation in six (7%).

TABLE 39–4. PATIENT SURVIVAL RATE AFTER FIRST REDO BYPASS*

Interval (mo)	No. at Risk	No. Died	No. Withdrawn	Interval Survival Rate	Cumulative Survival Rate	SE
0	82	3	3	0.96	0.96	0.021
6	76	17	6	0.77	0.74	0.050
12	53	8	3	0.85	0.62	0.057
24	42	10	1	0.76	0.47	0.060
36	31	12	3	0.59	0.28	0.056
48	16	3	3	0.79	0.22	0.053
60	10	4	2	0.56	0.12	0.047

* SE, standard error.

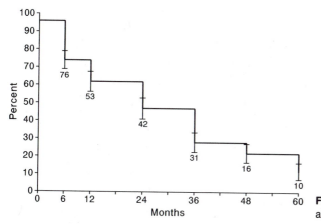

Figure 39–3. Life Table patient survival after the first redo bypass.

TABLE 39–5. PRIMARY PATENCY OF MOST RECENT MULTIPLE REDO GRAFT*

Interval (mo)	No. at Risk	No. Occluded	No. Withdrawn	Interval Patency Rate	Cumulative Patency Rate	SE
0	85	6	8	0.926	0.926	0.0273
6	71	5	14	0.922	0.854	0.0387
12	52	3	13	0.934	0.798	0.0497
24	36	0	12	1.000	0.798	0.0598
36	24	0	8	1.000	0.798	0.0732
48	16	0	11	1.000	0.798	0.0897

* SE, standard error.

No significant difference in primary patency was observed between bypass grafts using arm vein compared with vein grafts from alternative sources. Prosthetic primary patency did not differ statistically from vein graft patency, albeit 18 prosthetic grafts was too small a number for meaningful comparison. Primary bypass patency in women equaled that in men. Similarly, the primary patency rate of 93% at 4 years in the 16 patients with diabetes was not significantly different from the 75% primary patency rate at 4 years observed in patients without diabetes ($P > .05$). The primary patency in surveillance-detected graft revisions using separate Life Tables was similar to the primary patency rate of entirely new grafts, 77% at 4 years ($P = NS$).

TABLE 39–6. LIMB SALVAGE RATE AFTER MOST RECENT MULTIPLE REDO GRAFT*

Interval (mo)	No. at Risk	No. Amputated	No. Withdrawn	Interval Survival Rate	Cumulative Survival Rate	SE
0	50	2	7	0.957	0.957	0.0297
6	41	4	7	0.893	0.855	0.0551
12	30	2	8	0.923	0.789	0.0677
24	20	2	6	0.882	0.696	0.0859
36	12	0	3	1.000	0.696	0.0859
48	9	0	6	1.000	0.696	0.0859

* SE, standard error.

TABLE 39–7. PATIENT SURVIVAL RATE AFTER MOST RECENT MULTIPLE REDO BYPASS*

Interval (mo)	No. at Risk	No. Died	No. Withdrawn	Interval Survival Rate	Cumulative Survival Rate	SE
0	81	1	8	0.987	0.987	0.0125
6	72	5	10	0.925	0.913	0.0317
12	57	2	15	0.960	0.876	0.0409
24	40	2	11	0.942	0.825	0.0546
36	27	1	7	0.957	0.790	0.0697
48	19	2	9	0.862	0.681	0.0882

* SE, standard error.

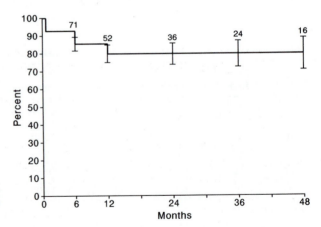

Figure 39–4. Life Table primary patency of the most recent multiple redo graft.

DISCUSSION

A specific number of treatment options are available for a patient with a failed or failing leg bypass. These include primary amputation, graft thrombolysis or thrombectomy (with or without revision), repeat bypass preferably with autogenous vein, or repair of the patent but failing graft.

Amputation in the presence of reconstructible vessels is not an acceptable option. Compared with leg bypass, it has equal or greater mortality and morbidity coupled

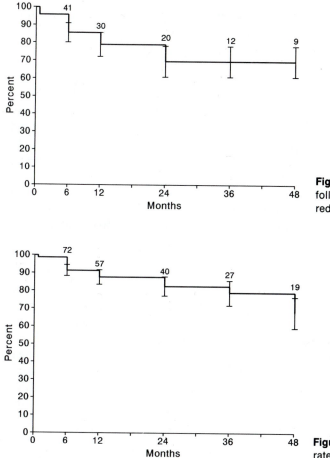

Figure 39–5. Life Table limb salvage following the most recent multiple redo graft.

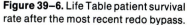

Figure 39–6. Life Table patient survival rate after the most recent redo bypass.

with an unacceptably large percentage (over 50%) of amputees who never regain ambulatory status.[13] Many authors have shown that limb revascularization is cost-effective compared with amputation and that it ultimately provides superior quality of life when successful.[14–16]

Thrombolysis of occluded grafts, even when followed by graft revision, is associated with a 1-year average primary patency rate of 30% to 40%.[17,18] Although this may yield an advantage over blind operative thrombectomy or be deemed suitable for patients with insufficient distal outflow in whom a bypass cannot be constructed, it does not compare with our own reported series of repeat limb bypass after a single graft failure in which we found a 79% and 57% primary patency rate at 1 and 5 years, respectively.[11] Similarly, balloon catheter thrombectomy (with or without revision) has resulted in poor long-term patency rates, ranging from 65% at 3 years for above-knee grafts to 12% at 3 years for below-knee popliteal and infrapopliteal grafts using polytetrafluoroethylene (PTFE). Combining multiple series including both vein and prosthetic conduits, the average patency rate has been disappointingly less than 20% at 3 years.[17–19] The failure of amputation, graft thrombolysis, and thrombectomy to provide acceptable results in patients with failed leg bypasses underlies our philosophical approach of aggressive repeat revascularization.

Historically, poor results led several authors to question whether repeat bypass should be performed at all on patients who have had graft occlusion.[8] Unfortunately, most reports leading to this conclusion included many patients who underwent reoperations on failed prosthetic bypasses or reoperations using prosthetic conduit. In 1968, Sautot[20] retrospectively reviewed results for bypass grafts after failed reconstructions. A disappointing 1-year limb salvage rate of 50% was observed. Craver et al[21] reported on 98 infrainguinal grafts that occluded within 1 month after operation. Life Table graft patency was 28% at 1 year. Szilagyi et al[22] followed in 1974 with a review of 169 secondary operations for lower extremity ischemia following graft failure. Although no calculation of Life Table patency was performed, the authors commented that their results were inferior to those of secondary aortoiliac reconstructions. In 1978, Painton et al[23] reviewed the effectiveness of reoperation after late failure of infrainguinal bypass. Five of 13 patients required amputation within 2 weeks. In 1978, Tyson et al[24] reported similar results. In the late 1970s and early 1980s, a number of reports described results of reoperative procedures for failed infrainguinal bypass grafts.[9,10,25–30] Whereas prosthetic reconstructions were reported to have patencies as low as 0.0% at 3 years and limb salvage rates of only 50% at 5 years, vein bypasses were reported to have patencies as high as 46% at 5 years.

Overall, past reports of repeat limb bypass after a single graft failure have demonstrated average patency rates of less than 30% at 5 years and poor limb salvage rates. These poor results form the basis for the opinion of some authors that amputation may be preferable to repeat bypass surgery or at least that revascularization should be reserved for critical limb-threatening ischemia.[8] Though primary patency of repeat leg bypass is clearly lower than that of first time bypasses, we have reported repeat bypass after a single prior failure to yield a primary patency rate of 57% at 5 years.[11] Interestingly we have described primary patency after two or more ipsilateral leg bypass failures of nearly 80% at 4 years.[12] Limb salvage rates in both the first-time redo and multiple redo groups at 4 to 5 years has been 69% to 90% and has resulted both from careful follow-up and good primary patency. Because of our favorable experience with regrafting after both single and multiple failed ipsilateral leg bypasses,[11,12] we continue to maintain an aggressive surgical policy of repeat infraguinal revascularization whenever possible, regardless of the number of prior graft failures. This policy is based on a strong commitment to autogenous vein. This decision for aggressive revascularization is supported by the observation that many elderly amputees remain nonambulatory, require nursing home care, and experience rapidly progressive decline and death.[31–34]

For us, complete graft replacement for the treatment of a failed graft fares far better than alternative management strategies. In our opinion the important reasons for improved results include a strong commitment to autogenous reconstruction coupled with general improvement in the outcome of leg bypass surgery resulting from improved anesthetics and postoperative management. This includes restoration of pulsatile flow at the most distal possible limb level to aid the healing of foot ulcers,[35] use of alternative autogenous vein when saphenous vein is unavailable,[5] and intraoperative techniques including Doppler scanning, electromagnetic flow measurements, and arteriograms to ensure technical adequacy.[36] We prefer to avoid previously dissected arteries if an acceptable downstream site for distal anastomosis exists, even if this requires using a pedal artery. Postoperative examinations including ultrasonic graft surveillance are performed every 3 months for the first year and then every 6 months for life. Graft surveillance includes ABI measurements and duplex ultrasound–determined graft flow velocities.[37,38]

Nearly 80% of repeat leg bypasses in our experience were constructed from autogenous vein. No statistical difference in patency occurred between patients receiving arm vein compared with other sources of autogenous vein. Because of the small number of prosthetic grafts, no statistical difference was observed between prosthetic and autogenous conduit. Prosthetic conduit was preferentially avoided, constituting less than 21% of grafts. In comparison, only 6% of our primary leg bypass grafts were prosthetic. This commitment is based on the disappointing 46% 1-year primary prosthetic patency of tibial bypasses.[8,39,40]

Although results after a graft failure are superior to those previously reported for repeat bypass grafting, the primary patency of first time redo grafts following a single graft failure is significantly less than our patency with first time bypasses. This would appear to be associated with the patient population selected by graft failure. Because the 30-day primary patency is 90% to 96% in this group, early technical errors have nearly been eliminated as a cause for graft failure.

As noted, patients who underwent revascularization after a single graft failure have a disappointingly low 5-year survival rate of 12%. Most previous reports regarding reoperative lower extremity bypass grafting have not addressed the issue of long-term survival.[9,10,22–24,27,30] Authors who have reported this information have noted disparate values, which range from 52% at 3 years to 80% at 5 years.[7,8] Increasingly, current studies of lower extremity ischemia are recognizing the inverse relationship between the severity of lower extremity occlusive disease and long-term survival. Patients requiring reoperation for bypass failure may be considered to have especially severe lower extremity ischemia, particularly if the original procedure was performed for limb salvage. Therefore, the long-term survival rate for group reoperated on after a single graft failure is significantly less than patients undergoing primary bypass grafting. Surprisingly, it is also less than that for patients who undergo revascularization after two or more ipsilateral leg bypass failures.

Primary patency after the third, fourth, or fifth leg bypass is nearly 80% at 4 years. This is similar to results for patients without prior graft failure in whom the primary patency rate at 5 years generally has been in the range of 75% to 85%.[1,41] Excluding revisions detected by graft surveillance, the primary patency rate is still over 77% at 4 years. The 68% Life Table patient survival rate at 4 years continues to be the most amazing difference between these two groups of patients. It is remarkably higher than the 12% 5-year survival among patients who undergo repeat leg bypass after a single graft failure. The obvious question is, why do these patients who undergo multiple operations fare so much better than those who do not?

Interestingly, patients admitted for revascularization after multiple failed bypasses form a distinct subgroup demographically dissimilar to those admitted after a single graft failure. It appears that a large portion of patients in the first time redo leg bypass group lose either life or limb before entering the multiple failure ($\geq$2) patient subgroup.

Patients reoperated on after two or more failed bypasses appeared to be more durable than those in the one-time group probably because this subgroup contained no patients with renal failure or renal insufficiency and only 20% with diabetes.[42] Prior series have documented renal failure in as many as 11% of leg bypass patients, and in our patients operated on after a single graft occlusion there were twice as many diabetics (40%).[1,11] Earlier reports of leg bypass patients with renal failure revealed an 18% survival rate at 3 years.[43,44] Patients with both diabetes and renal insufficiency have a reported 5-year survival rate of only 21%.[34]

The survival rate in the subgroup operated on for the third, fourth, or fifth time nearly equaled that of patients with claudication, who experience a reported 5-year survival rate of 70% to 80%.[45] Notably, more than 60% of the patients in this subgroup had their first bypass placed for claudication, not limb-threatening ischemia. These patients clearly displayed the same trend in survival as patients with claudication despite their need for repeat surgery predominately for limb salvage after prior leg bypass failure. In fact, 70% limb salvage at 4 years was not strikingly different from results obtained in our series of primary leg bypasses, which had a 5-year limb salvage rate of 93%. By attrition, these patients have selected themselves as heartier and demographically quite different from patients in both primary and secondary bypass series. In survival terms, they remain on the curve generated by the indication for their first bypass, a finding of considerable interest.

Operative mortality and morbidity for both groups following reoperation for graft failure are similar to most primary bypass series using either vein or prosthesis.[6,46] The mortality of 3.5% is well within the range of the 2% to 7% reported in other primary and repeat bypass series.[2,10,24] Of note is the observation that the average mortality risk for amputation is significantly higher at 6%.[13] It does not appear that failure following repeat bypass attempts increases amputation level. In our most recent series of reoperations following multiple graft failure, 70% of amputations were performed below the knee. This ratio is no different from that in other series of both primary and repeat limb bypass failures,[41] a finding noted by others.[13,48] Theoretically, reoperation might be associated with greater wound morbidity; however, this was not observed in either of our series. An overall morbidity rate of less than 25% is nearly the same as that reported after infrapopliteal bypass (22%, major and minor complications) in both primary and repeat limb bypass series.[42,47]

In the past, our position has been that patients with leg bypass failure as a group are at higher risk for future graft failure. The new information reported herein has modified our position. Although patients who had had a single graft failure are at slightly higher risk for future graft failure and have an exceptionally low 5-year survival rate, patients operated on after two or more bypass failures are not. They have both an exceptionally long survival time and a high primary patency rate. We suspect that, in addition to reflecting a very select patient group, these results reflect in part both commitment to autogenous conduit use and intensive graft surveillance.[49] Graft flow velocity surveillance has been more successful at outflow preservation than no surveillance and treatment after graft occlusion. Failure to treat a failing graft results in a high incidence of thrombosis and increased need for a complicated reoperation that yields lower graft patency and limb salvage. Between 25% and 80% of patients, depending on initial operative indication, have their circulatory status worsened compared with their preoperative condition following graft failure.[9]

Optimal care of patients with limb-threatening ischemia after single or multiple failed infrainguinal bypasses in our opinion consists of aggressive revascularization. Current results of repeated bypass surgery demonstrate primary patency and limb salvage rates that are sufficiently good to make repeat bypass our choice following graft failure. We continue to avoid thrombolysis, thrombectomy, and balloon angioplasty because the results to date are markedly inferior to those achieved by repeat leg bypass. With resolute commitment an all-autogenous reconstruction can be achieved in more than 80% of patients who undergo repeat bypass. Although the 5-year survival rate among patients who have had a single graft failure is disappointingly low, the 5-year survival rate among patients operated on after two or more bypass failures is quite good. These two patient groups are quite dissimilar. The latter is a very durable select subgroup that has an exceptionally low incidence of both diabetes and renal insufficiency. However, repeat leg bypass can be performed on either of these groups with low mortality, acceptable morbidity, and with the expectation that primary patency will be distinctly superior to that obtained after treatment with thrombolysis, thrombectomy, or balloon angioplasty (with or without revision). Repeat limb bypass provides excellent palliation and allows most patients to remain ambulatory for the duration of life.

Acknowledgment
Supported by Grant RR00331, CRC Branch, National Center for Research Res NIH.

REFERENCES

1. Taylor LM Jr, Hamre D, Dalman RL, Porter JM. Limb salvage vs amputation for critical ischemia: the role of vascular surgery. *Arch Surg.* 1991;126:1251–1258.
2. Veith FJ, Gupta SK, Samson RH, et al. Progress in limb salvage by reconstructive arterial surgery combined with new or improved adjunctive procedures. *Ann Surg.* 1981; 194:386–401.
3. Green RM, Ouriel K, Ricotta JJ, et al. Revision of failed infrainguinal bypass graft: principles of management. *Surgery.* 1986;100:646–653.
4. Harris RW, Andros G, Salles-Cunha SX, et al. Totally autogenous venovenous composite bypass grafts. *Arch Surg.* 1986;121:1128–1132.
5. Harris RW, Andros G, Salles-Cunha SX, et al. Alternative autogenous vein grafts to the inadequate saphenous vein. *Surgery.* 1986;100:822–827.
6. Ascer E, Collier P, Gupta SK, et al. Reoperation for polytetrafluoroethylene bypass failure: the importance of distal outflow site and operative technique in determining outcome. *J Vasc Surg.* 1987;5:298–310.
7. Bartlett ST, Olinde AJ, Flinn WR, et al. The reoperative potential of infrainguinal bypass: long-term limb and patient survival. *J Vasc Surg.* 1987;5:170–179.
8. Dennis JW, Littooy FN, Greisler HP, et al. Secondary vascular procedures with polytetrafluoroethylene grafts for lower extremity ischemia in a male veteran population. *J Vasc Surg.* 1988;8:137–142.
9. Brewster DC, LaSalle AJ, Robison JG, et al. Femoropopliteal graft failures: clinical consequences and success of secondary procedures. *Arch Surg.* 1983;118:1043–1047.
10. Whittemore AD, Clowes AW, Couch NP, Mannick JA. Secondary femoropopliteal reconstruction. *Ann Surg.* 1981;193:35–42.
11. Edwards JM, Taylor LM Jr, Porter JM. Treatment of failed lower extremity bypass grafts with new autogenous vein bypass grafting. *J Vasc Surg.* 1990;11:13–45.
12. De Frang RD, Edwards JM, Moneta GL, et al. Repeat bypass after multiple prior bypass failures. *J Vasc Surg.* 1994;19:268–277.
13. De Frang RD, Taylor LM Jr, Porter JM. Basic data related to amputations. *Ann Vasc Surg.* 1991;5:202–207.
14. Hickey NC, Thomson IA, Shearman CP, et al. Aggressive arterial reconstruction for critical lower limb ischemia. *Br J Surg.* 1991;78:1476–1478.
15. Stern PH. Occlusive vascular disease of lower limbs: diagnosis, amputation surgery, and rehabilitation. *J Phys Med Rehab.* 1988;88:145–154.
16. Nehler MN, Moneta GL, Taylor LM, Jr., et al. Surgery for chronic lower extremity ischemia in patients 80 years old or older: operative results and assessment of quality of life. (Abstract.) *J Vasc Surg.* 1993;17:226–227.
17. Graor RA, Risius B, Young JR, et al. Thrombolysis of peripheral arterial bypass grafts: surgical thrombectomy compared with thrombolysis, a preliminary report. *J Vasc Surg.* 1988;7:347–355.
18. Gardiner GA Jr, Harrington DP, Koltun W, et al. Salvage of occluded arterial bypass grafts by means of thrombolysis. *J Vasc Surg.* 1989;9:426–431.
19. Veith FJ, Ascer E, Gupta SK, et al. Management of the occluded and failing PTFE graft. *Acta Scand Chir.* 1987;538:117–124.

20. Sautot J. Possibilities and limitations of repeated restorative surgery in secondary and delayed failures. *J Cardiovasc Surg [Torino].* 1988;34:481–501.

21. Craver JM, Ottinger LW, Darling RC, et al. Hemorrhage and thrombosis as early complications of femoropopliteal bypass grafts: causes, treatment, and prognostic implications. *Surgery.* 1973;74:839–845.

22. Szilagyi DE, Elliot JP, Smith RF, et al. Secondary arterial repair: the management of late failures in reconstructive arterial surgery. *Arch Surg.* 1975;110:485–493.

23. Painton JF, Avellone JC, Plecha FR. Effectiveness of reoperation after late failure of femoropopliteal reconstruction. *Ann J Surg.* 1978;135:235–237.

24. Tyson RR, Grosh JD, Reichle FA. Redo surgery for graft failure. *Am J Surg.* 1978;136:165–170.

25. Burnham SJ, Flanigan DP, Goodreau JJ, et al. Nonvein bypass in below-knee reoperation for lower limb ischemia. *Surgery.* 1978;84:417–424.

26. Raithel D. Long-term results of femoro-popliteal/tibial bypasses with special references to reoperation in former femoro-popliteal procedures. *J Cardiovasc Surg [Torino].* 1980;21:541–546.

27. Baker WH, Hadcock MM, Littooy FN. Management of polytetrafluoroethylene graft occlusions. *Arch Surg.* 1980;115:508–513.

28. O'Mara CS, Flinn WR, Johnson ND, et al. Recognition and surgical management of patent but hemodynamically failed arterial grafts. *Ann Surg.* 1981;193:467–476.

29. Kacoyanis GP, Whittemore AD, Couch NP, Mannick JA. Femorotibial and femoropopliteal bypass vein grafts. *Arch Surg.* 1981;116:1529–1534.

30. Flinn WR, Harris JP, Rudo ND, et al. Results of repetitive distal revascularization. *Surgery.* 1982;91:566–572.

31. Whitehouse JW, Jurgenson C, Block MA. The later life of the diabetic amputee: another look at the fate of the second leg. *Diabetes.* 1968;17:520–577.

32. Little JM. Successful amputation—by whose standards? *Am Heart J.* 1975;90:806–807.

33. Little JM, Petritsi-Jones D, Zylstra P, et al. A survey of amputation for degenerative vascular disease. *Med J Aust.* 1973;1:329–332.

34. Whittemore AD, Donaldson MC, Mannick JA. Infrainguinal reconstruction for patients with chronic renal insufficiency. *J Vasc Surg.* 1993;17:32–41.

35. Dalman RL, Taylor LM Jr, Moneta GL, et al. Simultaneous operative repair of multilevel lower extremity occlusive disease. *J Vasc Surg.* 1991;13:211–221.

36. Taylor LM Jr, Porter JM. Technique of reversed vein bypass to distal leg arteries. In: Bergan JJ, Yao JST, eds. *Techniques in Arterial Surgery.* Philadelphia, Pa: Saunders; 1990:109–122.

37. Bandyk DF, Cato RF, Towne JB. A low flow velocity predicts failure of femoro-popliteal and femorotibial bypass grafts. *Surgery.* 1985;98:799–809.

38. Le MC, Luscombe JA, Figg-Hoblyn L, et al. Decreased graft flow velocity is a reliable early indication of impending failure of reversed vein grafts. *J Vasc Technol.* 1988;12:133–137.

39. Killewich LA, Bartlett ST. The all autogenous tissue policy for infrainguinal reconstruction questioned. *Am J Surg.* 1990;160:552–555.

40. Dalman RL, Taylor LM Jr. Basic data related to infrainguinal revascularization procedures. *Ann Vasc Surg.* 1990;4:309–312.

41. Taylor LM Jr, Edwards JM, Porter JM. Present status of reversed vein bypass: long-term results of a modern series. *J Vasc Surg.* 1990;11:193–206.

42. Taylor LM Jr, Edwards JM, Phinney ES, Porter JM. Reversed vein bypass to infrapopliteal arteries: modern results are superior to or equivalent to in-situ bypass for patency and for vein utilization. *Ann Surg.* 1987;205:90–97.

43. Edwards JM, Taylor LT Jr, Porter JM. Limb salvage in end-stage renal disease (ESRD): comparison of modern results in patients with and without ESRD. *Arch Surg.* 1988;123:1164–1168.

44. Chang BB, Paty PSK, Shah DM, et al. Results in infrainguinal bypass for limb salvage in patients with end stage renal disease. *Surgery.* 1990;108:742–747.

45. Taylor LM Jr., Porter JM. Natural history of chronic lower extremity ischemia. *Semin Vasc Surg.* 1991;4:182–187.

46. Davis RK, Bosher LP, Brown PW, et al. Lower extremity arterial revascularization with autogenous ectopic vein. In: Veith FJ, ed. *Current Critical Problems in Vascular Surgery.* St. Louis, MO: Quality Medical, 1989:52–57.

47. Silverman SH, Flynn TC, Seeger JM. Secondary femoral-distal bypass. *J Cardiovasc Surg.* 1991;32:121–126.

48. Tsang GMK, Crowson MC, Hickey NC, Simms MH. Failed femorocrural reconstruction does not prejudice amputation level. *Br J Surg.* 1991;78:1479–1481.

49. Bandyk DF. Postoperative surveillance of infrainguinal bypass. *Surg Clin North Am.* 1990;70:71–82.

X

Thrombolytic Therapy in Ischemia of Lower Extremities

40

Thrombolysis for Native Arterial Occlusive Disease

Robert A. Graor, MD

HISTORICAL DEVELOPMENT

Although intra-arterial thrombolysis has been used for more than 30 years, it is only in the past decade that the method has become widely accepted as a legitimate treatment of arterial and venous thrombotic disease. Tillett and Garner discovered streptokinase in 1933, but it was not until 1959 that its clinical use was suggested.[1] The experience with thrombolysis in the 1960s was not encouraging because of the need for high doses because of the relative impurity of the agents and the dramatic hemorrhage and allergic complications.[2] It was clear that these agents could lyse thrombus, but the risks seemed excessive.

In 1971, Chesterman et al described the use of low-dose intra-arterial streptokinase for a case of small-vessel thrombosis following a vascular injury.[3] Subsequently, a single case report by Dotter with a detailed description of the method of thrombolysis was published in the early 1970s.[4]

Problems still remain, despite several decades of use of thrombolytic agents. The long-term benefits of this treatment have not been fully assessed. Throughout the years, we have reported thrombolysis as a powerful diagnostic and therapeutic tool and one that has been a part of the overall strategy for the management of arterial or bypass graft occlusion. The quest for better methods of treating arterial occlusion arise from multiple sources. The results of arterial reconstruction, although improving, are not uniformly successful and certainly not without considerable risk. Second, by the year 2010, the mean age of the largest population will be the sixth decade of life. Age is a dominant risk factor for vascular disease, as are diabetes and smoking. For all these risk factors, there are no strong data that prove that the current efforts to alter dietary and smoking habits will have an effect on the prevention of complications of arterial disease already established in the adult population.

Only a small proportion of those with vascular disease will need thrombolysis or other invasive treatments. It has been argued that intervention is too frequent among patients in certain areas of the United States. In fact, some data suggest that interventional and endovascular treatment such as thrombolysis and angioplasty have had no effect on the number of amputations done for ischemic limbs.

The burden of vascular disease is increasing in our aging population, and valid evidence of the effect of thrombolysis on the quality of life is needed before a judgment about cost and benefit is possible. The increasing popularity of thrombolysis and endovascular treatments may or may not reduce the number of patients who require vascular surgery, but at least temporarily, it enhances the quality of life for many individuals. An endovascular approach to treatment of patients with vascular disease has proven to be successful in the short term. Evaluating the long-term results is like trying to hit a moving target because the techniques of treatment have changed and evolved, making results of older standard therapies obsolete. One of the most important aspects of evaluating endovascular procedures, including thrombolysis, will be the resources available or the limitations of these resources. Although these treatments appear to be less invasive, the issue of costs may be no less intrusive.

RESULTS OF NATIVE ARTERIAL THROMBOLYSIS

There are very few data available strictly evaluating the intra-arterial use of thrombolysis for thrombotic occlusion of native arteries. It is clear that among patients who have acute limb ischemia in general, the mortality may be as high as 40%.[5,6] These reports of high mortality are associated with prolonged hospitalizations and rehabilitation and frequently associated with diminished self-sufficiency from amputation or ischemic neuropathies. Because of the high morbidity and mortality associated with acute limb ischemia, most clinicians argue that immediate balloon thromboembolectomy, with or without vascular reconstruction, is necessary to restore flow and maintain life and limb. Others contend that the immediate use of thromboembolectomy is highly dangerous, and they emphasize an in-hospital mortality in excess of 25% and an associated overall amputation rate of 33%.[7,8]

There is no doubt that in some highly specialized vascular centers, the morbidity and mortality associated with acute limb ischemia are significantly lower. However, experienced interventionalists report promising results of nonsurgical intervention.

McNamara et al described their experience with the use of thrombolysis as the initial treatment for 63 patients with acute limb ischemia.[9] Their results indicated a markedly lower mortality of only 1.6% and had an amputation rate of 8.5% among the survivors. Eighty-two percent of the patients in the study had critically threatened or irreversible limb ischemia.

Importantly, the approach to treatment utilizing thrombolysis initially did not preclude subsequent prompt surgical treatment when necessary and in some cases it clearly reduced the amount of surgery required to successfully revascularize the patients. There was an associated reduction in the need for urgent surgery and a simplified approach when thrombolysis produced a patent arterial bed. Thrombolysis did not adversely affect the subsequent surgical procedures since it was noted that only 2.8% of patients had clinically significant bleeding.

The lower mortality associated with an initial thrombolytic approach has been previously reported in seven publications reporting on 160 patients demonstrating a cumulative mortality of 1.9%. Although it is difficult to fully evaluate whether all 160 patients had acutely and critically ischemic limbs, the overall mortality is impressively low, and this experience supports the impression that a thrombolytic approach is tolerated better than emergency surgery.

Another aspect of the use of endovascular and thrombolytic procedures is the issue of cost and cost-benefit considerations. Although few data are available to strictly evaluate cost, two important components of the costs associated with a thrombolytic form of treatment include the average hospital stay and the cost of the thrombolytic agent. In the data collected by McNamara et al the average length of stay for patients treated with thrombolysis as an initial approach was 3.5 days, and the wholesale cost of the urokinase used as the thrombolytic agent was $1,575. Although wholesale costs do not reflect actual patient cost, which may be twice as high as the wholesale cost, it does represent a substantial reduction when compared with intensive care and operating room time associated with the treatment of these patients.

Ouriel et al found that patients randomized to surgery or thrombolysis as the primary treatment of peripheral arterial or bypass graft occlusion had similar outcomes with regard to the limb salvage (82%).[10] Of interest, they noted that the in-hospital complication rate and mortality was significantly lower for thrombolysis treated patients (84% vs 58%, $P = .01$), predominantly attributable to an increased frequency of cardiopulmonary problems in the surgical group. They also noted no difference in the duration of hospital stay and a modest increase in hospital cost in the thrombolytic arm (median cost $15,672 vs $12,253, $P = .02$).

The STILE (Surgery Versus Thrombolysis-Ischemia of the Lower Extremity) study was designed to evaluate intra-arterial thrombolytic therapy versus surgery in the treatment of nonembolic arterial and graft occlusions.[11] Clearly, this trial evaluated patients with chronic ischemia, and only a small percentage of these patients had acute limb ischemia. The primary outcome for these patients included death, major amputation, recurrent ischemia, and major morbidity.

When thrombolysis of native arterial occlusions and bypass grafts were compared, there were no differences in the clinical outcome, although patients who underwent surgery as their initial form of therapy had significantly fewer episodes of recurrent ischemia than the thrombolysis group. Surgical patients had a higher mortality than the native arterial thrombolysis group.

Although the overall patency results supported a primary surgical approach to patients with occluded native arteries, a subgroup of patients who had relatively acute ischemia, that is, less than 14 days of ischemia, faired better with an initial thrombolytic approach. Surgical patients had more major amputations (17.9%) than those who underwent primary thrombolysis (5.5%).

The design of this trial and the number of patients enrolled with chronic ischemia resulted in a not surprising benefit of surgery over thrombolysis. Yet, there was an advantage of thrombolysis over surgery for patients who had less than 14 days of ischemia. Data from this trial supported the impression of McNamara et al that patients with relatively acute ischemia, limb-threatening or not, had a lower amputation rate with thrombolysis as their initial approach than did those who underwent surgical revascularization. However, among patients with more chronic ischemia, a trend toward reduction and major amputation and significant reduction and recurrent ischemia occurred among the patients who had a primary surgical approach.

Sixth-month follow-up data provide important information on the treatment strategy and their long-term perspective. Although there was no overall difference in mortality or major amputation at 6 months, there appeared to be a difference when the results were separated according to the duration of ischemia. In acutely ischemic patients, there was a higher amputation-free survival rate among patients who underwent thrombolysis than among surgical patients. However, the converse was true for chronically ischemic patients, who had a better limb salvage rate when treated with a primary surgical approach.

Again considering costs, among patients enrolled in this trial who had acute limb ischemia (0 to 14 days of ischemia), the surgical patients had a mean hospital stay of 14.3 days, whereas thrombolysis patients had a mean hospital stay of only 9.7 days ($P = .04$). Patients with chronic limb ischemia did not demonstrate a difference in length of hospital stay. Therefore, it appears that simply on the basis of hospital stay, thrombolysis appears to be a more cost-efficient method of treating patients with acute limb ischemia.

TECHNICAL CONSIDERATIONS OF NATIVE ARTERIAL THROMBOLYSIS

Catheter placement is critical to the success of native arterial thrombolysis. Successful single-wall puncture of the common femoral artery, usually from the contralateral side, provides easy access around the aortic bifurcation to the occluded limb segment. If prior arteriographic evaluation has been undertaken, following a suitable waiting period, antegrade cannulation for distal segmental occlusions may be appropriate. After arterial cannulation, traversing the occlusion with a guide wire and appropriately placing a catheter across the arterial occlusion yields the highest rate of success. It is technically more difficult to cross a long segment of occlusion than to simply place a catheter at the proximal extent of the occluded segment, but ultimately the results appear to be better with full traversal of the thrombolytic infusion catheter.

The technique of thrombolytic infusion varies considerably. Data are available to support continuous infusions of urokinase at 4000 U/minute over the first 2 to 4 hours, followed by 2000 U/minute until complete thrombus resolution occurs. A higher-dose regimen with a bolus or lower-dose regimens have also been tried and have resulted in successful outcomes. The use of recombined tissue plasminogen activator has been explored in clinical trials, and it appears that 0.05 mg/kg per hour will result in rapid and complete thrombolysis. The predominant benefit of recombinant tissue plasminogen activator is more rapid thrombolysis, with average opening occurring after 5 to 7 hours of infusion, compared with urokinase, with which opening occurs after 18 to 24 hours.

Meticulous attention needs to be paid to the vascular entrance sites because they are the most common area of bleeding complications. The use of a vascular sheath is important if multiple catheter exchanges are required.

Careful selection of appropriate patients for treatment with intra-arterial thrombolysis and using proven techniques and careful monitoring will result in successful outcomes. Avoidance of thrombolytic complications is important to maintain a good morale among nursing and other medical staff.

The use of adjunctive medications during thrombolysis can be divided into three phases. These phases include medications used during lysis, which frequently include antiplatelet agents and anticoagulants. The second phase is during the secondary procedure that follows thrombolysis and generally drugs administered include both antiplatelet and anticoagulants. The third phase is the late phase, which is predominantly to prevent late reocclusion. Medications used in this phase include antiplatelet agents, predominantly aspirin, and in some cases anticoagulants. The efficacy of anticoagulation during thrombolysis has not been clearly delineated, but it appears to be important for the prevention of pericatheter thrombosis and maintenance of patency of small vessels during the thrombolytic process.

CONCLUSION

Considering the first important investigations into peripheral thrombolysis began more than a decade ago, tremendous advances in knowledge have been made. Intra-arterial thrombolysis has now become a widely applied method of initial therapy for patients with peripheral arterial and bypass graft occlusions. Some data are now available to prove its efficacy as the primary initial approach to patients who have acutely ischemic limbs. Fascinating data are also available to indicate a lower mortality associated with this initial therapy with adequate initial long-term results.

The technical considerations of thrombolysis are important to produce highly successful outcomes, but this is not an area of practice for the uninitiated or inexperienced. Knowledge of all aspects of anticoagulation and thrombolysis are important, as is a solid understanding of the underlying etiologies and associated conditions, complications, and alternatives associated with thrombotic peripheral arterial occlusion.

Careful consideration of the use of thrombolysis should be applied to patients with acutely ischemic limbs (less than 14 days of ischemia) to achieve a highly effective and cost-efficient method of therapy. Further studies of these groups of patients are necessary to define the optimal patients and to yield the best of outcomes.

REFERENCES

1. Tillet WS, Garner RL. The fibrinolytic activity of hemolytic streptococci. *J Exp Med.* 1933;58:485–502.
2. Johnson AJ, McCarty WR. Lysis of artificially induced clots in man by intravascular infusion of streptokinase. *J Clin Invest.* 1959;38:1627–1643.
3. Chesterman CN, Nash T, Biggs JC. Small vessel thrombosis following vascular injury: successful treatment with a low dose intra-arterial infusion of streptokinase. *Br J Surg.* 1971;58:582–588.
4. Dotter CT, Rosch J, Seaman AJ, et al. Streptokinase treatment of thromboembolic disease. *Radiology.* 1972;102:283–290.
5. Blaisdell FW, Steele M, Allen RE. Management of acute lower extremity arterial ischemia due to embolism and thrombosis. *Surgery.* 1978;84:822–834.
6. Jivegard LE, Arfvidsson B, Holm J. Selective conservative and routine early operative treatment in acute limb ischemia. *Br J Surg.* 1987;74:798–801.
7. Fogarty TJ, Cranley JJ, Krause RJ, et al. A method for extraction of arterial emboli and thrombi. *Surg Gynecol Obstet.* 1963;241–244.
8. Kendrick J, Thompson BW, Read RC, et al. Arterial embolectomy in the leg: results in a refferal hospital. *Am J Surg.* 1981;142:739–743.
9. McNamara TA, Bomberger RA, Merchant RF. Intra-arterial urokinase as initial therapy for acutely ischemic lower limbs. *Circulation.* 1991;83 (Suppl 1):1-106–1-119.
10. Ouriel K, Shortell CK, DeWeese JA, et al. A comparison of thrombolytic therapy with operative revascularization in the initial treatment of acute peripheral arterial ischemia. *J Vasc Surg.* 1994;19:1021–1030.
11. The STILE trial investigators. Results of a prospective randomized trial evaluating surgery versus thrombolysis for ischemia of the lower extremity. *Ann Surg.* 1994;220:251–268.

41

Thrombolytic Therapy in the Management of Peripheral Arterial Occlusion

Kenneth Ouriel, MD

Traditionally, operative revascularization has been the mainstay of therapy in the setting of lower extremity ischemia.[1] Although operative bypass, endarterectomy, and thromboembolectomy all have been utilized quite successfully to restore arterial circulation and salvage the threatened limb, these results have been tempered by an extraordinarily high patient mortality.[2–4]

Thrombolytic therapy is gaining increasing acceptance as a treatment modality performed as an adjuvant or alternative to operation in patients with acute peripheral arterial occlusion. Administration of these clot-dissolving agents provides a potentially less invasive means of restoring arterial continuity. As such, the goal of thrombolytic therapy is to lessen the morbidity and mortality associated with acute lower extremity ischemia while maintaining the excellent limb salvage results achieved with operative revascularization.

HISTORY OF THROMBOLYSIS

Thrombolytic agents have been used clinically since the late 1940s.[5] The early pharmacologic preparations were obtained from impure isolates of streptococcus bacterium and contained streptodornase and other foreign protein contaminants in addition to the active agent streptokinase.[6] These contaminants were responsible for a variety of untoward systemic effects and forced investigators to limit the use of thrombolytic agents to extravascular disease processes, specifically, to dissolve the fibrinous septae of loculated hemothoraces.

In 1956, Cliffton and Grossi reported successful preliminary results with a mixture of plasminogen and streptokinase and 1 year later Cliffton reported an experience with direct intra-arterial infusions in two patients with peripheral arterial occlusions.[7,8] These historical insights confirm that although Dotter et al must be credited with promulgating the use of catheter-directed peripheral arterial thrombolysis in 1974,[9] Cliffton pioneered the use of this technique 17 years earlier.

A useful classification of the severity of lower extremity ischemia is provided within a Society for Vascular Surgery/International Society for Cardiovascular Surgery report that places patients into one of three classes: viable and nonthreatened, viable but threatened, and nonviable.[10] In this schema, class II patients are generally the most appropriate candidates for thrombolysis; class I do not usually manifest sufficient symptoms to warrant the risks attendant thrombolytic therapy, and class III are, by definition, irretrievable with any treatment modality.

The etiology of acute arterial occlusion can be divided into two categories: thrombosis and embolism. Thrombotic etiologies are observed more frequently by a ratio of four-to-one in most series of acutely compromised lower extremities.[11,12] Irrespective of etiology, the initial occlusive process is rapidly followed by prograde and retrograde propagation of thrombus to the next large collateral channel. The development of propagated thrombus attains significance in the setting of pharmacologic thrombolysis; thrombus within small tibial and pedal arteries may be difficult to remove with operative, mechanical techniques. Similarly, the red-cell rich, platelet-poor secondary thrombus is easy to lyse, but the occluding head of platelet-rich thrombus or older embolus is relatively resistant.[13]

OPERATIVE THERAPY IN ACUTE ARTERIAL OCCLUSION

Despite technical advances and the resultant decreases in the amputation rate associated with operative treatment of acute lower extremity ischemia, limb salvage has been achieved at the cost of an alarmingly high perioperative mortality, approaching 25% in the review of Blaisdell et al,[2] 20% in a series of Jivegård et al,[4] and 15% in a more recent study by Yeager et al.[14] These observations suggest that acute limb ischemia develops in a medically compromised subpopulation, a group that may be further jeopardized by invasive reconstructive procedures. It is on this background that the advent of effective thrombolytic agents provided some hope for a treatment modality that would maintain the excellent limb salvage rates associated with immediate operation concurrent with a decreased periprocedural mortality.

PHARMACOLOGY OF THROMBOLYTIC AGENTS

All thrombolytic agents represent "plasminogen activators," converting fibrin-bound plasminogen to fibrin-bound plasmin, which subsequently degrades the fibrin thrombus to soluble endproducts (Table 41–1).[15] Interestingly, the administration of exogenous plasmin has very little, if any, thrombolytic activity, suggesting that plasmin itself may not bind effectively to fibrin.[16] Thrombolytic agents, when present in the systemic circulation, convert plasminogen to plasmin. Free plasmin then degrades plasma fibrinogen to its degradation products. The generation of fibrinogen degradation products by plasmin comprises the "systemic proteolytic state."

There exist four thrombolytic agents currently approved by the United States Food and Drug Administration: streptokinase, urokinase, recombinant tissue plasminogen activator (rt-PA), and acylated plasminogen streptokinase activator complex (APSAC). Streptokinase is a purified isolate from streptococcus bacteria and is an inactive single-chain 46,000-dalton protein. It forms a complex with plasminogen or plasmin, and this complex requires an additional streptokinase molecule to convert plasminogen to plasmin. Urokinase, clinically employed in both high molecular weight (54,000 dalton) and low molecular weight (31,000 dalton), is a two-chain compound present

TABLE 41–1. PROPERTIES OF COMPONENTS OF THE THROMBOLYTIC SYSTEM[a]

Component	Molecular Weight	Structure	Plasma Half-life
Streptokinase	46,000	Single-chain	11 minutes
Urokinase	54,000	Two chains	10 minutes
rt-PA	70,000	One or two chains	5 minutes
APSAC	131,000	lys-plasminogen-SK	70 minutes
Pro-urokinase	53,000	Single-chain	6 minutes
Plasminogen	88,000	Single-chain	2.2 days
Plasmin	88,000	Two chains	0.1 sec
α_2-antiplasmin	70,000	Single-chain	2.6 days
PAI	40,000	Single-chain	Unknown

rt-PA, recombinant tissue plasminogen activator; APSAC, acyclated plasminogen streptokinase activator complex; PAI, plasminogen activator inhibitor.
[a] Adapted from Marder VJ. The use of thrombolytic agents: choice of patient, drug administration, laboratory monitoring. *Ann Intern Med.* 1979;90:802–812.

in urine. Unlike streptokinase, urokinase directly activates plasminogen without the need for initial binding to an additional plasminogen molecule. rt-PA is a single- or two-chain 70,000 dalton molecule containing two kringle structures, one of which is important in the binding of rt-PA to fibrin.[17] Thus, rt-PA has been promoted as an agent with "fibrin specificity" and a low potential for systemic fibrinogen degradation. This contention has not been substantiated in the clinical setting, similar decreases in plasma fibrinogen concentration following systemic administration of urokinase or rt-PA.[18] APSAC consists of an equimolar complex of streptokinase and plasminogen, originally developed to hasten fibrinolysis by eliminating the initial step of plasminogen binding. In practice, the benefits of APSAC may be related to its increased half-life rather than plasminogen supplementation.

The plasminogen activators differ in their relative rate of fibrin dissolution and in their fibrin-specificity.[19] An ideal agent would manifest a high degree of fibrinolytic activity with a low potential for systemic fibrinogen degradation. Reputedly, streptokinase has the lowest activity and is not fibrin-specific. Urokinase is intermediate, but rt-PA has been reported to be associated with the highest rate of fibrinolysis and the greatest degree of fibrin specificity. Unfortunately, these contentions are based on *in vitro* data, and significant differences have not been consistently observed in clinical investigations.

The widespread belief that rt-PA is a fibrin-specific agent unassociated with significant fibrinogenolysis has not been substantiated in several clinical reports. Meyerovitz et al documented more rapid clot lyais in patients treated with rt-PA but systemic fibrinogen levels were significantly lower than those in patients treated with urokinase.[20] A retrospective analysis of 465 patients with peripheral arterial occlusion reported by Graor et al documented successful clot lysis in 94% of patients treated with rt-PA, 89% of patients treated with urokinase, but only 72% of patients treated with streptokinase.[21] Systemic fibrinogenolysis was observed in all groups; even the rt-PA treated patients experienced a decrease in fibrinogen levels to 66% of baseline.

TECHNIQUE OF ARTERIAL THROMBOLYSIS

At the outset, the most important caveat of arterial thrombolysis relates to the goal of therapy. Thrombolysis is designed to rid the arterial tree of occluding thrombus, uncovering the anatomic lesion responsible for the occlusive event when one exists. Operation or endovascular interventions are subsequently employed to correct the unmasked lesion.[22-25] It is only in a few patients without demonstrable anatomic defects that successful thrombolytic therapy can be employed without subsequent operative revascularization or balloon angioplasty. Thus, studies designed to document the effectiveness of thrombolysis are flawed when the primary outcome measure is avoidance of operation, since the goal of arterial thrombolysis is to uncover and clearly define the etiologic mechanism and lessen the magnitude of a subsequent remedial intervention.[26]

Irrespective of the agent employed, arterial thrombolysis is best accomplished by means of a catheter-directed approach, with the delivery of activator agent directly into the substance of the thrombus.[27] In contrast to the setting of acute coronary artery occlusion, intravenous routes of administration have been entirely unsatisfactory in the periphery. Intravenous streptokinase attained popularity in the 1960s but was associated with successful lysis in a minority of patients.[28]

The difference in the success rate of intravenous thrombolysis in the coronary and peripheral arterial setting is presumably a result of the larger size of peripheral thrombi, with an inability of thrombolytic agent to diffuse into the substance of the larger clots. The numerous side branches of coronary arteries also may aid in the efficiency of intravenous thrombolytic therapy. The short length of thrombus between the head of the thrombus and the next side branch is easily lysed, followed by washout of the by-products of the process through the side branch (Fig. 41–1). Fresh blood containing lytic agent and plasminogen then comes in contact with the new thrombus head just beyond the side branch. Thus, short segments of thrombus are dissolved in a sequential manner from side branch to side branch until the coronary artery is completely open. By contrast, thrombolysis of a long length of thrombus within a branchless peripheral artery or bypass graft is impeded by the absence of washout between branches. Clot dissolution can proceed only through diffusion of new lytic agent through the meniscus of by-products at the head of the clot, explaining the poor success rates with intravenous (systemic) thrombolysis of peripheral arterial thrombi.

Direct, intra-arterial infusion of thrombolysis provides a method to achieve high local doses of activator agent. Dotter et al in 1974[9] reintroduced catheter-directed thrombolysis, using a low-dose streptokinase regimen. Hess et al reported the results of catheter-directed thrombolysis, with successful clot dissolution in 69% of patients.[29] Subsequently, McNamara and Bomberger employed a high-dose urokinase regimen and observed complete clot lysis in 77% of infusions.[30] My associates and my studies have corroborated findings of McNamara and Bomberger. We observed a successful lytic result (greater than 80% clot lysis) in 70% of 57 patients randomized to urokinase therapy for acute limb ischemia.[12] These data, however, must be analyzed in the content of patient selection and the definition of successful lysis, both of which vary from study to study.

Both antegrade and contralateral catheter insertion techniques have been successfully employed in catheter-directed peripheral arterial thrombolysis. The contralateral route is safest, especially in inexperienced hands, because failure to accomplish antegrade access may leave the patient with multiple needlestick holes in the ipsilateral femoral artery, which may bleed during subsequent thrombolytic infusion through a contralateral approach. There is a tendency for thrombus to form on the wall of the catheter during any protracted intra-arterial procedure, and embolization of this "pericatheter thrombus" may occur as the thrombus is sheared off the catheter at the

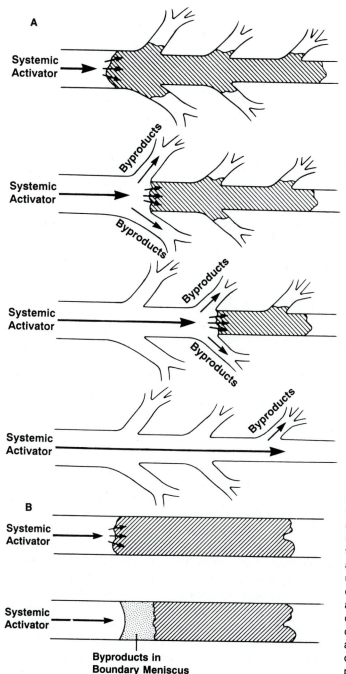

Figure 41–1. Thrombus within arterial segments containing frequent side branches are more susceptible to lysis through an intravenous route of administration, since the side branches allow washout of the by-products of thrombolysis. (**A**) The coronary arterial tree is an example of such a system. (**B**) By contrast, long, branchless conduits require a catheter-directed approach to achieve adequate contact between the lytic agent, plasminogen, and the fibrin clot.

time of removal. The frequency of complications can be minimized through the use of small-bore catheters and concurrent heparin or aspirin therapy. An increase in the risk of hemorrhagic complications with systemic anticoagulation or antiplatelet agents, however, has forced some practitioners to avoid these adjuvants and rely on low-dose heparin flushes through the infusion sheath alone.

The procedure of intra-arterial thrombolysis is begun with an adequate diagnostic arteriogram, generally through the contralateral femoral artery with suitable views of

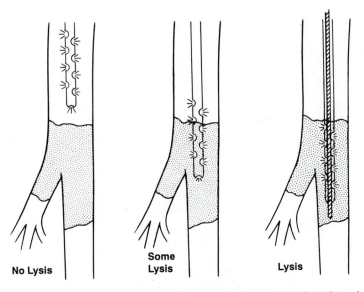

Figure 41–2. It is most important to place all catheter infusion holes into the substance of the thrombus, since the infused agent tends to flow through the path of least resistance. When the infusion holes are not within thrombus, lysis is rare. All of the infusion holes should be embedded within the thrombus and a tip-occluding guide wire can be positioned to force the thrombolytic agent through the side holes of the catheter.

the abdominal aorta and both lower extremities to the foot level. Once adequate diagnostic information has been obtained, the diagnostic catheter may be replaced with an infusion catheter. The infusion catheter is threaded around the aortic bifurcation and into the occluded bypass graft or native artery. Alternatively, an antegrade approach through the ipsilateral common femoral artery may be attempted when the diagnostic arteriogram reveals an appropriate anatomic situation. Specifically, an antegrade approach is applicable when a sufficient length of proximal superficial femoral artery is patent to allow an adequate distance between the site of common femoral cannulation and the exit of lytic agent from the catheter.

The choice of infusion catheter is important to assure accurate and thorough distribution of the lytic agent. A catheter diameter of 5-F is usually best. "Multi–side-hole" catheters with a series of ports spaced along the distal portion of the catheter are commonly employed. One must choose an appropriate length so that the first and last holes are positioned within the proximal and distal portions of the thrombus, respectively (Fig. 41–2). A tip-occluding wire is helpful when using multi–side-hole catheters, since the bulk of the thrombolytic agent tends to flow out the end hole rather than the smaller side holes. The lack of a means of occluding the end hole of multihole diagnostic flush catheters makes these catheters inappropriate substitutions for the specialized multi–side-hole infusion catheters. Coaxial systems with infusion through an outer catheter and inner "infusion wire" may be useful to split the dose of lytic agent when infusion into two anatomically separate sites is advantageous. A single–end-hole catheter may be required when small thrombi are encountered, especially in cases of emboli without proximal or distal clot propagation. Introducing sheaths are usually employed in sizes approximating the outer diameter of the infusion catheter. Replacement of the initial sheath with a larger sheath may be required during the course of thrombolysis, since catheter manipulation may cause enlargement of the arterial puncture site and produce seepage of blood around the sheath.

TABLE 41–2. PROTOCOL FOR INTRA-ARTERIAL THROMBOLYTIC INFUSION (OURIEL-MARDER)[12]

Urokinase Treatment Protocol
325 mg aspirin on presentation
Catheter positioned into substance of thrombus
Urokinase infusion, 4,000 IU/min for 2 hours (5,000 IU/mL, in 5% dextrose)
Decrease to 2,000 IU/min, continue for 2 hours
Decrease to 1,000 IU/min, continue to a maximum of 48 hours' total therapy

Several methods of infusion of thrombolytic agents are in routine use. A "pulse-spray" technique has been utilized, bolusing the thrombolytic agent through a multiholed catheter along the length of the occlusive thrombus, potentially increasing the rate of dissolution. "Lacing" refers to the infusion of large amounts of agent along the length of the thrombus as the catheter is withdrawn, in an effort to attain even and complete distribution of lytic agent throughout the thrombus. "Burst therapy" refers to the intermittent infusion of thrombolysis, discontinuing therapy for a period of hours to allow hepatic repletion of total body plasminogen. Despite theoretic advantages, no consistent benefits have been documented with the use of one technique over another.[31] At present, the method of thrombolytic administration should be based on the experience of the patient care team and the needs of the specific clinical situation. Continuous infusions of thrombolytic agent are most commonly employed, usually beginning with a larger dose (e.g., 4,000 IU urokinase per minute for 4 hours)

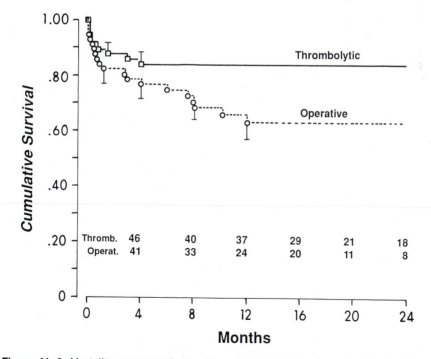

Figure 41–3. Mortality among patients with acute limb ischemia randomized to initial therapy with urokinase or operation. (*Modified from Ouriel K, Shortell CK, DeWeese JA, et al. A comparison of thrombolytic therapy with operative revascularization in the treatment of acute peripheral arterial ischemia. J Vasc Surg. 1994;19:1021–1030.*)

and tapering thereafter (Table 41–2). It is important to follow the progress of thrombolysis with serial arteriographic studies. Catheter manipulation is necessary in most instances, with repositioning of the infusion holes to keep them within the substance of the unlysed thrombus. A maximum duration of lytic administration of 48 hours is recommended, since a prime correlate of complications appears to be the duration of infusion. Moreover, if no degree of reperfusion has been achieved after 12 to 18 hours of intrathrombus infusion of lytic agent, further attempts are unlikely to be successful.[12]

Distal embolization is a well-known complication of thrombolysis and is heralded by acute deterioration in the status of the foot. My colleagues and I have coined the phrase *secondary embolization* to describe this event. The process occurs as the trailing portion of a thrombus is lysed and the remaining bits of undissolved clot travel distally with the resumption of normal arterial flow. Large prosthetic grafts appear to be prone to secondary embolization and the techniques of bolusing and lacing may increase this risk. Patients in whom secondary embolization of thrombotic debris develops should not be taken immediately to the angiographic suite or the operating room. Rather, a period of observation is warranted because the process fortunately is treatable with continuation of infusion, sometimes with an increase in the thrombolytic dose. Repositioning of the catheter into the distal emboli is not always immediately necessary, because small particles of embolized material are usually sensitive to upstream administration of lytic agent. Thus, secondary embolization represents one of the few exceptions to the caveat of infusing agent directly into the substance of the thrombus, possibly because the embolized material has been presaturated with lytic agent. However, if clinical improvement does not occur within 1 to 2 hours, arteriography and catheter repositioning into the tibial vessels may be necessary.

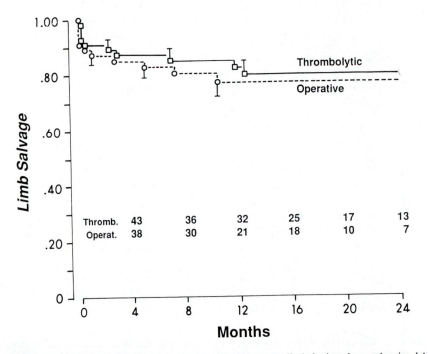

Figure 41–4. The amputation rate of patients with acute limb ischemia randomized to initial therapy with urokinase or operation. (*Modified from Ouriel K, Shortell CK, DeWeese JA, et al. A comparison of thrombolytic therapy with operative revascularization in the treatment of acute peripheral arterial ischemia. J Vasc Surg. 1994;19:1021–1030.*)

Monitoring of coagulation parameters during thrombolytic therapy remains controversial. Fibrinogen concentration, thrombin time, and other laboratory tests have been advocated as measures with which to gauge the risk of distant bleeding complications, but there does not exist conclusive evidence in this regard.[15,32] Bleeding complications almost always result from defects in vascular integrity, usually at the site of arterial cannulation. These events bear little or no correlation with abnormalities in the coagulation tests, but accumulating evidence indicates that the duration of thrombolytic infusion may be an important predictor of hemorrhage.

Intracranial hemorrhage is one of the most dreaded complications of thrombolytic therapy. Other devastating bleeding complications include retroperitoneal hemorrhage and massive gastrointestinal blood loss. These life-threatening bleeding complications are treated with immediate termination of lytic infusion and replacement of fibrinogen and other clotting proteins with fresh frozen plasma or cryoprecipitate when they are depleted. Epsilon amino caproic acid can be infused intravenously to arrest ongoing fibrinolysis in cases of severe bleeding.

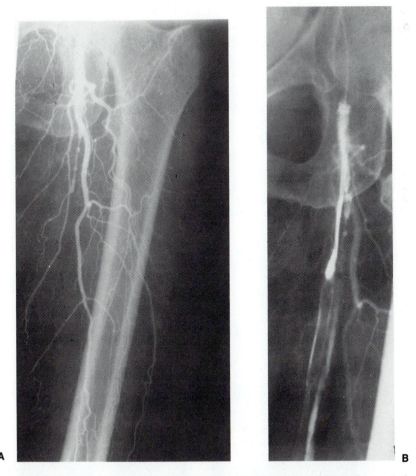

Figure 41–5. A patient who had a femoral-to-above-knee popliteal polytetrafluoroethylene (PTFE) placed for a toe ulceration 2 years before presentation. The graft thrombosed and the patient was left with rest pain. (**A**) The diagnostic arteriogram showing the profunda femoris outflow. The graft is not visualized. (**B**) The graft has been cannulated through a contralateral femoral approach and a small amount of contrast material outlines thrombus within the PTFE graft. (*Figure continues*)

RESULTS OF THROMBOLYSIS IN ACUTE PERIPHERAL ARTERIAL OCCLUSION

Large, retrospective series of patients treated with intra-arterial thrombolytic therapy began to appear in the early 1980s.[11,33–35] Success was reported in more than 90% of cases over a mean duration of infusion of 6 to 12 hours. Amputation rates averaged less than 10%, with early mortalities of less than 5% and bleeding complications in 5% to 10% of patients. Urokinase and rt-PA were argued to be safer and more efficacious than streptokinase. There were, however, severe limitations with these studies and their conclusions are not entirely justified by the data. Streptokinase, for example, was utilized early in the course of each series, usually at a time when the medical team had little experience in thrombolytic treatment. Patients with acute and chronic limb ischemia were included in many of the studies, precluding meaningful comparison with data on truly threatened extremities. Moreover, outcome measures were frequently subjective, bearing little clinical relevance to limb salvage or mortality.

These early series triggered several contradictory reports, all retrospective and somewhat anecdotal.[26,36,37] The data generated by these studies argued against the

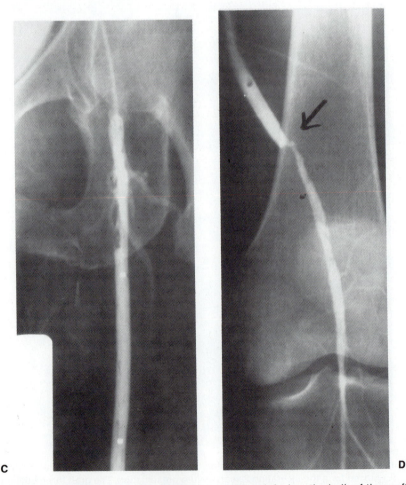

C   **D**

Figure 41–5. *(continued)* **(C)** After 3 hours of urokinase infusion, the bulk of the graft is open, with residual thrombus lining the walls of the graft. **(D)** A tight stenosis at the distal anastomosis is unmasked. *(Figure continues)*

use of thrombolytic agents in acute arterial occlusion, principally on the basis of poor patency rates associated with sole therapy and the frequent need for concurrent operative intervention to achieve an acceptable result. The goal of thrombolysis, however, is not to replace or eliminate surgery. Rather, thrombolytic therapy should be employed in an effort to diminish the magnitude of required interventions and thereby decrease the frequency of morbid and mortal events. Studies that failed to tabulate long-term survival and limb-salvage as primary end points predictably indicted thrombolysis as a useless therapeutic endeavor.

More recent trials have avoided these limitations by employing a randomized, prospective design and objective, clinically relevant end points.[22] In peripheral arterial occlusion, two major issues have been addressed by clinical trials: (a) a comparison of the efficacy of different thrombolytic agents and (b) a comparison of thrombolytic and operative treatment modalities.

To date, there exist three completed prospective comparisons of thrombolysis and operative management of peripheral arterial occlusion. The first published trial was a small series from Sweden. Thrombolysis with intra-arterial rt-PA was constrasted with surgical treatment in 20 ischemic limbs. The small number of patients in this series precluded any meaningful conclusions.

The STILE trial (Surgery Versus Thrombolysis for Ischemia of the Lower Extremity) randomized more than 300 patients with acute and subacute peripheral arterial

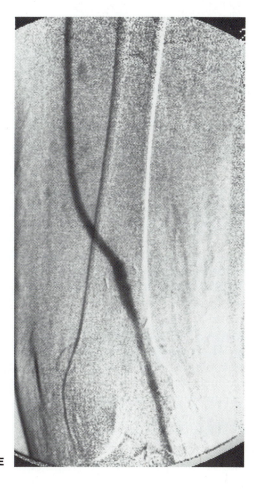

Figure 41–5. (*continued*) (**E**) A digital arteriogram following an operative patch angioplasty of the distal stenosis, performed 1 week after the procedure.

E

TABLE 41–3. FACTORS PREDICTIVE OF SUCCESS IN A MULTIVARIATE ANALYSIS (STEPWISE LINEAR REGRESSION) OF 103 PERIPHERAL ARTERIAL AND BYPASS GRAFT OCCLUSION TREATED WITH THROMBOLYTIC THERAPY

Predictive Factor	Percentage of Patients	Success Rate (%)
Catheter into Thrombus		
Yes	86	88
No	14	0
Guide Wire Traversed Thrombus		
Possible	82	89
Impossible	18	16
Conduit Involved		
Vein graft	18	55
Prosthetic graft	34	80
Native artery	48	78
No. of Arterial Segments Involved		
One	51	88
Two	33	71
Three	16	40
Diabetes Mellitus		
Present	29	49
Absent	71	80

Adapted from Ouriel K, Shortell CK, Green RM, DeWeese JA. Differential mechanisms of failure of autogenous and nonautogenous bypass conduits: an assessment following successful graft thrombolysis. *Cardiovasc Surg.* [in press].

occlusion to one of three treatment groups: operation, intra-arterial rt-PA, or intra-arterial urokinase. Improvement in the rate of limb salvage was observed in the surgical arm. The results, however, were confounded by an inability to place the catheter into the thrombus in a large percentage of patients randomized to thrombolysis. The third completed trial of operation versus thrombolysis was conducted at the University of Rochester and comprised 114 patients with ischemia of 7 days' duration or less.[12] Intra-arterial urokinase was compared with operation in the *initial* management of the patients in the realization that thrombolysis would need to be followed by operative intervention in many of the thrombolytic patients with underlying anatomic lesions responsible for the thrombotic process. A 62% reduction in 1-year mortality occurred in the thrombolytic group (Fig. 41–3). This difference was attributed to a lower requirement for surgery concurrent with a decrease in the frequency of cardiopulmonary complications in the patients randomized to thrombolysis. No increment in the requirement for amputation was observed, with 1-year limb salvage rates of approximately 20% in each treatment arm (Fig. 41–4). The conclusion of the study was that thrombolysis with or without subsequent operation was superior to operation alone in the treatment of the acutely ischemic limb, presumably as a result of a reduction in the incidence of in-hospital cardiopulmonary complications in the operative group.

It is likely that different patient categories will benefit from one form of therapy over another. Anecdotal experience suggested that some patients will be best served with thrombolysis, while others will benefit most from immediate operative interven-

TABLE 41–4. ECONOMIC COSTS OF THROMBOLYTIC VERSUS OPERATIVE INTERVENTION IN THE INITIAL MANAGEMENT OF ACUTE PERIPHERAL ARTERIAL OCCLUSION

Costs	Thrombolysis (n = 57)	Operation (n = 57)
Hospital Cost	$22,171	$19,775
Professional Fees	$2,445	$3,517
Total Costs	$24,616	$23,292
One-year Survival Rate Percent	58	84
Cost per Life Saved	$29,305	$40,158

Modified from Ouriel K, Shortell CK, DeWeese JA, et al. A comparison of thrombolytic therapy with operative revascularization in the treatment of acute peripheral arterial ischemia. *J Vasc Surg.* 1994;19:1021–1030.

tion (Figure 41–5). In a multivariate analysis of patients treated with intra-arterial thrombolysis, five variables were found to be predictive of successful arteriographic dissolution (Table 41–3).[39] Technical factors appeared most important. Successful lysis was seldom achieved if the infusion catheter could not be threaded into the thrombus or if a guide wire could not be passed through the occlusive process. Several clinical factors also attained significance as independent predictors of arteriographic success. Vein grafts were less likely to undergo successful lysis than prosthetic grafts or native arteries. Lysis was more frequently achieved in nondiabetics than diabetics and in patients with fewer arterial segments involved.

The economics of thrombolysis have attained increased importance with the recent emphasis on the cost of health care. Thrombolysis appears to be associated with a similar length of hospital stay when compared with operative intervention.[12] The cost of hospitalization may be somewhat greater when thrombolytic therapy is employed, principally as a result of the cost of the lytic agent (Table 41–4).[38] When professional fees are considered, however, these differences vanish. Clear advantages to the use of thrombolysis are realized when the cost data are expressed in relation to the dollars expended per life saved.

REFERENCES

1. Green RM, DeWeese JA, Rob CG. Arterial embolectomy before and after the Fogarty catheter. *Surgery.* 1975;77:24–33.
2. Blaisdell FW, Steele M, Allen RE. Management of acute lower extremity arterial ischemia due to embolism and thrombosis. *Surgery.* 1978;84:822–834.
3. Edwards JE, Taylor LM Jr, Porter JM. Treatment of failed lower extremity bypass grafts with new autogenous vein bypass grafting. *J Vasc Surg.* 1990;11:136–145.
4. Jivegård L, Holm J, Schersten T. Acute limb ischemia due to arterial embolism or thrombosis: influence of limb ischemia versus pre-existing cardiac disease on postoperative mortality rate. *J Cardiovasc Surg.* 1988;29:32–36.
5. Tillett WS, Sherry S. The effect in patients of streptococcal fibrinolysin (streptokinase) and streptococcal desoxyribonuclease on fibrinous, purulent, and sanguinous pleural exudations. *J Clin Invest.* 1949;28:173.
6. Tillett WS, Sherry S, Christensen LR. Streptococcal desoxyribonuclease: significance in lysis of purulent exudates and production by strains of hemolytic streptococci. *Proc Soc Exp Biol Med.* 1948;68:184.
7. Cliffton EE, Grossi CE. Investigations of intravenous plasmin (fibrinolysin) in humans: physiologic and clinical effects. *Circulation.* 1956;14:919.

8. Cliffton EE. The use of plasmin in humans. *Ann N Y Acad Sci.* 1957;68:209–229.

9. Dotter CT, Rösch J, Seaman AJ. Selective clot lysis with low-dose streptokinase. *Radiology.* 1974;111:31–37.

10. Rutherford RB, Flanigan DP, Gupta SK, et al. Suggested standards for reports dealing with lower extremity ischemia. *J Vasc Surg.* 1986;4:80–94.

11. McNamara TO, Fischer JR. Thrombolysis of peripheral arterial and graft occlusions: improved results using high-dose urokinase. *Am J Roentgenol.* 1985;144:769–775.

12. Ouriel K, Shortell CK, DeWeese JA, et al. A comparison of thrombolytic therapy with operative revascularization in the treatment of acute peripheral arterial ischemia. *J Vasc Surg.* 1994;19:1021–1030.

13. Jang IK, Gold HK, Ziskind AA, et al. Differential sensitivity of erythrocyte-rich and platelet-rich arterial thrombi to lysis with recombinant tissue-type plasminogen activator: a possible explanation for resistance to coronary thrombolysis. *Circulation.* 1989;79:920–928.

14. Yeager RA, Moneta GL, Taylor LM Jr, et al. Surgical management of severe acute lower extremity ischemia. *J Vasc Surg.* 1992;15:385–393.

15. Marder VJ. The use of thrombolytic agents: choice of patient, drug administration, laboratory monitoring. *Ann Intern Med.* 1979;90:802–812.

16. Alkjaersig N, Fletcher AP, Sherry S. The mechanism of clot dissolution by plasmin. *J Clin Invest.* 1959;38:1086.

17. Agnelli G, Buchanan MR, Fernandez F, Hirsh J. The thrombolytic and hemorrhagic effects of tissue type plasminogen activator: influence of dosage regimens in rabbits. *Thromb Res.* 1985;40:769–777.

18. Goldhaber SZ, Heit J, Sharma GVRK, et al. Randomized controlled trial of recombinant tissue plasminogen activator versus urokinase in the treatment of acute pulmonary embolism. *Lancet.* 1988;2:293–298.

19. Kane KK. Fibrinolysis: a review. *Ann Clin Lab Sci.* 1984;14:443–449.

20. Meyerovitz MF, Goldhaber SZ, Regan K, et al. Recombinant tissue-type plasminogen activator versus urokinase in peripheral arterial and graft occlusions: a randomized trial. *Radiology.* 1990;175:75–78.

21. Graor RA, Olin J, Bartholomew JR, et al. Efficacy and safety of intraarterial local infusion of streptokinasae, urokinase, or tissue plasminogen activator for peripheral arterial occlusion: a retrospective review. *J Vasc Med Biol.* 1990;2:310–315.

22. Nilsson L, Albrechtsson U, Jonung T, et al. Surgical treatment versus thrombolysis in acute arterial occlusion: a randomized controlled study. *Eur J Vasc Surg.* 1992;6:189–193.

23. McNamara TO. Thrombolysis as an alternative initial therapy for the acutely ischemic lower limb. *Semin Vasc Surg.* 1992;5:89–98.

24. Gardiner GA Jr, Sullivan KL. Catheter-directed thrombolysis for the failed lower extremity bypass graft. *Semin Vasc Surg.* 1992;5:99–103.

25. Allen DR, Smallwood J, Johnson CD. Intra-arterial thrombolysis should be the initial treatment of the acutely ischaemic lower limb. *Ann R Coll Surg Engl.* 1992;74:106–108.

26. Faggioli GL, Peer RM, Pedrini L, et al. Failure of thrombolytic therapy to improve long-term vascular patency. *J Vasc Surg.* 1994;19:289–297.

27. McNamara TO, Bomberger RA, Merchant RF. Intra-arterial urokinase as the initial therapy for acutely ischemic lower limbs. *Circulation.* 1991;83 [Suppl I]:I-106–I-119.

28. Hess H. Thrombolytische therapie. In: *Symposion der Deutschen Gesellschaft fur Angiologie.* Stuttgart, Germany: Springer-Verlag; 1967:91–108.

29. Hess H, Ingrisch H, Mietaschk A, Rath H. Local low-dose thrombolytic therapy of peripheral arterial occlusions. *N Engl J Med.* 1982;307:1627–1630.

30. McNamara TO, Bomberger RA. Factors affecting initial and 6 month patency rates after intraarterial thrombolysis with high dose urokinase. *Am J Surg.* 1986;152:709–712.

31. Kandarpa K, Chopra PS, Aruny JE, et al. Prospective, randomized comparison of forced periodic infusion and conventional slow continuous infusion. *Radiology.* 1993;188:1–7.

32. Marder VJ, Sherry S. Thrombolytic therapy: current status (II). *N Engl J Med.* 1988; 318:1585–1595.

33. Graor RA, Risius B, Young JR, et al. Low-dose streptokinase for selective thrombolysis: systemic effects and complications. *Radiology.* 1984;152:35–39.

34. Krings W, Roth FJ, Cappius G, Schmidtke I. Catheter-lysis: indications and primary results. *Int Angiol.* 1985;4:117–123.
35. Graor RA, Risius B, Lucas FV, et al. Thrombolysis with recombinant human tissue-type plasminogen activator in patients with peripheral artery and bypass graft occlusions. *Circulation.* 1986;74:I-15–I-20.
36. Sicard GA, Schier JJ, Totty WG, et al. Thrombolytic therapy for acute arterial occlusion. *J Vasc Surg.* 1985;2:65–78.
37. Ricotta J. Intra-arterial thrombolysis: a surgical view. *Circulation.* 1991;83:I-120–I-121.
38. Ouriel K, Shortell CK, Green RM, DeWeese JA. Differential mechanisms of failure of autogenous and nonautogenous bypass conduits: an assessment following successful graft thrombolysis. *Cardiovasc Surg.* [in press].

XI

Arterial Injury to the Lower Extremity

42

The Role of Color-Flow Duplex Ultrasonography in the Management of Arterial Injuries in Penetrating Trauma

Jonathan B. Towne, MD, and Janis Edwards, RN, RVT

The role of vascular assessment in patients with extremity limb trauma remains one of the more controversial areas in trauma vascular surgery. In most instances, a thorough clinical examination detects the presence and location of both major arterial and venous injury and directs surgical management correctly.[1] Immediate operation is indicated for patients with absent distal pulses, distal ischemia, expanding hematoma, and active hemorrhage. When the site of arterial injury is obvious, modalities to examine the site of the injury only delay operation and do not contribute to the care of the patient. The area of greatest controversy is the evaluation of a patient who has an injury close to a major blood vessel without any signs of a serious vascular injury.

Throughout the past several decades the pendulum has swung from routine exploration to routine angiography, which has evolved into selective angiography.[2–5] Routine exploration has been associated with a high rate of negative explorations. Sirinek et al,[2] in a 5-year study of 390 patients who were explored for suspected vascular injury, had a negative exploration rate of 64%.[2] Negative exploration was associated with a 5% morbidity and a 0.4% mortality, indicating that this is not a totally risk-free procedure. Since arteriography has been used in place of exploration for injuries close to major blood vessels, there has been a high incidence of negative arteriograms. Reid et al, in a study of 507 patients with 534 asymptomatic penetrating extremity injuries, all of which were evaluated with arteriography, demonstrated a 6.7% incidence of abnormal angiograms.[3] Of these abnormal findings, 1.9% were later determined to be false-positive angiograms on subsequent surgical exploration. Of importance is that arteriography was associated with a 2.6% incidence of complications.

The value of arterography in decreasing the negative exploration rate was demonstrated by Geuder et al.[5] In a study in which all patients with potential vascular injuries were explored, the negative exploration rate was 84%, which decreased to

2.4% when angiography was used in the initial evaluation of injuries close to major blood vessels. In a study by Hessel et al, which was a review of radiologists from 514 hospitals reporting a total of 118,000 examinations, the angiography complication rate was 1.7% for transfemoral, 2.89% for translumbar, and 3.29% for transaxillary approach.[6] The investigators noted a mortality of 0.3%, indicating that angiography is safe but not totally risk free.

Because of the persistent false-positive rate with angiography, which is about 2%, as well as the small but measurable morbidity related to arteriography and its cost, there has been an increasing interest in developing surveillance techniques that are more efficient both in terms of time and cost. Duplex ultrasound (US) is uniquely qualified for this. It is noninvasive and allows follow up to be done easily. This chapter deals with the usefulness in evaluation and technique of duplex US examinations.

Duplex US scanning is the combination of two US techniques to obtain anatomic and hemodynamic information from the peripheral, cerebrovascular, and abdominal vasculature. These systems combine high-resolution real-time US imaging for assessment of vessel wall anatomy and pulsed Doppler spectral analysis to yield information about blood flow characteristics. Color-flow imaging provides two-dimensional displays composed of real-time flow superimposed on gray-scale anatomic scans,[7] which are able to display Doppler-shifted echoes as various shades of color. Imaging is used to locate vessels and evaluate wall characteristics and morphologic changes. Pulsed Doppler spectral analysis measures blood flow velocities at precise points within the visualized vessel and provides diagnostic information regarding normal or turbulent flow.

Duplex US has become the standard technique for determining the presence and severity of disease in the carotid arteries and is gaining widespread use for diagnostic, intraoperative, and postoperative evaluation of all vascular systems.

The feasibility for using duplex US to evaluate arterial injury was demonstrated in the laboratory by Panetta et al, who produced a laceration, blunt injury, and arteriovenous (AV) fistulas in the femoral and carotid arteries of dogs and then evaluated these by duplex US and biplane arteriography to determine the accuracy of duplex US in detecting arterial injury.[8] They found the duplex US was more sensitive (90.1% vs 80.2%) at detecting arterial injury. It was particularly better at identifying lacerated arteries. Arteriography had a greater specificity (94.7% vs 68.4%) and was more accurate in identifying normal arteries. The authors noticed that the validity of duplex US increased in the latter half of the study, demonstrating, very importantly, that there was a learning curve.

Following this work our group performed a prospective study comparing color-flow duplex US scanning with arteriography in 67 patients who sustained 75 penetrating injuries to the extremity without obvious arterial injury.[9] All patients brought to our medical center with penetrating extremity trauma in the area between the clavicle and the wrist or between the inguinal ligament and the ankle were eligible for the study. Patients with ongoing hemorrhage, obvious limb ischemia, vessel occlusion, or expanding hematoma were taken immediately to the operating room for vascular surgical repair and were excluded from further study. Patients without obvious vascular injury but with diminished pulses, neurologic deficit, nonexpanding hematoma, or a history of hemorrhage that was controlled at the time of the initial examination were eligible for the study. Patients with a wound close to a major artery but no other physical findings were also eligible. Proximity was assessed by the surgical staff member, a vascular surgery fellow, or a senior fifth-postgraduate-year surgical resident. It was defined as entry, exit, or wound track thought to have passed through or within 1 cm of a major conduit vessel. Eligible patients underwent biplane intra-arterial digital subtraction angiography generally within 24 hours of admission. Patients were also offered color-flow duplex US examinations of the affected extremity.

The duplex US examinations were performed by registered vascular technologists or a vascular surgical fellow specializing in vascular US. The vascular laboratory is a full-time noninvasive vascular laboratory directed by a vascular surgeon and accredited by the Intersocietal Commission for Accreditation of Vascular Laboratories. Most examinations were performed by a single vascular nurse specialist or by a vascular fellow. These examinations were performed either in the vascular laboratory or in the intensive care unit. With a 3- or 5-to-10-MHz tranducer, scans were performed with longitudinal and transverse views with imaging of the entire arterial segment thought to be at risk. The vessel contour, compressibility, and presence of fluid collections were assessed. Doppler waveforms, spectral analysis of segments at risk, and segments proximal and distal to the area in question gave information regarding the direction of flow, spectral configuration, turbulence, phasicity, and presence of flow in adjacent fluid collection. When possible, duplex US scanning was performed before arteriography. At no time were results seen on arteriogram made known to those performing or interpreting the duplex US images until the duplex US examination had been completed and interpreted.

Positive examinations were defined as those demonstrating injury that warranted surgical repair, including AV fistulas, pseudoaneurysms, intimal flaps, or occlusions of major conduit vessels. Negative examinations were defined as those that were not positive, that is, normal, as well as any with mild abnormalities that did not appear to warrant surgery (spasm narrowing, perivessel hematoma, pseudoaneurysm or occlusion of small branch vessels, and any venous injury. The decision to intervene surgically was made by the attending trauma surgeon and the consulting vascular surgeon and based on the physical findings and arteriographic results. Patients with negative examination were discharged after recovery from arteriography unless wound care or other injuries warranted further hospitalization.

The 75 penetrating injuries in 67 patients included 63 gunshot wounds, nine stab wounds, and three shotgun wounds. Physical findings demonstrated negative examinations of 85% of the patients, a hematoma in 11%, neurologic deficit in 3%, and decreased distal pulse in one patient. Ninety-six percent of the color-flow duplex US examinations were negative; 4% were positive. Color-flow duplex US scanning was successful in all patients, although the presence of open wounds, tender soft tissue, and hematomas made performance of the duplex US scanning more challenging than in other clinical settings. The arterial segments examined are shown in Table 42–1. The incidence of positive angiograms was 5.3%.

TABLE 42–1. ARTERIAL SEGMENTS EXAMINED WITH ARTERIOGRAPHY AND COLOR-FLOW DUPLEX ULTRASONOGRAPHIC SCANNING

Arterial Segment	No.	Percentage
Axillary	8	10.6
Brachial	7	9.3
Radial/ulnar	1	1.3
Common femoral	3	4.0
Superficial/deep femoral	44	58.7
Popliteal	5	6.7
Tibioperoneal/anterior/posterior tibial/peroneal	7	9.3

All arteriographic abnormalities were confirmed at subsequent surgical procedures. Two of these were demonstrated on color-flow duplex US examinations. Two of the patients who had positive arteriograms had negative color-flow duplex US examinations and thus had false-negative examinations. They both had small pseudoaneurysms—one at the mid humeral level in a radial artery that originated well above the elbow and the second in the axillary area (Fig. 42–1).

Seventy negative color-flow duplex US examinations were confirmed by negative arteriography. These included some that were slightly abnormal but either demonstrated minor injuries that did not merit surgical repair or were not believed to demonstrate injuries at all. One positive color-flow scan read as showing a popliteal artery-pseudoaneurysm actually showed a pseudoaneurysm originating from the genicular artery (Fig. 42–2). Because this injury was not believed to require surgical repair and because of the location of the pseudoaneurysm was slightly different from that indicated by the color-flow duplex US scan, we categorized this a false-positive result.

Pseudoaneurysms were detected on color-flow imaging by loss of vessel wall integrity and by a contiguous, rounded fluid-filled cavity (Fig. 42–3). Turbulent flow with accompanying spectral broadening was demonstrated in the cavity and the adjacent vessel. Pseudoaneurysm cavity size correlated well with that estimated by arteriography. AV fistulas are characterized by continuous diastolic flow in the proximal arterial segment and turbulent flow at the injury site and in the proximal venous

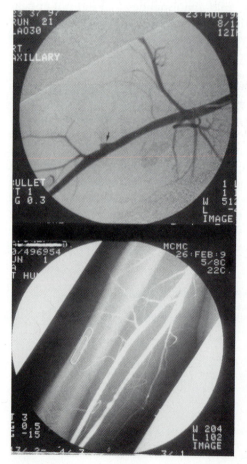

Figure 42–1. *Top,* axillary artery pseudoaneurysm missed on US imaging. *Bottom,* pseudoaneurysm at midhumeral level of an aberrant radial artery originating just distal to the axilla that was missed on US imaging. (*Reprinted with permission from Bergstein JF, Blair JF, Edwards J, Towne JB, et al. Pitfalls in the use of color-flow duplex ultrasound for screening of suspected arterial injuries in penetrated extremities. J Trauma. 1992;33:395–402.*)

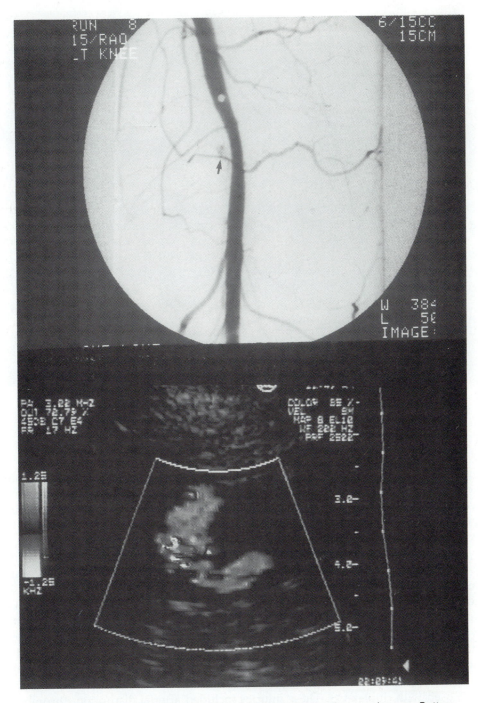

Figure 42–2. *Top,* pseudoaneurysm of genicular artery (arrow) on angiogram. *Bottom,* same vessel seen on color-flow duplex US scan. Note appearance of contiguous flow between popliteal artery (below) and pseudoaneurysm (above). This was considered a false-positive color-flow duplex US study. (*Reprinted with permission from Bergstein JF, Blair JF, Edwards J, Towne JB, et al. Pitfalls in the use of color-flow duplex ultrasound for screening of suspected arterial injuries in penetrated extremities. J Trauma. 1992; 33:395–402.*)

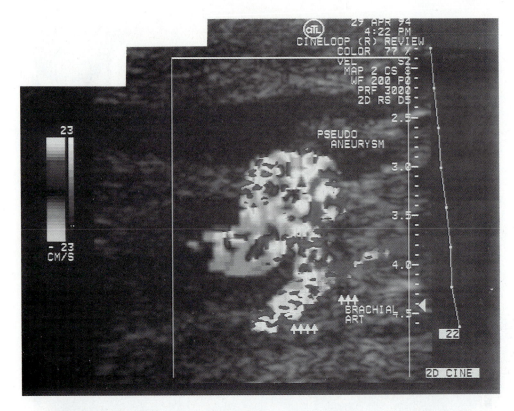

Figure 42–3. Color-flow duplex US image demonstrating pseudoaneurysm obtained after angiogram was obtained by means of catheterization of brachial artery.

segment with arterialization to the venous signal (Fig. 42–4). Spectral broadening indicative of turbulent flow was also present. Our final results were 72 negative, two positive, two false-negative, and one false-positive examinations, resulting in a specificity of 99%, sensitivity of 50%, positive predictive value of 66%, negative predictive value of 97%, and an overall accuracy of 96%.

The utility of duplex US evaluation in extremity trauma was evaluated by Bynoe et al.[10] They evaluated 198 consecutive trauma patients with one or more potential vascular injuries who were prospectively studied by the use of standard duplex US techniques. Patients with obvious signs of arterial injury were excluded and taken directly to the operating room. These authors identified vascular injury with a sensitivity of 95% but, more important, excluded vascular injuries with a specificity of 99% with an overall accuracy of 98%. One advantage of duplex US examination noted by these authors was the ability to depict venous injuries. Their series included thrombosis, AV fistulas, and venous disruption (Fig. 42–5). All major arterial injuries were diagnosed with duplex US. These injuries included arterial disruption, thrombosis, intimal flap, pseudoaneurysms, AV fistulas, and shotgun pellet arterial puncture with distal embolization. For the 20 major vascular injuries, 13 of the repairs were performed on the basis of duplex US alone without the need for confirmatory arteriography. Injuries missed by the duplex US scan included two minor shotgun pellet arterial punctures. One patient had a shotgun wound in the thigh near his superficial femoral artery and a fluctuating dorsal pedal pulse that prompted arteriography. No superficial femoral artery injury was seen, but the shotgun pellet had embolized distally in the

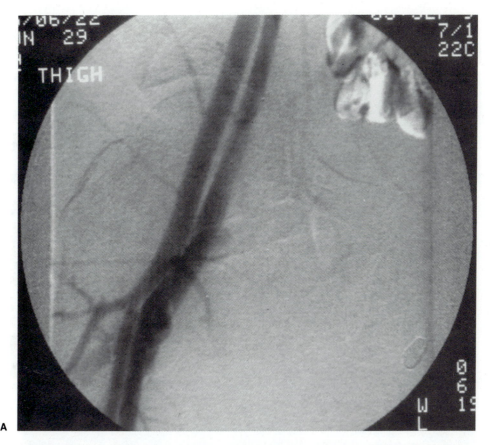

Figure 42–4. Femoral AV fistula after gunshot wound. Angiogram (**A**) and color duplex US scan (**B**). (*Reprinted with permission from Bergstein JF, Blair JF, Edwards J, Towne JB, et al. Pitfalls in the use of color-flow duplex ultrasound for screening of suspected arterial injuries in penetrated extremities. J Trauma. 1992;33:395–402.*) (*Figure continues*)

dorsal pedal artery. A second patient had a shotgun pellet that was found imbedded in the wall of the superficial femoral artery during surgical debridement. The only false-positive finding in this study was a carotid plaque that was atherosclerotic in origin and was interpreted as an intimal flap.

Meissner et al evaluated duplex US as a screening tool for arterial trauma in 89 patients with 93 injuries, mostly of the extremities.[11] Among the 60 scans performed solely because of wound proximity to nearby vascular structures, 6.7% were positive, as compared to 68% in patients with clinical indications of vascular injury. There were four false-negative duplex US scans, for an incidence of 4.3%; however, no major arterial injuries were missed and no false-positive studies were noted. Of the 6.7% abnormal studies in proximity-only injuries, the authors demonstrated occlusion of posterior tibial arteries, anterior tibial arteries, and internal carotid arteries as well as a large hematoma without other vascular abnormalities. Four patients had abnormal angiograms in the presence of normal duplex US studies. These included demonstrations of an occluded costocervical trunk, a brachial artery intimal flap, and an occluded distal profunda femoris artery (deep femoral) branch in the superficial femoral artery spasm.

The role of duplex US arterial imaging in patients with penetrating arterial trauma was studied by Knudson et al.[12] They evaluated 86 extremities in 77 patients who

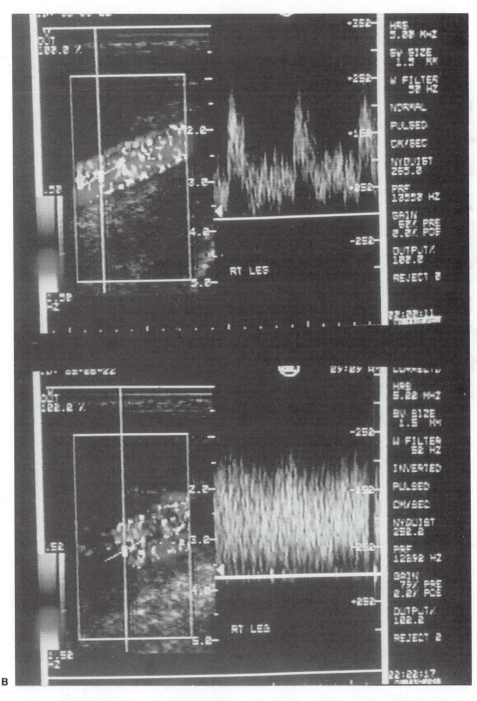

Figure 42–4. (*continued*)

did not have definitive signs of arterial injury, for example, expanding or pulsating hematoma, absent or distal pulses, bruit throw, or hemorrhage from the wound. Five percent of these patients had abnormal duplex US examinations and underwent arteriography. In all of the patients, the injury suggested by the duplex US scan was confirmed at arteriography. These included small intimal defect, a peripheral AV

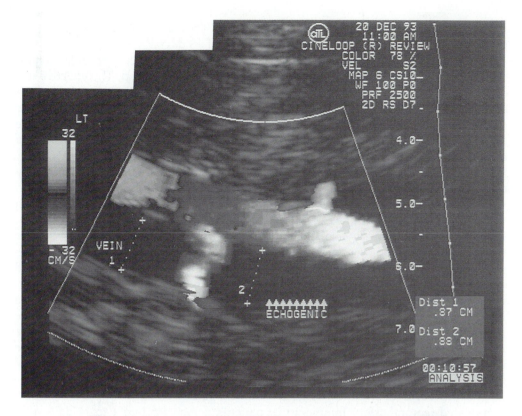

Figure 42–5. Superficial femoral vein thrombosis after gunshot wound.

fistula, and a popliteal AV fistula. None of the patients who had negative duplex US examinations had signs or symptoms of vascular injury in clinical follow-up.

As a result of these studies, duplex US examination can be used for screening of patients with proximity-only indications. There are several caveats. First, duplex US scanning is technician-dependent. Only experienced technicians should perform this test. Ideally, these technicians should be certified and work in a laboratory that participates in an ongoing quality assurance program to document the validity of their findings.

Several pitfalls may affect the examination. In the head and neck region in muscular people, it is sometimes difficult to visualize the vascular structures beneath the clavicle. If these structures cannot be adequately visualized, arteriography is indicated. Second, the technicians have to be aware of commonly-occurring anatomic variations. This was the cause of errors in two of our patients. These variations most commonly involve bifurcation of the brachial artery and bifurcation of the popliteal artery. Finally, none of these tests are 100% accurate, emphasizing the need for careful follow up of these patients. In the trauma setting, follow up is often difficult, but attempts should be made to accomplish it.

An important role of duplex US examination is the evaluation and treatment of complications following femoral artery catheterizations for most cardiac interventional procedures. Sheikh et al evaluated 25 patients referred to the US laboratory for evaluation of possible femoral complications related to recent cardiac catheterization.[13] Five patients had normal examinations and in the remaining 20 patients there were 14 pseudoaneurysms and nine AV fistulas. Johns et al used duplex US scans to evaluate small false aneurysms after arterial catheterization. They demonstrated that many of these false aneurysms had resolved after a mean of 18 days.[14]

An effective use of duplex US scanning is the obliteration of catheter-related false aneurysms and AV fistulas with pressure applied by the scan head. The effective use of this technique precludes surgical intervention in a large number of cases. Feld et al used US-guided compression to occlude pseudoaneurysms in the groin following cardiac catheterization in 16 of 18 patients, cerebral angiography in one, and multiple femoral punctures to retrieve blood samples in one.[15] Their technique included a careful search to identify the neck of the pseudoaneurysm or the site of the AV fistula. Under direct sonographic monitoring, the neck of the pseudoaneurysm was manually compressed with the duplex US transducer, which interrupted flow into the lesion without compromising flow in the underlying or adjacent vasculature. Compression was maintained for 10 minutes, 20 minutes in patients who received anticoagulation. Pressure was then slowly released and flow was reassessed. Compressions were repeated for the same time increments if necessary until a successful outcome was obtained. On occasion, this procedure was attempted on subsequent days. In the 18 patients evaluated, three false aneurysms spontaneously thrombosed. In the remaining 15 patients, successful thrombosis was obtained in 56%. Three of the patients in whom the initial trial of compression failed had spontaneous thrombosis of the pseudoaneurysm after anticoagulation was reduced or withdrawn. Compression times ranged from 10 minutes to as long as 150 minutes of intermittent pressure. The average compression time was 53 minutes. Included was one single patient who had an AV fistula that responded to compression.

Fellmeth et al reported a 93% success with US-guided compression of catheterization-related femoral artery injuries in 29 patients detected 6 hours to 14 days after catheterization.[16] This is an effective technique that can limit the morbidity associated with treatment of this complication.

REFERENCES

1. Turcotte JK, Towne JB, Bernhard VB. Is arteriography necessary in the management of vascular trauma of the extremities? *Surgery*. 1978;84:557–562.
2. Sirinek KR, Levine BA, Gaskill III HV, Root HD. Reassessment of the role of routine operative exploration in vascular trauma. *J Trauma*. 1981;21:341–344.
3. Reid JDS, Weigelt JA, Thal ER, Francis HF III. Assessment of proximity of a wound to major vascular structures as an indication for arteriography. *Arch Surg*. 1988;123:942–946.
4. Menzoian JO, Doyle JE, LoGerfo FW, et al. Evaluation and management of vascular injuries of the extremities. *Arch Surg*. 1983;118:93–95.
5. Geuder JW, Hobson II RW, Padberg FT Jr et al. The role of contrast arteriography in suspected arterial injuries of the extremities. *Am Surg*. 1985;2:89–93.
6. Hessel SJ, Adams DF, Abrams HL. Complications of angiography. *Diag Radiol*. 1981;138:273–281.
7. Kremkau FW. *Doppler ultrasound: principles and instruments*. Philadelphia, PA: WB Saunders; 1990:114.
8. Panetta TF, Hunt JP, Buechter KJ, et al. Duplex ultrasonography versus arteriography in the diagnosis of arterial injury: an experimental study. *J Trauma*. 1992;33:627–636.
9. Bergstein JF, Blair JF, Edwards J, et al. Pitfalls in the use of color-flow duplex ultrasound for screening of suspected arterial injuries in penetrated extremities. *J Trauma*. 1992;33:395–402.
10. Bynoe RP, Miles WS, Bell RM, et al. Noninvasive diagnosis of vascular trauma by duplex ultrasonography. *J Vasc Surg*. 1991;14:346–352.

11. Meissner M, Paun M, Johansen K. Duplex scanning for arterial trauma. *Am J Surg.* 1991;161:552–555.
12. Knudson MM, Lewis FR, Atkinson K, Neuhaus A. The role of duplex ultrasound arterial imaging in patients with penetrating extremity trauma. *Arch Surg.* 1993;128:1033–1038.
13. Sheikh KH, Adams DV, McCann R, et al. Utility of Doppler color flow imaging for identification of femoral arterial complications of cardiac catheterization. *Am Heart J.* 1989;117:623–628.
14. Johns JP, Pupa Jr LE, Bailey SR. Spontaneous thrombosis of iatrogenic femoral artery pseudoaneurysms: documentation with color Doppler and two-dimensional ultrasonography. *J Vasc Surg.* 1991;14:24–29.
15. Feld R, Patton GM, Carabasi RA, et al. Treatment of iatrogenic femoral artery injuries with ultrasound-guided compression. *J Vasc Surg.* 1992;16:832–840.
16. Fellmeth BD, Roberts AC, Bookstein JJ, et al. Postangiographic femoral artery injuries: nonsurgical repair with US-guided compression. *Radiology.* 191;178:671–675.

43

Compartment Syndrome

William D. Turnipseed, MD

Compartment syndrome is a clinical condition that results in compromised perfusion to neuromuscular structures within confined myofascial spaces of the upper or lower extremities.[1-3] The underlying pathology resulting in impaired tissue perfusion is compartmental hypertension. Acute increases in myofascial compartment pressure may result from blunt[4] or penetrating injuries,[5] associated long-bone fractures[6] or vascular trauma,[7] severe soft-tissue crush injury,[8] delayed treatment of sudden arterial occlusions,[9] thermal burns, extrinsic muscle compression,[10] or accidental extravasation of caustic chemicals into subcutaneous tissues.[11] These insults can trigger a cascade of physiologic events that left unchecked result in neuromuscular injury, permanent disability, and possibly amputation.

One of the earliest modern descriptions of acute compartment syndrome (ACS) was made by Richard Von Volkmann in 1881.[12] He correlated the development of permanent flexion and contracture of the hand with the use of rigid casting in the treatment supracondylar humeral fractures in adolescents. These patients experienced unremitting forearm pain, hand edema, progressive muscular dysfunction, hyperesthesia, and permanent flexion contracture of the hand. Bardenheuer, in 1911, was the first to propose and successfully use fasciotomy in the treatment of this condition.[13] Since that time surgical release procedures have been widely used in the treatment of ACS. Diagnosis of this condition can usually be made on the basis of progressive motor sensory limb dysfunction associated with provocative trauma, and the onset of common clinical findings such as tense swelling and edema of compartment muscles, disproportionate muscle pain aggravated by passive extension, decreased peripheral pulses, and slow capillary refill.[14] Despite a general awareness of this condition, the diagnosis of ACS is often delayed or missed because there has been no consistent agreement as to indications, timing, and method of treatment.

The diagnosis of ACS should be suspected clinically when blunt or penetrating trauma is followed by limb swelling, motor-sensory dysfunction, and vasomotor instability. Surgery should be performed when these conditions exist. Clinical diagnosis of ACS may be more difficult to confirm in a comatose or confused patient and may require compartment pressure measurements for confirmation. Compartment pressures can be measured with a Wick catheter,[15] the Whitesides needle method,[16] or by use of a handheld computerized needle transducer (Stryker, Kalamazoo, Mich). There is no absolute pressure associated with clinical development of compartment syndrome.[14] Normal resting pressure in the lower leg compartment is less than 15 mm Hg. Circulatory impairment begins to occur when compartment pressure increases to within 30 mm Hg of normal diastolic pressure.[15] When this happens, normal venous drainage is impaired, aggravating further edema and soft-tissue swelling. When clinical symptoms of ACS coexist with resting compartment pressures that exceed 30 mm Hg, open fasciotomy should be performed. Patients in shock may have swelling at lower pressures. Transcutaneous Doppler venous flow has been used in conjunction with serial measurement of compartment pressures to more accurately diagnose impending acute compartment syndromes. Loss of phasic flow is the first Doppler change that occurs, and these changes correlate with pressures that exceed 25 mm Hg. Loss of venous flow augmentation correlates with pressures exceeding 30 mm Hg.[17] Although there is no predictable clinical relationship between the development of compartment symptoms and pressure measurements between 30 and 60 mm Hg, ischemic symptoms uniformly develop when pressures exceed 60 mm Hg.[18]

In general, its safer to err on the side of commission and to perform compartment release surgery when clinical signs and symptoms are present even though pressure measurements may not be striking. Early decompressive fasciotomy frequently averts ischemic complications and prevents permanent disability and/or amputation. The only treatment of ACS is *open* fasciotomy and/or fasciectomy. There is no place for subcutaneous fasciotomy in these patients because skin and subcutaneous tissue have a limited ability to stretch.[19]

Several techniques for compartment release have been described. The double-incision technique first described by Mubarek and Owen[19] is the most widely used procedure and is performed using a linear incision on the anterior lateral surface of the lower leg half way between the anterior border and the lateral border of the fibula. Fasciotomy and/or fasciectomy can be used to release the anterior and lateral compartments through this approach. A medial incision is made just posterior to the tibia at the medial calf and used to relieve both the superficial and deep posterior compartments. It is necessary to take down the medial tibial attachments of the soleus muscle to completely relieve the deep posterior compartment. Anterolateral, posterior superficial, and distal posterior deep compartment releases can be performed using local anesthesia. Proximal deep posterior compartment release requires spinal or general anesthesia.

Alternative methods of surgically decompressing the four muscle compartments of the lower extremity include fibulectomy-fasciotomy and lateral four-compartment fasciotomy without the use of fibulectomy. Fibulectomy was originally proposed by Kelly and Whitesides in 1967.[20] This technique has not been widely accepted because of concern regarding impaired limb function and valgus deformity of the foot. Fibulectomy actually can be very effective in accomplishing complete decompression of the distal lower extremity without considerable morbidity. The fibula has no weight-bearing function in adults and exists primarily as a strut for muscle and ligamentous attachments. However, the distal fibula is important for maintaining stability of the ankle joint and preventing valgus deformity. Although an intact fibula can be used to stabilize adjacent tibial fractures, in most cases when trauma is severe enough to cause an associated compartment syndrome both bones are broken, and excision of the fibula carries with it very little additional morbidity.

Fibulectomy is performed by making a skin incision two fingerbreadths below the fibular head that is carried distally to a point approximately four fingerbreadths above the lateral malleolus. This incision is carried down to the fascia of the lateral compartment. The intermuscular septum between the lateral and posterior superficial compartment can be identified distally if the finger is inserted posterior to the peroneus longus tendon. The intermuscular septum is split the entire length of the incision, releasing the posterior superficial compartment. The fibular periosteum is then excised and the fibula transected 10 cm above the lateral malleolus distally and proximally approximately at the fibular neck. The deep posterior compartment is entered by an incision in the medial wall of the periosteal bed. The anterior compartment can be entered through a periosteal incision anterior and parallel to the previous incision (Fig. 43–1). Fibulectomy-fasciotomy is a good technique but reservations about its use are hard to dispute. This method does seem to be appropriate when a crush injury is associated with multiple lower bone fractures, since the fibula plays no important part in functional orthopedic repair of these injuries.[21]

A modification of the fibulectomy approach was described by Nghiem and Bolan in 1980[22] and by Rollins et al in 1981.[9] This technique allows complete myofascial decompression of the distal lower extremity without fibulectomy. It is performed by making a lateral skin incision over the fibula, extending from the neck to approximately 4 cm above the lateral malleolus. The incision is carried down to the overlying lateral compartment fascia, which is open its entire length. The anterior fascia is exposed by retracting the skin and using a separate long, parallel fascial incision to decompress the extensor muscles of the foot. The skin and subcutaneous tissue overlying the posterior superficial compartment are retracted, and fascia is incised along the entire length of the gastrocnemius and soleus muscles. The attachments of the soleus muscle to the fibula are divided so as to expose the deep posterior compartment. Fascia investing the deep flexors can be incised by epimysiotomy of the individual muscle bellies if necessary. This technique is effective, assures complete selective decompres-

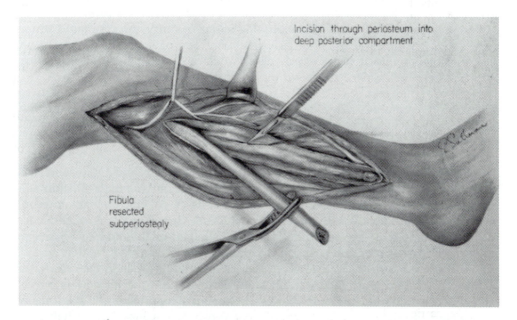

Figure 43–1. Surgical decompression of all four compartments in the distal lower extremity can be released through a lateral incision. Surgical decompression is facilitated by partial resection of the fibula. The deep posterior compartment release is performed by incising the medial wall of the fibular periosteal tube. (*Reprinted with permission from Ernst CB, Kaufer H. Fibulectomy-fasciotomy. J Trauma. 1971;2:368–380.*)

sion of each compartment, avoids possible functional consequences of fibulectomy, and can be performed with one incision.

ACUTE COMPARTMENT SYNDROMES

ACSs most commonly affect the lower extremity and may be caused by penetrating gunshot wounds, blunt trauma, or by delayed treatment of acute thromboembolic arterial occlusions. Less common causes include severe crush injury and extrinsic muscle compression associated with drug or alcohol abuse. Iatrogenic causes of ACS include use of military antishock trousers (MAS) in the treatment of trauma victims;[23,24] prolonged pelvic surgery operations with patients in the lithotomy position;[25,26] intramuscular hemorrhage associated with the use of oral anticoagulation,[27] reperfusion injury following the use of thrombolytic drugs, and extravasation of caustic intravenous drugs into subcutaneous tissues.

Low-velocity gunshot wounds do not usually cause enough soft-tissue damage to result in an ACS unless coexistent arterial and/or venous injuries occur. In a review of post-traumatic lower extremity complications following gunshot injuries, Feleciano et al demonstrated that 80% of all patients in whom ACS developed had angiographic evidence of isolated arterial injury (40%)[5] or combined arterial and venous trauma (40%). Shah et al confirmed this observation. They noted that compartment problems often developed when patients experienced more than 6 hours of ischemia.[28] Femoral and/or popliteal arterial injuries combined with venous occlusion resulting from ligation or failed venous repair frequently caused an acute ischemic compartment syndrome. As a consequence, prophylactic fasciotomy is recommended by both groups of authors when dual vascular injuries occur and when restoration of circulation to an ischemic limb has been delayed more than 6 hours. The most common cause of amputation among patients with penetrating vascular injury and resultant compartment syndrome is the delay in surgical treatment and/or incomplete compartment release. Patients with neuromuscular defects demonstrated before surgical release almost uniformly had permanent significant postoperative residuals.[28]

A similar pattern of associated vascular injury has been observed in nearly half of patients in whom ACSs develop after blunt trauma. Tibial fractures are commonly associated with such complications and usually involve the anterolateral and/or posterior compartments. Symptoms of impending ischemic injury to anterolateral neuromuscular structures include weakened dorsiflexion of the ankle, exaggerated muscle discomfort with passive toe flexion, muscle swelling, foot drop, and diminished sensation in the first web space. Fasciotomy is essential for preserving limb function when these symptoms occur. Because fasciotomy converts closed fracture sites into open ones, rigid stabilization with intramedullary nails or external fixator is usually necessary. Fasciotomy incisions should be placed so as to allow skin and muscle coverage of vascular anastomoses and sites of orthopedic fracture repair.[1]

ACS is much less likely to develop in the thigh muscles than in the calf muscles because the thigh compartments are much larger in volume and blend anatomically with muscles of the hip and buttocks. Compartment symptoms in the thigh usually are a result of crush injury or high-velocity vehicular crashes. Nearly half of the patients have ipsilateral femoral fractures and multiple associated injuries to the head, thorax, and abdomen. These patients are very ill and have an average trauma score of greater than 32 points. Most patients with massive thigh trauma have myoglobinuria (60%) and may experience renal failure unless aggressively treated with fluids, diuretics, and systemic alkalinizing agents. The mortality may be as high as 50%. Conscious patients often complain of thigh pain, swelling, and muscle weakness. Factors associated with the development of the thigh compartment syndrome include internal fixation of the femur with consequent reduction in the anterior compartment size, coagulopathies with intramuscular hemorrhage, hypotension, and extrinsic muscle compression. Prolonged use of MAST (>2 hours) for these patients should be avoided whenever possible, particularly when hypovolemic shock requiring large volumes of fluid resuscitation occurs. Extrinsic compression from the MAST may precipitate acute muscle ischemia in these circumstances.

The thigh has three myofascial compartments (anterior, medial, posterior). The anterior thigh compartment contains the quadriceps muscle along with the femoral artery, nerve, and vein. Passive flexion of the knee with the hip in full extension causes pain and decreased sensation in the medial thigh, suggesting an anterior thigh compartment syndrome. The posterior compartment contains the hamstring muscles and the sciatic nerve. Posterior compartment symptoms can be elicited by passive extension of the knee with the hip in full flexion. The medial compartment contains the abductor muscle groups and the cutaneous branch of the obturator nerve and is rarely involved. The anterior and posterior compartment symptoms are most commonly associated with acute thigh injury. Surgical release of both anterior and posterior compartments can be achieved using a single laterally placed incision. Fasciotomy should be performed even when open fractures occur, because trauma to the fascial envelope does not assure adequate decompression.[29,30]

Crush syndrome due to limb compression may concurrently result in significant muscle injury and the development of secondary compartment syndromes. The crush syndrome was originally described by Waters and Beall in 1941.[31] Civilian victims of aerial bombardments in London whose extremities were crushed by debris frequently presented with swollen limbs, hypotension, dark urine (myoglobinuria) and acute renal failure. The mortality among these patients was extremely high.

Mubarek and Owen in 1975 described the relationship between compartment syndrome and the crush syndrome.[8] They appropriately referred to the crush syndrome as systemic manifestations of muscle necrosis including acidosis, hyperkalemia and shock, with cardiac and renal failure. The compartment syndrome refers to local manifestations of neuromuscular ischemia due to increased pressure within the myofascial compartments.[8] The most common cause of crush syndrome is prolonged limb compression caused by abnormal positioning of an obtunded, comatose, or drugged patient. Limb swelling is the most common physical finding. There may be evidence of superficial skin injury such as blistering, erythema, and venous congestion. Peripheral pulses are usually intact. Signs of compartmental hypertension are variable and usually include, pain, muscle tenderness, and hypesthesia, with muscle weakness and/or paralysis. Compartmental pressure measurements may be helpful in identifying compartmental hypertension following crush injuries in obtunded patients. Compartment hypertension is associated with significant third-space fluid loses into myofascial spaces. Resultant muscle necrosis causes significant elevations of creatine kinase, production of myoglobinuria, secondary acidosis, hyperkalemia, and even cardiac arrhythmias.

The treatment of crush syndrome includes proper ventilation and control of the airway, particularly for the comatose or obtunded patients. Hypotension requires volume replacement, preferably with isotonic fluid. If urine checks are positive for myoglobin, a forced alkaline diuresis can be achieved with the use of bicarbonate, furosemide, and mannitol. Alkalinized urine makes hematin pigment and myoglobin more soluble in urine and assists in its excretion. Renal failure is usually temporary, but almost always requires dialysis. Isolated limb perfusion, to wash out myoglobin from the injured extremity, may be effective in reducing the magnitude or onset of renal failure. Open fasciotomy should be performed as soon as the diagnosis is made. There is a high incidence of Volkmann-type nerve injury with prolonged compartment hypertension in crush injury patients. When fasciotomy is performed within 12 hours of the onset of symptoms, permanent morbidity is reduced significantly.[18]

Iatrogenic injury has been implicated in the development of ACSs, which adversely affect morbidity statistics in health care centers. Common causes of iatrogenic compartment injuries include use of compression devices such as MAST or orthopedic casts, prolonged lithotomy positioning during lower abdominal and pelvic operations, extravasation of caustic chemicals into subcutaneous tissues, and the use of thrombolytic agents in patients with ischemically threatened limbs. As stated previously, the use of MAST in the treatment of hypovolemic shock may be associated with significant ischemic muscle injury when high compression is maintained for more than 2 hours. MAST compression should be applied no longer than absolutely necessary, and complete deflation and removal of the devices should be accomplished before surgery. MAST must be inflated and deflated in proper sequence, which means that the leg segment should be inflated first, then the abdominal portions, and the decompression sequence reversed. Current guidelines for MAST application outlined by the American College of Surgeons Advanced Trauma Life Support Protocols document a low incidence of the compartment syndrome with proper use.[23]

Closed induction of distal lower extremity fractures and tight application of a rigid cast can result in ischemic injury and secondary myonecrosis due to compartmental hypertension. Patients complain of pain and tightness and may notice dusky cyanosis of the foot and digits. Casts should be split to relieve these symptoms and allow reperfusion to the ischemic limb. Reperfusion is often associated with secondary muscle edema and third-space fluid loss, potentiating further limb swelling. Fiberglass casts, unlike plaster ones, will not give if only one split line is made. The result of incomplete extrinsic pressure release may be further neuromuscular injury. Fiberglass casts should be bivalved and temporarily converted to an open posterior splint. Pulses should be checked, and if absent or diminished, compartment pressures and possibly arteriography should be performed to differentiate intrinsic from extrinsic vascular occlusion. Fasciotomy may prevent myonecrosis and permanent injury if performed soon after the onset of symptoms. If it is not, permanent neuropraxia and/or amputation all too often occur.

Although civilian trauma such as supracondylar fractures, comminuted forearm fractures, thermal injury, soft-tissue compression, and arterial injury are the common causes of ACSs in the upper extremity, iatrogenic injury often is overlooked as a cause and may actually have worse clinical outcomes because patients are often unconscious or obtunded. Accidental extravasation of intravenously administered drugs is the most common mechanism of injury. The most frequent agents associated with such iatrogenic compartment syndromes are phenytoin and doxorubicin.[11] Pressured administration of blood and blood products during surgery can also result in compartment syndrome if extravasated into the soft tissues of the arm. As in the lower extremity, pain unrelieved by immobilization and aggravated by passive stretch of the respective compartment muscles, along with weakness in the flexion of the hand, are strongly suggestive of impending compartment syndrome.

There are two major forearm compartments: the volar and dorsal compartments. The volar compartment is divided into a superficial, intermediate, and deep layer.

The median and ulnar nerves and their respective arteries occupy this compartment as do the flexors of the forearm and hand. The dorsal compartment contains the wrist and finger extensors. When clinically significant forearm and hand swelling develops along with clinical symptoms of pain and motor sensory loss, confirmation of compartment syndrome can be made by measuring compartmental pressures. As in the lower extremity, pressures greater than 30 mm Hg are considered abnormal and when associated with the signs and symptoms of compartment syndrome mandate surgical decompression.

Volar fasciotomy is performed using a long curvilinear incision from the medial epicondyle to the midpalm. Often the volar release is adequate, and dorsal decompression may not be necessary. Dorsal release, if indicated, can be performed by making a straight dorsal incision from the elbow to the midarm. Hand swelling may require decompression surgery to assure protection of the intrinsic muscles and neurovascular components of the digits. Surgical decompression of the hand is performed using straight incisions on the dorsum of the hand over the second and fourth metacarpals. Additional incisions over the first and fifth metacarpals may be necessary to decompress the thenar or hypothenar spaces, respectively.[3]

Vascular surgeons have learned that re-establishing blood flow to an ischemically threatened limb may result in a reperfusion syndrome that impairs neuromuscular function and predisposes the patient to acute compartment hypertension. Compartment decompression is routinely performed at the time of embolectomy or arterial reconstruction to prevent permanent disability in patients who have prolonged ischemic events. When acute ischemia is relieved in less than 6 hours, close observation for clinical symptoms (swelling, pain, decreased neuromuscular function) and careful monitoring with serial compartment pressures, transcutaneous Doppler measurements of tibial vein flow, and assessment of arterial perfusion may help to identify patients who need urgent secondary release procedures.[7]

With the advent of thrombolytic drugs (streptokinase, urokinase) and their use in the treatment of patients with ischemically threatened but viable extremities, the risk for secondary compartment syndromes has greatly increased. This is because of prolonged ischemia times and gradual reperfusion of the ischemic limb. Not uncommonly, these patients are attended by nonsurgical staff. Unless the staff is trained to recognize the problem, an evolving ACS can be missed, risking further neuromuscular injury and seriously jeopardizing functional recovery. Compartment syndromes that develop as a result of thrombolytic therapy are difficult to treat because of the potential for excessive blood loss at the time fasciotomy is performed. This complication occurs in about 5% of all patients treated with thrombolytic drugs.

The lithotomy position is currently used for exposure during distal colon procedures, gynecologic operations, and urologic surgery. Complications associated with lithotomy positioning have been described sporadically. They include arterial thromboses, myonecrosis, neuropraxia, and compartment syndromes. The mechanism of development of the compartment is not precisely understood. One important factor, however, seems to relate to the length of the operation. Most patients who have these complications have operating times that exceed 5 hours. Leg elevation decreases arterial perfusion, and the dead weight of the calf against the limb cradle produces direct pressure against the anterior, lateral, and posterior calf muscles, contributing to direct muscle necrosis and local nerve injury. Venous congestion and subsequent distal venous hypertension associated with extreme hip flexion and flexion of the knees also may aggravate swelling and edema and potentiate development of a compartment syndrome. Peroneal nerve injury can occur in the absence of a compartment syndrome because of the effects of compression on the intermuscular septum. Again, the length of operative time seems to be the most important factor; most procedures that result in this complication last longer than 5¹/₂ hours. Padding to protect the leg apparently does not have any effect on prevention. Clinical experience with this sequence of complications would suggest that the most important means of prevention is to minimize the time in the lithotomy position. If a prolonged operation is expected, it may be best to perform as much of the procedure with the patient in the supine position and place the legs in the cradle only when the procedure requires lithotomy positioning. Delayed diagnosis in the postoperative period is associated with permanent injury. When patients recovering from pelvic surgery complain of calf pain, an immediate compartment pressure measurement should be performed, and fasciotomy completed when resting pressures exceed 30 mm Hg. If symptoms persist for more than 12 hours, without decompression of the compartment, meaningful recovery of function is uncommon.[25]

CHRONIC COMPARTMENT SYNDROMES

The chronic or exertional compartment syndrome is defined as a condition in which exercise increases intramuscular compartment pressure to a point where ischemic pain develops.[32] Chronic compartment syndrome (CCS) was first described by Mavor in 1956.[33] Making the diagnosis of CCS can be challenging because clinical symptoms are not uniformly reproducible and often mimic other musculoskeletal ailments and because physical examination is frequently unimpressive. In general, the patients are young (mean age 22 years) with long-standing symptoms (>2 years) that abate or disappear with extended rest only to recur again with exercise. The most prevalent complaint is claudication (90%), which differs from classic "intermittent claudication" because of the long exercise distances required to unmask symptoms.[34] These symptoms occur without clinical evidence of arterial occlusive disease or venous insufficiency. Muscle tightness and swelling specific to identifiable myofascial compartments are often diagnostic and may persist for hours after exercise stress (60%). Paresthesias are less common (25%) and usually occur in patients with symptomatic anterior or distal deep posterior compartment syndromes. These symptoms tend to be less reproducible, and although somewhat uncommon, are most worrisome for the patient and usually bring the person to formal medical evaluation.

The diagnosis of CCS is usually based on clinical history. In order of clinical prevalence, symptoms most commonly occur in the distribution of the anterolateral, distal deep posterior, proximal deep posterior, and superficial posterior compartments. Symptoms commonly associated with the anterolateral compartment include pain and tightness in the affected muscle groups, sensory changes on the dorsum of the foot, and, on rare occasions, weakness of the foot extensors. Symptoms that affect the distal deep posterior compartment include claudication with muscle tightness behind the tibia and intermittent numbness and paresthesia on the medial and plantar surface of the foot. CCS is most commonly associated with overuse injury in well-conditioned athletes, particularly runners and athletes exposed to great impact stress to the lower extremity (basketball, football, gymnastics, track).[35] Less common causes of CCS include intramuscular hemorrhage secondary to blunt trauma, venous hypertension, and soft-tissue tumor expansion. Unlike ACSs, chronic syndromes rarely cause permanent neuromuscular injury, probably because discomfort restricts the patient's activity enough to prevent a prolonged increase in compartmental pressures.

Diagnosis

Confirmation of the diagnosis is usually made by demonstrating elevated compartment pressures. Compartment pressure measurements can be performed using a number of techniques. I prefer to use a handheld Stryker digital computer system because it provides very accurate information in a cost-efficient and user-friendly way. Normal resting pressures in the lower extremity compartments are usually less than 15 mm Hg. Resting pressures between 16 and 20 mm Hg are suggestive of CCS, and pressures above 25 mm Hg are markedly abnormal and uniformly consistent with this diagnosis.[36] When a patient has symptoms that suggest CCS and borderline pressure measurements at rest, repeat measurements should be performed after the patient has undergone treadmill stress or has run until symptoms develop. It is much easier to have patients actually go outside to run until they develop symptoms and then have them come back into the laboratory for measurements, because claudication distances are often quite long, requiring 20 or 30 minutes of exercise time on a treadmill, causing a severe bottleneck in a busy diagnostic laboratory. Compartment pressures normally increase after exercise to a peak two or three times the resting pressure and quickly return to baseline values within 6 to 10 minutes after exercise. Patients with incipient CCS show much more dramatic postexercise increases in compartment pressure (three to five times base pressure) and a prolonged return to baseline values (>10 minutes). Postexercise criteria used for defining as CCS may vary between centers, but most authors agree with guidelines established by Pedowitz et al and Shyssis et al suggesting that resting pressure greater than 15 mm Hg, 1-minute postexercise pressure greater than 30 mm Hg, and a 5-minute postexercise pressure greater than 20 mm Hg establishes the diagnosis of this condition at the 95% confidence level.[37,38]

Noninvasive testing should be used to selectively rule out vascular disorders that may occur in young adults and mimic CCS. These include premature atherosclerosis, popliteal entrapment, and chronic venous insufficiency. Resting and postexercise pulse volume recordings provide plethysmographic and segmental pressure data that can be used to screen for intrinsic arterial occlusive disease and to screen for popliteal entrapment. Popliteal entrapment screening is performed by having the supine patient extend the knee with forced plantar flexion of the foot (Fig. 43–2). Color-flow duplex ultrasonic scans and magnetic resonance imaging are routinely used at my institution to evaluate patients with positive entrapment screens. These studies allow confirmation of the location of popliteal artery compression and differentiation between anatomic and functional forms of entrapment.[39]

Duplex ultrasonic testing is helpful in evaluating symptoms of CCS when limb edema is present. In addition, abnormalities in tibial veinflow have been documented

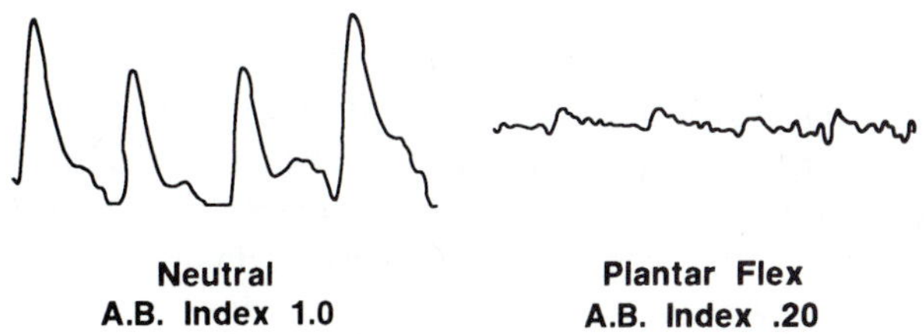

Neutral
A.B. Index 1.0

Plantar Flex
A.B. Index .20

Figure 43–2. Positive screening for popliteal artery compression in a patient with calf claudication. The waveform and ankle–brachial (AB) index is normal with the knee in extension and the foot in neutral position. With forced plantar flexion there is blunting of the arterial waveform and a fall in the AB index to a level of critical ischemia, suggesting vascular entrapment. PVR, pulse volume recording.

using this technique in patients with symptomatic ACS (absent phasic venous flow, decreased venous augmentation), which normalizes after surgical release. These findings support observations by Jones, Perry, and colleagues that impaired tibial vein drainage is associated with the development of ACS.[17]

The use of electromyelography and nerve conduction testing along with diabetic screening is appropriate when patients complain of paresthesias in order to rule out peripheral neuropathy or nerve impingement. Bone scans should be performed when bone pain is associated with muscle compartment complaints because periostitis and/or stress fractures frequently co-exist with compartment syndromes in patients with overuse injuries. Occasionally magnetic resonance imaging can be helpful when symptoms of CCS develop in the absence of rigorous physical activity, particularly when there is a history of blunt trauma and a suspicion of intramuscular hematoma or when a diagnosis of soft-tissue tumor is suspected.[35]

Treatment

Surgical treatment of CCS is indicated when athletically induced symptoms persist despite aggressive medical management or when the severity of claudication complaints worsen to a point that daily activities are adversely affected. The onset of paresthesias and the development of resting pressures in excess of 25 mm Hg also are indications for prompt release. Recreational athletes who have CCS symptoms are usually encouraged to change their sport or modify the intensity and duration of their training as an alternative to surgery. Most people involved in competitive athletics are unwilling or unable to accept behavior modification or training modification as a permanent means of controlling their symptoms.

The most common surgical technique used to treat CCS is the extended subcutaneous fasciotomy. Subcutaneous fasciotomy can be performed using limited transverse skin incisions placed over the proximal and distal portions of the compartment affected by symptoms. Compartment fascia is incised by subcutaneously passing scissors or cutting devices between the two incisions and extending them proximally and distally.[36,40] Open fasciectomy is performed using one linear incision over the medial one-third of the anterior lateral surface of the leg (Fig. 43–3). An ellipse of fascia approximately 6 cm long and 2 cm wide is removed from the anterior and lateral compartments, leaving a strip of fascia over the intermuscular septum to protect the superficial peroneal nerve from direct injury or scar adherence. Extended compartment release can be achieved by proximal and distal subcutaneous fasciotomy performed under direct vision.[35]

I have used both surgical methods for treating CCS and now recommend use of fasciectomy (Fig. 43–4 and 43–5) for managing both anterolateral and posterior compartment syndromes because it appears to be a safer and more effective treatment. Open fasciectomy has fewer postoperative complications and fewer recurrences than blind subcutaneous fasciotomy. Open fasciectomy is done through a skin incision made parallel to the long axis of the muscle compartment, which improves exposure and makes identification of anatomic structures more precise. This exposure allows for direct control of bleeding points and reduces the hazards of intraoperative trauma to neurovascular structures.

At my institution intraoperative or early postoperative complications occurred in 11% of all patients treated using the subcutaneous fasciotomy technique. The most common problems were wound hematomas and superficial wound infections, which occurred in approximately 5% of patients. The most bothersome problems were cutaneous sensory nerve injuries to the superficial peroneal nerve, saphenous nerve,

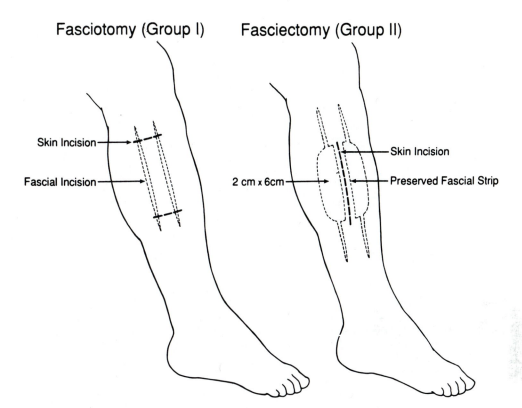

Figure 43–3. Surgical techniques for release of chronic anterolateral compartment syndrome include subcutaneous fasciotomy (left) and open fasciectomy with extended subcutaneous fasciotomy (right). Subcutaneous fasciotomy is performed using transverse skin incisions over the proximal and distal elements of the compartment and passing scissors or cutting devices blindly through the subcutaneous spaces to cut the fascia. Open fasciectomy is performed using one linear incision, in the medial one-third of the anterolateral surface of the leg. An ellipse of fascia approximately 6 cm long and 2 cm wide is removed from the interior and lateral compartment leaving a protective strip of fascia over the intermuscular septum. Extended subcutaneous fasciotomy, both proximally and distally, can be performed under direct vision. (*Reprinted with permission from Turnipseed W, Detmer DE, Girdley F. Chronic compartment syndrome: an unusual cause for claudication. Ann Surg. 1989;210:557–563.*)

and/or sural nerve. Other complications included thrombophlebitis, lymphocele, and seroma. One-third of all complications occurred within the first 3 postoperative months and were related to postoperative hematomas. The other complications occurred within 1 year of the operation and resulted from dense scarring at the site of fasciotomy or scar fixation of muscle to the margins of the fasciotomy site with subsequent herniation of muscle into the fasciotomy defect. Interestingly, most of the symptomatic recurrences developed in the anterolateral compartments, as opposed to the posterior compartment releases, and were successfully treated by open fasciectomy. Dense myofascial scarring was noted throughout the middle-third of the compartment. It appeared to be unrelated to the previous fasciotomy site.

Our clinical success with the use of fasciectomy in treating recurrent compartment syndromes led us to conclude that this technique may be clinically superior as a primary means of treatment. Our subsequent experience has borne this out by virtue of the fact that our complication rate has dropped from 11% to 5% and that no vascular

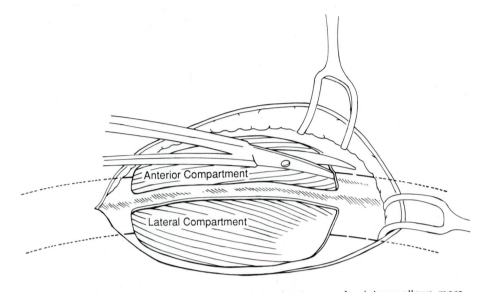

Figure 43–4. Open fasciectomy with extended subcutaneous fasciotomy allows more complete and precise decompression of the compartments and reduces the likelihood of scar recurrence. Bleeding complications and neurovascular injuries have been significantly reduced because of better exposure through the linear skin incision. (*Reprinted with permission from Turnipseed W, Detmer DE, Girdley F. Chronic compartment syndrome: an unusual cause for claudication.* Ann Surg. *1989;210:557–563.*)

or cutaneous sensory nerve injuries have been incurred since this approach was implemented. In our last 300 operations, only two patients have developed peripheral neuropathy, which was associated with wound scar entrapments. Two patients had recurrent symptoms in the distribution of the deep posterior compartment.

We now routinely use fasciectomy in the release of anterolateral compartments and both the superficial and deep posterior compartments. When the deep proximal or distal compartment releases are done through a medial approach, the tibial attachments of the gastrocnemius fascia are taken down and a large ellipse of fascia from the medial belly of the gastrocnemius is excised before the soleal attachments to the tibia are released. Soleal insertions to the tibia must be taken down from the posterior medial surface of the bone before the deep compartment can be entered (Fig. 43–6). The coalescent fascial insertions of these two muscles must be cut back and excised along the entire length of this insertion, or fixation to bone will recur. When the proximal deep posterior compartment is being released, excision of the soleal band and the anterior fascia of this muscle is necessary to prevent recurrent fixation to the tibia (Fig. 43–7). Our recurrence rate of 2% is much better than that recorded in the literature (>20%).[35]

Research into Chronic Compartment Syndrome

Mechanical and biochemical evaluation of fascial specimens removed at the time of surgery along with data from our vascular laboratory have helped us to better understand the physiologic mechanisms that predispose some individuals to clinical CCS. Fascia taken from patients with symptomatic CCS was compared with fascia from age-group controls that was removed from traumatically amputated limbs or was excised because of acute post-traumatic compartment syndrome. Fascia from the patients with CCS was thicker and structurally stiffer than control fascia. When the collagen content was evaluated, there were no significant differences between patho-

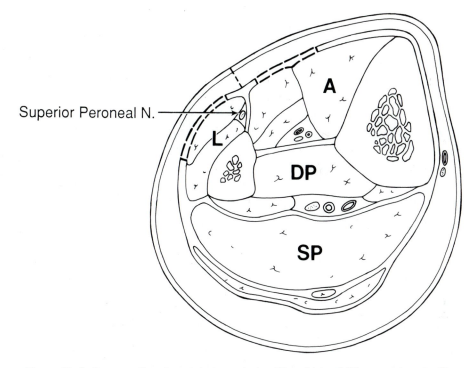

Superior Peroneal N.

Figure 43–5. Cross-section demonstrates anterior (A) and lateral (L) compartments. The broken lines demonstrate the incision placement and locations of fascial excision necessary for release of the anterior and lateral compartments. DP, deep posterior compartment; SP, superficial posterior compartment. (*Reprinted with permission from Turnipseed W, Detmer DE, Girdley F. Chronic compartment syndrome: an unusual cause for claudication.* Ann Surg. *1989;210:557–563.*)

logic and normal fascia.[41] The clinical observation that extensive myofascial scarring occurs in patients with symptoms of CCS but not in compartments without symptoms suggests that microtrauma and inflammation may be important factors in compartmental hypertension.

Previous studies and our own experience with duplex ultrasonic evaluation of tibial venous flow in patients with chronic anterior compartment syndrome suggest that mild elevations in compartment pressure can significantly impair venous drainage from myofascial compartments.[17] This combination of myofascial scarring, fascial thickening, and impaired venous drainage may explain why CCS develops in some patients. These findings further support the logic of performing fasciectomy in the treatment of CCS and may explain why recurrence rates are higher among patients treated with fasciotomy.

We initially had some concerns about whether functional performance would be adversely affected when fasciectomy was performed. We have performed extensive CYBEX and exercise stress testing on patients who have had compartment syndromes treated by fasciectomy or fasciotomy. There have been no significant differences in strength, flexibility, or endurance between patients treated with successful fasciotomy and those treated with fasciectomy. Despite technical differences in the extent of the surgery, there were no significant recovery differences between the two techniques in uncomplicated cases. Patients returned to work or school and were ambulatory within 48 hours. Postoperative swelling was common and required elastic compression support for 10 days to 2 weeks. Patients began stretching exercises on discharge from the hospital and were encouraged to abandon crutch support within 4 to 5 days of the operation. Once skin incisions were healed, rehabilitation started in the swimming

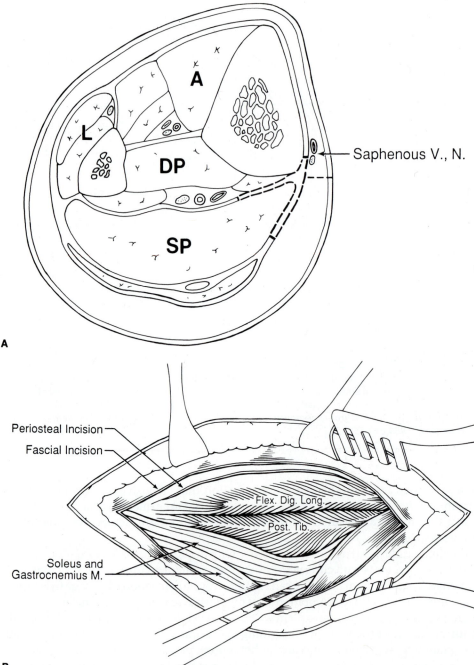

Figure 43–6. (A) Cross-section of lower leg shows the medial approach and fascial excisions necessary for release of the distal deep posterior (DP) compartment. The skin incision should be placed posterior to the saphenous vein and nerve and dissection around these structures avoided to reduce the probability of intraoperative trauma or postoperative scar entrapment. A, anterior compartment; L, lateral compartment; SP, superficial posterior compartment. (*Reprinted with permission from Turnipseed W, Detmer DE, Girdley F. Chronic compartment syndrome: an unusual cause for claudication. Ann Surg. 1989;210:557–563.*) **(B)** Surgical decompression of the distal deep posterior compartment requires excision of the fascial attachments of the gastrocnemius and distal soleus muscles to the posterior medial surface of the tibia. Confirmation of deep space entry is made by visualizing the posterior surface of the tibia, the flexor digitorum longus, and the posterior tibialis muscles.

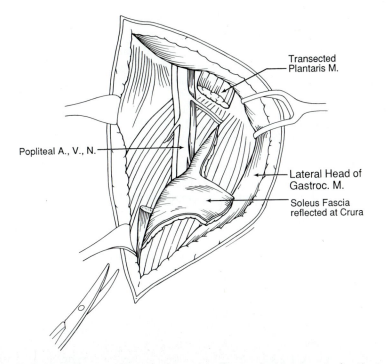

Transected
Plantaris M.

Popliteal A., V., N.

Lateral Head of
Gastroc. M.

Soleus Fascia
reflected at Crura

Figure 43–7. Medial approach routinely used in the surgical treatment of patients with claudication symptoms arising from the proximal deep posterior compartment (soleus compartment). Decompression of this compartment is performed by taking down medial attachments of the soleus muscle to the tibia by excising the dense fascial sling of the soleus from the tibia medially and from the fibula laterally. The fascia over the popliteus muscle is often excised as well, making it more difficult to have dense scar adhesion to neurovascular structures that pass between the two muscles. (*Reprinted with permission from Turnipseed WD, Pozniak M. Popliteal entrapment as a result of neurovascular compression by the soleus and plantaris muscles. J Vasc Surg. 1992;15:285–294.*)

pool with a kickboard and in the gym with a stationary bicycle. At approximately 3.5 to 4 weeks, the patients began an injured running program and generally returned to full athletic capacity within 2 to 3 months of the operation.[35,36]

In conclusion CCS is underdiagnosed and should be considered in young adults with claudication and normal vascular studies. CCS most commonly results from overuse injury in well-conditioned athletes, particularly runners. This condition rarely causes permanent neuromuscular injury, probably because discomfort restricts activity enough to prevent a prolonged increase in compartment pressures. Surgery is the only appropriate treatment of this condition. Open fasciectomy is associated with fewer complications and fewer recurrences than closed subcutaneous fasciotomy and should be considered as the surgical procedure of choice in treating this condition.

REFERENCES

1. Bourne RB, Rorabeck CH. Compartment syndromes of the lower leg. *Clin Orthop.* 1989;240:97–104.
2. Matsen FA, Krugmire RB Jr. Compartment syndromes. *Surg Gynecol Obstet.* 1978;147: 943–949.

3. Wienstein SM, Herring SA. Nerve problems and compartment syndromes in the hand, wrist, and forearm. *Clin Sports Med.* 1992;11:161–187.

4. Lagerstrom GF, Reed RL II, Rowlands BJ, Fischer RP. Early fasciotomy for acute clinically evident posttraumatic compartment syndrome. *Am J Surg.* 1989;158:36–39.

5. Feliciano DV, Creese PA, Spjut-Patrinely V, et al. Fasciotomy after trauma to the extremities. *Am J Surg.* 1988;156:533–538.

6. Gershuni DH, Mubarak SJ, Yaru NC, Lee YF. Fracture of the tibia complicated by acute compartment syndrome. *Clin Orthop.* 1987;217:221–227.

7. Patman RD, Thompson JE. Fasciotomy in peripheral vascular surgery: report of 164 patients. *Arch Surg.* 1970;101:663–672.

8. Mubarak SJ, Owen GA. Compartmental syndrome and its relation to the crush syndrome: a spectrum of disease. *Clin Orthop.* 1975;113:81–89.

9. Rollins DL, Bernhard VM, Towne JB. Fasciotomy: an appraisal of controversial issue. *Arch Surg.* 1981;116:1474–1481.

10. Owen CA, Mubarak SJ, Hargens AR, et al. Intramuscular pressures with limb compression. *N Engl J Med.* 1979;300:1169–1172.

11. Rao VK, Feldman PD, Dibbell DG. Extravasation injury to the hand by intravenous phenytoin. *J Neurosurg.* 1988;68:667–696.

12. Von Volkman R. Die schamisehen muskellohmungen undkontrakturen. *Zentralbl Chir.* 1881;8:801–803.

13. Bardenheuer L. *Dstch Z Chir.* 1911;108:44.

14. Matsen FA III, Winquirst RA, Krugmire RB Jr. Diagnosis and management of compartment syndromes. *J Bone Joint Surg* [*Am*]. 1980;62:286–291.

15. Mubarak SJ, Owen CA, Hargens AR, et al. Acute compartment syndromes: diagnosis and treatment with the aid of the Wick catheter. *J Bone Joint Surg* [*Am*]. 1978;60:1091–1095.

16. Whitesides TE Jr, Haney TC, Morimoto K, et al. Tissue pressure measurements as a determinant for the need of fasciotomy. *Clin Orthop.* 1975;113:43–51.

17. Jones WG, Perry MO, Bush HL Jr. Changes in tibial venous blood flow in the evolving compartment syndrome. *Arch Surg.* 1989;124:801–804.

18. Kikta MJ, Meyer JP, Bishara RA, et al. Crush syndrome due to limb compression. *Arch Surg.* 1987;122:1078–1081.

19. Mubarek SJ, Owen CA. Double-incision fasciotomy of the leg for decompression in compartment syndromes. *J Bone Joint Surg* [*Am*]. 1977;59:184–187.

20. Kelly RP, Whitesides TE Jr. Transfibular route for fasciotomy of the leg. *J Bone Joint Surg.* 1967;49:1020–1023.

21. Ernst CB, Kaufer H. Fibulectomy-fasciotomy. *J Trauma.* 1971;2:368–380.

22. Ngheim DD, Boland JP. Four compartment fasciotomy of the lower extremity without fibulectomy: a new approach. *Ann Surg.* 1980;July 414–417.

23. Kunkel JM. Thigh and leg compartment syndrome in absence of lower extremity trauma following MAST application. *Am J Emerg Med.* 1987;5:118–120.

24. Brotman S, Brouner BD, Cox EF. MAST trousers improperly applied causing a compartment syndrome in lower extremity trauma. *J Trauma.* 1982;22:598–599.

25. Fowl RJ, Allers DL, Kempczinski RF. Neurovascular lower extremity complications of the lithotomy position. *Ann Vasc Surg.* 1992;6:357–361.

26. Adler LM, Loughlin JS, Morin CJ, Henning RU Jr. Bilateral compartment syndrome after a long gynecologic operation in the lithotomy position. *Am J Obstet Gynecol.* 1990;162:1271–1272.

27. Hay SM, Allen MJ, Barnes MR. Acute compartment syndromes resulting from anticoagulant treatment. *Br Med J.* 1992;305:1474–1475.

28. Shah PM, Wapnir I, Babu S, et al. Compartment syndrome in combined arterial and venous injuries of the lower extremity. *Am J Surg.* 1989;158:136–141.

29. Schwartz JT, Brumback RJ, Lakatos RL, et al. Acute compartment syndrome of the thigh. *J Bone Joint Surg* [*Am*]. 1989;71:392–400.

30. Winternitz WA, Metheny JA, Wear LC. Acute compartment syndrome of the thigh in sports related injuries not associated with femoral fractures. *Am J Sports Med.* 1992;20:476–478.

31. Waters EGL, Beall D. Crush injuries with impairment of renal function. *Br Med*. 1941; 1:427–432.
32. Fronek J, Mubarak SJ, Hargens AR, et al. Management of chronic exertional anterior compartment syndrome of the lower extremity. *Clin Orthop*. 1987;220:217–227.
33. Mavor GE. The anterior tibial syndrome. *J Bone Joint Surg*. [Br] 1956;38:513–517.
34. Rorabeck CH, Fowler PJ, Nott L. The results of fasciotomy in the management of exertional compartment syndrome. *Am J Sports Med*. 1988;16:224–227.
35. Turnipseed WD, Detmer DE, Girdley F. Chronic compartment syndrome: an unusual cause for claudication. *Ann Surg*. 1989;219:557–563.
36. Detmer DE, Sharpe K, Seefit R, Girdley F. Chronic compartment syndrome: diagnosis, management, and outcomes. *Am J Sports Med*. 1985;13:162–170.
37. Pedowitz RA, Hargens SJ, Mubarek SJ, et al. Modified criteria for the objective diagnosis of chronic compartment syndrome of the leg. *Am J Sports Med*. 1990;18:35–40.
38. Shyssis AA, Mortini D, Corgett M. Surgical management of exertional compartment syndrome of the lower leg: long-term followup. *Am J Sports Med*. 1993;21:811–817.
39. Turnipseed WD, Pozniak M. Popliteal entrapment as a result of neurovascular compression by the soleus and plantaris muscle. *J Vasc Surg*. 1992;15:285–294.
40. Mubarak SJ, Hargens AR. Diagnosis and management of compartment syndromes. AAOS Symposium on Trauma to the Leg and its Sequelae. St. Louis, Mo: Mosby;1981.
41. Hurschler C, Vanderby R, Martinez DA, et al. Mechanical and biochemical analyses of tibial compartment fascia in chronic compartment syndrome. *Ann Biomed Eng*. [In press].

44

Management of Iatrogenic Arterial Injury in the Lower Extremity

Elliot L. Chaikof, MD, PhD, and Robert B. Smith III, MD

Galen was called in consultation by a young and inexperienced surgeon who had opened the artery at the bend of the elbow instead of the vein, and blood spurted out *"clarus, rubens, lucidus et caid."* "I took the situation at once; there happened to be an elderly physician with me, so we prepared a medicine, viscid, conglutmable, and obstructive, and placing it strongly against the lips of the wound bound over it a soft sponge. The surgeon who had opened the artery wondered, but said nothing. When we went out [note the professional touch!] I said to the surgeon that he had opened the pulsating vessel, and charged him not to dress the wound before the fourth day, and not without me." The cure was complete, and Galen remarks that this was his only successful case of the kind, as in all others aneurysm had followed.

> William Osler. Remarks on arterio-venous aneurysm. *Lancet.* 1:949, 1915.

Descriptions of accidental arterial injury during the course of medical treatment have been a part of our recorded surgical heritage since the writings of Galen in the first century. Although aneurysm formation after injury was a frequent subject of the early medical literature, it was not until 1757 that William Hunter first described two cases of arteriovenous fistula (AVF). Again, both injuries were produced accidentally in the course of therapeutic bloodletting.[1,2] Nearly 200 years latter, Daniel C. Elkin noted perceptively at the 1947 Annual Meeting of the Southern Surgical Association that while "blood letting has long passed into oblivion, the re-introduction on a large scale of both venous and arterial puncture as a diagnostic and therapeutic measure will probably be followed by an increased number of aneurysms and fistulas."[3]

In the 1990s, our efforts in continuous monitoring, precise diagnosis, and recent improvements in catheter-based international technology have led to the verification of Elkin's prediction. Reports dealing with iatrogenically induced arterial complications have proliferated though the spectrum of clinical presentation, and options for management remain remarkably similar. Prevention remains the first rule of management. Nevertheless, as in Galen's era, if accidental arterial injury should occur, early detection and correction can minimize both the clinical sequelae and the potential legal implications.

MECHANISMS OF INJURY AND CLINICAL MANIFESTATIONS

> This man had a left inguinal hernia repaired on May 13, 1946. He was told after the operation that a blood vessel had been injured. His surgeon stated that he "encountered some bleeding when a stitch was placed to unite the conjoined tendon to the inguinal ligament, but the bleeding was easily controlled by a ligature." Two months following operation, the patient noticed in the left inguinal region a small firm mass which gradually increased in size over a period of four months, and then suddenly enlarged causing severe pain in this region. . . .
>
> C.M., Emory University Hospital 1166-936. Elkin CD. *Ann Surg.* 127:774, 1948.

Iatrogenic arterial trauma may be an unintended consequence of (a) general surgical or orthopedic procedures; (b) inadvertent intra-arterial injections; or (c) arterial catheterizations. Major vascular injuries after inguinal herniorrhaphy are infrequent but have been documented and attributed to the proximity of the iliac artery to Poupart's ligament. Elkin's patient appears to be both the first reported case and successful repair of an external iliac aneurysm following herniorrhaphy (Fig. 44–1).[3] Elkin performed a preliminary left lumbar sympathectomy followed by closure of the arterial opening with four silk sutures. In a more recent review, Shamberger et al suggested that incorporation of the femoral sheath in stitches placed close to the medial part of the internal inguinal ring risks puncture or laceration of the external iliac artery or one of its branches.[4] As in Elkin's report, the injury may be compounded by additional "blind" suture placement prompted when bleeding from the floor of the hernia repair is observed. Both arterial occlusion and pseudoaneurysm formation following hernia repair have been reported.[5]

Although it remains difficult to comprehend the accidental ligation or stripping of a principal arterial trunk during the course of varicose vein surgery, such injuries have been described.[6–8] Because we have been unable to find the description of this complication in the recent literature, we presume (and hope) that this surgical error is of historical interest alone.

The case reports of arterial injury following orthopedic surgery are numerous and are often complicated by compartment syndrome. Excluding cast-related injuries, the femoral and popliteal arteries have been injured during a variety of hip and knee repairs (Fig. 44–2).[5,9,10] Although both are rare events, the former is more common. The use of external fixators for the treatment of grade 2 or 3 open fractures involves the insertion of medial and lateral pins for bony transfixion. Many large series have not observed vascular injury in association with this procedure, but Paul et al believe these iatrogenic injuries to be under-reported.[11] In their recent review, a 3.3% incidence of vascular injury was observed during a 5-year period in which 121 fractures were treated (Fig. 44–3). Arterial occlusion, pseudoaneurysm formation, and erosion of the arterial wall in vessels were documented both above and below the knee. All required surgical intervention. Although diagnostic angiography confirmed the presence of these injuries, they were manifest clinically by either ischemia or hemorrhage.

The accidental intra-arterial infusion of anesthetic agent, saline solution, and sclerotherapy solutions has been described in the literature. On occasion, ischemia may be reversible. More often, tissue necrosis is the end result of vasospasm and arterial thrombosis. Natali and Benhamou described 32 arterial injuries following sclerotherapy for varicose veins.[5] Skin necrosis occurred in 24 cases, and amputations were required by an additional four patients.

The increase in frequency and complexity of percutaneous transcatheter techniques for diagnosis and treatment of coronary artery and valvular heart disease has been accompanied by a concomitant rise in iatrogenic femoral artery injuries (Fig.

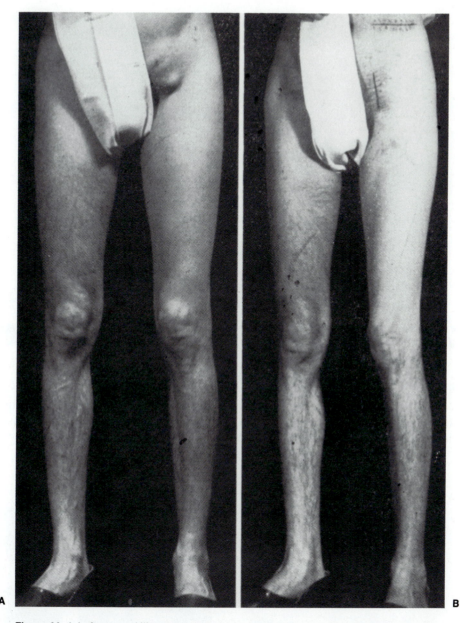

Figure 44–1. Left external iliac artery pseudoaneurysm following an inguinal herniorraphy. Pre- and postoperative photographs. (*From Elkin CD. Aneurysm following surgical procedures: report of five cases. Ann Surg. 1948;127:769–779.*)

44–4). At Emory University Hospital several retrospective studies have examined the frequency of complications and etiologic factors.[12–15] Whereas the incidence of arterial complications following diagnostic cardiac catheterization is relatively low (0.05% to 0.7%),[16,17] the frequency is much higher after percutaneous transluminal angioplasty (0.7% to 9.0%)[12,17,18] and higher still after coronary arthrectomy, intracoronary stent placement, aortic valvuloplasty, and intra-aortic balloon pump insertion (5% to 17%).[19–21] Our own analysis confirmed that, in general terms, older, obese women are at higher risk for postcatheterization complications.

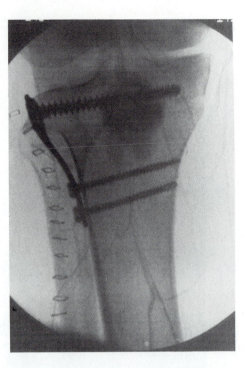

Figure 44–2. Popliteal artery pseudoaneurysm following bony transfixion of the tibial plateau.

In prior studies, thrombotic complications predominated. The presumed mechanism of injury was either the development of intimal flaps during arterial puncture, the stripping off of a fibrin sleeve following catheter removal, or simply the occlusion of arterial outflow by an indwelling catheter.[22,23] In our own experience, bleeding

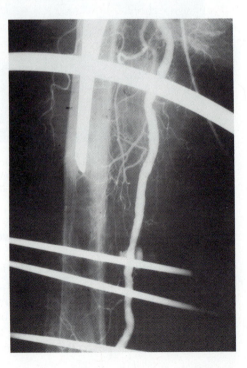

Figure 44–3. Pseudoaneurysm of the superficial femoral artery caused by an external fixator.

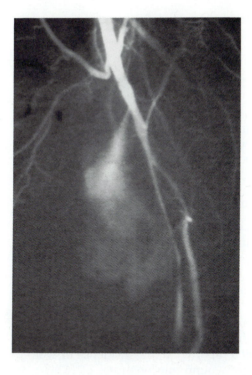

Figure 44–4. Large femoral artery pseudoaneurysm as a complication of cardiac catheterization.

problems and pseudoaneurysms currently outnumber arterial occlusions (84% vs 3.1%) (Table 44–1).[15] We believe this change in pattern reflects the more aggressive use of anticoagulants and, in some instances, the larger diameters of some of the newer devices. Among 95 consecutive patients operated on during an 18-month period, anticoagulation followed the initial percutaneous procedure in nearly 85%. Catheter insertion at sites other than the common femoral artery has been considered a risk factor for groin complications. We have found a higher incidence of AVF formation with punctures of the profunda femoris (deep femoral) artery. In addition, retroperitoneal hematomas are clearly more common in patients with aberrant arterial puncture above the inguinal ligament. Without doubt, this is the most morbid complication of femoral arterial injury, and it should be suspected in a patient with an

TABLE 44–1. TYPES OF COMPLICATIONS FOLLOWING PERCUTANEOUS CARDIAC PROCEDURES REQUIRING SURGICAL INTERVENTION

Diagnosis	Percentage of All Complications
Pseudoaneurysms	61.2
Hematoma	11.2
Arteriovenous fistula	10.2
External bleeding	6.1
Retroperitoneal hematoma	5.1
Thromboses	3.1
Groin abscess	2.0
Mycotic aneurysm	1.0

Reproduced with permission from Lumsden AB, Miller JM, Kozinski AS, et al. A prospective evaluation of surgically treated groin complications following percutaneous cardiac procedures. *Am Surg.* 1994;60:132–137.

unexplained drop in hematocrit and with motor or sensory deficits in the distribution of the femoral nerve.[14]

OPERATIVE PRINCIPLES

> Run you bistoury upwards and downwards, so as to slit up the tumour quickly; plunge your hand suddenly down towards the bottom; turn out the great clots of blood with your fingers, till having reached the bottom entirely, you begin to feel the warm jet of blood; and directed by that, clap your finger on the wounded point of the artery; as it has but a point your finger will cover it directly, and your feeling the beating of the artery assures you that all is now safe.
>
> John Bell. *Discourses on Nature and Cure of Wounds*. Edinburgh, 1800, vol. i, p. 75.

Bell was likely the first to demonstrate the effectiveness of direct surgical intervention for pseudoaneurysm repair. This description is all the more remarkable when one considers the absence of anesthetic, suction, or incandescent lighting. Two centuries later, the rationale for prompt surgical treatment of iatrogenic arterial injury is still based on the low incidence of spontaneous resolution, the risk for further complications, and the low risk of repair.[16,24,25] Although effective, surgery does carry a high incidence of local wound complications, particularly when performed for acute complications of percutaneous cardiac procedures. Lumsden et al in a recent review of our experience at Emory University Hospital reported an 8% incidence of wound bleeding or lymph leak.[15] Others have reported wound infection rates of 16%.[26]

There remain many proponents of Bell's original direct approach of arterial control and repair, primarily for the femoral artery pseudoaneurysm. We, however, believe that initial proximal arterial control ultimately results in a more expeditious repair, which is more easily tolerated in the locally anesthetized patient. Exposure of the anterior and lateral walls of the femoral artery at the level of the inguinal ligament allows control and provides an anatomic landmark. It is all too easy to mistakenly identify a hole in the deep fascia as being the source of bleeding or to wander to an obese thigh searching for a femoral artery that has been displaced into an unusual anatomic position. We do not systemically heparinize, and drains are placed in all anticoagulated patients. In a rare patient, control of the external iliac artery is required through a suprainguinal extraperitoneal incision. Although preoperative duplex ultrasonic (US) imaging is discussed in greater detail elsewhere in this text, we emphasize that it is a helpful adjunct that provides technically useful information with regard to (a) the depth of the pseudoaneurysm from the skin; (b) the site of the arterial puncture; and (c) the presence of more than one arterial jet.

AVFs are repaired by separating the respective artery and vein, followed by local suture repair. We typically monitor the Doppler signal within the vein and continue the dissection until the fistula is identified and arterialization based on the venous Doppler signal is eliminated.

CONSERVATIVE STRATEGIES: NATURAL HISTORY OF FEMORAL ARTERY PSEUDOANEURYSMS AND ARTERIOVENOUS FISTULAS

Few would argue about the need for prompt surgical intervention when faced with an ischemic extremity, enlarging hematoma, or symptomatic pseudoaneurysm of AVF. However, several centers have recently adopted a conservative approach based on preliminary studies of the natural history of femoral artery pseudoaneurysms and

AVF. Together, these injuries currently constitute the majority of iatrogenic vascular injuries. There is increasing evidence that within a few weeks of injury, some AVFs may close and many small pseudoaneurysms will spontaneously thrombose.[18,27] Rivers et al reported that six of seven pseudoaneurysms (1.3 to 4.0 cm maximum diameter) thrombosed within 4 weeks and six of nine AVFs closed within an initial period of observation.[28] Likewise, Kresowik et al followed seven pseudoaneurysms (1.3 to 3.5 cm maximum diameter), all of which thrombosed within 4 weeks.[18] Three AVFs persisted during an 8-week follow-up period. Similar results have been reported by Kent et al.[27] Size or volume as determined by duplex US scanning may be important in the selection of patients for nonoperative management.[27] The small numbers of patients treated in this way currently precludes hard and fast rules. The influence of concurrent anticoagulation on this approach is unknown, but we believe it would reduce the likelihood of success; therefore, we strongly advocate surgical repair for such patients.

ULTRASOUND-GUIDED COMPRESSION OF FEMORAL ARTERIAL INJURIES

The indications are to imitate the natural modes of cure. . . . In some cases a common four-pound weight may be placed over the artery in the groin, with a pad intervening; or the pressure may be effected by the fingers. The advantages of compression are, that it can be discontinued in a moment should it appear expedient . . . and that should it fail, the knife can still be resorted to, without deterioration or disadvantage in the condition of the parts. The objections which have been urged against it are, that in some cases the patient, from irritability of system, cannot bear it for a sufficient length of time to produce a cure. . . .

Robert Druitt, *A Surgeon's Vade Mecum: A Manual of Modern Surgery.* London, 1865, p. 346.

Compression devices have long been a part of the medical armamentarium for the treatment of peripheral arterial pseudoaneurysms (Fig. 44–5). Recently, US guidance has provided a modern flavor to this approach.[26,29,30] A US probe can be used to identify a high-velocity jet from the femoral artery into the pseudoaneurysm or AVF. Pressure is increased until the jet is obliterated, while the flow in the native vessel is maintained. Typically, compression is continued for 20-minute periods until thrombosis occurs. Compression times are variable, averaging 22 to 53 minutes, but may require up to 150 minutes.[30,31] Follow-up scanning is necessary in 48 to 72 hours to assure continued obliteration, since recurrence has been reported.[31] Use of intravenous narcotics, sedation, and epidural anesthesia has increased the likelihood of success by improving patient tolerance of prolonged compression. Some centers have claimed a pseudoaneurysm thrombosis rate of 56% to 93%.[31] Failure rates have been high among anticoagulated patients.

NOVEL APPROACHES

Various modes of cure have been from time to time proposed on the principle of causing coagulation of the blood in the sac. The most hopeful of these, is the injection of a solution of basic perchloride of iron. . . .

M. Pravaz, *Lancet.* 1853, vol. 1, p. 561.

Several hemostatic compounds are currently under investigation for the closure

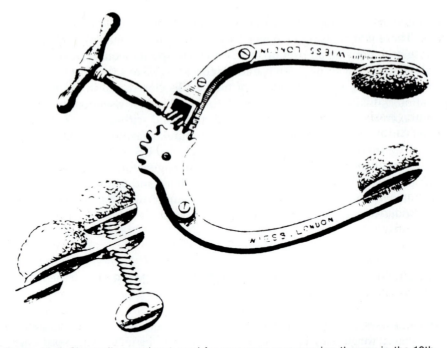

Figure 44–5. Sigoroni's tourniquet used for aneurysm compression therapy in the 19th century. (*From Robert Druitt.* A Surgeon's Vade Mecum: A Manual of Modern Surgery. *London;1865:347*).

of arterial puncture sites following catheterization. Angio-Seal, developed by the Kensey Nash Corporation, Exton, PA, consists of a bioresorbable anchor that lies along the inner arterial surface, a collagen plug located on the outside of the artery, and a suture that secures these two components against the puncture site. In a phase I study, successful device deployment was achieved in the majority of patients who had undergone cardiac catheterization. In fact, primary hemostasis was achieved in most without any manual compression. In the remaining patients seeping was noted at the puncture site, but rapid or pulsatile bleeding was absent. There have been no cases of arterial thrombosis or device embolization.

SPECIAL CONSIDERATIONS IN THE NEONATE AND PEDIATRIC AGE GROUP

The management of iatrogenic arterial thrombosis in infants and children warrants special comment because in all but the busiest of pediatric trauma centers, catheterization procedures are currently the most common cause of lower extremity arterial injury for which surgical consultation is obtained. Despite the advent of smaller and more flexible catheters, the application of duplex US imaging has demonstrated that arterial thrombosis continues to be surprisingly common in the pediatric population, occurring in 20% to 40% of children following femoral artery catheterization.[32,33] In contradistinction to femoral artery occlusion in the adult, most of these injuries in the pediatric age group are asymptomatic. Only rarely does the viability of a limb become truly threatened.

Characteristically, once vascular consultation has been sought, the presence of a cool, mottled, pulseless extremity is noted on physical examination, associated with the absence of insonated peripheral arterial signals. A history of recent catheter-associated trauma is usually found, but careful questioning about failed past catheterizations, recent long-term indwelling catheters, and arterial or venous blood drawing should be sought. Accidental intra-arterial infusion must be considered in a limb with rapidly progressive ischemia (Fig. 44–6).

Options for the management of an ischemic extremity abound, though few are supported by results of prospective trials. Removal of the offending catheter and systemic heparinization has become the initial standard of care, based on the experience of Freed et al.[34] In a prospective trial, Flanigan et al[32] evaluated heparin therapy for children with palpable femoral pulses, but absent distal palpable pulses, and Doppler evidence of impaired perfusion (ankle–brachial index (<0.9). Ankle–brachial indices returned to normal in 11 of 12 (93%) patients. Of note, a similar presentation was observed in eight children who could not be heparinized: ankle–brachial indices normalized in five of eight (63%). Heparin is usually administered with a 100 U/kg bolus dose followed by a constant infusion at 25 U/kg per hour.[35] In neonates there is no proven safe and therapeutic range. However, bleeding complications are reduced if the platelet count is maintained above 50×10^9/L and fibrinogen levels are above 150 mg/dL. Doses are adjusted to the low end of the adult therapeutic range of the activated partial thromboplastin time or heparin level. Typically, the risks of coumadin therapy outweigh the benefits in this age group, and, as a consequence, heparinization often lasts longer in neonates, averaging 7 to 14 days.

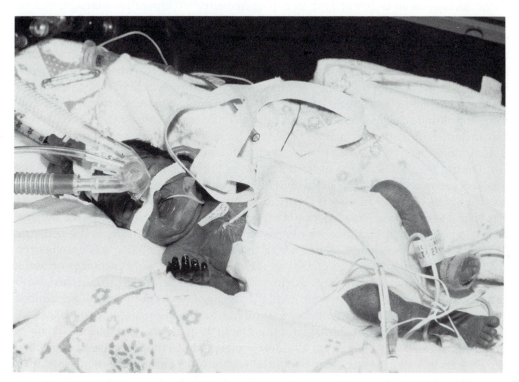

Figure 44–6. Upper extremity ischemia with associated digital necrosis. This injury followed inadvertent catheterization of the brachial artery with infusion of a hypertonic saline solution.

Thrombolytic therapy has been most frequently applied in the treatment of neonates with aortoiliac thrombosis, but successful management of femoral arterial occlusion also has been reported.[36–40] Ino et al[41] reviewed the outcome of 45 pediatric patients who required treatment for femoral artery thrombosis following cardiac catheterization. Heparin therapy was successful in 32 patients. Of the 13 in whom heparin therapy failed, 11 were successfully treated with thrombolytic therapy, and two required surgical thrombectomy. The recommended loading and maintenance doses for urokinase are 4,400 U/kg and 4,400 U/kg per hour, respectively.[42] Contraindications to thrombolytic therapy include recent surgery or active bleeding. Intramuscular injections, arterial or venous catheterizations, rectal temperatures, and the use of antithrombotic agents must be avoided during lytic therapy. Further, blood drawing may be performed only from indwelling catheters or superficial veins. Although the fibrinogen level should be maintained at 100 mg/dL or higher during urokinase infusion, no single test establishes a safe therapeutic range. Nonetheless, the prothrombin time, activated partial thromboplastin time, fibrinogen levels, and thrombin time are routinely monitored every 4 to 6 hours during the first 24 hours and every 12 hours thereafter. The optimal duration of therapy is uncertain, although a response should be seen within 6 to 12 hours. At the completion of thrombolytic therapy, heparin should be instituted without a bolus (20 U/kg per hour) once the fibrinogen level is greater than 100 mg/dL. We advocate a cautious approach to the widespread adoption of thrombolytic therapy given the absence of established pediatric success rates, the risks of hemorrhage, and the potentially catastrophic effect of further delays in treatment.

Steady improvements in microsurgical techniques and materials have culminated in the salvage of an ischemic limb in a 1-kg neonate.[43–46] Operative management of the occluded femoral artery usually includes simple balloon catheter thrombectomy with a 2-F Fogarty catheter with primary or vein-patch closure or resection and end-to-end anastomosis. Perioperative heparinization, magnification, topical papaverine, and microsurgical techniques are all important in arterial reconstruction. Notwithstanding the increasing frequency of reports documenting excellent outcomes, other centers have had far less encouraging results.[47,48] In our experience, arterial thrombectomy is not uniformly successful, but it can be considered a safe procedure with very rare instances of tissue loss even in patients who weigh less than 5 kg. Revascularization of more distal injury sites is indeed difficult and rarely needed.

During the past 30 years, indications for surgical intervention in the infant have evolved, along with our knowledge of the sequelae that follow acute arterial thrombosis. The ability of collateral vessels to provide compensatory flow after arterial occlusion has been a tenet of vascular surgery since John Hunter's historic ligation of the femoral artery in 1785. Catheterization experiences have verified this principle in the pediatric population. The uncommon occurrence of threatened limb viability was emphasized by Smith and Green,[47] who as of 1981 could document only eight instances of tissue loss secondary to arterial trauma. Klein et al[49] reported an 8-year experience, with tissue loss in six of 33 injuries; four involved the upper extremity and two produced intestinal infarction. Intermittent claudication has been an unusual late complication; Taylor et al[33] reported this finding in only one of 19 patients. Our recent review of an 11-year period at the Egleston Children's Hospital at Emory University revealed only seven infants younger than 6 months with arterial thrombosis that warranted surgical intervention.[50]

Controversy has generally centered on the tissue of prophylactic vascular repair and its proper timing, particularly as it applies to the phenomenon of limb growth abnormalities. In the 1960s, Bassett et al reported limb shortening in 86% of catheterized lower extremities.[51] These figures were sharply moderated by reports in the 1970s from Rosenthal et al,[52] Hawker et al,[53] and Jacobsson et al.[54] In part, the dissimilarity among clinical reports was related to the lack of a standardized approach to assess leg length as well as the absence of data concerning normal leg asymmetry in children. In 1981, the potential importance of this problem was again highlighted by a study that compiled 15 cases of angiographic or operative confirmation of arterial thrombosis in children younger than 2 years, all of whom subsequently had significant limb length disparities. It was concluded that ". . . a child with thrombosis of a femoral artery is virtually certain to suffer growth retardation of the affected leg."[47] Taylor et al[33] placed this tissue into perspective by emphasizing that gait disturbance in adults is common only when the anticipated leg asymmetry at maturity will be greater than 2 cm. Through the use of growth charts, Taylor et al determined that the incidence of clinically significant projected limb retardation in children catheterized before the age of 5 years was 8%. Although current data suggest that the presence of an occluded femoral artery in a child with no other symptoms is not an indication for repair, pediatricians should be informed of the need to periodically assess leg lengths and gait in children with arterial occlusion confirmed by duplex US examination. It must be emphasized that the presence of pedal pulses does not ensure the absence of major arterial occlusion. As recommended by Taylor et al,[33] bone-length radiographs should be obtained when the child is 5 years of age. If a discrepancy greater than 1.0 cm is noted, follow-up radiographs are warranted on a yearly basis. Several authors have reported the correction of leg length discrepancies following arterial repair in adolescents.[32,49,55]

The clinical experience of any single institution is limited by the infrequent presentation of the ischemic extremity in an infant or child. We believe that the decision to intervene surgically should be dictated primarily by the immediate threat of irreversible tissue damage. Remote growth abnormalities occur in only a small minority of children. In the nonthreatened extremity, systemic heparinization for a 6- to 12-hour trial continues to have a role and may obviate surgical intervention. However, when palpation and Doppler examination both fail to reveal a proximal femoral arterial pulse, prolonged "conservative" heparin therapy is rarely warranted. Further, the persistent absence of a palpable proximal pulse, even in the presence of a Doppler signal, is sufficient evidence to indicate exploration in many cases. Finally, in a limb with a palpable proximal pulse, but absent distal Doppler signals, the judgment whether to operate is never clear-cut, but associated mottling of the skin and absence of capillary refill are ominous signs that justify catheter thrombectomy, in our view.

REFERENCES

1. Hunter W. Medical observations and inquiries. *Soc Phys London.* 1757;1:323.
2. Hunter W. Medical observations and inquiries. *Soc Phys London.* 1762;2:390.
3. Elkin DC. Aneurysm following surgical procedures: report of five cases. *Ann Surg.* 1948;127:769–779.
4. Shamberger RC, Ottinger LW, Malt RA. Arterial injuries during inguinal herniorrhaphy. *Ann Surg.* 1984;200:83–85.
5. Natali J, Benhamou AC. Iatrogenic vascular injuries. *J Cardiovasc Surg.* 1979;20:169–176.
6. Eger M, Golcman L, Torok G, Hirsh M. Inadvertent arterial stripping in the lower limb: problems of management. *Surgery.* 1973;73:23–27.

7. Liddicoat JE, Bekassy SM, Daniell M, DeBakey ME. Inadvertent femoral artery stripping surgical management. *Surgery.* 1975;77:318–320.

8. Luke JC, Miller GG. Disasters following the operation of ligation and retrograde injection of varicose veins. *Ann Surg.* 1948;127:426.

9. Dorr L, Corraty J, Hohl R. False aneurysm of the femoral artery following total hip surgery. *J Bone Joint Surg.* 1974;56:1059–1062.

10. Hirsh SA, Robertson H, Gorniowsky M. Arterial occlusion secondary to methylmethacrylate use. *Arch Surg.* 1976;3:204.

11. Paul MA, Patka P, van Heuzen EP, et al. Vascular injury from external fixation: case reports. *J Trauma.* 1992;33:917–920.

12. Oweida SW, Roubin GS, Smith RB, Salam AA. Postcatheterization vascular complications associated with percutaneous transluminal angioplasty. *J Vasc Surg.* 1990;12:310–315.

13. Miller JS, Dodson TF, Salem AA, Smith RB III. Vascular complications following intra-aortic balloon pump insertion. *Am Surg.* 1992;58:232–238.

14. Sreeram S, Lumsden AB, Miller JS, et al. Retroperitoneal hematoma following femoral arterial catheterization: a serious and often fatal complication. *Am Surg.* 1993;59:94–98.

15. Lumsden AB, Miller JM, Kozinski AS, et al. A prospective evaluation of surgically treated groin complications following percutaneous cardiac procedures. *Am Surg.* 1994;60:132–137.

16. Babu SC, Piccorelli GO, Shah PM, et al. Incidence and results of arterial complications among 16,350 patients undergoing cardiac catheterization. *J Vasc Surg.* 1989;10:113–116.

17. Messina LM, Brothers TE, Wakefield TW, et al. Clinical characteristics and surgical management of vascular complications in patients undergoing cardiac catheterization: interventional versus diagnostic procedures. *J Vasc Surg.* 1992;13:593–600.

18. Kresowik TF, Khoury MD, Miller BV, et al. A prospective study of the incidence and natural history of femoral vascular complications after percutaneous cardiac transluminal coronary angioplasty. *J Vasc Surg.* 1991;13:328–335.

19. Sheikh KH, Adams DB, McCann R, et al. Utility of Doppler color flow imaging for identification of femoral arterial complications of cardiac catheterization. *Am Heart J.* 1989;117:623–628.

20. Muller DWM, Shamir KJ, Ellis SG, Topol EJ. Peripheral vascular complications after conventional and complex percutaneous coronary procedures. *Am J Cardiol.* 1992;69:63–68.

21. Schatz RA, Baim DS, Leon M, et al. Clinical experience with the Palmaz-Schatz coronary stent. *Circulation.* 1991;83:148–161.

22. Seidenberg B, Hurwitt ES. Retrograde femoral (Seldinger) aortography: surgical complications in 26 cases. *Ann Surg.* 1966;163:221–226.

23. Bourassa MG, Nobel J. Complication rate of coronary arteriography: a review of 5250 cases studied by a percutaneous femoral technique. *Circulation.* 1976;53:106–114.

24. Mills JL, Wiedman JE, Robinson JG, Hallett JW. Minimizing mortality and morbidity from iatrogenic arterial injuries: the need for early recognition and prompt repair. *J Vasc Surg.* 1986;4:22–27.

25. Hallett JW, Wolk, SW, Cherry KJ, et al. The femoral neuralgia syndrome after arterial catheter trauma. *J Vasc Surg.* 1990;11:702–706.

26. Steinsapir ES, Coley BD, Fellmeth BD, et al. Selective management of iatrogenic femoral artery injuries. *J Surg Res.* 1993;55:109–113.

27. Kent KC, Mcardle C, Kennedy B, et al. The natural history of femoral pseudoaneurysms and arteriovenous fistulae induced by arterial puncture. *J Vasc Surg.* 1993;17:125–133.

28. Rivers SP, Lee ES, Lyon RT, et al. Successful conservative management of iatrogenic femoral arterial trauma. *Ann Vasc Surg.* 1992;6:45–49.

29. Khoury MD, Batra S, Berg RA, et al. Influence of arterial access sites and interventional procedures on vascular complications after cardiac complication. *Am J Surg.* 1992;164:205–209.

30. Feld R, Patton GM, Carabasi RA, et al. Treatment of iatrogenic femoral artery injuries with ultrasound-guided compression. *J Vasc Surg.* 1992;16:832–840.

31. Fellmeth BD, Barron SB, Brown PR, et al. Repair of postcatheterization pseudoaneurysms by color flow ultrasound guided compression. *Am Heart J.* 1992;123:547–551.

32. Flanigan DP, Keifer TJ, Schuler JJ, et al. Experience with iatrogenic pediatric vascular injuries. Incidence, etiology, management, and results. *Ann Surg.* 1983;198:430–442.
33. Taylor LM, Troutman R, Feliciano P, et al. Late complications after femoral artery catheterization in children less than five years of age. *J Vasc Surg.* 1990;11:297–306.
34. Freed MD, Keane JP, Rosenthal A. The use of heparinization to prevent arterial thrombosis after percutaneous cardiac catheterization in children. *Circulation.* 1974;50:565–569.
35. Schmidt B, Andrew M. Report of scientific and standardization subcommittee on neonatal hemostasis: diagnosis and treatment of neonatal thrombosis. *Thromb Haemostasis.* 1992; 67:381–382.
36. Rubenson A, Jacobsson B, Sorensen SE. Treatment and sequelae of angiographic complications in children. *J Pediatr Surg.* 1979;14:154–157.
37. Krueger TC, Neblett WW, O'Neill JA, et al. Management of aortic thrombosis secondary to umbilical artery catheters in neonates. *J Pediatr Surg.* 1985;20:328–332.
38. Strife JL, Ball WS Jr, Towbin R, et al. Arterial occlusions in neonates: use of fibrinolytic therapy. *Radiology.* 1988;166:395–400.
39. Pettenazzo A, Gamba P, Salmistraro G, et al. Peripheral arterial occlusion in infants: a report of two cases treated conservatively. *J Vasc Surg.* 1991;14:220–224.
40. Smith PK, Miller DM, Lail S, Mehta AV. Urokinase treatment of neonatal aortoiliac thrombosis caused by umbilical artery catheterization: a case report. *J Vasc Surg.* 1991;14:684–687.
41. Ino T, Benson LN, Freedom, RM, et al. Thrombolytic therapy for femoral artery thrombosis after pediatric cardiac catheterization. *Am Heart J.* 1988;115:633–639.
42. Andrew M. Anticoagulation and thrombolysis in children. *Texas Heart Inst J.* 1992;19:168.
43. LaQuaglia MP, Upton J, May JW Jr. Microvascular reconstruction of major arteries in neonates and small children. *J Pediatr Surg.* 1991;26:1136–1140.
44. Chicarilli ZN. Pediatric microsurgery: revascularization and replantation. *J Pediatr Surg.* 1986;21:706–710.
45. Gaul JS III, Nunley JA. Microvascular replantation in a seventh-month-old girl: A case report. *Microsurgery.* 1988;9:204–207.
46. Kay S, Gilpin DJ. Combined microsurgical and thrombolytic salvage of an ischaemic lower limb in a 1079 gram preterm neonate. *Br J Plast Surg.* 1991;44:310–311.
47. Smith C, Green RM. Pediatric vascular injuries. *Surgery.* 1981;90:20–31.
48. Whitehouse WM, Coran AG, Stanley JC, et al. Pediatric vascular trauma: manifestations, management, and sequelae of extremity arterial injury in patients undergoing surgical treatment. *Arch Surg.* 1976;111:1269–1275.
49. Klein MD, Coran AG, Whitehouse WM Jr., et al. Management of iatrogenic arterial injuries in infants and children. *J Pediatr Surg.* 1982;17:933–939.
50. Chaikof, EL, Dodson, TF, Salam, AA, et al. Acute arterial thrombosis in the very young. *J Vasc Surg.* 1992;16:428–435.
51. Bassett FH III, Lincoln CR, King TD, Canent RV. Inequality in the size of the lower extremity following cardiac catheterization. *South Med J.* 1968;61:1013–1017.
52. Rosenthal A, Anderson M, Thomson SJ, et al. Superficial femoral artery catheterization: Effect on extremity length. *Am J Dis Child.* 1972;124:240–242.
53. Hawker RE, Palmer J, Bury RG, et al. Late results of percutaneous retrograde femoral arterial catheterization in children. *Br Heart J.* 1973;35:447–449.
54. Jacobsson B, Carlgren LE, Hedvall G, Sivertsson R. A review of children after arterial catheterization of the leg. *Pediatr Radiol.* 1973;1:96–99.
55. Bloom JD, Mozersky DJ, Buckley CJ, Hagood CO. Defective limb growth as a complication of catheterization of the femoral artery. *Surg Gynecol Obstet.* 1974;138:524–526.

45

Transluminally Placed
Endovascular Stented Graft Repair
for Arterial Trauma

Michael L. Marin, MD, Luis A. Sanchez, MD,
Frank J. Veith, MD, and Jacob Cynamon, MD

Civilian trauma has been steadily increasing with a dramatic rise in handgun injuries. Penetrating trauma to the vascular system from these high-velocity missiles can lead to the formation of arterial occlusions, pseudoaneurysms, and arteriovenous (AV) fistulas. The optimal management of these vascular injuries has been described in wartime and civilian trauma experiences.[1-6] Severe injuries that demonstrate pulse deficits and severe ischemia or expanding hematomas and active hemorrhage require urgent surgical exploration and vascular repair. The direct surgical repair of these injuries may be complicated by several factors, including inaccessibility of the vascular lesion when trauma occurs to central vessels. In addition, false aneurysms and AV fistulas may distort local anatomy and induce venous hypertension, increasing the challenge of a standard surgical repair with considerable blood loss. If the patient's condition remains stable after the vascular trauma, an alternative treatment using catheter-directed techniques may reduce procedural risks. One such therapy employs endovascular stented grafts to directly repair the injured vessel from the luminal surface.[7-9] These devices allow minimally invasive arterial repairs to be performed from easily accessible sites in the vasculature that are remote from the area of arterial trauma. This chapter describes the development and clinical experience with the placement of stented grafts for the treatment of arterial pseudoaneurysm and AV fistula.

TECHNIQUES AND DEVICES

Transluminally placed stented grafts for treating traumatic arterial lesions were conceptualized by Dotter in 1969,[10] and the first clinical procedure was performed by Volodos et al[11] using a Dacron graft and a self-expanding stent. Experimental and clinical experience has shown that a wide range of devices may be used for treating

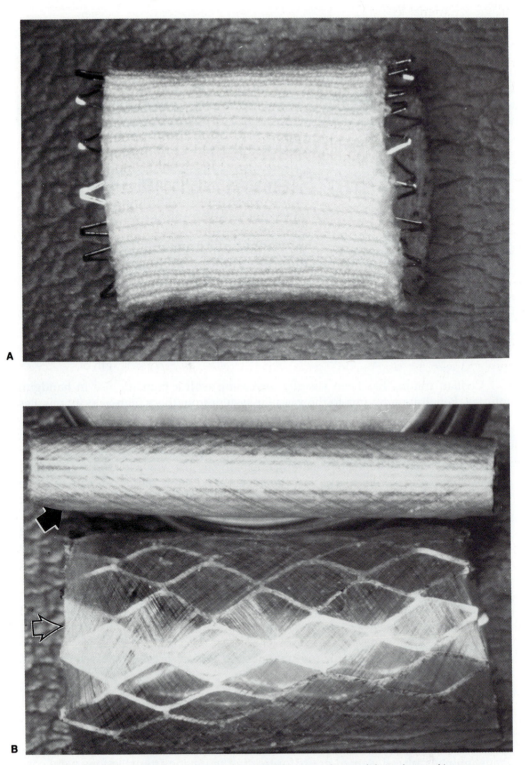

Figure 45–1. Endovascular covered stents. (**A**) Dacron graft material may be used to cover the balloon expandable stents. (**B**) Polyurethane can be fabricated directly onto a stent. This material has "elastic" properties that allow a closed stent (arrow) to remain well covered after deployment (open arrow). (*Figure continues*)

traumatic arterial lesions[7,12] (Fig. 45–1). The external covering on the stent does not appear to be critical to stent graft function in the treatment of traumatic lesions.

At the Montefiore Medical Center, we have used the Palmaz balloon expandable stent in conjunction with thin-walled polytetrafluoroethylene (PTFE) material to perform arterial repair of pseudoaneurysms and AV fistulas (Fig. 45–2). The stents varied between 2 cm and 3 cm in length and were fixed inside 6-mm Gore-Tex grafts (W.L. Gore and Associates, Flagstaff, AZ) by two U stitches (Fig. 45–3A). The stent graft was then mounted on a balloon angioplasty catheter that contains a tapered dilator tip (Fig. 45–3B). The entire device was loaded into a 12-F delivery system, prepared for over-the-wire insertion through an arterial cutdown or percutaneously.

RESULTS

As shown in Table 45–1, eight patients received eight stented grafts to treat traumatic arterial lesions. The mean age of the patients receiving these grafts was 40 years (range, 18 to 78 years). Seven patients were men. Five injuries occurred as a result of gunshot wounds (Fig. 45–4). One knife wound and two iatrogenic needle catheterization injuries constituted the remaining cases (Figs. 45–5 and 45–6). All injuries were associated with a surrounding pseudoaneurysm. In two instances the arterial injury formed a fistula to an injured adjacent vein. Associated injuries were present in six patients with traumatic arterial injuries and one of the two patients with iatrogenic injuries (Table 45–1). With these stented graft repairs, in-hospital length of stay aver-

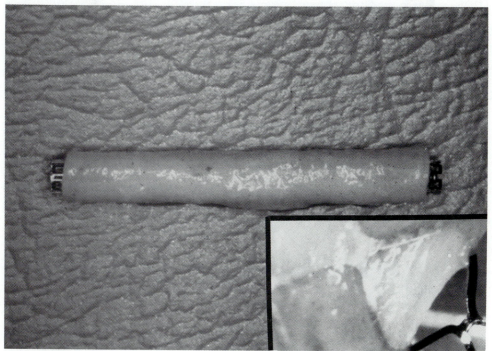

C

Figure 45–1. (*continued*) (**C**) Auogenous vein can be used to cover stents, creating biological stented grafts. The collapsed stent graft assumes a small profile, which effectively covers the struts of the stent following deployment (inset).

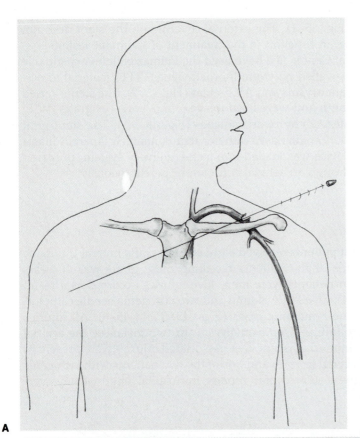

A

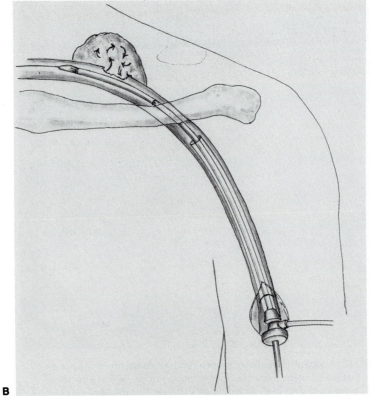

B

Figure 45–2. Stented graft repair of an arterial injury. (**A**) A bullet wound partially disrupts the wall of the vessel. (**B**) The stent graft device is delivered to the site of injury via a remote arteriotomy. (*Figure continues*)

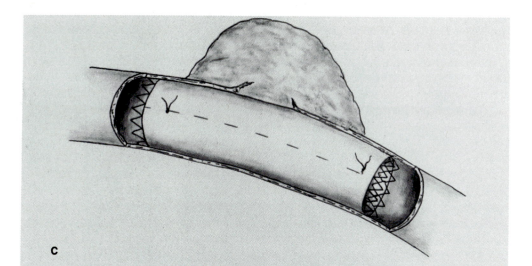

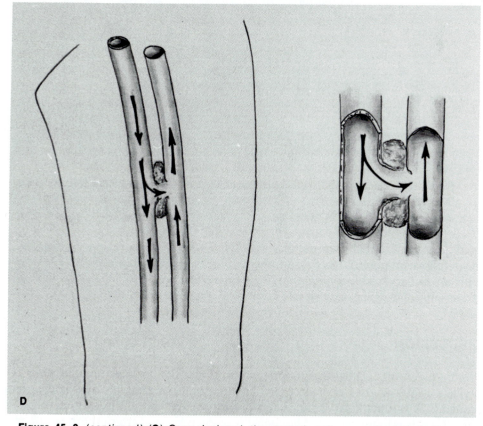

Figure 45–2. (*continued*) (**C**) Once deployed, the stented graft covers the hole in the vessel. (**D**) When an arteriovenous fistula forms after a vascular injury, the same principles apply for stented graft repair. In this example, the stent graft device is inserted In the superficial femoral artery at a site remote from the arterial injury. (*Figure continues*)

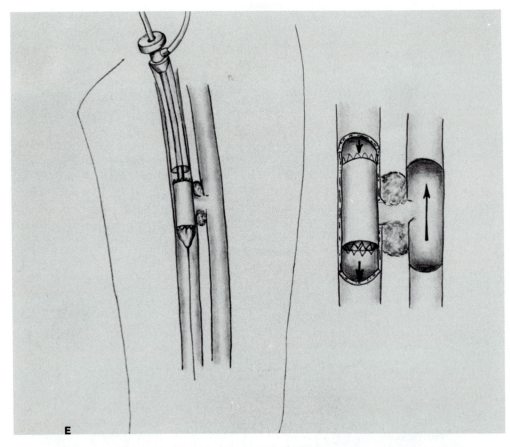

Figure 45–2. (*continued*) (**E**) After deployment, the stented graft occludes the arteriovenous fistula.

aged 5.5 days. Stented graft patency was 100% with no early or late occlusions. The mean follow-up period was 8.0 months with a range of 2 to 16 months. One patient with an axillary pseudoaneurysm required a vein patch to repair the site of the arteriotomy. No other early or late complications were encountered.

DISCUSSION

Prompt diagnosis and treatment of penetrating vascular trauma are required to avoid the late sequelae that may occur when important injuries are not appropriately treated.[13-16] Traumatic AV fistulas and pseudoaneurysms that involve non-essential vessels, such as branches of the hypogastric or deep femoral arteries, can be effectively treated by catheter-directed arterial embolization.[17,18] Long-term follow-up of coil-treated lesions has been favorable. Injuries to vital arteries traditionally have required direct surgical repair of the damaged vessel employing lateral repairs of grafts to restore critical arterial flow and to avoid delayed complications.

Endovascular methods are rapidly evolving to treat a variety of vascular disorders, including arterial trauma.[18] Similar endovascular treatment using balloon angioplasty of large vessels such as the iliac arteries appears to be a safe and effective alternative

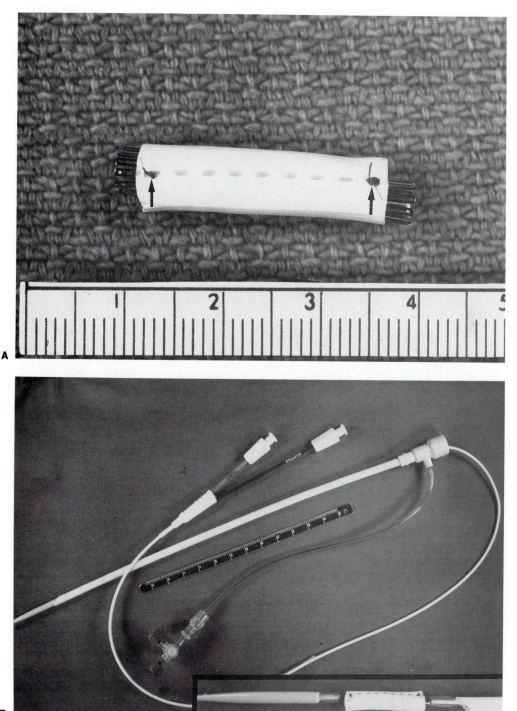

Figure 45–3. (A) An endovascular stented graft. A segment of PTFE is attached to a stainless steel slotted balloon-expandable (Palmaz) stent using two 5–0 polypropylene U stitches (arrows). **(B)** The stent graft is mounted on an angioplasty balloon and placed into a sheath before insertion. The dilator tip at the end of the balloon catheter provides a smooth taper within the catheter (inset).

TABLE 45–1. STENTED GRAFTS FOR ARTERIAL TRAUMA

Sex/ Age (y)	Mechanism of Injury	Vessel Involved	Pseudo- aneurysm	Arterio- venous Fistula	Associated Injuries	Injury to Repair Time Interval	Stent Graft Length (cm)	Access	Hospital Stay (days)	Patency Period (mo)	Balloon Diameter (mm)
M/20	Bullet	LSFA LSFV	Yes	Yes	Soft tissue buttock	36 h	3	LSFA percutaneous	5	14	8
M/28	Bullet	RSFA	Yes	No	Left open femur fracture	12 h	3	RSFA arteriotomy	9	11	7
M/22	Bullet	LSFA	Yes	No	Soft tissue right thigh; left deep venous thrombosis	12 h	3	LSFA arteriotomy	6	2[a]	8
M/24	Knife	LASA	Yes	No	Pneumo- thorax; hemothorax	4 h	3	Left brachial arteriotomy	7	9	8
M/35	Bullet	RASA	Yes	No	Brachial plexus	3 wk	3	Right brachial arteriotomy	4	5	7
F/78	Catheteri- zation	RSA	Yes	No	Hemothorax	24 h	3	Right brachial arteriotomy	8 wks[b]	3	8
M/78	Catheteri- zation	LCIA	Yes	No	None	4 mo	2	LCFA arteriotomy	2	2	10
M/18	Bullet	RSA	Yes	Yes	Hemothorax	48 h	3	Right brachial artery	4	2	6

[a] Died 2 months after procedure (homicide).
[b] Hospitalized for multiple medical problems.
LSFA, left superficial femoral artery; LSFV, left superficial femoral vein; RSFA, right superficial femoral artery; LASA, left axillary subclavian artery; RASA, right axillary subclavian artery; RSA, right subclavian artery; LCIA, left common iliac artery; LCFA, left common femoral artery.

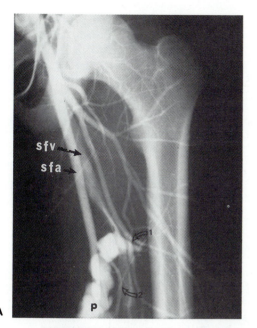

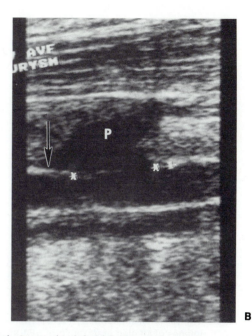

Figure 45–4. (A) Femoral arteriogram after gunshot wound to left thigh. An arteriovenous fistula associated with a large pseudoaneurysm is seen between the left superficial femoral artery (SFA) and the superficial femoral vein (SFV). Selective catheterization of the deep femoral artery and the SFA branch showed that these vessels were not injured (p = pseudoaneurysm). **(B)** Duplex ultrasonographic scan of SFA depicted in **A.** Loss of the intimal stripe (arrow) and associated pseudoaneurysm (p) is seen. Arterial defect measures approximately 13 mm (distance between Xs). (*Figure continues*)

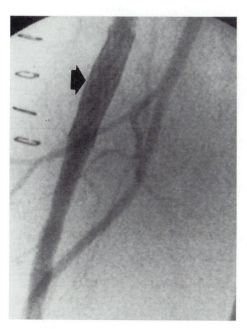

Figure 45–4. (*continued*) **(C)** Completion arteriogram demonstrates patency of the SFA, proper positioning of the stented graft (arrow) and no evidence of the arteriovenous fistula or extravasation. Metal clips were placed in the skin before the procedure to facilitate fluoroscopic localization of the arteriovenous fistula and proper placement of the stented graft. (*Figure continues*)

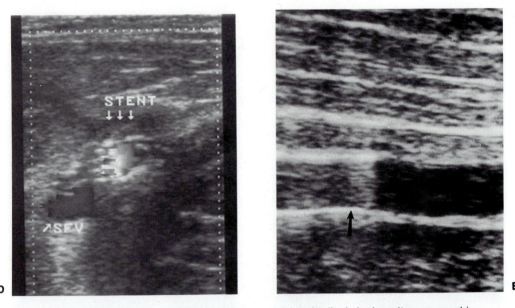

D   **E**

Figure 45–4. (*continued*) (**D, E**) Transverse and longitudinal duplex ultrasonographic images of stented graft repair of SFA after 3 months. (**D**) Transverse image of artery and vein at level of stent can be identified with evidence of normal flow in arteries. (**E**) Longitudinal duplex ultrasonogram identifies stented graft within artery (arrow). Minimal changes in peak systolic velocities are appreciated between the native SFA and that portion of the vessel that is covered by the stented graft.

to surgery for some forms of stenotic and occlusive vascular disease.[19] This form of therapy may be successfully extended to more complex lesions by the use of intra-arterial stents.[20] The blending of intravascular stent and prosthetic graft technologies has resulted in the evolution of new devices (stented grafts) with a wide range of potential applications in the vascular system. Early feasibility studies of these devices have shown them to be technically capable of excluding experimentally created arterial aneurysms with the potential for treating other lesions.[21–23]

One of the first clinical experiences with stented grafts was reported by Parodi et al for the treatment of patients with abdominal aortic aneurysms.[24] Parodi et al extended this experience to the first successful treatment of AV fistulas following a traumatic vascular injury.[7]

This chapter describes a preliminary experience with stented grafts for the treatment of traumatic arterial lesions. Follow-up of these patients lasted 16 months. In this series, device insertion was accomplished with uniform technical success. Satisfactory repair of the arterial lesion has been maintained in all cases (mean, 8.0 months), with preservation of the arterial flow through the injuried critical segment. Distal embolization did not occur.

PTFE grafts combined with balloon expandable (Palmaz) stents inserted from a remote site in the arterial tree have several advantages over conventional repairs. Compared with standard operative repair of similar lesions, stented grafts appear to be associated with less blood loss and a reduced requirement for anesthesia and dissection in the traumatized field. These advantages are particularly important in patients with large, central vessel injuries or truncal AV fistulas with venous hyperten-

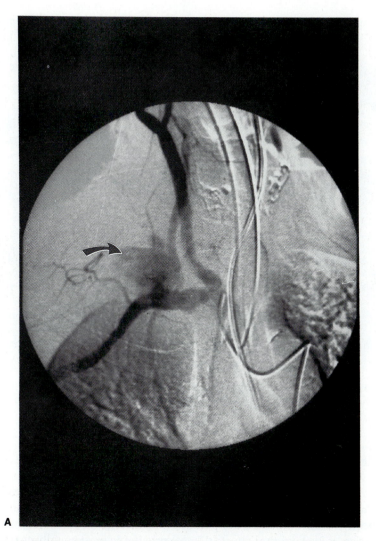

Figure 45–5. (A) Arteriogram shows a large pseudoaneurysm of the subclavian artery (arrow) just distal to the right vertebral artery, which occurred after an attempted subclavian vein catheter insertion. (*Figure continues*)

sion. Standard surgical repair of such lesions is notoriously difficult and associated with considerable blood loss. Stented graft repair of these central or truncal artery false aneurysms avoids the need for extensive operations through major body cavities. These advantages are also important in patients who are critically ill from other coexisting injuries or major medical co-morbidities. In these dire circumstances, the use of stented grafts already appears justified to treat some traumatic lesions of major, critical arteries.

Controversy exists regarding the best conduit for management of extremity arterial trauma distal to the subclavian and common femoral arteries, and this concern extends to the use of prosthetic stented grafts. Autogenous vein is preferred by most surgeons, with excellent early and late patency rates.[25] Autogenous veins have also been used to fashion stented grafts for the treatment of arterial trauma in infected

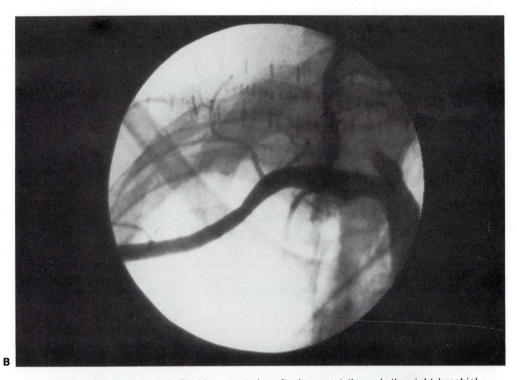

B

Figure 45–5. (*continued*) (**B**) After stented graft placement through the right brachial artery, the pseudoaneurysm was excluded. Vertebral artery flow was maintained.

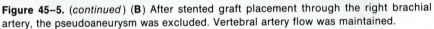

fields as well as to repair arterial injuries located in the carotid circulation where mural thrombosis would present the greatest risk for embolization. Some authors have achieved satisfactory results with conventional surgery using prosthetic grafts for extremity arterial wounds.[26] Although long autogenous grafts for arteriosclerotic ischemia have been associated with better patency than arterial reconstructions performed with prosthetics, it is likely that short (≤3 cm) prosthetic graft segments will function satisfactorily in the axillary and superficial femoral arteries. However, this premise remains to be proven by longer patient follow-up. Even if late failure of stent grafts in these locations occurs, a subsequent elective vein graft bypass could then be performed in a field free of traumatized tissue and contamination and when the status of the venous circulation in a traumatized limb is known. If the function of prosthetic stented grafts in the superficial femoral and axillary arteries is poor, an autogenous vein–covered stent could be considered as an alternative.

One theoretic problem with stented graft repairs involves the potential for stimulating intimal hyperplasia at the stent graft–arterial junction. Although any form of traumatic injury to an artery may induce a hyperplastic response in the cells that compose the arterial wall, the Palmaz intra-arterial stent has been shown to cause only limited intimal hyperplasia in experimental studies as well as in the treatment of stenotic or occluded iliac arteries in patients.[20] In the latter setting, prolonged patency has been the rule.[20]

Despite the potential disadvantages of using a thrombogenic stented graft device that could stimulate intimal hyperplasia to treat a traumatic lesion of the axillary or femoral arteries, the advantages of minimally invasive deployment, decreased blood

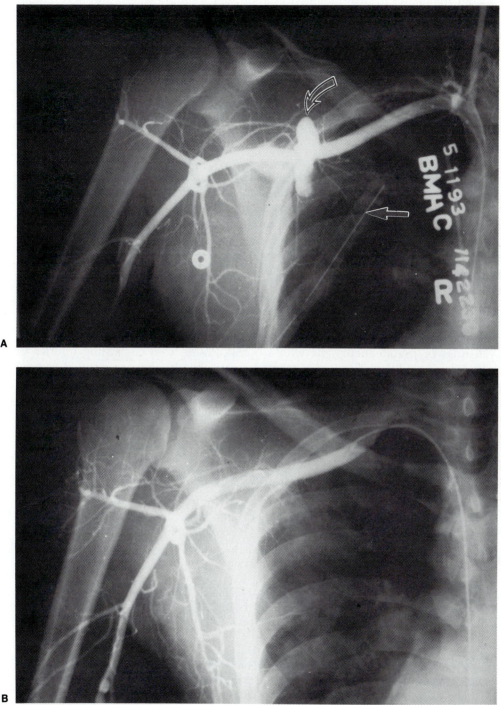

Figure 45–6. (**A**) Axillary–subclavian artery arteriogram of a large pseudoaneurysm (open arrow) after a stab wound to the chest resulted in a hemopneumothorax (arrow = chest tube). (**B**) After transluminal insertion of the stent graft device, the pseudoaneurysm was repaired and flow was restored.

loss, and the ability to insert stented grafts under local anesthesia through remote sites make this endovascular technique for repair of penetrating vascular injuries a potentially important tool for more widespread use. This is already true for multiple trauma and critically ill patients with central artery injuries. Long-term follow up of these repairs will be necessary to fully evaluate the safety and efficacy of these devices in extremity arteries and in other less critical circumstances.

CONCLUSION

Intravascular stents have become important tools for the management of vascular lesions; however, stents in combination with vascular grafts have only recently reached clinical application. This chapter describes an experience with stented grafts for the treatment of penetrating arterial trauma. Eight transluminally placed stented grafts were used to treat 2 AV fistulas and six pseudoaneurysms. These grafts were successfully inserted percutaneously or through open arteriotomies that were remote from the site of vascular trauma. The devices were composed of balloon expandable, stainless steel stents (Palmaz) covered with PTFE grafts. Patency up to 16 months was achieved (mean follow up, 8.0 months). The use of stented grafts appears to be associated with decreased blood loss, a less invasive insertion procedure, reduced requirements for anesthesia, and a limited need for an extensive dissection in the traumatized field. These advantages are particularly important in patients with central AV fistulas or pseudoaneurysms who are critically ill from co-existing injuries or medical co-morbidities. The use of stented grafts already appears justified to treat traumatic arterial lesions in these circumstances. Although the early results with the eight patients in this report are encouraging, documentation of long-term effectiveness must be obtained before these devices can be recommended for widespread or generalized use in the treatment of major arterial injuries.

Acknowledgments
Supported by grants from the U.S. Public Health Service (HL 02990-01), the James Hilton Manning and Emma Austin Manning Foundation, The Anna S. Brown Trust, and the New York Institute for Vascular Studies.

REFERENCES

1. Drapanas T, Hewitt RL, Weichert RF, Smith AD. Civilian vascular injuries: a critical appraisal of three decades of management. *Ann Surg*. 1970;172:351–360.
2. Burnett HF, Parnell CL, Williams GD, Campbell GS. Peripheral arterial injuries: a reassessment. *Ann Surg*. 1976;183:701–709.
3. Perry MO, Thal ER, Shires GT. Management of arterial injuries. *Ann Surg*. 1971;173:403–408.
4. Feliciano DV, Bitondo CG, Mattox KL, et al. Civilian trauma in the 1980s: a 1-year experience with 456 vascular and cardiac injuries. *Ann Surg*. 1984;199:717–724.
5. Jahnke EJ, Jr, Seeley SF. Acute vascular injuries in the Korean war: an analysis of 77 consecutive cases. *Ann Surg*. 1953;138:158–177.
6. Rich NM, Spencer FC. *Vascular Trauma*. Philadelphia: WB Saunders, 1978.
7. Parodi JC, Barone HD, Schonholz C. Transfemoral endovascular treatment of aortoiliac aneurysms and arteriovenous fistulas with stented Dacron grafts. In: Veith FJ, ed. *Current Critical Problems in Vascular Surgery*. Vol 5. St. Louis, MO: Quality Medical; 1993:264.
8. Marin ML, Veith FJ, Panetta TF, et al. Percutaneous transfemoral insertion of a stented graft to repair a traumatic femoral arteriovenous fistula. *J Vasc Surg*. 1993;18:299–302.

9. May J, White G, Waugh R, et al. Transluminal placement of a prosthetic graft-stent device for treatment of subclavian artery aneurysm. *J Vasc Surg.* 1993;18:1056–1059.

10. Dotter CT. Transluminally-placed coilspring endarterial tube grafts. Long-term patency in canine popliteal artery. *Invest Radiol.* 1969;4:329–332.

11. Volodos NL, Karpovich IP, Troyan VI, et al. Clinical experience of the use of self-fixing synthetic prostheses for remote endoprosthetics of the thoracic and the abdominal aorta and iliac arteries through the femoral artery and as intraoperative endoprosthesis for aorta reconstruction. *Vasa [Suppl].* 1991;33:93–95.

12. Rivera FJ, Palmaz JC, Encarnacion CE, et al. Aneurysm and pseudoaneurysm balloon expandable stent/graft bypass: clinical experience. (Abstract). *J Vasc Intervent Radiol.* 1994;5:19.

13. Feliciano DV, Cruse PA, Burch JM, Bitondo CG. Delayed diagnosis of arterial injuries. *Am J Surg.* 1987;154:579–584.

14. Richardson JD, Vitale GC, Flint LM Jr. Penetrating arterial trauma: analysis of missed vascular injuries. *Arch Surg.* 1987;122:678–683.

15. Ben-Menachem Y. Vascular injuries of the extremities: hazards of unnecessary delays in diagnosis. *Orthopedics.* 1986;9:333–338.

16. Escobar GA, Escobar SC, Marquez L, et al. Vascular trauma: late sequelae and treatment. *J Cardiovasc Surg.* 1980;21:35–40.

17. Rosch J, Dotter CT, Brown MJ. Selective arterial embolization: a new method for control of acute gastrointestinal bleeding. *Radiology.* 1972;102:303–306.

18. Panetta TF, Sclafani SJA, Goldstein AS, Phillips TF. Percutaneous transcatheter embolization for arterial trauma. *J Vasc Surg.* 1985;2:54–64.

19. Johnston KW, Rae M, Hogg-Johnston SA, et al. 5-Year results of a prospective study of percutaneous transluminal angioplasty. *Ann Surg.* 1987;206:403–413.

20. Palmaz JC, Laborde JC, Rivera RJ, et al. Stenting of the iliac arteries with the Palmaz stent: experience from a multicenter trial. *Cardiovasc Intervent Radiol.* 1992;15:291–297.

21. Mirich D, Wright KC, Wallace S, et al. Percutaneously placed endovascular grafts for aortic aneurysms: feasibility study. *Radiology.* 1989;170:1033–1037.

22. Laborde JC, Parodi JC, Clem MF, et al. Intraluminal bypass of abdominal aortic aneurysm: feasibility study. *Radiology.* 1992;184:185–190.

23. Balko A, Piasecki GJ, Shah DM, et al. Transfemoral placement of intraluminal polyurethane prosthesis for abdominal aortic aneurysm. *J Surg Res.* 1986;40:305–309.

24. Parodi JC, Palmaz JC, Barone HD. Transfemoral intraluminal graft implantation for abdominal aortic aneurysms. *Ann Vasc Surg.* 1991;5:491–499.

25. Keen RR, Meyer JP, Durham JR, et al. Autogenous vein graft repair of injured extremity arteries: early and late results with 134 consecutive patients. *J Vasc Surg.* 1991;13:664–668.

26. Feliciano DV, Mattox KL, Graham JM, Bitondo CG. Five-year experience with PTFE grafts in vascular wounds. *J Trauma.* 1985;25:71–82.

Index